Neurocutaneous Diseases

Neurocutaneous Diseases
A Practical Approach

EDITED BY

Manuel Rodriguez Gomez, M.D.

PROFESSOR OF PEDIATRIC NEUROLOGY, MAYO MEDICAL SCHOOL, AND
CONSULTANT, SECTION OF PEDIATRIC NEUROLOGY, DEPARTMENT OF
NEUROLOGY, MAYO CLINIC, ROCHESTER, MINNESOTA

FOREWORD BY

Raymond D. Adams, M.D.

BULLARD PROFESSOR OF NEUROPATHOLOGY, EMERITUS, HARVARD MEDICAL
SCHOOL, AND SENIOR NEUROLOGIST, MASSACHUSETTS GENERAL HOSPITAL,
BOSTON, MASSACHUSETTS

With 40 Contributing Authors

Butterworths

Boston   London   Durban   Singapore   Sydney   Toronto   Wellington

Every effort has been made to ensure that the drug dosage schedules within this text are accurate and conform
to standards accepted at time of publication. However, as
treatment recommendations vary in the light of continuing research and clinical experience, the reader is advised
to verify drug dosage schedules herein with information
found on product information sheets. This is especially
true in cases of new or infrequently used drugs.

Library of Congress Cataloging-in-Publication Data

Neurocutaneous diseases.

   Includes bibliographies and index.
   1. Neurocutaneous disorders.   I. Gomez, Manuel R.,
1928–   . [DNLM: 1. Nervous System Diseases—
complications.   2. Skin Diseases—complications.
WR 140 N494]
RL701.N48   1987   616.8   87–670
ISBN 0–409–90018–4

Butterworth Publishers
80 Montvale Avenue
Stoneham, MA 02180

10 9 8 7 6 5 4 3 2 1

Printed in the United States of America

Contents

Contributing Authors

FELICIA B. AXELROD, M.D.
Professor of Pediatrics, New York University School of Medicine, New York, New York

ELIZABETH M. BEBIN, M.D.
Resident in Pediatric Neurology, Mayo Graduate School of Medicine, Rochester, Minnesota

BRUCE O. BERG, M.D.
Professor of Neurology and Pediatrics and Director, Child Neurology, University of California Medical Center, San Francisco, California

ELENA BODER, M.D.
Clinical Professor of Pediatrics, University of California, Los Angeles, UCLA School of Medicine, Los Angeles, California

STUART B. BROWN, M.D.
Clinical Associate Professor of Neurology and Pediatrics, University of Miami School of Medicine, Miami, Florida

ENRIQUE CHAVES-CARBALLO, M.D.
Professor of Neurology, Eastern Virginia Medical School, Norfolk, Virginia

WILLIAM A. DE BASSIO, PH.D., M.D.
Clinical Assistant Professor of Neurology, Boston University School of Medicine, Boston, Massachusetts

W. EDWIN DODSON, M.D.
Professor of Pediatrics and Neurology, Washington University School of Medicine, St. Louis, Missouri

PAUL R. DYKEN, M.D.
Professor and Chairman, Department of Neurology, University of South Alabama College of Medicine, Mobile, Alabama

B. RAFAEL ELEJALDE, M.D.
Professor of Obstetrics/Gynecology and Medicine, University of Wisconsin Medical School—Milwaukee Clinical Campus, Milwaukee, Wisconsin

MARIA-MERCEDES DE ELEJALDE
Director of Genetics Services, Mount Sinai Medical Center, Milwaukee, Wisconsin

MARVIN A. FISHMAN, M.D.
Professor of Pediatrics and Neurology, Baylor College of Medicine; Chief, Neurology Service, Texas Children's Hospital, Houston, Texas

ROBERT J. GORLIN, M.D.
Regents' Professor and Chairman, Department of Oral Pathology and Genetics; Professor, Departments of Pathology, Dermatology, Pediatrics, Obstetrics/Gynecology, and Otolaryngology, Schools of Dentistry and Medicine, University of Minnesota, Minneapolis, Minnesota

MAKOTO GOTO, M.D.
Assistant Professor, Departments of Internal Medicine and Physical Therapy, Faculty of Medicine, University of Tokyo; Associate Professor, Rheumatology Center, Tokyo Women's Medical College, Tokyo, Japan

DONALD J. HAGLER, M.D.
Associate Professor of Pediatrics, Mayo Medical School, Rochester, Minnesota

WILLIAM G. JOHNSON, M.D.
Associate Professor of Clinical Neurology, Columbia University—College of Physicians and Surgeons, New York, New York

RICHARD A. KING, M.D., PH.D.
Professor of Medicine, University of Minnesota Medical School—Minneapolis, Minneapolis, Minnesota

JOHN H. MENKES, M.D.
Professor of Neurology and Pediatrics, University of California, Los Angeles, UCLA School of Medicine, Los Angeles, California

VIRGINIA V. MICHELS, M.D.
Associate Professor of Medical Genetics, Mayo Medical School, Rochester, Minnesota

BRIAN P. O'NEILL, M.D.
Associate Professor of Neurology, Mayo Medical School, Rochester, Minnesota

ROBERTA A. PAGON, M.D.
Associate Professor of Pediatrics, University of

Washington School of Medicine, Seattle, Washington

IGNACIO PASCUAL-CASTROVIEJO
Professor of Pediatric Neurology, Hospital Infantil "La Paz," Madrid, Spain

JOHN PEARSON, M.D.
Professor of Pathology, New York University School of Medicine, New York, New York

MICHEL PHILIPPART, M.D.
Professor of Psychiatry, Neurology, and Pediatrics, University of California, Los Angeles School of Medicine, Los Angeles, California

ARTHUR L. PRENSKY, M.D.
Allen P. and Josephine B. Green Professor of Pediatric Neurology, Department of Pediatrics, Washington University School of Medicine, St. Louis, Missouri

SIGVALD REFSUM, M.D., PH.D., F.R.C.P.
Professor Emeritus and former Head, Department of Neurology, Rikshospitalet University of Oslo, Oslo, Norway

VINCENT M. RICCARDI, M.D.
Professor of Medicine, Baylor College of Medicine, Houston, Texas

JAY H. ROBBINS, M.D.
Senior Investigator, Dermatology Branch, National Cancer Institute, National Institutes of Health, Bethesda, Maryland

N. PAUL ROSMAN, M.D.
Professor of Pediatrics and Neurology, Tufts University School of Medicine, Boston, Massachusetts

RAMON RUIZ-MALDONADO, M.D.
Professor and Chairman, Department of Dermatology, National Institute of Pediatrics, Mexico City, Mexico

EIJIRO SATOYOSHI, M.D.
Director, National Center for Nervous, Mental, and Muscular Disorders, Kodaira, Tokyo, Japan

JAMES R. SCHIMSCHOCK, M.D.
Assistant Clinical Professor, Oregon Health Sciences University, Portland, Oregon

GUNNAR B. STICKLER, M.D., PH.D.
Professor of Pediatrics, Mayo Medical School, Rochester, Minnesota

ODDVAR STOKKE, M.D., PH.D.
Professor of Clinical Biochemistry; Head, Department of Clinical Chemistry, Rikshospitalet, University of Oslo, Oslo, Norway

NOBUHIKO SUNOHARA, M.D.
Chief, Division of Clinical Neurology, National Center for Nervous, Mental, and Muscular Disorders, Kodaira, Tokyo, Japan

HERBERT M. SWICK, M.D.
Professor of Neurology and Pediatrics, Medical College of Wisconsin, Milwaukee, Wisconsin

PHILIP VAN HALE, M.D.
Fellow, Department of Oncology, Los Angeles County–University of Southern California Medical Center; Instructor, Department of Medicine, University of Southern California School of Medicine, Los Angeles, California

HANS-RUDOLF WIEDEMANN, M.D.
Professor Emeritus and former Head, Children's Clinic, University of Kiel, Kiel, Federal Republic of Germany

BRIAN R. YOUNGE, M.D.
Associate Professor of Ophthalmology, Mayo Medical School, Rochester, Minnesota

DONALD ZIMMERMAN, M.D.
Assistant Professor of Pediatrics, Mayo Graduate School, Rochester, Minnesota

Foreword

It can hardly be claimed that there is any lack of authoritative treatises on diseases of the nervous system or diseases of the skin. But hitherto there has been no systematic presentation limited to diseases that affect both of these parts of the human organism.

Such diseases are numerous and beguiling, as the reader will discover in perusing this volume. They are of theoretical and practical importance. A knowledge of common embryogenesis offers explanations of developmental anomalies that are manifest in both the neuraxis and its osseous and cutaneous integuments. The intricacies of dermal innervation shed light on peripheral neurocutaneous relationships; indeed, one must be reminded that there are infinitely more nerve fibers in the skin than in all other organs combined. Moreover, specialized cutaneous receptors in the skin are the source of impulses which inform us constantly of the contacts of our bodies to our physical environment. And finally, a less-explored aspect of theoretical neurocutaneous relationships will probably be found in the similarities of histologic structure and chemistry that underlie susceptibilities to diseases affecting skin and nervous cells concomitantly.

Clinical experience divulges other relationships between the nervous system and the skin. The skin regularly undergoes important changes that are purely secondary to disease of the nervous system. A diversity of examples comes to mind, such as anhidrosis and hyperhidrosis from paralysis or overactivity of the autonomic nervous system; trophic ulcerations and other changes from denervation; factitious ulceration in the hysteric or malingerer. Then too, the skin may be the primary source of a disease that has its major impact on the nervous system. Examples of these cutaneo-nervous relationships are the diphtheritic wound that yields a toxin that causes a sensorimotor polyneuropathy and the dermal tetanus infection that causes muscle spasms by activating motor neurons.

From the more practical side, the neurologist and dermatologist will find knowledge of these diseases of real clinical value. Many of the diseases described in these pages do not affect the skin and nervous system simultaneously. The appearance of a particular skin lesion may offer a means of predicting the later appearance of a neurologic defect, or vice versa. For example, the diagnosis of incontinentia pigmenti in early infancy foretells a severe degree of mental retardation at an age when immaturity of the nervous system makes this prognosis impossible. Or a few ash-leaf-shaped white spots in the skin prognosticate that a few infantile spasms are the forerunner of tuberous sclerosis.

Dr. Gomez and his colleagues have placed in our hands a work that will be of service to both dermatologists and neurologists. And, the many diseases which they present, mostly not well understood, may stimulate new lines of scientific inquiry, for understanding of a pathologic change in easily accessible dermal cells promises to clarify a more recondite brain disease.

Raymond D. Adams

Preface

For almost a century, diseases affecting both the skin and the nervous system have interested clinicians and puzzled students while inflicting pain and other forms of suffering on patients and their families. The ectodermal origin of the skin and nervous system appeared to justify studying all these diseases under a common name. Ben W. Lichtenstein said forty years ago at a postgraduate course given by the Chicago Medical Society: "The skin is a great mirror in that it reflects a variety of physical and mental abnormalities. Since both the epidermis and the nervous system have common ancestry in the ectoderm, and since both are protected and nourished, so to speak, by a mesenchymal derivative composed of vascular connective tissue, it is only logical that there be a number of disorders in which both the skin and the nervous system show abnormalities" [1].

The neurocutaneous syndromes in Lichtenstein's time were only a handful, and were grouped under different labels. Yakovlev and Guthrie [2] called them congenital ectodermosis while van Bogaert [3] preferred congenital neuro-ectodermal dysplasias. Some authors accepted van der Hoeve's term phakomatoses [4], originally introduced to encompass only tuberous sclerosis and neurofibromatosis. That attractive new term was derived from the Greek *phakos,* meaning "lens," "lentil," or "mother-spot." The common characteristic of patients with this order of diseases is that some of their otherwise normal organs harbor groups of cells with excessive growth potential. The spot or *phakos* in tissues as different as the skin, heart, kidneys, and brain is a hamartoma made up of benign cells that may or may not slowly grow, behaving like a true tumor. This requisite was lost when disorders such as Sturge–Weber disease and incontinentia pigmenti were included under the label of phakomatoses instead of simply being called neurocutaneous diseases. As MacDonald Critchley explains: ". . . various other rare disorders embracing lumps, rashes and fits were squeezed . . ."

into one group [5]. Even Jules François, in his introduction to the volume on Phacomatoses in the *Handbook of Clinical Neurology,* writes: "It must be recognized that in its true sense the concept of van der Hoeve is a little obscure and perhaps even a little artificial" [6], as Dr. Critchley reminds us [5]. In this volume, the term phakomatoses has been avoided principally because if it is to be used at all, it should include only tuberous sclerosis, neurofibromatosis, von Hippel–Lindau disease, and nevoid basal cell carcinoma syndrome.

Although our purist intention was to encompass in this book all the neurocutaneous diseases, it became a difficult task to do within a reasonable number of pages. There are many disorders so rare that only one case has been published. Reports on obscure disorders are often incomplete or have been made under different names a few times each. More needs to be known about some "new" disease entities, if indeed they *are* new diseases.

Certain maladies included in this volume are characterized by involvement of the hair but not of the skin. Two of them, von Hippel–Lindau and cerebrotendinous xanthomatosis, have no ectodermal component at all, but we thought it appropriate to include them because they are often listed with the other neurocutaneous diseases described in this book. Most of the more than forty neurocutaneous diseases described in full here are well-established clinical and pathologic entities; others, although uncommon, are biochemical entities. Little is known about some of them, or the knowledge is so scattered in a variety of medical specialty journals and books as to justify the editor's motivation to undertake this book.

The great majority of diseases presented in this volume are grouped according to the type of mendelian inheritance. Those in the last section are not firmly established as hereditary in nature. They are congenital vascular anomalies, perhaps with multifactorial etiology, possibly of autosomal recessive or autosomal dominant inheritance, but associated with failure to reproduce.

.The great number of physicians, researchers, and scholars who have contributed chapters to this book have the praise and gratitude of the editor. Ms. Nancy Megley, medical editor of Butterworths, has given encouragement and support without which the book would not have been produced. Ms. Marge Hinze has responded when needed to prepare my manuscripts and to collect and sometimes retype those of my coauthors. Therefore she has been very instrumental in getting the work done.

M.R.G.

References

1. Lichtenstein BW. Neurocutaneous syndromes. Chicago Med Soc Bull, April 9, 1949.
2. Yakovlev PI, Guthrie RH. Congenital ectodermosis (neurocutaneous syndromes) in epileptic patients. Bourneville tuberous sclerosis (epiloia). Arch Neurol Psychiatry 1931;26:1145–1194.
3. Van Bogaert L. Les dysplasies neuroectodermiques congénitales. Rev Neurol (Paris) 1935;63:354–398.
4. Van der Hoeve J. Eye symptoms in tuberous sclerosis of the brain and in Recklinghausen disease. Trans Ophthalmol Soc UK 1923;45:534–541.
5. Critchley M. Foreword. In Gomez MR. Tuberous Sclerosis. New York: Raven Press, 1979:vii–ix.
6. François J. A general introduction. In: Vinken PJ, Bruyn GW, eds. Handbook of clinical neurology. New York: Elsevier, 1972;14:1–18.

Chapter 1
Genetic Principles

WILLIAM G. JOHNSON

An understanding of the principles of medical genetics is helpful both in diagnosing neurocutaneous diseases and in working with patients and families after the diagnosis has been made. In addition, the genetic basis of a disorder is of critical importance in understanding its cause and developing effective specific treatment.

This chapter focuses on the patterns of inheritance that characterize these disorders and on how the clinician can contribute to localization of the genes that cause these disorders.

Inheritance Patterns for Human Genetic Disorders

Autosomal Dominant Inheritance

Pattern of Transmission

Inheritance of a disorder transmitted in autosomal dominant fashion is vertical, that is, through successive generations, from parent to child to grandchild. Dominant inheritance, in the older terminology, is "hereditary" rather than "familial." Males and females are affected with equal frequency and equal severity. There is no increased frequency of parental consanguinity as in autosomal recessive inheritance. Children of an affected parent have a 50% risk of receiving the harmful gene and therefore a 50% risk of being affected (see Penetrance and Expressivity, below). Half sibs through the affected parent have the same risk of being affected as full sibs, in sharp contrast to the situation in autosomal recessive diseases where the risk to half sibs is very small. Male-to-male transmission occurs in autosomal dominant inheritance and should always be looked for. Male-to-male transmission cannot occur in X-linked dominant pedigrees and may not occur in small autosomal dominant pedigrees simply by chance.

Definitions of Dominance— Genotypes vs. Phenotypes

Critical to the understanding of the differences between autosomal dominant and autosomal recessive inheritance is the concept of genotype and phenotype.

Genotype is a shorthand statement of whether an individual's two gene copies are normal or abnormal. A gene is normally found at a particular spot or place (locus) on a particular choromosome. Genes have different forms (alleles) that may be normal (often called *wild type*) or abnormal; a gene may have several or even many abnormal forms or abnormal alleles. Since an individual has only two copies of a particular gene (two chromosomes with one copy each), there are only four possible genotypes: (a) the individual has two normal alleles (normal homozygote), (b) the individual has one normal and one abnormal allele (heterozygote), (c) the individual has two abnormal alleles (abnormal homozygote), or (d) the individual has one each of two different abnormal alleles ("compound heterozygote or genetic compound").

The phenotype, on the other hand, is a property of the system in which the gene operates: usually this system is the individual patient or family member. The phenotype is either normal or abnormal. For example, the patient may have the abnormal phenotype because he or she complains of symptoms of the disorder, because the patient has the physical findings of that disorder, or because the results of clinical testing methods such as roentgenography or electromyography are abnormal.

This work was supported by grants from the National Institutes of Health (NS-15281 and NS-11766), the Muscular Dystrophy Association (H. Houston Merritt Clinical Research Center for Muscular Dystrophy and Related Diseases), the March of Dimes Birth Defects Foundation, and a generous gift from the Alexander Rapaport Foundation.

The difference between autosomal dominant and autosomal recessive inheritance can be easily explained. In both autosomal dominant and autosomal recessive inheritance patterns, normal homozygotes have the normal phenotype and abnormal homozygotes have the abnormal phenotype. The difference between the dominant and recessive patterns results from the phenotype of the heterozygote: if the heterozygote has the abnormal phenotype, the disorder is dominant; if the heterozygote has the normal phenotype, the disorder is recessive.

Dominant Lethals

This group of dominant disorders is mentioned separately because its inheritance pattern is different. Dominant lethal disorders are those in which an affected individual does not reproduce. The disorder is not necessarily lethal to the patient. However, because the patients do not reproduce, the disease cannot be transmitted from parent to child. Therefore all cases (in fact, nearly all cases) are sporadic and result from new mutation of a gamete. When one searches the literature and finds that all published cases of a disorder are sporadic, it is not reasonable to conclude that the disorder is nongenetic. A fortunate and practical result of this situation, however, is that recurrence risk for the next pregnancy is (nearly) zero for parents who have had a child affected with a dominant lethal disorder.

Penetrance and Expressivity

These features are especially characteristic of dominant rather than recessive inheritance. In individuals who are known to carry the abnormal gene but who have the normal phenotype, the abnormal gene is said to be nonpenetrant. Penetrance refers to the fraction of individuals with an abnormal allele who actually have the abnormal phenotype. The vast majority of individuals affected with dominant disorders in human populations carry a single rather than a double dose of the abnormal gene; that is, they are heterozygotes rather than abnormal homozygotes. Because of this, other factors in addition to the abnormal gene (such as the second, normal, copy of the gene; the individual's other genes at other loci; and environmental factors) can play a greater role in determining the phenotype. Obviously, whether an individual is "affected" can be defined or determined in different ways. Different ways of determining the abnormal phenotype will give different numerical values for penetrance. If, for example, in a group of individuals carrying the gene for neurofibromatosis,

only individuals with multiple neurofibromas are said to be affected, the penetrance will be rather low. If a careful search for café-au-lait spots is made, additional affected individuals will be uncovered. If axillary freckles and iris Lisch nodules are carefully searched for, additional affected individuals will be found. Finally, if procedures such as magnetic resonance imaging (MRI) of the spinal cord, examination for scoliosis or bony deformities, or complete autopsy are carried out, nearly all the individuals carrying the abnormal gene will be detected and the penetrance of the disorder will be high.

Expressivity is the degree of clinical involvement in an individual with the abnormal gene. It is especially characteristic of dominant disorders that two individuals, perhaps sibs in the same family, who carry the same abnormal gene may vary greatly in the severity of their disease. Obviously, nonpenetrance is an extreme form of variable expressivity.

The Sporadic Case

The most common presentation for genetic disorders in (small) human families is probably the sporadic case. If the clinician waited for a second case in a family before suspecting a genetic disorder, most genetic disorders would escape diagnosis. The following is a partial list of diagnostic possibilities for the sporadic case:

- Autosomal dominant (reduced penetrance).
- Autosomal dominant (new mutation).
- Autosomal recessive.
- X-linked recessive.
- X-linked dominant.
- Multifactorial–threshold inheritance.
- Polygenic inheritance.
- Nonpaternity.
- Adopted child.
- Nongenetic (phenocopy).

Autosomal Recessive Diseases

Pattern of Transmission

Inheritance of a disorder transmitted in autosomal recessive fashion is horizontal rather than vertical. Affected individuals are usually seen only in a single sibship (or "family," accounting for the older name "familial") in which the parents are unaffected but are both heterozygotes for the harmful gene. Collateral sibships are occasionally affected. Of course, disorders occurring in a sibship are not necessarily genetic; infectious disorders may cluster in a sibship. Males and females are affected with equal frequency and with equal severity in autosomal recessive conditions.

Unlike dominant disorders, autosomal recessive disorders have an increased incidence of parental consanguinity. In general, the rarer the disorder, the greater the fraction of families with parental consanguinity. A corollary of this is that rare recessive disorders are most likely to be found in inbred genetic isolates. Recessive disorders also frequently show striking ethnic predilections, a fact that is helpful in diagnosis. A corollary is that heterozygotes for some autosomal recessive disorders have increased frequency in specific ethnic groups, a fact that has made possible carrier testing for such disorders as Tay-Sachs disease, thalassemia, and sickle cell disease.

Couples at risk, that is, those where both parents are heterozygotes, are usually ascertained only after the birth of the first affected child. Further children of a couple at risk have a 25% chance of being affected and a 50% chance of being heterozygous carriers. Unaffected sibs of an affected individual have a 67% chance of being heterozygous carriers if they are old enough to be sure that they are not themselves affected. Couples at risk for having children affected with autosomal recessive disorders can be detected before the birth of the first child if a carrier test is available and if the heterozygous carriers are common or at least common in a defined ethnic group. Voluntary carrier testing for Tay-Sachs disease in individuals of Ashkenazi Jewish background has been highly successful, and classical infantile Tay-Sachs disease is now rarely seen because of amniocentesis. Half sibs of an affected individual with an autosomal recessive disease have a small chance of themselves being affected, a sharp contrast to the situation in autosomal dominant diseases in which the risk to half sibs through the affected parent is the same (50%) as that of full sibs.

Definitions of Recessive—Genotypes vs. Phenotypes

Definitions of genotypes and phenotypes are the same as those discussed above in Definitions of Dominance—Genotypes vs. Phenotypes for autosomal dominant diseases. However, recessive diseases are those in which the heterozygote is unaffected, that is, the heterozygote has the normal phenotype.

In plant or animal genetics the definitions of dominant inheritance may be somewhat different. Not only must the heterozygote be affected with a trait or disease, but the phenotype of the affected heter-

ozygote and the affected abnormal homozygote must be identical or indistinguishable. As already mentioned, in human populations that are relatively small, abnormal homozygotes are rarely encountered and individuals affected with autosomal dominant diseases are nearly always heterozygotes.

Compound heterozygotes, that is, individuals with two different abnormal alleles at a locus, are particularly important for autosomal recessive diseases. A genetic compound may have a phenotype quite different from that of either corresponding abnormal homozygote. Consequently, in taking the family history of an apparently autosomal recessive disorder, care must be taken not to ignore a cousin or perhaps more distant collateral relative who is affected but appears to have a disorder different from that of the patient; both affected individuals may have different forms of the same disorder, perhaps an enzyme deficiency, one individual being an abnormal homozygote, the other being a genetic compound. A genetic compound may also have a phenotype identical with that of either corresponding abnormal homozygote. In fact, many or even most individuals who are apparently abnormal homozygotes with autosomal recessive disorders may in fact be genetic compounds, except where there is parental consanguinity or where the parents are part of a genetic isolate or members of a defined population where heterozygote frequency for that disorder is high. It is important to recognize genetic compounds, where possible, since carrier testing or prenatal diagnosis in that family may be difficult or impossible without special testing.

Other Features of Autosomal Recessive Disorders

Variable penetrance and variable expressivity are far less important for autosomal recessive disorders than for autosomal dominant disorders. Nonpenetrance is quite unusual, and variation in expressivity tends to be much smaller. When major differences in expressivity are seen, other explanations, such as the presence of a genetic compound, should be considered.

X-Linked Diseases

Pattern of Inheritance

X-Linked Dominant Inheritance. X-linked dominant pedigrees show vertical transmission and look like autosomal dominant pedigrees except that in X-linked dominant pedigrees: (a) male-to-male transmission does not occur, (b) all daughters of an affected male are affected, (c) females are more frequently affected than males, (d) females are less severely affected than males, (e) occasional female heterozygotes show nonpenetrance (probably as a result by chance of preponderant Lyon inactivation of the X chromosome carrying the abnormal gene).

Since X-linked dominant pedigrees look so much like autosomal dominant pedigrees, X-linked dominant inheritance can easily be overlooked unless every apparently autosomal dominant pedigree is carefully examined for the features just mentioned.

X-Linked Recessive Inheritance. X-linked recessive inheritance somewhat resembles autosomal recessive inheritance especially when only a single sibship is considered. However, in larger pedigrees the appearance is different from either [autosomal recessive] or autosomal dominant inheritance. Transmission is "diagonal" rather than vertical or horizontal; affected males are connected on the pedigree through unaffected females. Only males are affected, but no male-to-male transmission occurs. Occasional female heterozygotes may be affected (probably as a result of preponderant Lyon inactivation by chance of the X chromosome carrying the normal gene).

X-Linked Diseases—Genotypes vs. Phenotypes

Definition of phenotypes is the same for X-linked disorders as for autosomal disorders; and the phenotype is either normal or abnormal (affected). For females, the possible genotypes are the same as for autosomal disorders: the normal homozygote, the heterozygote, the abnormal homozygote, and the genetic compound or compound heterozygote are defined as above. However, definition of the genotypes is somewhat different for males. Since males have only a single X chromosome, they are hemizygotes; depending on whether their X chromosome carries the normal or abnormal allele, the male is a normal or abnormal hemizygote.

The Lyon Hypothesis

A body of knowledge has accumulated about the peculiar behavior of the X chromosome in mammalian females following the hypothesis of Mary Lyon. X-inactivation in the mammalian female has the following features. Early in development (about 15 to 20 days in humans) one of the female's two X chromosomes is inactivated. The choice of which X chromosome is inactivated is random, although some

disease states may affect that choice or at least the final result in the adult (for example, X-autosome translocations and some single genes such as that causing adrenoleukodystrophy). The X-inactivation is stabile, and subsequent progeny of each X-inactivated cell have the same X chromosome inactivated. Germ cell X chromosomes are not inactivated. A small part of the inactivated X chromosome remains active (or not inactivated). This concept of X-inactivation has been well documented by a large body of work. Among other things it explains why some female heterozygotes are unaffected in X-linked dominant diseases, and why some female heterozygotes are affected in X-linked recessive diseases as mentioned in X-Linked Recessive Inheritance, above.

Metabolic Interference

Metabolic interference is a postulated mechanism in which two alleles at a locus or two alleles of genes at different loci cause a harmful effect only when they are present together in the same individual. That is, in the simple form of metabolic interference, only the heterozygote is affected; both of the corresponding homozygotes are unaffected. The pedigrees that result from this are in some instances rather conventional: for example, any apparently autosomal dominant pedigree could in fact result from metabolic interference. In some instances, however, these pedigrees are strikingly unusual: for example, (a) a disorder limited to females, apparently dominant or recessive, especially a disorder passed to affected females through unaffected males; (b) a disorder occurring in all members of a large sibship with normal parents; (c) a disorder occurring in all members of a large sibship with one parent similarly affected; (d) an apparently dominant disorder with females more severely affected than males; or (e) an apparently X-linked dominant disorder in which males are not more severely affected.

A number of pedigrees have been reported that are explained by the metabolic interference hypothesis but are not easily explained by any other known pattern.

Multifactorial–Threshold Diseases

Mechanism of Multifactorial–Threshold Inheritance

These diseases are rather common in the population with frequencies of approximately 1 per thousand (0.1 to 5 per thousand births). However, they are often not recognized to be genetic because recurrence risks in a family are in the range of 0.5 to 20 per thousand, far lower than those for any of the mendelian disorders discussed above.

The mechanism involves the interaction between a continuous variable (the genetic factor) and a discontinuous variable (an environmental factor). The genetic factor may be thought of as a susceptibility to the disease; quantitatively, the degree of susceptibility is distributed in the population roughly according to the normal distribution curve. A threshold then operates on this susceptibility such that if the susceptibility is below the threshold, the phenotype is normal. However, if the susceptibility is above the threshold, the phenotype is abnormal. The presence of a threshold converts the continuous variation into discontinuous variation. Examples of disorders that fit this model are neural tube defects, cleft lip, cleft palate, psoriasis, and pyloric stenosis.

Pattern of Inheritance

As just mentioned, the pattern of inheritance is quite different from the mendelian patterns just discussed. In mendelian pedigrees, the risk to the next child is independent of the number of affected children. However, in a family with a multifactorial disease, the risk that the next child will be affected increases with the number of children in the family who are already affected. The reason is that parents are likely to have higher genetic susceptibility if two children have crossed the threshold and are affected than if only one child has crossed the threshold and is affected. Thus parents with two affected children are likely to transmit a greater genetic susceptibility to their next child than parents with one affected child. In addition, in mendelian pedigrees, the risk to the next child is independent of the disease's severity in a relative. However, in a family with a multifactorial disease, the risk that the next child will be affected increases if the affected relative is severely affected rather than mildly affected. This is because parents are likely to have higher genetic susceptibility if a child is severely affected than if a child is mildly affected. Thus, parents of a severely affected child are likely to transmit a greater genetic susceptibility to their next child than parents of a mildly affected child.

The frequency of the multifactorial diseases characteristically varies between the sexes, different ethnic groups, and different geographical areas. For example, the incidence of pyloric stenosis is five times as great in males as in females. For anencephaly, the male to female incidence ratio is 0.6. Neural tube defects have increased incidence in Wales and Ireland.

A surprising result of these features is that risk for a multifactorial disease to relatives of a patient with that disease is higher if the patient is of the less frequently affected sex. For example, the risk of pyloric stenosis for the son of an affected father is 5.5 per thousand, while the risk to the son of an affected mother is 18.9 per thousand. The reason is that females, who are less frequently affected, must carry a greater genetic susceptibility than males in order to cross the threshold and have the normal phenotype. Therefore, an affected female is likely to carry a greater genetic susceptibility than an affected male and is likely to transmit a greater genetic susceptibility to her offspring than an affected male.

How the Clinician Can Help to Localize Genes

Molecular genetics is rapidly changing the approach to genetic diseases. This discussion focuses on disorders with unknown gene product since it is relatively straightforward to localize a gene on the genome once the gene product is known.

Gene Mapping by Restriction Fragment Length Polymorphisms

Restriction fragment length polymorphisms (RFLPs) have revolutionized human gene mapping in recent years, yet in principle the technique is little different from gene mapping using earlier markers. The two features that account for the difference are the greatly increased number of informative polymorphic markers that are becoming available for human gene mapping, and the fact that mapping with all of these markers is done with the same methods and the same equipment, that is, in the same laboratory.

Restriction Fragment Length Polymorphisms

Restriction endonucleases are bacterial enzymes that cut DNA in a sequence-specific way. These enzymes, numbering about 300 to date, have nothing to do with human DNA, but seem to be involved with the survival of one bacterial strain versus another. However, these enzymes are able to cut human DNA like other kinds of DNA, and they do this by recognizing a particular DNA sequence that they then cut. Thus these enzymes can recognize and localize certain DNA sequences, usually of four to eight base pairs.

Restriction fragments are the pieces that result after a restriction endonuclease has cut a length of DNA. The DNA that is cut may have been a small DNA fragment, phage DNA, a human chromosome, or the entire human genome. Whatever the starting material, the result is a mixture of DNA fragments of a wide variety of lengths.

Restriction fragment lengths can be determined and restriction fragments of different sizes can be separated by means of sodium dodecyl sulfate polyacrylamide gel electrophoresis (SDS–PAGE). Specific DNA sequences can be found on such a gel if the complementary sequence (the probe) is available and is radiolabeled. The gel is blotted to get the restriction fragments out of the polyacrylamide and onto the flat surface of a nitrocellulose or nylon filter. Then the filter is soaked under specific conditions (hybridized) with a solution containing radiolabeled probe, which will bind to its complementary sequence somewhere on the filter. The location of the probe (determined by autoradiography) on the filter gives the location on the original gel of the DNA fragment it recognizes and therefore the length of the original DNA fragment, since distance of migration on SDS–PAGE is related to the size of DNA.

Restriction fragment length polymorphisms are simply polymorphic variants of restriction fragment lengths. A polymorphism is a common genetic variant that is present in some members of a population but not others. A polymorphism may be a phenotypic variant, a variant in activity or electrophoretic mobility of an enzyme, a variant in DNA sequence, or other genetic variant. A genetic variant is considered common if it is present in 1% of genes; because each individual has two copies of each autosomal gene, a variant present in 1% of genes will be present in 2% of individuals. A polymorphism, then, is a genetic variant present in a least 2% of individuals. However, a useful polymorphism should have a higher frequency with 10 to 40% of individuals carrying the minor allele. Finally, individuals carrying the polymorphic variant will have the normal phenotype in nearly all cases. The reason for this is that harmful alleles will rapidly be eliminated from the population by natural selection and brought down to frequencies of well below 1%. Therefore polymorphic variants are not likely to be harmful. A RFLP results when a polymorphic variant in a specific DNA base sequence eliminates or adds a restriction endonuclease site. If the variant sequence is in the region recognized by a known probe, then the number or position of bands recognized by the probe will be different in the variant sequence than in the normal sequence (by convention, the "variant" sequence usually is the one with the smaller population frequency).

Use of Restriction Fragment Length Polymorphisms for Gene Mapping

Gene mapping using RFLPs is little different in principle than gene mapping using other kinds of markers. The basic procedure is (a) to collect a kindred affected with the particular disorder, (b) to determine by clinical examination whether each individual carries the disease and by DNA blotting whether each individual carries the normal allele, the variant allele, or both, and finally (c) to compare the distribution in the pedigree of the clinical disorder and in the DNA markers to see if linkage is present.

Each time an individual produces progeny, the two copies of each gene are separated at the first meiotic division of gametogenesis and go into different cells; only one copy from that parent can be transmitted to each child. Genes on different chromosomes assort randomly during meiosis. Because of the crossing-over that takes place at the first meiotic division, genes that are far apart on the same chromosome also assort randomly. Genes that are close together on the same chromosome do not assort randomly, that is, they show linkage. However, before this process can be followed, the two copies of each of the genes being tested for linkage must be marked so that the transmission of each copy from parent to child can be followed. The "informative" individual is informative precisely because each of the two alleles of the two genes being tested for linkage (the disease gene and the RFLP) has been marked since the individual is heterozygous at each of the two loci.

An informative individual is one whose two alleles can be distinguished for the genes being considered. An affected individual, a heterozygote in the usual situation in which the gene for a dominant disease gene is being mapped, has one abnormal allele (causing the disease) and one normal allele and is therefore informative at the disease gene locus. To be informative for the RFLP being tested for linkage, the individual must be heterozygous at this locus, having one copy of the normal RFLP allele and one copy of the variant RFLP allele.

A final requirement is that the phase be established for that individual: that is, if the disease gene and the marker RFLP are linked, is the variant RFLP allele located on the chromosome that carries the abnormal allele of the disease gene or on the chromosome that carries the normal allele of the disease gene? Knowing the phase makes possible the construction of haplotypes (a shorthand statement of which alleles of the considered genes sit on the same chromosome of a chromosome pair) for the individual; in general, however, this is usually established only by examining the pedigree as a whole.

After the clinical state (affected or not) and the genotype of the RFLP being tested for linkage have been determined for each member of the kindred, the frequency of recombination between the disease gene locus and the RFLP gene locus is determined: 50% recombination is expected if the two gene loci are on different chromosomes or far apart on the same chromosome; 0% recombination would suggest very tight linkage between the two loci, especially if the pedigree were large so that there were many opportunities for recombination to occur.

In practice, tables or a computer program are used to calculate the logarithm of the odds ratio (LOD) at different postulated recombination frequencies from the pedigree data. The logarithm of the odds ratio is the ratio of the odds for linkage to the odds against linkage. Recombination frequency (theta) is successively assumed to be 0%, 5%, 10% . . . 50%, for example, and LOD is calculated at each theta. The result is a plot whose abscissa is recombination frequency and whose ordinate is the LOD. A plot in which linkage is present gives a curve with a peak at some value of theta. The height of the peak gives the LOD at the most likely recombination frequency. For example, a curve with a peak of 2 at a recombination frequence of 10% is evidence for linkage of the two loci tested at a recombination frequency of 10%; at that recombination frequency, the odds ratio is 100:1 in favor of linkage. This sounds impressive: there seems little likelihood that the result is mere coincidence. Nonetheless a LOD score of 3, an odds ratio of 1,000:1 in favor of linkage, is the usual minimum requirement for general acceptance of a linkage claim.

Since gene loci that are farther apart have a higher recombination frequency, the distance between two gene loci can be measured using recombination frequency; gene loci that have a 1% recombination frequency are 1 centimorgan apart. The distance in centimorgans is approximately linear with recombination frequency for small distances, but not with larger distances because of increasing frequency of double cross-overs. The distance in centimorgans does not show linear correlation with chromosomal length measured morphologically with banded chromosome preparations because cross-overs are more frequent near the ends of chromosomes than near the centromere.

Once linkage testing for a disease locus and an RFLP is completed, it is important to remember that any linkage established is between the two loci and not between any of the specific alleles at these two loci. Association between specific alleles is a different phenomenon called linkage disequilibrium.

If linkage was established, testing can be done with new RFLPs known to be linked to the first RFLP for more accurate mapping. If linkage was not established because the peak of the LOD curve was less than 3, then new families can be studied with the same RFLP. Since the LOD scores from the old and new families are all in the form of logarithms, the old and new data (for the same values of theta) can simply be added to give new LOD scores. When the peak of the LOD curve passes 3, linkage has been established. Of course the new families studied must all have the same disease as the original family; if some of the families appear to have the same disease but in fact have a disease not caused by the same gene, the situation will become more confused rather than more clear with the addition of new families.

If, on the other hand, linkage was not established because there was no peak of the LOD curve, then new RFLPs need to be tested for linkage.

Importance of Large Kindreds

In general, it is easier to do gene mapping with one very large family than with several large families and easier with several large families than with many small families. Therefore, the clinician should be alert for large families. Since large kindreds are relatively uncommon they are a valuable resource for research. When such a large family is ascertained, a laboratory interested in gene mapping should be contacted so that the family may have a chance to participate in research of direct benefit to them.

Gene Mapping by Chromosomal Abnormalities

Patients with genetic disorders have one or more damaged copies of a particular gene. The damage can come about in a number of ways. One way is that a DNA point mutation in a gene's coding region can lead to an amino acid substitution in the protein gene product. Another is that a small deletion can remove part or all of a gene's DNA sequence. A larger deletion may remove all of the DNA sequence of the gene in question plus that of one or more neighboring genes. Such a deletion may be large enough to be visible on a banded chromosome preparation. Another possibility is that the gene may be damaged when one breakpoint of a chromosome translocation cuts through the gene's DNA sequence. Such a translocation is likely to be visible on a banded chromosome preparation.

It is likely that a subgroup of patients with nearly every genetic disease has that disease because of chromosome damage significant enough to be visible in banded chromosome preparations. Although this group is not large, it is extremely important because the site of chromosome damage gives the chromosomal location of the disease gene directly. Moreover, there are strategies for using the abnormal chromosomes from patients to clone the gene for the disease even though the gene product is unknown. Therefore, it is important to study patients with genetic disease for chromosome morphology, especially when there is something atypical about their disease. And it is important to bring such patients to the attention of medical geneticists.

References

1. Emery AEH. An introduction to recombinant DNA. New York: John Wiley & Sons, 1984.

2. Johnson WG. Principles of genetics in neuromuscular disease. In: Kelley VC, ed. Practice of pediatrics. New York: Harper & Row, 1979;14.

3. Johnson WG. Metabolic interference and the $+/-$ heterozygote. A hypothetical form of simple inheritance which is neither dominant nor recessive. Am J Hum Genet 1980;32:374–386.

4. Nora JJ, Fraser FC. Medical genetics: principles and practice. Philadelphia: Lea & Febiger, 1981.

5. Old RW, Primrose SB. Principles of gene manipulation. An introduction to genetic engineering. Berkeley: University of California Press, 1981.

6. Rosenberg RN. Neurogenetics: principles and practice. New York: Raven Press, 1986.

7. Vogel F, Motulsky AG. Human genetics. Problems and approaches. New York: Springer-Verlag, 1979.

8. Watson JD, Tooze J, Kurtz DT. Recombinant DNA: a short course. New York: WH Freeman, 1983.

PART ONE

DISEASES WITH AUTOSOMAL DOMINANT INHERITANCE

Chapter 2
Neurofibromatosis

VINCENT M. RICCARDI

Neurofibromatosis (NF) is the disorder par excellence to introduce and focus attention on neurocutaneous disorders. On the positive side, NF epitomizes the combined involvement of the skin and various parts of the nervous system, central and peripheral, and it exemplifies general features shared with other neurocutaneous disorders, such as a genetic etiology, a frequent concern for the embryonic neural crest having a role in pathogenesis, and a frequent, if not consistent presence of benign or malignant tumors during the course of the disease. On the negative side, however, emphasis on "neurocutaneous" as such tends to detract from the fact that these disorders are almost always much more pleiotropic, requiring a pathogenetic explanation that goes far beyond the skin and nervous system.

In the following discussion, the emphasis is on a practical approach, in keeping with the title and intention of this book. For a more encyclopedic and general discussion, the reader is referred to the recent work of Riccardi and Eichner [1]. The material presented here derives in large part from the experiences recorded in that book, as well as from previous publications, particularly reviews such as those by Borberg [2], Crowe et al. [3], Brasfield and Das Gupta [4], Wander and Das Gupta [5], Holt [6], Riccardi [7], Samuelsson [8], and Sorensen et al. [9], plus additional data from the entire array of some one thousand patients with or at risk for NF seen through the Baylor College of Medicine NF Program from March 1978 through January 1986.

Definition and Heterogeneity

Before proceeding to what NF is, however, it must be made clear the one thing NF is not. *Neurofibromatosis is not a single disorder.* That is, the unqualified use of the term *neurofibromatosis* designates a spectrum of disorders that share many features, although no one feature or set of features is shared by all of them. On the other hand, the term neurofibromatosis is often taken to specify the disorder described in 1882 by von Recklinghausen [10]. This latter, more specific syndrome will be referred to here as NF–I [1,7,11], and it will be given the most attention, because it accounts for at least 85% of all NF cases. The converse is equally important: with as many as 15% of NF cases not being adequately characterized by the details of NF–I, any reasonably complete discussion must consider all types or forms of the disorder. Put another way, heterogeneity is a cardinal element of NF.

Neurofibromatosis in the broadest sense has come to mean the presence of multiple neurofibromas or multiple café-au-lait spots, and is to be distinguished from solitary neurofibromas and nonspecific hyperpigmentation (although either of these two distinctions may not always be easy or straightforward). The specific type of NF may be apparent from the timing of the appearance of neurofibromas or their total number and distribution over the body, although often, especially in younger patients, the presence of other features, especially various types of tumors, will indicate the type of NF that is present in an individual or a family. Iris Lisch nodules [12], optic gliomas (and other intracranial astrocytomas), or pseudarthroses appear to be reasonably specific for NF–I. Intracranial and spinal schwannomas and meningiomas ordinarily indicate another form of NF, the prototypic one being the "acoustic" form reported on extensively by Eldridge [13]. The point here is that any realistic discussion of NF immediately engenders the notion of heterogeneity. However, the pitfall in dealing with heterogeneity prematurely is that the distinctions seem to be mere "hairsplitting." Thus, while heterogeneity is critical in the definition of NF, this is largely a function of the consistency of the most common form (regarding progression with age and largely unknown factors that determine expressivity). Thus, at this point we specifically address NF–I, and only later consider the other forms.

Itemization of NF–I Features

The features that characterize NF–I are best considered from two vantage points, structural (or anatomic) and functional.

Structural NF–I Features

Benign Tumors and Pigmentation

Neurofibromas can occur in all parts of the body and anywhere on the skin surface, except perhaps for the glans penis. They may also arise at sensory and autonomic ganglia, and on dorsal nerve roots, primary and secondary plexus radicles, and major, intermediate, minor, and terminal nerve components. There are basically three varieties: (a) cutaneous tumors (that is, tumors that move when the skin is moved) that are often violaceous or red in color at the surface, soft and fleshy, and sessile or pedunculated (Figure 2.1); they vary in size from several millimeters to well over a meter in circumference; they are generally not painful or tender; (b) subcutaneous neurofibromas (that is, ones that do not move when the skin above is moved) that are oval in shape (Figure 2.2), have the consistency of a hard rubber eraser, and may be painful or tender; they vary in size from several millimeters to 3 to 4 cm in their longest diameters; (c) plexiform neurofibromas, which combine elements of cutaneous and subcutaneous elements, and characteristically insinuate into adjacent normal tissue as the tumor grows, not infrequently to massive proportions; often the overlying skin demonstrates hyperpigmentation (distinct from café-au-lait spots) [14,15], or hypertrichosis (Figure 2.3). Neurofibromas may be present at birth and develop at any time thereafter, generally with a steady increase in number and size with age. Both adolescence and pregnancy appear to increase the likelihood of new neurofibromas appearing and previous ones growing. The sexually mature adult female nipple and areola are especially likely to manifest cutaneous neurofibromas (at least 85% at age 21). (More will be said about neurofibromas below.)

Café-au-lait spots are one of the characteristic types of NF–I hyperpigmentation (Figure 2.4). Size varies with age, but they are present at almost all ages, though they often are not as readily visible in infancy as they are later. Ordinarily, by 1 year of age at least six or so café-au-lait spots are apparent,

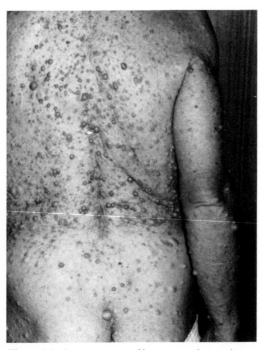

Figure 2.1. Cutaneous neurofibromas on the trunk.

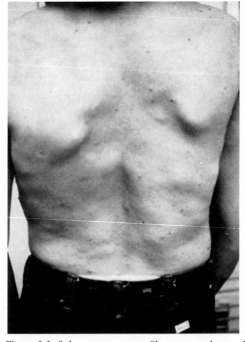

Figure 2.2. Subcutaneous neurofibromas on the trunk.

Figure 2.3. A diffuse plexiform neurofibroma with overlying hyperpigmentation on the arm.

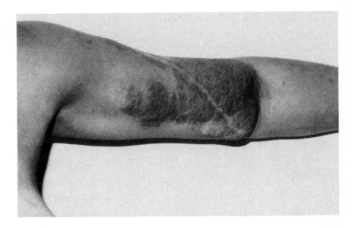

Figure 2.4. Typical NF–I café-au-lait spots about the neck.

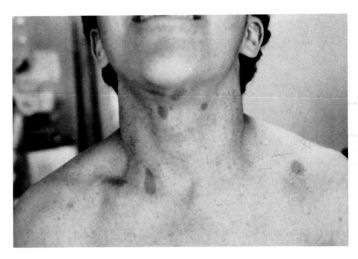

ranging in size from 15 to 150 mm or more in diameter. Most often the edges are well defined and the pigmentation is more or less uniform throughout the lesion. Freckling, that is, very small (1 to 3 mm) hyperpigmented macules present at birth, is indistinguishable by color from café-au-lait spots; congenital freckling is most commonly seen in the axillae (Figure 2.5). Freckling may also develop after birth in any of the intertrigenous regions (including the axillae), and anywhere that there is skinfold apposition (for example, in the inframammary region and in obesity skinfolds) or constant rubbing, as from underwear or persistent scratching of itching. Hyperpigmentation overlying and contiguous with the borders of a plexiform neurofibroma [15] may be the earliest indication that the neurofibroma is present. When such hyperpigmentation approaches or crosses the midline, neurofibroma involvement of the neuraxis should be presumed unless proved otherwise. In some NF–I patients the entire skin surface manifests a distinctive, somewhat darker hue than is

expected on the basis of the ethnic background and skin coloration of the parents, siblings, or offspring.

Iris Lisch nodules [12,16] are pigmented hamartomas [17] (Figure 2.6) that appear to be unique to NF–I (with the exception of at least one patient with a more localized form of NF [18]). Their presence and number is a function of age: at age 6 years only about 10% of NF–I patients manifest them; at 29 years the proportion reaches 50%, and by the mid-sixties 100% of patients show them. Other than indicating the presence of the mutant NF gene, Lisch nodules are uninformative about the course of the disease in general. At least one case has been reported with Lisch nodules as the only expression of the mutant gene [19]. Certainly, every adult at risk for NF must have a slit-lamp ocular examination to look for these lesions before a conclusion is drawn that the gene is not present. For children, the absence of Lisch nodules is less compelling as evidence against the diagnosis because of the age differential noted above.

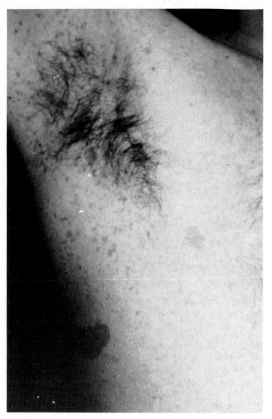

Figure 2.5. Axillary freckling typical of NF–I.

Neurofibromas of the skin can be of minimal or trivial importance, or their numbers or location can cause a variety of problems, the most common one being cosmetic. Neurofibromas, particularly the plexiform variety, occurring elsewhere than on the skin can cause a number of problems, reflecting both the size of the tumor and disruption of the integrity of adjacent normal tissue. Discrete neurofibromas of larger nerves may lead to peripheral neuropathies. Oral (including lingual) neurofibromas may disrupt phonation, respiration, and deglutition. Diffuse plexiform neurofibromas of the face tend to be of two distinct types, though occasionally there are patients with a combination of distributions. About 5% of NF youngsters show an orbital/periorbital plexiform tumor with resultant proptosis and, sometimes, visual compromise. Other facial plexiform neurofibromas tend to have an alternative distribution, that is, below the zygomatic arch, with invasion into the buccal pad, gingivae, lingual, pharyngeal, retropharyngeal, and laryngeal regions. Infants with this type of tumor may develop sudden respiratory compromise, even if there are few or no outward signs of the tumor. For this reason, all infants with, or at risk for, NF–I should have a radiographic examination of their cervical and mediastinal anatomy. Paraspinal neurofibromas can cause problems from the pressure exerted on adjacent structures, direct invasion of the thecal space about the spinal cord, compromise of dorsal and ventral nerve roots, and erosion

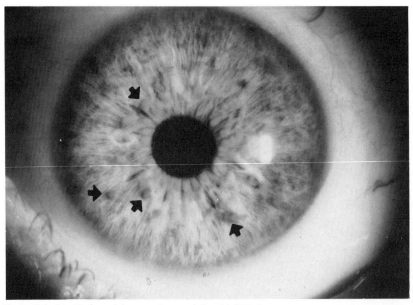

Figure 2.6. Iris Lisch nodules seen in an adult with NF–I.

of vertebrae, with a resultant collapse and further disruption of spinal cord and nerve root function. Paraspinal neurofibromas in the cervical region can invade the retropharyngeal/laryngeal regions; in the thoracic region, compromise of mediastinal and other intrathoracic structures is possible, if not likely; in the lower thoracic, lumbar, and sacral regions, extensive growth in the retroperitoneal space is a potential complication; in additon, sacral neurofibromas may extend into the perineal region, distorting both the appearance and function of the internal and external genitalia, the ureters, bladder, and terminal bowel. Plexiform neurofibromas of the limbs may assume gigantic proportions, even to the point of requiring surgical amputation as the only reasonable treatment approach. Neurofibromas of the viscera may also occur, the most frequent sites being at the renal hilum, leading to one form of renovascular compromise, and the entire length of the bowel, leading to bowel obstruction or gastrointestinal bleeding. Schwannomas may rarely occur as part of NF–I, and when they do, they ordinarily only involve peripheral nerves.

Central nervous system tumors tend to be restricted to astrocytomas, the most common one being optic glioma (or pilocytic astrocytoma). Optic gliomas appear to occur in more than 15% of NF–I patients, but cause problems in only about one-third (5% of the total)[1]. Optic gliomas as part of NF–I warrant special emphasis: they result in a series of serious complications that can be prevented by the use of routine computerized radiographic (CT) or magnetic resonance (MRI) scanning and they appear to be a hallmark of this particular form of NF (Figure 2.7). That is, I am totally unaware of any patient with NF–I having an acoustic neuroma (schwannoma) or meningioma, which are the key features of other forms of NF. Simply put, we have never seen an instance of an optic glioma (or any other intracranial astrocytoma) in association with an acoustic neuroma or meningioma. Optic gliomas may be confined to either or both of the optic nerves in their intraorbital segments, or may extend into the optic chiasm. Alternatively, the chiasm may be involved and the intraorbital components spared. Chiasmal involvement may also extend into the optic tracts and radiations. Although the observations are currently incomplete, non-optic-pathway intracranial astrocytomas may be more common among patients with optic gliomas [9]. This possibility is distinct from the relatively frequent, though unaccounted-for, abnormal findings (suggestive of multiple astrocytomas) seen on MRI scans of patients studied because of an optic glioma. Central nervous system spinal

cord tumors, distinct from paraspinal neurofibromas, are most unusual among NF–I patients.

Pheochromocytomas are more frequent among NF–I patients than in the general population, with an estimated incidence of about 1 in 200 if all ages are considered. However, they are virtually unheard of among children (with or without NF–I), and thus the incidence of pheochromocytoma is presumably somewhat higher among adults with NF–I. Nonadrenal locations, particularly the organ of Zuckerkandl at the aortic bifurcation, must always be considered.

Other types of benign tumors, particularly other types of neural crest–derived tumors such as ganglioneuromas, as well as glomus tumors may occur as part of NF–I.

Malignant Tumors

Malignancy as a complication of NF–I is particularly important. On the one hand, it is one of the definite contributors to the disorder's mortality, with respect to both its frequency, about 6% (i.e. somewhat above 5%), and its resistance to all treatment modalities except timely total surgical extirpation. On the other hand, it is reasonable to presume that elucidating the cellular and molecular mechanisms that ultimately explain this complication will contribute to our understanding of malignant transformation in the other genetic conditions that predispose to cancer as well as to carcinogenesis in the general population. The most characteristic and most com-

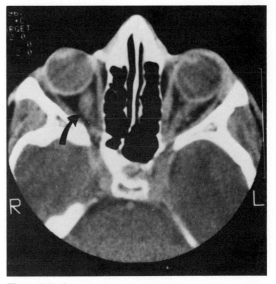

Figure 2.7. Computed tomograph (CT) scan showing a right intraorbital optic glioma.

mon type of NF–I malignancy is neurofibrosarcoma (also known as malignant schwannoma or malignant nerve sheath tumor) [20,21]. Its histologic appearance, however, may not always be that of a typical neurofibrosarcoma, alternative forms being angiosarcoma [22], malignant fibrous histiocytoma [21], liposarcoma, and so on [23]. Embryonal malignancies also appear to occur more frequently, particularly in Wilms' tumor and rhabdomyosarcoma; data are less clear for neuroblastoma [20]. Leukemia, particularly juvenile chronic myelogenous leukemia, is much more frequent among NF–I patients than can be explained by coincidence [20,24].

Although the risk for neurofibrosarcoma is relatively modest, in the neighborhood of 5%, this still represents a much greater risk than that which exists for the general population, and it behooves all clinicians providing any level of health care for NF patients to be aware of this risk and to be prepared to carry out the proper diagnostic procedures necessary to minimize the serious morbidity and untimely death due to this complication. Any unexplained development of pain, especially if referred pain is a component, a sudden increase in tumor (that is, neurofibroma) size, or the new or rapid worsening of any type of neuropathy should raise the suspicion of a neurofibrosarcoma or related tumor. Most often, a neurofibrosarcoma develops in a previous neurofibroma, usually but not always of the plexiform variety. The most common sites generally reflect their propensity for plexiform neurofibromas: paraspinal and retroperitoneal. More than one neurofibrosarcoma or similar tumor may develop in a given patient. Neurofibrosarcomas are extremely rare (if they occur at all) in NF–I youngsters less than 10 years of age. The most effective means of therapy is total surgical extirpation, including amputation if deemed appropriate to the circumstances. Limited resection, radiotherapy, and chemotherapy have limited and uncertain utility.

Ocular Abnormalities

In addition to iris Lisch nodules, the ocular globes are also directly affected by an NF–I mutation. Hypertrophic corneal nerves are not infrequent. It is of interest that this feature of NF–I is also seen in the multiple mucosal neuroma syndrome, or multiple endocrine neoplasia (MEN) IIb. Choroidal hamartomas are also distinctive characteristics of NF–I. One devastating complication of NF–I is congenital glaucoma, leading as it does to buphthalmos and not infrequently to loss of the involved eye. This com-

plication may be seen in about 0.5 to 1% of NF–I infants.

Skeletal Abnormalities

Short stature is not uncommon among NF–I patients of all ages [1,7]. The mechanism(s) responsible for this recently recognized clinical disturbance has yet to be clarified, though a simple hormonal (e.g. growth hormone) deficiency appears not to obtain. A more widespread direct skeletal (i.e growth center) disturbance is more likely.

Macrocephaly has long been known as a component of the NF–I spectrum of skeletal disturbances. At least 16% of NF–I patients have head circumference at or above the 98th centile, adjusted for age and sex.

Craniofacial dysplasia is a relatively frequent feature of NF–I, affecting at least 5% of patients of all ages. Virtually all portions of the cranial vault may be involved, but most commonly it is the occipital regions and bones contributing to the orbit, especially the greater wing of the sphenoid bone (Figure 2.8). The sphenoid wing dysplasia may be associated with an orbital/periorbital plexiform neurofibroma, but often there is no local evidence of tumor, leaving a mechanistic explanation of the sphenoid wing abnormality totally unclear. Of importance is the fact that this is a progressive lesion, with the posterior orbital wall deficit enlarging as the patient gets older. Other types of facial skeletal aberrations may also be present, and are usually secondary to the effects of a growing plexiform neurofibroma.

Vertebral dysplasia may also be present to varying degrees. The recent recognition that aberrant hair whorls may be seen overlying localized vertebral dysplasia, with or without accompanying neurofibromas, emphasizes the embryonic onset of some of the lesions of NF–I and adds legitimacy to the notion of dysplasia in a strict sense as part of the overall clinical picture of NF–I. The minimal vertebral involvement is posterior scalloping of the lumbar vertebrae as seen on spine radiographs. The pathogenetic explanation for these lesions is not always apparent. That is, while neurofibromas may also be seen in the region of the scalloping, this is not always the case. More severe involvement of the spinal column is based on varying degrees of vertebral dysplasia (as considered above) and the presence of paraspinal neurofibromas, the growth of which can lead to erosion of adjacent vertebrae and even to their collapse. This latter complication is seen most frequently in the cervical and upper thoracic spine,

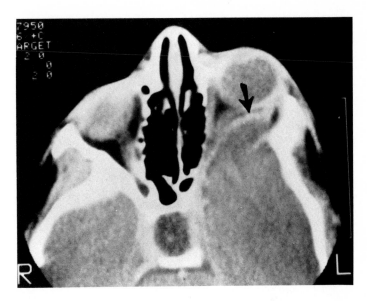

Figure 2.8. A cranial CT scan showing left sphenoid wing dysplasia.

nd to a lesser extent in the lower lumbar and upper sacral spine. Of course, scoliosis may accompany any of these vertebral distortions and may occur in the absence of any other localized abnormality. Prototypic NF–I scoliosis involves the lower cervical and upper thoracic spine and has a strong kyphotic component; it is progressive, often leading to major neurologic and cardiorespiratory complications. Onset is almost invariably in the second half of the first decade. Lesser degrees of simple lateral scoliosis may be seen in many NF–I patients, and in some there may be a minor to moderate rotatory component as well.

Pseudarthrosis is a major characteristic feature of NF–I; so much so that any newborn with evidence of pseudarthrosis must be presumed to have NF–I until it is established otherwise. However, it is not true that all cases of pesudarthrosis require the diagnosis of NF–I. Most commonly the pseudarthrosis involves the distal portion of one tibia, but other tubular bones may be affected as well, including the fibula, radius, ulna, humerus, and clavicle, among others. Localized neurofibromas do not account for this complication of NF–I; its pathogenesis remains a mystery. The severity of the lesion and its consequences vary tremendously, ranging from mild bowing of the involved bone to disruptions for which the only effective therapeutic approach is amputation.

Genu valgum and genu varum (Figures 2.9 and 2.10) have only recently been recognized to be relatively frequent in NF–I [1]. Again, the range of severity extends from the trivial, to distortion sufficient enough to warrant bracing or surgical correction. In

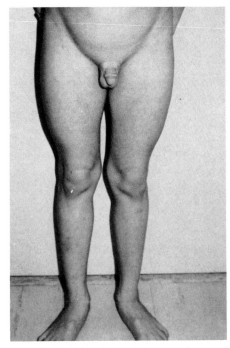

Figure 2.9. Moderate genu valgum in NF–I patient.

the neighborhood of 15 to 20% of NF–I patients may manifest this feature.

Pectus excavatum, characteristically involving only the lower half of the sternum (Fig. 2.11), is also seen in upward of about 20% of NF–I patients. It may be minimal, merely a casual finding, or it may be more severe, distorting the entire chest and medias-

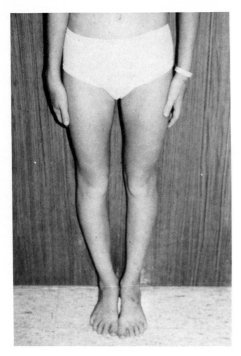

Figure 2.10. Moderate genu varum in NF–I patient.

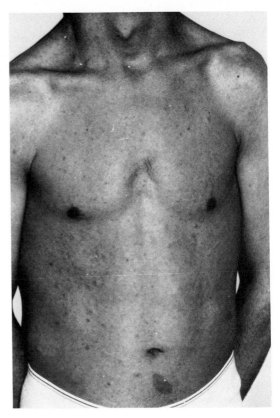

Figure 2.11. Lower sternal pectus excavatum, characteristic of NF–I.

tinum. When more severe, there is often associated flaring of the lower ribs.

Other less-frequent osseous complications may also be seen in NF–I, although the causal relationship may not always be clear. Benign osseous cysts apparent only by radiographic study have been variously claimed to be a feature of NF–I, but the picture is far from complete.

Other Structural Abnormalities

Ganglioneuromatosis of the large bowel, distinct from diffuse plexiform neurofibroma involvement, is a feature of NF–I that is (along with hypertrophied corneal nerves) also seen in multiple endocrine neoplasia (MEN) IIb. This anatomic lesion leads to varying degrees of decreased bowel motility and, therefore, varied functional problems, and accounts for at least a portion of the 10 to 15% of NF–I patients with constipation or obstipation.

Xanthogranulomas of the skin have only recently been recognized as a feature of NF–I [1]. They may be important for several reasons, including the following. First, they may be the presenting symptom in young children. Second, it is not at all apparent as to why these lesions should be considered a part of NF–I; certainly they do not neatly fit into the neural crest approach to pathogenesis. Thus, clari-

fying the origin of these lesions in NF–I is likely to be particularly revealing about overall NF–I pathogenesis. Third, these lesions may be associated with some of the leukemias that develop in NF–I.

Angiomas of the skin have been emphasized [25] as a feature of NF. Certainly, they do occur with significant frequency among NF–I patients, and angiomas may occur as a central feature of the disorder in some alternate forms of NF, suggesting that these lesions are an instructive feature of NF–I. Another reason to focus on these microvascular lesions is because endothelial cells do comprise a major portion of neurofibromas; indeed, even some of the sarcomas that develop in NF–I are angiosarcomas [22].

Various types of intrinsic and extrinsic lesions of middle-size and major arteries occur in at least 5% of NF–I patients if all ages are taken into account. There are numerous well-documented instances of arterial aberrations involving the kidney [26], the brain [27], and the gastrointestinal tract [28]. In addition to extrinsic distortions from adjacent neurofibromas, there are (more frequently) intrinsic, that is, intramural lesions, seen as localized annular constrictions, gradual fusiform constrictions, or aneurysms of various types. Slow, progressive changes may even lead to the angiographic image of moyamoya.

Dilation of the intracerebral cerebrospinal fluid (CSF) space, particularly the third ventricle, and frank hydrocephalus are not infrequent features of NF–I [1]. Varying degrees of third ventricle dilation may be discovered incidentally at the time of cranial CT scanning, or it may develop acutely as a consequence of brain tumor (most usually an astrocytoma) or on the basis of aqueductal stenosis, the mechanism of which is obscure.

Dural ectasias and pseudomeningoceles or arachnoid cysts are not uncommon features of NF–I. The cerebral arachnoid cysts are usually discovered coincidentally on CT scans and are not associated with any clinical features. On the other hand, although spinal dural ectasias or pseudomeningoceles may be coincidental, they are usually appreciated at the time of spinal computerized imaging [MRI] or myelography that may be performed in evaluating advancing scoliosis.

Excessive dental caries sometimes appear to be more frequent among NF–I patients. And since the entire tooth other than the enamel is derived from the neural crest, the possibility of direct dental involvement as part of NF–I is worth exploring. However, this is such a common clinical problem, with numerous genetic and environmental contributions, that it will be some time before the association is clarified.

Other anatomic/structural lesions may also occur in association with NF–I, but their relation to the disorder as a whole is problematic, either because of a low frequency of association or because of the potential of reporting bias. The purported association of parathyroid adenomas with NF–I [29] falls in this category. Pulmonary interstitial disease [30] also can be considered here, although its true frequency in NF–I is a matter of controversy—while some authors consider it to be relatively frequent [30] others have considered it to be distinctly unusual.

Functional NF–I Features

Some clinical abnormalities are best catalogued and organized in terms of functional distortions, especially since it is often in these terms that patients present for clinical assistance, and the problem as a whole may involve more than one body segment or multiple anatomic structures or domains.

Cosmetic Disfigurement

Cosmetic disfigurement is one of the outstanding clinical problems of NF–I patients. For all but a small portion there is some degree of cosmetic compromise, and for at least one-third of patients this is likely to be a major element of their overall clinical picture. Surgical approaches applied after the lesions have developed represent the only realistic treatment modality at the present time, and usually the results are suboptimal and the likelihood of recurrence, to at least some degree, is substantial.

Hypertrophy

Hypertrophic overgrowth of a body segment, with both cosmetic distortions and functional disturbances, complicates the course of at least several percent of NF–I patients. The weight of the lesion (plexiform neurofibroma), destruction of bone supporting elements, vascular compromise, and nerve compression all contribute to the disability that may develop. Surgical reductions of the tumor mass (debulking) often provides only temporary relief and is associated with further cosmetic distortion or neurologic compromise (from iatrogenically interrupted nerves). Amputation of an involved limb is not uncommon.

Neurologic and Psychiatric Features

Various types of neurologic dysfunction may develop in the course of NF–I, each having at least the potential of more than one contributing factor. Included here are such items as general incoordination (often seen in association with developmental delay and learning disability); weakness, paresis, or frank paralysis (for example, from cerebrovascular involvement, paraspinal neurofibromas, and peripheral nerve neurofibromas); varying degrees of pain, especially in association with extensive paraspinal neurofibromas; seizures of all types, including infantile spasms, and other generalized seizure types; other neurologic problems, such as ataxia associated with acute hydrocephalus or a cerebellar astrocytoma; sensory deficits resulting from spinal roots, plexus, or peripheral nerve neurofibromas; or other lesions.

Electroencephalographic abnormalities that reflect brain abnormalities of an undefined type are seen in about 15% of NF–I patients [1], though only about one-fifth of them have an associated seizure disorder.

Strabismus may be more common than is seen in

the general population, but the observations are still preliminary [1].

Visual impairment may result from a variety of lesions, including optic gliomas, orbital/periorbital plexiform neurofibromas, cerebrovascular insults, and congenital glaucoma. Amblyopia secondary to strabismus is not uncommon, and thus attention to the question of strabismus, raised above, is of no small importance.

Hearing deficits may result from a variety of lesions, particularly neurofibromas obstructing the external auditory canal and extensive surgery to treat facial plexiform neurofibromas. At times the hearing deficit has no obvious cause, and under these circumstances may be purely coincidental, but more data are needed to clarify this point. The most common causes of hearing deficits among NF–I patients are coincidental to the NF, namely, recurrent otitis media and noise exposure. Note that acoustic neuromas are distinctly absent from this listing [1].

Speech impediments are frequently present, affecting at least 10% of the NF–I population. The specific mechanisms are unclear, though it is obvious that no one anatomic disturbance can explain all the cases and all the types of speech distortions that are seen. On the other hand, lingual neurofibromas and neurofibromas involving the recurrent laryngeal nerve are worth considering in individual cases.

Intellectual deficits over a wide spectrum characterize NF–I, ranging from minor developmental delay, through learning disabilities, to frank mental retardation. The most common problem is that of learning disabilities, affecting at least 40% of NF–I school-age patients [31]. The learning disabilities themselves generally involve an "attention deficit disorder," but are otherwise quite nonspecific, overlapping with the same type of problem seen in many other clinical settings. This set of problems, perhaps best referred to by the neutral phrase "school performance problems," is the single most common clinically disruptive element [31] in the NF–I population taken as a whole. And yet virtually nothing is understood about this component of NF–I at the pathogenetic, that is, the mechanistic level, the work of Rosman and Pearce [32] implicating cerebral heterotopias notwithstanding. Mental retardation, strictly defined, is seen in about 8% of NF–I patients, and it is not readily explained as a secondary consequence of brain tumors or hydrocephalus.

Psychiatric disturbances appear not to be more frequent among NF–I patients compared to other populations with chronic, potentially debilitating disorders, although Samuelsson (in a doctoral thesis [8]) considered there to be an excess of such problems among NF patients when compared to the Swedish population at large. On the other hand, the combination of intellectual deficits, the frustrations of actual and potential NF–I complications, and the lack of effective treatment certainly takes its toll in terms of adjustment problems, personality disorders, and aggravation of neuroses, a fact not to be ignored in the long-term planning of research efforts into this disorder.

Akin to this is the problem referred to as the psychosocial burden of NF–I. At the least, various degrees of cosmetic distortion will account for some significant portion of the NF–I population developing significant problems with social stigmatization, impaired self-esteem, and loss of self-confidence. From the patient's perspective, this is one of the most disheartening and burdensome elements of the disorder.

Other Functional Abnormalities

Headache is extremely common among NF–I patients, though most often it is of the "tension headache" variety, perhaps readily explained by the factors relevant to the psychosocial burden problems considered above. However, another type of headache also seems to be common among NF–I patients, perhaps affecting 5 to 10% of patients in or beyond their second decade. It appears to be a true migraine (i.e. vascular) type of headache and is usually of moderate severity, though at times it can be a patient's predominant symptom.

Puberty disturbances, involving either premature or delayed puberty, are frequently listed as cardinal features of NF–I; however, in actuality this type of complication involves only 1% or less of these patients. Perhaps trivial explanations, such as the confusion engendered by incomplete respect for heterogeneity and disfigurement from perineal/genital plexiform neurofibromas, contribute to the overstatements that abound with respect to this aspect of NF–I.

Pruritus is a significant symptom in at least 10% of NF–I patients. It is almost always associated with newly developing or rapidly growing neurofibromas and may even be a harbinger of their development or growth. It is aggravated by heat, either from the environment or from bodily exertion. For some patients it may be their most bothersome symptom. Its importance, however, transcends this latter fact, inasmuch as it has become the basis for developing a treatment strategy: to the extent that the pruritus may reflect mast cell secretions that contribute to neurofibroma development and growth, the possibility of interfering with mast cell secretion becomes a cogent treatment approach [7,14,15].

Constipation that significantly interferes with an NF–I patient's day-to-day activities and well-being occurs in about 5% of those with the mutant gene. In some instances it appears to be the result of the colon ganglioneuromatosis discussed above, but for other patients rectal biopsies fail to clarify the basis for this problem. In some youngsters (5 to 15 years old) who have constipation as a prominent symptom, there may be associated episodic fecal incontinence and urinary urgency, leading to serious disruptions of schooling and various social activities.

Gastrointestinal hemorrhage may occur with a frequency as high as 1 to 2 per 200 NF–I patients, almost always in adults. Usually it reflects erosions of intramural neurofibromas through the bowel mucosal surface, with some degree of involvement of a small artery when hemorrhage is massive. The neurofibromas that are the basis for the bleeding usually have been clinically inapparent up to the time of the hemorrhage, which may be massive. Any portion of the GI tract, from the lower esophagus to the rectum, may be involved, but most often the bleeding orginates in the small bowel, essentially reflecting the length of that portion of the tract. Prompt treatment, involving either local removal of the tumor or resection of a portion of the bowel, cannot only be life-saving in terms of the immediate problem, it can also obviate the problem indefinitely. The specific factors that predispose to bowel neurofibromas in large numbers or to their bleeding are not currently understood. It would be of interest to study the dietary habits and food ingestion patterns of such patients to determine whether identifiable environmental factors contribute to this important NF–I complication.

Systemic hypertension in NF–I may be due to several causes. First, it may be merely coincidental, reflecting both the general population risk and individual family histories. In other instances it may be a direct result of the NF–I mutation itself, either in terms of renovascular compromise or a pheochromocytoma, both of which have been discussed above. In any event, all NF–I patients at all ages, from infancy through advanced adulthood, must have their blood pressures monitored at all clinical encounters. Detecting a recent development of hypertension in an NF–I patient can be critically important in determining future health care, both immediately and over the long run.

Other types of functional problems can also develop in the course of NF–I, such as a hyperadrenergic state in at least some patients with massive cervical neurofibromas that apparently elaborate and secrete excessive amounts of catecholamines, particularly norepinephrine [1,33]. Another functional problem that may have a variety of origins is respiratory embarrassment; for example, that due to a restriction from severe kyphoscoliosis, or to diffuse interstitial/parenchymal involvement of the lungs themselves [30]. In addition, there is some sense in considering surgery as one of the functional complications of NF–I, respecting that probably at least one-third to one-half of all NF–I patients may require surgery at some time in their life and that surgical (and anesthetic) complications may supervene for any of a variety of reasons, some related directly to the NF itself and some to the surgical procedures.

Natural History and Age-related Progression

True "natural history" studies must involve essentially total ascertainment of the at-risk population and a long-term systematic prospective follow-up. No such natural history studies of NF–I have been carried out, even though the title of a published report may lead one to believe this [4]. One may presume that many aspects of the disorder's natural history have been revealed or at least touched on in a careful evaluation of a large number of patients whose past histories and current problems have been itemized and supplemented during years of follow-up [1,2,3,9]. From such reports the following facts do seem clear.

Neurofibromatosis in general, and NF–I in particular, is a progressive disease, becoming worse over time. Otherwise stated, the nature and severity of a given patient's NF is at least partly a function of the patient's age. This is important for the patient, and also for clinical investigators, since the frequency (or severity) of specific features or complications must take into account the age of the subjects under investigation: for example, neurofibrosarcomas or pheochromocytomas are virtually unheard of in the first decade of life, and, conversely, pseudarthrosis does not develop ab initio in an adult. One can readily glean from the available data that certain features or complications of NF–I are more likely in certain age groups [34].

Congenital or neonatal problems include the pseudarthroses, congenital glaucoma, sphenoid wing dysplasia, and plexiform neurofibromas (although these may be relatively subtle at the earliest ages).

Early childhood problems include developmental delay, embryonal tumors, compromise from the progression of certain strategically located plexiform neurofibromas (i.e. retropharyngeal, mediastinal, and so forth), and the presentation of symptomatic optic gliomas [35].

In the second half of the first decade we notice a significant number of optic gliomas, and instances of learning disabilities, and we begin to see considerably more frequent development of seizures, scoliosis (with or without kyphosis), and iris Lisch nodules [1,12], and the further worsening of plexiform neurofibromas; occasionally, patients begin to manifest relatively large numbers of cutaneous and subcutaneous neurofibromas.

In the second decade almost all patients begin to manifest at least a few cutaneous or subcutaneous neurofibromas, often in association with the onset of puberty; in this same time period hypertension and neurofibrosarcomas become obvious and scoliosis that will ultimately be severe declares itself so.

In adulthood, the main problems are continuation of the increase in the number or size of cutaneous and subcutaneous neurofibromas and the more frequent development of neurofibrosarcomas and pheochromocytomas.

In late adulthood (sixth decade and beyond), the disease is relatively quiescent except for the continued, but somewhat slower, progression of cutaneous and subcutaneous neurofibromas, and the ever-present possibility of neurofibrosarcomas.

Vascular compromise of the arterial trees of the brain, kidneys, and GI tract (see above) may present at any age, though it is less common in small children.

Specific factors that may contribute to the origin or aggravation of any of these features or their complications are largely unknown, although there may be some reason to consider that mechanical trauma may be a factor for at least some neurofibromas [1]. A specific or predictable adverse effect of environmental agents, such as ionizing radiation, chemotherapeutic agents and medications in general, and hormones (e.g. in birth control pills) remains to be established.

Laboratory, Radiologic, and Other Studies

Histopathology and Ultrastructure

The histologic and ultrastructural study of tumor and other tissue specimens from NF patients has not been fruitful for elucidating the primary defect in any form of the disease. On the other hand, such studies have made clear that there is nothing unique about any of the tumors that occur as part of a pleiotropic disorder known as NF in comparison to isolated tumors distinct from NF in any sense. Further, they have imposed limits and conditions that must be respected in more precise biochemical or cell culture (and other in vitro) studies. For example, Schwann cells comprise virtually all of the cells in schwannomas, but are only one of several cell types in neurofibromas; and vascular endothelial cells may be more important in neurofibromas than was previously thought [1]. On the other hand, the microscopic dissection of NF tumors has probably not been utilized to its full potential in ferreting out those facts that address cellular interaction as a key aspect of neurofibroma pathogenesis, although Peltonen and associates [36,37] have made some inroads in this regard. The use of cytochemical and immunocytochemical stains to characterize components of various NF tumors has been relatively limited, though when used [36–38] such stains have been very helpful in underscoring the multicellular, cooperative nature of these tumors. Certainly, additional research along these lines is critically important and is to be encouraged vigorously. Ultimately, even when the gene defect is known, the mechanisms to explain the tumor growth and afford some treatment rationale will still need to be sorted out. Studying the intact tumors, as well as cell culture derivatives therefrom, will be crucial in elucidating these mechanisms.

Although skin biopsies are not useful for routine diagnostic purposes, melanin production studied through the use of both bright-field optics combined with cytochemical staining and electron microscopy has provided the best data yet about an intracellular defect in NF. As demonstrated by a number of investigators [1,39,40], melanin macroglobules are characteristic of the skin melanocytes in NF and particularly NF–I. These distorted organelles derived from the Golgi–endoplasmic reticulum complex of the melanocyte–although not unique to NF, do suggest that the basic defect of NF is quite likely to involve this intracellular membrane system, perhaps as elaborated in the hypothesis proposed previously by Riccardi [11]. That is, if an intracellular defect is characteristic of one of the defining features of NF (i.e. café-au-lait spots and other skin pigmentation defects), it is likely to be relevant to the intracellular defect in the other cellular components of the various lesions of NF. It is of interest that relatively little has been done to extend the present observations to other disciplines, such as those of melanin biochemistry and somatic cell genetics.

Routine Blood and Urine Studies

Routine studies of blood and urine specimens have not been useful at all for identifying clues about NF pathogenesis or the basic defect. Studies of serum and urinary amino acids and urinary organic acids have been uniformly unrevealing, and likewise for studies of urinary catecholamines and melanin metabolites [1]. Systematic studies have not been carried out in CSF specimens of NF patients.

Radiologic Studies

Until the advent of CT radiologic studies of NF patients and NF lesions had done little more than add certain details to clinical descriptions. The extensive use of high-resolution CT scanning, however, has added a new dimension to characterizing the subtle and changing features of previously inaccessible lesions. For example, our reasonably complete appreciation of the frequency and range of variation in optic gliomas and other astrocytomas in NF–I, and the restriction of acoustic neuromas to forms of NF other than NF–I, was made possible for the first time with CT scanning. In addition, the details of the relationship between the superficial (i.e. integumentary) aspects of diffuse plexiform neurofibromas and deeper tissues became much clearer through the use of CT scans that characterize these tumors, for example, prior to surgery. And now nuclear magnetic resonance imaging [MRI or nuclear magnetic resonance (NMR)] scanning has broadened these horizons even more. Preliminary experience with MRI scanning of NF–I patients with optic gliomas already indicates that there may be more elements of abnormal pathology in the brains of these patients than had been obvious from the CT scans. In addition, MRI has become the standard for diagnosing acoustic neuromas and most types of spinal and paraspinal tumors. Certainly, research into further uses of this approach for understanding or minimizing the morbidity of NF should have high priority. Similarly, ^{32}P–NMR scanning and positron emission tomography are now available to explore not only the anatomy, but also the metabolism and function of the lesions and tissues in which the lesions occur. In addition, the use of various metabolites tagged with radionuclides might offer ways of studying NF lesions in their earliest or even incipient stages, as has been done for neuroblastomas and pheochromocytomas.

Electrophysiologic Studies

Electrophysiologic studies, particularly electromyography and nerve conduction velocity, electroencephalography, audiography/auditory brain stem response (ABR), and visual evoked response studies have probably not been utilized to the full extent in exploring subtle and changing tissue disturbances in the appropriate tissues of NF patients. For example, given that about 15% of NF–I patients have abnormal tracings by routine electroencephalographic studies, it is certainly conceivable that recent computerized digital electroencephalographic analysis would reveal much about the brain in NF–I.

Psychometrics

Because learning disability in one form or another is so frequent among NF–I youngsters (affecting 40% or more), routine testing of all children prior to entering school is appropriate, if not actually required. The point is not to label children, or to look for problems where there appear to be none, but to take action since learning disability is so common and has such disruptive effects if not countered vigorously with remediation and other special assistance. The exact nature of this learning disability has yet to be defined: it shares many features with other forms of learning disability, but it also has some distinction, particularly in the realm of visual/motor coordination and "motor planning" in general. Only about 8% or so of NF–I patients can be considered mentally retarded [31]. In contrast, as expected, several percent of NF–I patients have IQ scores well above average, though on the whole for age groups up to age 17 years the mean IQ scores are shifted to the left (85 to 90) [31]. Dealing with this aspect of NF–I is very time-consuming for the patient, family, teachers, and clinicians. Defining the extent and nature of the problem(s) through the judicious use of psychometric testing is well advised.

Growth Factors

Nerve growth factor (NGF), by virtue of its importance for the growth and differentiation of nervous system elements derived from the neural crest, particularly autonomic and sensory ganglia components, promised to provide a ready means of explaining NF pathogenesis, at least in part [41]. However, on the whole the data have been conflicting [42–44] or have failed to confirm a role for this substance in any simple explanation of NF pathogenesis [45]. On the other hand, the possibility that NGF-like substances or NGF receptors may play a role has not been discounted.

Except for a preliminary suggestion by Zelkowitz and Stambouly [46] and Zelkowitz [47] that epidermal growth factor (EGF) receptors may be abnormally regulated in cell cultures of skin biopsy fibroblasts from NF patients, neither EGF nor other specific growth factors have been implicated in NF pathogenesis. Seizinger et al. [48] have indicated that platelet-derived growth factor is not linked to NF–I, much as Darby et al. [49] have excluded linkage of beta-NGF from linkage to NF–I. On the other hand, Riccardi [50,51] has demonstrated a factor or factors that will enhance the growth of neurofibroma-derived cells in culture. A similar finding was noted by Krone et al. [52].

In Vitro Tumor Studies

Cell culture studies of NF tumors are a logical approach to understanding the disease's pathogenesis, and they have been, or are being attempted, in a dozen or more laboratories in the United States alone. However, in tumors that are relatively homogeneous, such as astrocytomas and schwannomas, getting the cells to grow is not as simple as it is for skin-derived fibroblasts. In addition, neurofibromas are notorious for giving rise to several different types of outgrowths. This means that a culture from a given tumor is not always comparable, in terms of morphology and general growth characteristics, to that of another neurofibroma, or even another segment of the same tumor. We often simply do not know the nature or origin of the cells comprising the outgrowth. Currently work must be done on clarifying the types of cells that can grow from neurofibroma explants and how the growth of certain cells can be enhanced while that of alternative cells is minimized. The utilization of transmission and scanning electron microscopy to study these cells, as well as the use of cytochemical and immunocytochemical stains (e.g. for S–100 protein, glial fibrillary acidic protein, fibronectin, laminin, neuron-specific enolase, collagen type IV) is currently a central focus. The overall point is to be able to culture the cells that are most likely to express the NF mutation, presumably in a manner that would reveal their behavior in vivo, and therefore reveal information about the mutation itself. Because cellular interaction is critical to the origin and dynamics of tumor growth in vivo, the ability to study the growth of these cells, both on their own and in combination with other cells or derivatives from other cells, should be given high priority.

Studying tumors directly without culturing has many advantages, and also disadvantages as well. One disadvantage has to do with size; if the amount of tumor is small, the ability to use all probes may be lost. For neurofibromas, however, an additional, more or less insurmountable problem for most studies is cellular heterogeneity: a DNA or RNA preparation of the entire tumor includes the nucleic acids from multiple cell types with divergent activities and then mixes them together in a single pool that represents an "average," so to speak, thus sacrificing information about specific cell components. And this latter, cell-specific information is likely to be the most useful over the long run. In situ cDNA probes for labeling individual cells is one way of approaching this problem. The use of cells cultured from a neurofibroma has the benefit of being more homogeneous (particularly after several passages) and providing relatively large amounts of material, but leaves open to question whether the "right" cell type is being studied.

Other types of tumors, including schwannomas, astrocytomas, and neurofibrosarcomas, are considerably more homogeneous, and whole-tumor nucleic acid preparations are likely to be more informative about the cell type comprising the major, if not critical, part of the tumor.

Of greatest interest in studies of this type are probes for known oncogenes, as well as those for growth factors and their receptors and for other gene products known or thought to have cell growth or differentiation regulatory functions. Ideally for such studies the following samples would be available from a single individual: malignant tumor (e.g. neurofibrosarcoma), benign tumor (for instance, neurofibroma, schwannoma, astrocytoma), and ostensibly normal tissue (such as white blood cells, skin, liver), plus cultured cells from each of these three types of tissue. Of special interest is the fact that four of four consecutive neurofibrosarcomas studied cytogenetically in one laboratory demonstrated multiple chromosome aberrations [23], a fact that must be taken into account in RNA and DNA studies.

Other studies on whole-tumor preparations and cell cultures from tumors (and on conditioned medium) can also be carried out, for example, identifying altered or aberrant production of growth factors.

Genetic and Epidemiologic Aspects of Neurofibromatosis

Population Genetics and Epidemiology

Epidemiologic and demographic research with respect to NF in general and NF–I in particular has been relatively poorly developed, owing to the high prevalence of the disease (making ascertainment, evaluation, and follow-up a tremendous logistic and strategic burden); its markedly variable manifestations, especially as a function of age; the high mobility of people in modern societies; and the lack of any sort of true registry for the disease. What surveys have been done have either emphasized largely the clinical elements (for instance, itemizing features but ignoring or minimizing the importance of considerations such as total ascertainment, biased ascertainment, and the like) or have emphasized population and demographic elements (attempting to estimate, for example, mutation rates but without full respect for critical clinical issues such as variable expressivity and clinical–genetic heterogeneity). There is clearly the need for additional studies, particularly as it now (or soon will be) possible to combine the strategies of the epidemiologist and demographer with the methodologies of the molecular biologist in attempting to identify the true incidence and frequency of NF and its various types, as defined on both clinical and gene-probe bases.

To date, only modest numbers of genetic studies have been carried out. From the standpoint of population genetics the emphasis has been on estimating prevalence, mutation rates, and fitness, which have led to relatively useful approximations, although they are imprecise for the reasons noted above. The works of Borberg [2], Crowe et al. [3] , Sergeyev [53], and Samuelsson [8] are the most useful in these areas, but all suffer to varying degrees from the same problems (i.e. those relating to ascertainment and heterogeneity). In any event, they have collectively established that the prevalence of NF is about 1 in 3,000 individuals (to be distinguished from the disorder's incidence, which is not known), that the mutation rate is approximately 1 mutation per 10,000 gametes per generation, and that the genetic fitness is about 0.85 (but with apparently significant sex differences). Improvements on these estimates are unlikely until registries and direct gene probes are utilized. A contribution of paternal age to the origin of some NF–I mutations seems clear [54], but this fact is of limited utility at the present time.

Genetic Linkage

The genetic linkage approach, which involves attempting to track a mutant NF gene with a gene product or DNA restriction fragment length polymorphism (RFLP), has been unsuccessful to date in identifying a linkage group or chromosomal locus. Published work by Ichikawa et al. [55], Spence et al. [56], DiLiberti and Rivas [57], Pericak–Vance [58], Dunn et al. [59], Huson et al. [60], and Darby et al. [49,61] has failed to provide specific genetic linkage clues, though some portions of the human genome have been effectively excluded or have made unlikely sites, including regions on chromosomes 1, 4, 6, 9, 13, 16, and 19. The possible linkage of NF–I to Steinert myotonic dystrophy [55,57] has stirred up interest in a possible assignment of NF–I to chromosome 19, but corroboration is lacking [59,60]. It is reasonable to expect that identification of the gene itself through genetic linkage studies will provide within the next few years, at the most, the opportunity to surmise, if not specifically designate, the intracellular biochemical defect.

In addition, direct genetic (i.e. DNA and RNA) analyses of NF tumors, particularly malignancies, may effectively complement the genetic linkage approach by identifying specific genes (e.g., oncogenes) that may be useful probes in the linkage studies. However, cellular heterogeneity of the tumors and the presence of multiple chromosome rearrangements in neurofibrosarcomas pose significant confounding problems that point to the genetic linkage approach as the most cogent and parsimonious. Chromosomal analyses of neurofibromas, schwannomas, optic gliomas, and other benign NF tumors [23,51] and of peripheral blood lymphocytes [62] have been unrevealing. No patient with a coincidental structural chromosome aberration suggesting a chromosomal site of the mutation has been identified, although mosaic trisomy 8 has been noted in one patient [63].

Genetic Counseling

Genetic counseling is still a key element of health care for NF–I patients and their families. Because NF–I is an autosomal dominant disorder with a high frequency of new mutations (i.e. 50% of index cases), the recurrence risks for siblings of a youngster with NF–I may be essentially those for the general population or may be as high as 50%, depending on whether a parent has the disorder. A full consideration of the genetic counseling aspects of NF–I and NF in general is beyond the scope of this presentation, but it should be clear to each and every clinician working with these patients and families that genetic counseling *must* be provided, preferably by someone with expertise in both genetics and NF; expertise in the latter is particularly crucial in view of the concerns about heterogeneity, reviewed below. Here especially, the significance of clinical and genetic heterogeneity becomes paramount.

Prenatal diagnosis is not possible at this time for any form of NF.

Heterogeneity

That there is more than one form of NF, at least from a clinical standpoint, seems reasonably well established, though the number of specific types and the defining features of each remains to be established or universally agreed on. The suggestion of one categorization scheme by Riccardi [1,11] is merely a starting point and is preliminary at best. In any event, even the most casual observer soon realizes that not all patients with what appears to be NF have the disorder described by von Recklinghausen. Similarly, patients with acoustic NF, who have been characterized so well by Eldridge et al. [13], do not adequately account for those remaining after NF–I has been excluded. For example, there is the so-called segmental form [64] and a form that appears to overlap substantially with Noonan's syndrome [65]. Suffice it to say that further delineation of heterogeneity is critical to (a) carrying out certain types of additional research, including genetic linkage studies and efforts to be specific about the precise nature of the intracellular defect studied in vitro, and (b) implementing genetic screening and prenatal diagnosis when a disease marker is eventually found.

Routine Health Care and Treatment

General Considerations

At least some portion of the health care of an NF patient should involve the services of an expert in this disorder, even if it is only through the use of telephone consultations or the use of a computer-based NF information service (NFormation, Houston, Texas). In general, although we all wish a mild course for any patient, the fact is that from many standpoints NF in general, and NF–I in particular, is a potentially serious disorder. I thus urge clinicians to approach the diagnosis of NF from that vantage point and yet not necessarily burden the patient and family with every minor suspicion. Until clinicians as a group approach NF as though it were potentially serious, problems in the early, possibly remediable stages will go unrecognized or unattended, but a sense of impending disaster need not be communicated to the patient and family. The use of information pamphlets, such as those provided by the Texas Neurofibromatosis Foundation, the National Neurofibromatosis Foundation, and the Baylor Neurofibromatosis Program [66] can be very useful. Finally, I wish to emphasize that earlier concerns about an adverse effect of a mother's NF–I on her offspring's own NF–I severity [67,68] have not been substantiated and by and large can be discounted [1].

Patient Ascertainment, Intake, and Baseline Evaluation

Neurofibromatosis–I patients are incorporated into the health-care system in many ways, and thus all clinicians must be alert to the presence and meaning of this disorder. Once the diagnosis has been entertained or established and the family history reviewed, an in-depth history-taking session is necessary, with special emphasis on vision, hearing, seizures, intellectual deficits, speech impediments, constipation, scoliosis and other skeletal problems, excessive itching, and the presence of tumors of any sort, especially those involving the face, trunk, and viscera. Additional baseline evaluation includes a detailed physical examination, with emphasis on the skin, eyes, ears, and musculoskeletal and nervous systems. The patient's intellectual capabilities are also evaluated. My own preference, based on our Baylor program experience, is to supplement these data with those derived from a cranial/orbital CT (or MRI) scan, plain radiographs of the skull, chest, and spine, electroencephalograms, audiogram and ABR, ophthalmologic examination (including slit-lamp biomicroscopy), and psychometric testing [1]. However, the patient's age, the total clinical picture, patient/family financial resources, and the availability of experts in NF need to be taken into account. In any case, patient and family concerns must be allayed through minimal "guesswork," and problems must be prevented or minimized through early recognition.

Routine Follow-up

Routine visits every 12 to 18 months suffice, given a cooperative patients and family, the absence of serious symptoms or recent progression, plus the patient's and family's understanding that they are being encouraged to call or return if any additional concerns develop.

Medical Treatment

There is now only one formal protocol for the medical treatment of NF. This project at the Baylor College of Medicine Neurofibromatosis Program has used the drug ketotifen (Zaditen, Sandoz Pharmaceuticals) to test the hypothesis that mast cells contribute both to the pruritus that is characteristic of NF (especially during growth of neurofibromas) and to the actual growth of the neurofibromas. The double-blind cross-over protocol using diminution or cessation of NF-associated itching has been completed, and data analyses are underway but are not otherwise available. The open-label protocol, which uses a decrease or cessation of neurofibroma growth as an end-point, will continue for approximately one more year.

The use of drugs that are routine for non-NF patients is rarely contraindicated by the NF mutation itself, though of course each patient must always be considered individually. Currently, the presence of NF–I is not an automatic contraindication to the use of birth control pills. There are no special considerations for anticonvulsants. Drug studies, particularly those exploring the influence of sex steroids on the course of NF or investigating improved chemotherapy for NF malignancies, particularly neurofibrosarcomas, are certainly in order, but apparently none are ongoing.

Surgical Treatment

Surgery is still the main approach to treating NF, but this means waiting for problems or complications to develop, and the results of surgery often are disappointing to both the surgeon and the patient. Nonetheless, since surgery will continue to be a therapeutic mainstay for many years, research into improved techniques warrants high priority. For example, exploration of the use of laser surgery, suction removal of tumor (i.e. neurofibroma) components, and microvascular techniques (e.g., for pseudarthroses) may be starting places.

Radiation Treatment

Likewise ionizing irradiation is a mainstay for the treatment of tumors that characterize NF, particularly optic gliomas and other astrocytomas, and neurofibrosarcomas. Further work on the value and consequences of current protocols and on the development of improved protocols is urgently needed. Given the large number of patients with these complications who present for treatment each year in the United States, carefully designed multi-institutional protocols could lead to useful results and new starting places in a very short time. In addition, such projects should include mechanisms for careful long-term follow-up to measure potential adverse effects of this treatment modality.

Multidisciplinary Referral Centers

It should be obvious from the foregoing that present and future research in NF requires close collaboration and mutual communication between patients and families, clinicians, clinical investigators, and laboratory investigators. The identification of specific problems warranting highest priority, the accumulation of research subjects, and the development of dedicated NF investigators are the functions of multidisciplinary regional NF referral centers. In addition, identifying and categorizing patients and families that are likely to benefit from specific research breakthroughs are the most important functions of such centers. The lessons learned from the efforts to implement the molecular biology identification of a gene near the Huntington disease locus must be respected. Identifying a gene, or establishing another sort of breakthrough (e.g. therapeutic) is only the beginning. Particularly in view of the variable expressivity of each form of NF, the critical importance of heterogeneity, and the overlap of NF with many other disorders and the normal population as well, there must be organizations and specific mechanisms in place to implement these findings in a logical, systematic, and compassionate manner. Given an NF population of at least 80,000 Americans, establishment of at least 20 such centers in the United States seems a reasonable immediate goal.

References

1. Riccardi VM, Eichner JE. Neurofibromatosis: phenotype, natural history, and pathogenesis. Baltimore: Johns Hopkins Press, 1986.

2. Borberg A. Clinical and genetic investigations into tuberous sclerosis and Recklinghausen's neurofibromatosis. Acta Psychiatr Neurol 1951;(suppl)71:1–239.

3. Crowe FW, Schull WJ, Neel JV. A clinical, pathological, and genetic study of multiple neurofibromatosis. Springfield, Il: Charles C Thomas, 1956:1–181.

4. Brasfield RD, Das Gupta TK. Von Recklinghausen's disease: a clinicopathological study. Ann Surg 1972;175:86–104.

5. Wander JV, Das Gupta TK. Neurofibromatosis. Curr Probl Surg 1977;14(2):1–81.

6. Holt JF. Neurofibromatosis in children. AJR 1978;130:615–639.

7. Riccardi VM. Von Recklinghausen neurofibromatosis. N Engl J Med 1981;305:1617–1627.

8. Samuelsson B. Neurofibromatosis (v. Recklinghausen's disease): a clinical-psychiatric and genetic study. Doctoral dissertation, University of Goteberg, Sweden, 1981.

9. Sorensen SA, Mulvihill JJ, Nielsen A. On the natural history of von Recklinghausen neurofibromatosis. Ann NY Acad Sci 1986;486:30–37.

10. Crump T. Translation of case reports, in Ueber die multiplen Fibrome der Haut und ihre Beziehung zu den multiplen Neuromen by F. V. Recklinghausen. Adv Neurol 1981;29:259–275.

11. Riccardi VM. Neurofibromatosis: clinical heterogeneity. Curr Probl Cancer 1982;7(2):1–34.

12. Lewis RA, Riccardi VM. Von Recklinghausen neurofibromatosis: prevalence of iris hamartomata. Ophthalmology 1981;88:348–354.

13. Eldridge R. Central neurofibromatosis with bilateral acoustic neuroma. Adv Neurol 1981;29:57–65.

14. Riccardi VM. The pathophysiology of neurofibromatosis: IV. Dermatologic insights into heterogeneity and pathogenesis. J Am Acad Dermatol 1980;3:157–166.

15. Riccardi VM. Cutaneous manifestations of neurofibromatosis: cellular interaction, pigmentation, and mast cells. Birth Defects Orig Art Ser 1981;17(2):129–145.

16. Lisch K. Uber Beteiligung der Augen, insbesondere das Vorkommen von Irisnotchen bei der Neurofibromatose (Recklinghausen). Z Augenheilkd 1937;93:137–143.

17. Perry HD, Font RL. Iris nodules in von Recklinghausen neurofibromatosis: electron microscopic confirmation of the melanocytic origin. Arch Ophthalmol 1982;100:1635–1640.

18. Weleber RG, Zonana J. Iris hamartomas (Lisch nodules) in a case of segmental neurofibromatosis. Am J Ophthalmol 1983;96:740–743.

19. Ritter J, Riccardi VM. Von Recklinghausen neurofibromatosis (NF–I): an argument for very high penetrance and a comparison of sporadic and inherited cases. Am J Hum Genet 1985;37:135A.

20. Hope DG, Mulvihill JJ. Malignancy in neurofibromatosis. Adv Neurol 1981;29:33–55.

21. Herrera GA, deMoreaes HP. Neurogenic sarcomas in patients with neurofibromatosis (von Recklinghausen's disease). Virchows Arch [A] 1984;403:361–376.

22. Riccardi VM, Wheeler TM, Pickard LR, et al. B. The pathophysiology of neurofibromatosis. II. Angiosarcoma as a complication. Cancer Genet Cytogenet 1984;12:275–280.

23. Riccardi VM, Elder DW. Multiple cytogenetic aberrations in neurofibrosarcomas complicating neurofibromatosis. Cancer Genet Cytogenet 1986;23:199–209.

24. Clark RD, Hutter JJ Jr. Familial neurofibromatosis and juvenile chronic myelogenous leukemia. Hum Genet 1982;60:230–232.

25. Wertelecki W, Superneau DW, Blackburn WR, et al. Neurofibromatosis: skin hemangiomas and arterial disease. Birth Defects 1982;18:29–41.

26. Salyer WR, Salyer DC. The vascular lesions of neurofibromatosis. Angiology 1974;25:510–519.

27. Taboada D, Alonso A, Moreno J, Muro D, Mulas F. Occlusion of the cerebral arteries in Recklinghausen's disease. Neuroradiology 1979;18:281–284.

28. Zochodne D. Von Recklinghausen's vasculopathy. Am J Med Sci 1984;287:64–65.

29. Chakrabarti S, Murugesan A, Arida EJ. The association of neurofibromatosis and hyperparathyroidism. Am J Surg 1979;137:417–420.

30. Unger PD, Geller SA, Anderson PJ. Pulmonary lesions in a patient with neurofibromatosis. Arch Pathol Lab Med 1984;108:654–657.

31. Riccardi VM. Neurofibromatosis as a model for investigating hereditary vs. environmental factors in learning disabilities. In: Arimd M, Suzuki Y, Yabuuchi H, eds. The developing brain and its disorders. Tokyo: University of Tokyo Press, 198:171–181.

32. Rosman NP, Pearce J. The brain in multiple neurofibromatosis (von Recklinghausen's disease): a suggested neuropathology basis for the associated mental defect. Brain 1967;90:829–837.

33. Rubenstein AE, Mytilineou C, Yahr MD, et al. Neurotransmitter analysis of dermal neurofibromas: implications for the pathogenesis on treatment of neurofibromatosis. Neurology 1981;31:1184–1188.

34. Riccardi VM. Neurofibromatosis in children. Cont Ed Fam Phys 1983;18:565–571.

35. Lewis RA, Riccardi VM, Gerson LP, et al. Von Recklinghausen neurofibromatosis: II. Incidence of optic-nerve gliomata. Ophthalmology 1984;91:929–935.

36. Peltonen J, Aho H, Halme T, et al. Distribution of different collagen types and fibronectin in neurofibromatosis tumors. Arch Pathol Microbiol Immunol Scand (sec A) 1984;92:345–352.

37. Peltonen J, Foidart J-M, Aho HJ. Type IV and V collagens in von Recklinghausen's neurofibromatosis. Virchows Arch [Cell Pathol] 1984;47:291–301.

38. Peltonen J. Collagens in neurofibromas and neurofibroma cell cultures. Ann NY Acad Sci 1986;486:260–270.

39. Benedict PH, Szabo G, Fitzpatrick TB, et al. Melanotic macules in Albright's syndrome and in neurofibromatosis. JAMA 1968;205:618–626.

40. Martuza RL, Phillipe I, Fitzpatrick TB, et al. Melanin

macroglobules as a cellular marker of neurofibromatosis: a quantitative study. J. Invest Dermatol 1985;85:347–350.

41. Schenkein I, Buecker ED, Helson L, et al. Nerve-growth factor in disseminated neurofibromatosis. N Engl J Med 1974;292:1134–1136.

42. Rubenstein AE, Mytilineau C, Yahr MD, et al. Neurological aspects of neurofibromatosis. Adv Neurol 1981;29:209–211.

43. Fabricant RN, Todaro T. Increased serum levels of nerve growth factor in von Recklinghausen disease. Arch Neurol 1981;38:401–405.

44. Fabricant RN, Todaro GT, Eldridge RE. Increased levels of a nerve growth factor cross-reacting protein in central neurofibromatosis. Lancet 1979;1:4–7.

45. Riopelle RJ, Riccardi VM, Faulkner S, et al.Serum neuronal growth factors in von Recklinghausen neurofibromatosis. Ann Neurol 1984;16:54–59.

46. Zelkowitz M, Stambouly J. Neurofibromatosis fibroblasts: slow growth and abnormal morphology. Pediatr Res 1981;15:290–293.

47. Zelkowitz M. Neurofibromatosis fibroblasts: abnormal growth and binding to epidermal growth factor. Adv Neurol 1981;29:173–189.

48. Seizinger BR, Tanzi RE, Gillian TC, et al. Genetic linkage of neurofibromatosis using DNA markers. Ann NY Acad Sci 1986;486:304–310.

49. Darby JK, Feder J, Selby M, et al. A discordant sibship analysis between beta-NGF and neurofibromatosis. Am J Hum Genet 1985;37:52–59.

50. Riccardi VM. A selective growth-promoting factor in crude extracts of neurofibromatosis (NF) neurofibromas. Am J Hum Genet 1984;36:206s.

51. Riccardi VM. Growth-promoting factors in neurofibroma crude extracts. Ann NY Acad Sci 1986;486:206–226.

52. Krone W, Fink T, Kling H, et al. Cell culture studies on neurofibromatosis (von Recklinghausen): characterization of cells growing from neurofibromas. Ann NY Acad Sci 1986;486:354–370.

53. Sergeyev AS. On the mutation rate of neurofibromatosis. Hum Genet 1975;28:129–138.

54. Riccardi VM, Dobson CE, Chakraborty R, et al.The pathophysiology of neurofibromatosis: IX. Paternal age effect on the origin of new mutations. Am J Med Genet 1984;18:169–176.

55. Ichikawa K, Crosley CJ, Culebras A, et al. Coincidence of neurofibromatosis and myotonic dystrophy in a kindred. J Med Genet 1981;18:134–138.

56. Spence MA, Bader JL, Parry DM, et al. Linkage analysis of neurofibromatosis (von Recklinghausen disease). J Med Genet 1983;20:334–337.

57. DiLiberti JH, Rivas M. Myotonic dystrophy and neurofibromatosis: probable linkage. Clin Res 1983;81:109A.

58. Pericak-Vance MA, Stajich JM, Conneally PM, et al. Genetic linkage analysis of myotonic dystrophy with complement component 3 (C3), secretor (Se), and Lewis (Le) loci on chromosome 19. Cytogenet Cell Genet 1984;37:156.

59. Dunn BC, Ferrell RE, Riccardi VM. A genetic linkage study of 15 families with von Recklinghausen neurofibromatosis. Am J Med Genet 1985;22:403–407.

60. Huson SM, Meredith AL, Sarfarazi M, et al. Linkage analysis of peripheral neurofibromatosis (von Recklinghausen disease) and chromosome 19 markers linked to myotonic dystrophy. J Med Genet 1986;23:55–57.

61. Darby JK, Goslin K, Riccardi VM, et al. Linkage analysis between NGFB and other chromosome 1p markers and disseminated neurofibromatosis. Ann NY Acad Sci 1986;486:311–326.

62. Kao YS, Kao-Shan CS, Knutsen T, et al. Neurofibromatosis: no chromosomal defect by prophasebanding technique. Cancer Genet Cytogenet 1984;13:281–282.

63. Palmer CG, Provisor AJ, Weaver DD, et al. Juvenile chronic granulocytic leukemia in a patient with trisomy 8, neurofibromatosis, and prolonged Epstein-Barr virus infection. J Pediatr 1983;102:888–892.

64. Miller RM, Sparkes RS. Segmental neurofibromatosis. Arch Dermatol 1977;113:837–838.

65. Opitz JM, Weaver DD. The neurofibromatosis–Noonan syndrome. Am J Med Genet 1985;21:477–490.

66. Riccardi VM, Valenta SH. Neurofibromatosis: a primer for patients and families. Houston: VM Riccardi, 1983.

67. Miller M, Hall JG. Possible maternal effect on severity of neurofibromatosis. Lancet 1978;2:1071–1074.

68. Hall JH. Possible maternal and hormonal factors in neurofibromatosis. Adv Neurol 1981;29:125–131.

Chapter 3
Tuberous Sclerosis

MANUEL R. GOMEZ

Tuberous sclerosis (TS), also called the tuberous sclerosis complex and in some countries better known as Bourneville's disease, is a malady that may affect almost any organ although is most often recognized by lesions in the skin, brain, retina, kidneys, heart, or lungs. Until recently it was regarded as a rare disease and yet the number of publications on its clinical, radiographic, genetic, epidemiologic, and pathologic aspects is in the thousands and has increased more rapidly in recent years. Increasing interest in this disease may be in part due to the ease of diagnosing it with the present technology for imaging organs such as ultrasound, computed tomography, and magnetic resonance imaging, all particularly useful in detecting asymptomatic subjects. Estimates of its prevalence based on data from institutionalized mentally handicapped patients are very low; however, these patients are often inadequately studied, with only a cursory if any examination of their direct relatives. Few population studies have been done since the newer methods of ascertainment became available [1,2].

The cause of TS remains unknown. It is of autosomal dominant inheritance. Linkage of the TS gene to a "marker" has not been found as yet. There is no known structural cell or organelle abnormality, enzyme deficiency, or molecular defect to identify affected individuals.

The diagnosis of this disease is still made by clinical, radiographic, or other forms of imaging or by pathologic examination of an involved organ. The standard statement in medical books and journals that "tuberous sclerosis is a rare disease characterized by seizures, mental retardation and adenoma sebaceum" in our experience is true in only one of three patients.

Tuberous sclerosis most often presents with seizures that presumably result from abnormal activity of bizarre neurons in cortical tuberosities, that is,

tubers. Mental retardation, the most serious neurologic manifestation, occurs only in those patients who have suffered generalized seizures in the first years of life. Cardiac, renal, pulmonary, and cerebral hamartomas may be small and cause no symptoms or may interfere with organ function either by obstruction [that is, blood, CSF] or parenchymal replacement. The diagnosis of TS can be made clinically when a subject has at least one of the characteristic lesions in the skin, retina, CNS, or kidneys and although the term tuberous sclerosis was coined for its cerebral pathology, the associated lesions found in other viscera, retina, or skin may be by themselves indicative of the disease. This is not to say that all patients with cerebral TS always have additional visceral involvement or, conversely, that all patients with dermic, renal, pulmonary, or cardiac lesions of TS have cerebral involvement. There are subjects with TS who have no evidence of CNS involvement. Thus, expressivity is very variable. Among patients with TS some are neurologically asymptomatic; in these individuals CNS involvement is demonstrable only by head CT scans, magnetic resonance imaging, or neuropathologic examination [3,4].

A definitive diagnosis of TS can be made on individuals who harbor at least one of the lesions listed in Table 3.1, preferably in multiple form. Facial angiofibroma should be multiple to be convincing. The organs more frequently involved—skin, brain, eyes, and kidneys—should, therefore, always be examined when the diagnosis of TS is under consideration. In individuals having any of the features listed in Table 3.2, the possibility of TS should be considered [5].

History

The earliest writing on TS is a brief necropsy description made by Friedrich Daniel von Reckling-

Table 3.1. Criteria for Definitive Diagnosis of Tuberous Sclerosis

Facial angiofibromas
Ungual fibroma
Retinal hamartoma
Cortical tuber
Subependymal glial nodule
Renal angiomyolipomas

Table 3.2. Criteria for Presumptive Diagnosis of Tuberous Sclerosis

Hypomelanotic macules
Shagreen patches
Peripapillary retinal hamartoma (drusen?)
Gingival fibromas
Dental enamel pits
Single renal angiomyolipoma
Multicystic kidneys
Cardiac rhabdomyoma
Pulmonary lymphangiomyomatosis
Radiographic "honeycomb" lungs
Infantile spasms
Myoclonic, tonic, or atonic seizures
Immediate relative with tuberous sclerosis

hausen in 1862 [6]: a newborn who had died "after taking a few breaths" had several "myomata" of the heart and many "scleroses" of the brain. Desiré–Magloire Bourneville in 1880 [7] reported the neuropathology of this disease and used the adjective "tuberous" (or "tuberose") to describe the potato-like firmness of widened hypertrophic cerebral gyri. The brain with TS of the circumvolutions was from a 15-year-old hemiplegic, epileptic, and mentally subnormal girl who had died in status epilepticus. On sectioning the brain Bourneville found white islands of glial tissue embedded in the striatum and nodules protruding into the lateral ventricles. The patient's face was covered with red papules not further described by Bourneville but classified as acne rosacea. Examination of the kidneys disclosed 3 small and 15 yet smaller tumors in the right kidney and fewer similar lesions in the left kidney.

Hartdegen in 1881 [8] reported the pathology of a 2-day-old infant who had died with convulsions. In addition to spina bifida, purulent meningitis, and sclerotic cerebral cortex, there were intraventricular tumors (from the walls of the lateral ventricles). Microscopic examination of the cortical lesions demonstrated the giant ganglion cells and glial hyperplasia that Hartdegen supposed to be a congenital gangliocellular glioma.

Between the years 1880 and 1900 Bourneville and his colleagues [9,10] reported on a total of ten pa-

tients and emphasized the association of cerebral TS with renal tumors. Balzer and Menetrier [11] in 1885 and Pringle [12] in 1890 described facial lesions that came to be known as adenoma sebaceum but did not recognize them as part of Bourneville's disease. Rayer's atlas of skin diseases published in 1835 [13] depicts a patient with facial lesions labeled *végétations vasculaires* that resemble those later known as "Pringle's adenoma sebaceum." There is no written description of the patient's symptoms or signs. Although Pringle's patient was mentally subnormal, nothing was said about seizures.

Perusini in 1905 [14] noted the association of cerebral, renal, cardiac, and cutaneous lesions of TS. Heinrich Vogt in 1908 [15] diagnosed TS apparently for the first time on a living patient who had seizures, mental retardation, and adenoma sebaceum, and thus this "triad" is named after him. In the first decades of the twentieth century the concept of a complete form of this disease with these three clinical features versus an incomplete type or forme fruste took shape following Schuster's report in 1914 [16] of a young man with seizures and adenoma sebaceum but no mental retardation. H. Berg in 1913 [17] reported on a family with afflicted members in three generations thus establishing the hereditary nature and autosomal dominant inheritance of this disease. The clinical manifestations varied from one individual to another: the propositus's grandfather who had normal intellect died of a renal tumor at the age of 60 years; the propositus's father had adenoma sebaceum and died at the age of 20 years from a renal tumor; and the propositus, a girl with seizures since age 4 years, died at age 8 with renal, cardiac, and cerebral TS. Berg also found retinal lesions in two members of this family, a finding previously reported by Campbell [18].

As the discrepancy between clinical manifestations begged for accurate nomenclature, in 1932 Critchley and Earl [19] in their classic paper proposed to adopt the term tuberose sclerosis for the fully manifested disease, reserving "epiloia," an unfortunate term introduced by Sherlock [20], for the most severe forms, and to designate "aborted monosymptomatic forms" or formes frustes by a descriptive label indicating the affected organ. Except for the obsolete term epiloia, current usage of terminology follows Critchley and Earl's recommendations. Thus, when either renal angiomyolipomas, cardiac rhabdomyomas, or cerebral giant cell astrocytoma is the only expression of the disease the term tuberous sclerosis is applied to patients with no other manifestations of this disease, as long as there is a direct relative with documented tuberous sclerosis.

In 1921, van der Hoeve, a Dutch ophthalmologist, brought attention to the retinal lesions [21] and introduced the term "phakomatoses" to encompass two neurocutaneous diseases, tuberous sclerosis and neurofibromatosis (NF). Later he added von Hippel–Lindau and Sturge–Weber syndromes to the list of phakomatoses (see the Preface).

In 1924 Marcus [22] described the roentgenographic intracranial calcifications, Dickerson [23] differentiated the areas of increased density within the calvarium (sclerotic plaques) from calcifications within the cerebrum in head radiographs, and Yakolev and Corwin [24] pointed out the two principal sites of intracranial calcification, the cortex and the periventricular regions. G. Berg and Vejlens [25] in 1939 described the pulmonary cysts. Critchley and Earl [19] first pointed out the hypomelanotic macules of the skin (white leaf-shaped macules or achromic patches), a feature that was subsequently emphasized by Gold and Freeman [26], Harris and Moynahan [27], and Fitzpatrick et al. [28].

Since the work of Gastaut et al. [29], Della Rovere et al. [30], and Pampiglioni and Pugh [31], the association of infantile spasms, hypsarrhythmia, and mental retardation known as West's syndrome is recognized as one of the most common manifestations of TS.

Lagos and Gomez [32] reported that 38 percent of patients with TS had average intelligence and that all mentally subnormal patients, but only 69% of patients with average intelligence, had previously had seizures.

With the introduction of CT of the head in 1973 and the widespread use of ultraviolet light to detect white spots in the skin, the diagnosis of cerebral or cutaneous TS in both symptomatic and asymptomatic individuals has increased considerably. Magnetic resonance imaging is proving to be even more practical than CT for identifying cortical tubers and white matter lesions.

Epidemiology

The hereditary nature of TS in an autosomal dominant manner is well established. There is no documented family with a skipped generation but the variation in gene expressivity between affected individuals, both from within the same family and from different ones, is notorious. There is no known selectivity, exemption, or preponderance, according to race, sex, or geographic location.

Tuberous sclerosis prevalence was estimated at 1 in 23,000 in Poland [33] by extrapolating the prevalence of TS among patients in institutions for the mentally subnormal and the epileptic on the prevalence of these disorders in the entire population. A more recent estimate of prevalence based on patients studied in the Oxford, England, region yielded a TS rate of 1 in 29,000 for persons under 65 years, 1 in 21,500 for those under 30 years, and 1 in 15,400 for children under 5 years of age [1]. Because not all individuals with TS are symptomatic these figures are low. Affected relatives are recognized only after a thorough examination for genetic counseling. Furthermore, patients who die very young with an obstructive cardiac rhabdomyoma or in renal failure from an angiomyolipoma, cystic kidneys, or both, or succumb in utero to cardiac failure (hydrops fetalis) are not always diagnosed and included in prevalence studies. Consequently, the prevalence must be greater than estimated. A pathologic study done in Switzerland [34] revealed six cases of TS in 49,402 autopsies over a period of 15 years, a prevalence of 12 in 100,000. Our study of prevalence and incidence in the limited population in Rochester, Minnesota, during the period 1950 through 1980 revealed eight patients, one of whom died and another was lost to follow-up [2] (Table 3.3). The point prevalence on December 31, 1980, was calculated as 10.6 cases per 100,000 persons, representing approximately 1 case

Table 3.3. Summary of Eight Cases of Tuberous Sclerosis in Rochester, Minn., 1950–1980

Characteristic	Number
Age at diagnosis	
<5	4
>5	4
Sex	
M	5
F	3
Family history of TS	2
Skin	
Hypomelanotic macules	8
Facial angiofibroma	4
Shagreen patch	2
Retinal phakoma	2
Central nervous system	
Seizures	4
Mental retardation	2
Spastic diplegia	1
Quadriplegia	1
CT scan abnormal[a]	6
Outcome (1983)[b]	
Alive	6
Dead	1

Source: adapted from Wiederholt et al. [2].
[a]Only six CT scans were done.
[b]One outcome unknown.

per 9,407 persons and an incidence of 0.56 cases for 100,000 person-years (Table 3.4). This estimate is also undoubtedly low because asymptomatic individuals, unless they have an affected and symptomatic relative who has been properly studied and diagnosed, may remain undetected.

Diagnostic Criteria

According to the value of the clinical data obtained it should be possible to discard the diagnosis of TS for lack of evidence or to arrive at one of two types of diagnosis of TS: (a) *definitive*, when the subject has at least one pathognomonic sign of TS, and (b) *presumptive*, when the subject has two or more non-pathognomonic clinical features frequently observed in patients with this disease.

The following findings are pathognomonic of TS (Table 3.1): facial angiofibromas, ungual fibromas, retinal hamartomas, cortical tubers or subependymal nodules, and multiple renal angiomyolipomas. The skin lesions and the retinal hamartomas are recognized by direct or indirect ophthalmoscopy with the aid of magnifying lenses but the cerebral lesions and the renal angiomyolipomas most often are discovered with imaging methods requiring interpretation. In rare instances the diagnosis is not confirmed until there is pathologic verification.

Each of the following features is alone insufficient but the presence of two of the following features allows a presumptive diagnosis of TS (Table 3.2): hypomelanotic skin macules; shagreen patches; a single peripapillary retinal hamartoma; gingival fibromas; congenital dental enamel pits; a single renal angiomyolipoma; multicystic kidneys; cardiac rhabdomyoma; pulmonary lymphangiomatosis or lymphangiomyomatosis; radiographic "honey-comb" lungs;

Table 3.4. Epidemiology of Tuberous Sclerosis in Rochester, Minn.

Cases identified: 8
Population
1980: 56,447 persons
1950 to 1980: 1,392,762 person-years
Point prevalence, December 31, 1980
10.6 cases/100,000 persons
(95% CI, 1.95 to 19.31)
Incidence, 1950 to 1980
0.56 cases/100,000 person-years
(95% CI, 0.16 to 0.96)

Source: adapted from Wiederholt et al. [2].
CI = confidence interval

infantile spasms; myoclonic, tonic, atonic, or akinetic seizures; and a first-degree relative with any of the pathognomonic findings shown in Table 3.1.

Clinical Features

Presenting Symptoms

Seizures are the most common presenting symptom of patients with TS. In children it is almost always the presenting complaint. Regardless of the presenting symptoms 90% of our 264 patients with TS had suffered seizures. However, in our more recently studied group of 158 individuals with TS that includes asymptomatic relatives, 82% had seizures.

Other presenting symptoms are mental subnormality or its equivalent (abnormal behavior, learning problems); facial rash or other skin lesion; symptoms of increased intracranial pressure; systemic hypertension (associated with renal disease); abdominal pain; hematuria; hypovolemic shock from a ruptured renal tumor; hydrops fetalis; neonatal cardiac failure; cardiac arrhythmia (from intramural rhabdomyoma); spontaneous pneumothorax; hemoptysis; respiratory failure (from pulmonary sclerosis and lymphangiomyomatosis); and a direct relative with TS. In brief, depending on the organ involved there is a wide variety of clinical expression. The interfamilial variability of presentation seems to be greater than the intrafamilial variability of presentation. The same can be said of expressivity.

Skin

The most frequent clinical feature of TS patients is one or more of several cutaneous signs. In patients selected according to the criteria for definitive diagnosis of TS (Table 3.1), 96% have one or more of the four skin lesions searched for (Table 3.5). The types of lesions listed in order of their frequency are the following: hypomelanotic macules, facial angiofibroma, periungual fibromas, and shagreen patches (Table 3.6). Other cutaneous lesions considered of no diagnostic value, such as brown spots (café-au-lait), molluscum pendulum (skin tags), and pigmented nevi, are less frequently seen and may not be found more often than in the population at large. Although their frequency is unknown, the fibrous plaques described below are of much diagnostic value if not pathognomonic. Facial angiofibroma (adenoma sebaceum) is present in only half of patients with TS. As one would expect, in the days when the Vogt triad was the only way of diagnosing TS, all

Table 3.5. Ratio of Clinical to Radiologic Features in Tuberous Sclerosis

Feature	Positive/ Total	% Positive
Skin: Angiofibromas, white spots, ungual fibromas, and shagreen patch	150/156	96
CT: Nodular incremental attenuation	124/140	89
Epileptic seizures	129/158	82
Retinal hamartoma	60/125	48
Mental subnormality	60/145	41

Table 3.6. Skin Lesions in 158 Patients with Tuberous Sclerosis

Skin Lesion	No. of Patients	%
Hypomelanotic macules	136	86
Facial angiofibromas	75	47
Ungual fibromas	31	20
Shagreen patches	30	19
None of the above	7	4
Incomplete skin examination	2	1

patients had facial angiofibroma. It is explained below that today less than half of patients with TS have facial angiofibroma, indicating that TS is now recognized at least twice as often as it was 20 years ago.

Hypomelanotic Macules

These white spots, also called depigmented or achromic patches or ash-leaf spots, are irregularly oval, lance-ovate, elliptic, round, or shaped like the leaf of mountain ash (Figure 3.1). Most of them measure 1 or 2 cm in length or in diameter but some may be only 2 mm or as large as 5 cm. They vary in number from one to more than one hundred. Although often

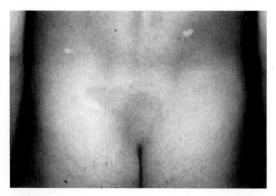

Figure 3.1. Two hypomelanotic macules and a shagreen patch in the lumbar and sacral areas of a young boy with tuberous sclerosis.

present at birth, they may not be recognized until the skin has been exposed to natural light long enough to produce sufficient melanin. When the patient has a fair complexion, it may be necessary to use the Wood's lamp (ultraviolet light of 360-nm wave length) to illuminate the skin in a dark room. Late appearance of these spots has been reported [35].

Histologic examination of a biopsy obtained from a hypomelanotic macule stained with hematoxylin and eosin is of no value for diagnosis. Electron microscopic examination of melanocytes may be necessary to differentiate a hypomelanotic macule from vitiligo, nevus depigmentosus, nevus anemicus, piebaldism, or Vogt–Koyanagi–Harada syndrome. Electron microscopic examination of the sections from a hypomelanotic macule reveals that the melanosomes in melanocytes and keratinocytes are reduced in number, in diameter, and in melanization [36]. Histologically, lesions of vitiligo display diminution or absence of melanocytes. In nevus depigmentosus, electron microscopic examination shows fewer melanosomes than in normal skin but they are normal in size and melanization [36]. In nevus anemicus, a functional vascular disorder, there is no pigment abnormality [36]. In piebaldism the white patches are located on the forehead and scalp, chin, mid-forearm, and mid-thigh, and histologic examination as in vitiligo reveals absent melanocytes [36]. Depigmentation in Vogt–Koyanagi–Harada syndrome also resembles vitiligo [36]. In Chediak–Higashi syndrome there is loss of pigment in hair and eyes and pigmentation of skin; the melanocytes have giant melanosomes [37].

Poliosis of the scalp in the shape of a hypomelanotic macule (Figure 3.2) or a few grouped canities are most often found over the occipital region or down toward the neck hairline [36]. Poliosis of the eyelashes has also been reported [38].

Although they are not specific for TS, hypomelanotic macules are the most frequent skin finding in patients with TS (Table 3.6). Screening of newborn infants for white spots has shown that 0.8% of all infants have hypopigmented nevi. The prevalence rate

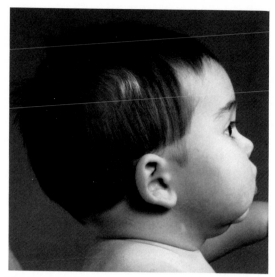

Figure 3.2. Patch of poliosis and a hypomelanotic macule in the neck of a young boy with tuberous sclerosis.

is 0.4% for white infants and 2.4% for black infants [39]. They may also be found in patients with neurofibromatosis or other neurocutaneous diseases.

The association of seizures in an infant with a few white spots, at least one of which is a typical hypomelanotic skin macule, is sufficient for making a presumptive diagnosis of TS. The demonstration of cerebral lesions by CT, or retinal lesions by ophthalmoscopy, confirms CNS involvement.

Facial Angiofibroma

Adenoma sebaceum is the name originally given by Balzer and Menetrier [11] to this lesion that is found in 47% of patients with TS. Many consider multiple facial angiofibromas in their typical symmetric facial distribution to be pathognomonic of TS, a view we have accepted since our experience has shown that whenever a subject with facial angiofibroma has been thoroughly examined, some other skin, cerebral, retinal, or renal lesion of TS is found.

Facial angiofibromas are hamartomas of the skin. They occupy symmetrical areas over cheeks, nasolabial folds, and chin, crossing the midline over the nasal bridge and the chin (Figure 3.3). They are rarely seen on the upper lip and are usually symmetric, although they may predominate on one side. The lesions first appear as small reddish spots at age 3 or 4 years, seldom after puberty, and very rarely in infancy. They have been seen even in newborns [32] and have appeared as late as 20 years of age [36]. Histologic examination of these lesions demon-

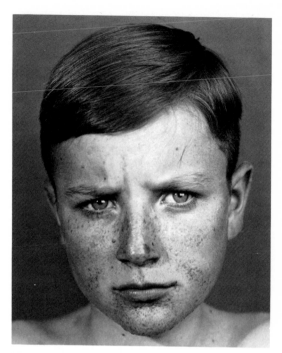

Figure 3.3. Facial angiofibroma occupying the nose, cheeks, chin, and lower lip in its classic distribution.

strates fibrosis of the dermal layer, dilated vessels surrounded by layered sclerotic collagen, and occasionally large stellate fibroblasts. An abundance of sebaceous glands is characteristic of the region of the skin in which this hamartoma grows.

The diagnosis of facial angiofibroma is made clinically, and there is seldom need for histologic examination of the lesion. However, multiple trichoepithelioma, also present as papules or nodules on the center of face and eyelids although different from the typical facial angiofibroma, also affect the scalp, neck, and trunk and are flesh-colored because they have no telangiectatic component [36]. Acne rosacea has a similar facial distribution and an erythematous telangiectatic component and thus may be mistaken for facial angiofibroma. When in doubt, a skin biopsy will demonstrate the pustules around the pilosebaceous units [36].

Fibrous Plaques

Fibrous plaques are usually found on the forehead and scalp (Figure 3.4). In the latter location there is associated alopecia that is sometimes surrounded by poliosis. The plaques are smooth elevations of the skin with the rubbery consistency of a fibroma, are yellowish-brown or flesh-colored, and are often seen

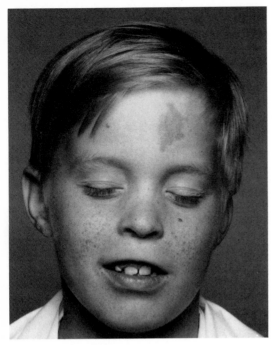

Figure 3.4. Fibrous plaque of the forehead and facial angiofibroma at an earlier stage than in Figure 3.3.

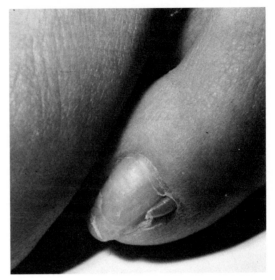

Figure 3.5. Periungual fibroma on the fifth toe of a young child with tuberous sclerosis.

in association with facial angiofibroma. They are sometimes found before the facial angiofibroma develops, that is, in the first 2 or 3 years of life, including the newborn period. They grow very slowly through the years, raising several millimeters over the skin surface, and may require cosmetic surgery. Histologically, fibrous plaques resemble angiofibromas and probably are also diagnostic.

Ungual Fibromas

Periungual or subungual fibromas, also pathognomonic lesions [36], are found in 20% of patients with TS. They are located around or under the fingernails or toenails (Figure 3.5) and arise from the skin of the nail groove or from the bed under the nail plate. They are more common on the toes than on the fingers, in females more than in males, and usually appear during or after puberty and continue to grow slowly. They may regrow after removal. Those located at the base of the nail may produce a longitudinal groove on the nail parallel to its axis.

Shagreen Patches

Shagreen patches (from the French *peau de chagrin*, "skin with the appearance of untanned leather") are

lesions usually found on dorsal body surfaces and particularly on the lumbosacral skin (Figure 3.1). It is rare to find them on the skin of the chest or abdomen. The lesion consists of a slightly elevated plaque of epidermis without color change or with a yellowish-brown discoloration. Their bumpy surface is reminiscent of orange skin. Most often they appear after puberty but may be found at a younger age. Histologically it is a hamartoma formed by the accumulation in the dermis of collagenous fibers, vascular structures, smooth muscle, and elastic and adipose tissue. Shagreen patches are found in 19% of all patients with cutaneous lesions of TS but by themselves are not diagnostic [36].

Other Skin Lesions

Café-au-lait or brown spots and molluscum pendulum or skin tags are found with more frequency in TS patients than in the general population. One or several subcutaneous nodules a few mm to as large as 2 cm in diameter that consist of homogeneous collagenous bundles and large abundant fibrocyte nuclei have been infrequently reported [40] and have been seen in only two of our patients.

In brief, 96% of all patients with TS and their affected relatives have at least one of the five above-described skin lesions, of which perhaps two are pathognomonic. A careful skin examination of individuals at risk for TS is the best and easiest method to make the diagnosis. It is still unknown how many affected individuals escape detection this way. When making the diagnosis of TS we should not depend solely on facial angiofibromas since only 47% of patients have this lesion. Hypomelanotic macules, on the other hand, are found in at least 86% of all patients with skin lesions. Examination of the skin of direct relatives is often necessary to substantiate the diagnosis on the propositus and should not be neglected.

Central Nervous System

Epileptic seizures, the most frequent presenting symptom, are also the second most common of the clinical features in patients with TS. Seizures occur in 82 to 90%, mental subnormality in 41 to 47% (Tables 3.5, 3.7), intracranial hypertension in less than 3%, and focal neurologic deficit in only 2% of all affected individuals.

Epileptic Seizures

Seizures in TS patients most often begin early in life. Further, since asymptomatic individuals with TS are not brought to medical attention early in life, the number of seizure-free children with TS is indeed small. Some but not all children presenting with cardiac, renal, and skin symptoms have in addition or subsequently develop seizures.

Of patients with seizures, 84% have generalized, 29% partial, and 15% both types [5]. The most common types of generalized seizures in children are infantile spasms and myoclonic seizures followed by tonic, atonic, and atypical absences. Tonic–clonic seizures are common only after the first year of life and are associated with or replace the other types. Infantile spasms are rare after the age of 4 years. In our experience typical absences or "pure petit mal" seizures do not occur as part of this disease. Atypical absences and partial seizures with complex symptoms, which may be mistaken for typical absences, however, are common. We know of only two patients reported to have petit mal seizures in associ-

ation with TS. The first one [19] was an 8-year-old girl who for many years had petit mal attacks and died after developing signs of increased intracranial pressure without localized motor signs. At postmortem examination, in addition to the characteristic cerebral lesions of TS, a "tumor the size of a walnut" was found in the posterior portion of the third ventricle. Although a complete clinical description of her seizures is not given and no EEG was done, it seems unlikely that the patient had a fortuitous association of absences and TS. It is more reasonable that she had partial seizures with complex symptoms. The second patient [41] is a good illustration of the fortuitous association of two unrelated disorders each inherited from a different parent: TS and petit mal seizures.

Mental Subnormality

In the Mayo Clinic experience 47% of patients have been found to be mentally subnormal (Table 3.8), a figure equal to the number of patients with average intelligence. The mental ability of 5% of patients is unknown. As more patients' direct relatives are examined with the newer imaging techniques, the number of asymptomatic affected individuals will undoubtedly grow. Whether they have CNS involvement without seizures and mental retardation or only extracerebral TS involvement, the rate of mental subnormality among all individuals with TS should fall below 47%.

There is a definite correlation between the occurrence of seizures early in life and the subsequent finding of mental subnormality. There are few reported instances of TS patients with mental subnormality who never had seizures, and these are not all well documented. Moreover, among the TS patients with seizures, the less frequent the seizures and the later in life was their onset, the smaller is the probability that the patient will be mentally subnormal [5]. In a group of 125 TS patients with average intelligence, 91 patients had and 34 did not have seizures (Table 3.9). In the group of 125 patients with subnormal intelligence all had had seizures. In this latter group of patients there was no correlation of

Table 3.7. Symptoms of Vogt Triad in 264 Patients with Tuberous Sclerosis

Symptom	No. of Patients	%
Facial angiofibroma	153	58
Seizures	238	90
Mental retardation	125	47
All three	78	30
None of the three	18	7

Table 3.8. Mentality of 264 Mayo Clinic Patients with Tuberous Sclerosis

Mentality	No. of Patients	%
Normal	125	47.3
Subnormal	125	47.3
Not known	14	5.3

Table 3.9. Mentality in Relationship to Seizures in 264 Patients with Tuberous Sclerosis

Mentality	No. of Patients		
	Without Seizures	With Seizures	Total
Normal	34	91	125
Subnormal	0	125	125
Not known	1	13	14
Total	35	229	264

the dermatologic findings with either previous occurrence of seizures or with mental subnormality.

Focal Neurologic Signs

Motor deficit has been infrequently recognized. Spastic diplegia usually in association with severe mental retardation, hemiplegia, monoplegia, triplegia, and atonic diplegia have all been reported [42]. Cerebellar signs are infrequent although it is not unusual to find extensive areas of cerebellar calcifications in head CT scans. Cerebellar hamartomas usually give no signs of cerebellar deficit. One exception to this rule has been reported [42]. Involuntary movements have been seen infrequently in patients with TS despite the selective location of the nodular hamartomas in the region of the basal ganglia. Choreoathetosis has been reported only once [43]. Cerebral embolism from intracardiac tumor has been proposed to occur but has not been verified pathologically (see Computed Tomography, below).

Patients with behavioral changes and other symptoms who may be grouped under the poorly defined labels of childhood schizophrenia, infantile autism, or related syndromes can show symptoms or signs of TS. Such children, thought to be normal at birth and through early infancy, later develop generalized seizures, usually infantile spasms, and gradually lose interest in their surroundings and their recently acquired social adaptation. They either regress or remain at a standstill. As these children's motor, speech, and language development fail, they become inattentive to parents and relatives and appear to intentionally ignore them, avoiding "eye contact" and behaving like other children classified as autistic. We have not seen these symptoms or similar behavioral changes in patients with TS who did not have seizures in the first years of life. It seems reasonable that only those autistic infants or children who have clinical seizures or epileptogenic electrographic abnormalities should be fully investigated to rule out TS.

Increased Intracranial Pressure

Obstruction of the CSF circulation at the foramina of Monro and of the third or fourth ventricle by a tumor probably results in intracranial hypertension in less than 3% of patients with TS. The tumor, a benign giant cell astrocytoma, is histologically similar to subependymal nodules (see Pathology and Pathogenesis of Central Nervous System Lesions, below) and retinal hamartomas characteristic of TS. When not calcified, the tumor may be visualized in the head CT scan only after injection of contrast material. Most often these tumors become symptomatic in patients between 5 and 18 years of age [44].

Ophthalmologic Findings

Retinal hamartomas or phakomas are found in at least one eye in almost 50 percent of all patients with TS [45]. Examination of the fundi yields the largest number of lesions by indirect ophthalmoscopy after mydriasis. The retinal hamartomas are astrocytic tumors with a tendency to calcify. They are round or oval in shape and when partially or fully calcified, they are opaque, pearly-white, and multinodular, resembling mulberries or tapioca grains. Before their calcification they are inconspicuous because they have poorly defined borders and are semitransparent or only slightly opaque and thus do not stand out from the background. Nonetheless, if they overlie a retinal vessel, they may be found by following the vessel from its emergence at the optic disc toward the periphery, looking for an interruption on it [45].

Retinal hamartomas when typical, multiple, and located far from the optic disc are pathognomonic for TS (Figure 3.6). Not so if they are found singly and peripapillary in location and thus very similar to the astrocytomas seen in neurofibromatosis. They can also be mistaken for retinoblastoma, particularly when the lesion is a single one and no other organ is involved. Follow-up examination to detect growth of a retinoblastoma at weekly intervals has been recommended to establish the correct diagnosis [45].

Retinal hamartomas are usually asymptomatic, seldom associated with a vitreous hemorrhage or with glaucoma and visual loss, and are never malignant. There is no effective way to treat them nor any need to do so [45].

Depigmented areas in the retina are also found in patients with TS [45], and hypopigmented iris spots have been said to be present before any other visible lesions of TS [46]. The iris spots, variable in size, are believed to be analogous to the cutaneous white spots.

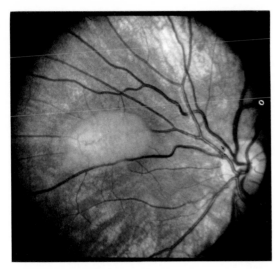

Figure 3.6. Uncalcified retinal hamartoma.

At least one patient has been reported to have poliosis of the eyelashes and depigmented areas in the retina.

Other eye findings infrequently reported in association with TS are cataracts; coloboma of the iris, lens, and choroid; corneal pannus; keratoconus, megalocornea; primary or secondary glaucoma; papilledema; optic atrophy; visual field defect; sixth cranial nerve paresis; strabismus; and vitreous hemorrhage [45]. Papilledema and sixth cranial nerve paresis are secondary to an intraventricular hamartoma obstructing the foramina of Monro or other sites along the CSF pathway to cause intracranial hypertension.

Kidneys

Two renal lesions occur in patients with TS: angiomyolipomas and renal cysts. Found independently or together, they may be unilateral, bilateral, single, or multiple [47,48].

In autopsy series all patients with TS have either renal angiomyolipoma, renal cysts, or both. In clinical–radiologic studies of 95 patients with TS only 51 (54%) had one or both renal lesions. Of these 51 patients only 14 (27%) had physical findings of renal disease [48].

Angiomyolipoma

Renal angiomyolipoma may be totally asymptomatic [48] and is usually clinically manifested by recurrent gross hematuria, flank or lumbar pain, and a palpable renal mass in patients older than 10 years of age. They also may present insidiously with progressive renal failure leading to uremia or abruptly with acute abdominal pain and hypovolemic shock after a massive retroperitoneal hemorrhage. Arterial hypertension caused by parenchymal loss, compression of the adjacent kidney, or fibromuscular dysplasia of the renal artery may be the only clinical feature.

Laboratory findings include microscopic hematuria, proteinuria, and elevation of serum calcium, urea, and creatinine.

Renal angiomyolipomas are found in 47% of patients when TS is investigated with the newer imaging methods. The tumors may be the only clinical–radiologic manifestation of the disease.

Angiomyolipoma as a single renal tumor occurs in patients with no other evidence of TS. Patients with multiple angiomyolipomas and no other signs of TS have been reported to have children with the full clinical picture of TS [49].

This tumor is benign and requires surgical removal only when it causes persistent hematuria with threat of massive hemorrhage or when there is renal artery compression.

Renal Cysts

Tuberous sclerosis with multiple renal cysts is not to be mistaken for polycystic disease of the kidneys, also an autosomal dominant disease. These cysts are found as the only renal lesion in 18% of patients and is associated with angiomyolipomas in 12% of TS patients who underwent renal CT scanning or ultrasonography [48]. The renal cysts are often asymptomatic, the presence of symptoms depending on the amount of parenchymal loss from the large size or number of the cysts. If large enough, the enlarged kidney may be palpable and in a young infant the abdomen may be distended. The cysts involve predominantly the superficial renal cortex and have a hyperplastic and eosinophilic epithelial lining that is unique to patients with TS and is therefore distinguishable from polycystic kidneys [47].

Hypertension and uremia may be caused by the cysts alone or may be associated with renal angiomyolipomas. Large cysts displacing renal parenchyma or obstructing the collecting system may need decompression.

Other Renal Findings

In recent years renal cell carcinoma has been found more frequently in TS patients, and a variety of renal malformations have been reported including pyeloectasis, large kidneys, double ureters, supernumerary kidneys, and a single kidney. These anomalies are probably incidental associations [50] with TS.

Heart

Although cardiac rhabdomyoma is the most common cardiac tumor in infants, it is still considered to be an unusual disorder. Yet 43% of 14 infants and children with TS who were consecutively examined at Mayo Clinic and studied with 2-D echocardiography had one or more cardiac rhabdomyomas [51]. Most of these patients were asymptomatic.

Cardiac symptoms develop through one of three possible mechanisms: (a) obstruction of blood flow by an intracavitary tumor in the outflow tract of the right or left ventricle; (b) cardiac arrhythmia caused by a septal myoma interrupting the conduction system; and (c) impairment of ventricular wall contractility resulting from myocardial replacement by noncontractile intramural tissue [52].

Clinical features of left ventricular outflow tract obstruction simulate subvalvular aortic stenosis. Obstruction also may be found in the right ventricular outflow tract and the tricuspid or mitral valves.

Intrauterine cardiac failure may be the cause of hydrops fetalis [53], stillbirth [54], or neonatal death [55]. Congestive heart failure due to intramural tumors replacing a large portion of the ventricular wall may be mistaken for a cardiomyopathy.

With the aid of echocardiography and angiography, patients have been diagnosed early and successfully treated by removal of the obstructing tumor. Magnetic resonance imaging and CT of the heart are other useful methods for the diagnosis of rhabdomyoma. Cardiac rhabdomyoma has been detected by echocardiography in a fetus at 22 weeks' gestation and pathologically confirmed after terminating the pregnancy. A previous echocardiogram at 18 weeks' gestation had been normal [56].

Cardiac arrhythmias associated with rhabdomyoma include atrial or ventricular tachycardia, Wolff–Parkinson–White syndrome, junctional ectopic beats, complete heart block, and ventricular fibrillation [57].

Cardiac rhabdomyomas have a pale tan to white color and are well demarcated, although instead of a true capsule they have a pseudocapsule formed by compressed myocardial fibers.

Lungs

Cystic disease of the lungs and pulmonary lymphangiomyomatosis are the two possible manifestations of TS in the lungs [58]. It almost always affects women but occurs in less than 1% of women with

TS and is generally curiously confined to those with few or no signs of other organ involvement; these individuals are said to have the forme fruste.

Cystic Lung Disease

The symptoms vary according to the mechanisms involved and may be the result of (a) spontaneous pneumothorax, (b) pulmonary failure with hyperinflation of the lungs, and (c) pulmonary hypertension and cor pulmonale.

Spontaneous pneumothorax is recurrent and is manifested by sharp chest pain often associated with blood-streaked sputum. A chest radiograph will reveal a partial pneumothorax, and there may be increased markings in a reticulate pattern that gives a honeycomb appearance to the pulmonary parenchyma.

Lymphangiomyomatosis

Pulmonary fibrosis with loss of tissue elasticity progresses to respiratory failure giving the false appearance of obstruction. The patient is dyspneic and has a distended thorax; the vital capacity and forced expiratory volume gradually diminish, and the residual volume and total lung capacity increase. There is hypoxemia, first associated with hypocapnia, then normocapnia, and finally hypercapnia [59].

The proliferation of smooth muscle cells from the wall of pulmonary arterioles distorts small airways, venules, and lymphatic vessels, increases the pulmonary vascular resistance, and leads to pulmonary hypertension and cor pulmonale. The patient is dyspneic but as the disease progresses, pulmonary hyperinflation develops and radiographic studies reveal cyst-like spaces, an image known as "honeycomb lung."

The diagnosis is confirmed by the characteristic radiographic appearance of the lungs and additionally cytologic examination is performed to search for the hemosiderin-laden macrophages in the bronchoalveolar lavage fluid that are indicative of secondary hemosiderosis. A lung biopsy specimen will show distortion of the pulmonary architecture with fibrosis of the trabecula or interstitium, including vessels and small airways. There is an increment of interstitial fibrous and smooth muscle tissues or leiomyomatous hyperplasia [59].

Liver

The incidence of liver involvement in TS is unknown. Chiefly from autopsy findings different types of hamartomas have been described: racemose angiomas, adenomas, and lipomyomas and mesenchymatous fatty tumors [60]. An 8-year-old had multiple hamartomas of portal origin, some composed of only fat tissue, others of bile ducts, and still others of mixed mesodermal and endodermal tissues. The bile duct hamartomas were similar to those seen in polycystic disease of the liver [61]. With selective angiography of the celiac artery the hamartomas are demonstrable. Magnetic resonance imaging or CT scan of the liver with contrast is likely to show these asymptomatic lesions. We have observed small cysts in the CT scan of the liver in patients with TS.

Spleen

Splenic hemangioma is a rare manifestation of TS. In a review of 43 cases of splenic hamartoma there was only one patient with TS [62]. There are only five patients recorded with this association [60]. In three the splenic hemangioma was an incidental postmortem finding. One was an infant who had died of cardiac failure at the age of 4 days and who also had a cardiac rhabdomyoma and cerebral TS. Two symptomatic patients were 12- and 14-year-old boys with seizures, mental retardation, and skin lesions of TS who presented with abdominal pain and an enlarging abdominal mass. They both underwent splenectomy. The enlarged spleen of each patient contained a hamartoma that was predominantly vascular and that distorted the splenic architectural pattern. There were no malpighian corpuscles but cystic blood-filled spaces with the appearance of a cavernous angioma were present [60].

Ancillary Studies

Electroencephalography

The EEG of patients with or without seizures may demonstrate epileptiform abnormalities. Although of importance for the diagnosis and treatment of seizures, this test is unnecessary for the diagnosis of TS since the abnormalities are nonspecific [63,64].

Associated with infantile spasms, tonic–clonic, tonic, or atonic seizures, the EEGs of infants and young children contain characteristic wave patterns with generalized or multifocal abnormalities: hypsarrhythmia or modified hypsarrhythmia often accompanies infantile spasms; generalized spike and wave discharges associate with tonic–clonic seizures; and generalized sharp and slow-wave complexes are found with tonic or atonic seizures. The latter as-

sociation corresponds to the electroclinical diagnosis of Lennox–Gastaut syndrome and the infantile spasms and hypsarrhythmia to West's syndrome.

Focal abnormalities in the EEG consist of localized sharp waves or spike discharges in association with partial motor seizures or partial seizures with complex symptomatology. Other focal patterns may consist of slow-wave abnormalities associated with tubers or tumors or a projected rhythm associated with increased intracranial pressure due to obstruction of the CSF circulation [63].

Roentgenography

Since the advent of CT, ultrasound, and MRI, plain radiographs are no longer used to detect intracranial calcifications in patients with TS. The calcifications are in the subependymal nodules, in hamartomas (giant-cell astrocytomas), or within the white matter.

Radiography is still necessary to detect areas of osteomatous thickening within the skull (cranial vault sclerosis), vertebral spine, pelvis, and long bones and for the cystic lesions in the metacarpals and metatarsals that may or may not be associated with periosteal new bone formation. None of these images is pathognomonic of TS. Plain radiographs are still most useful for revealing a "honeycomb" appearance of the lung in cases of pulmonary TS (Figure 3.7). Since this type of involvement is most commonly seen in women in the third and fourth decades of life, chest radiographs should be part of the examination of

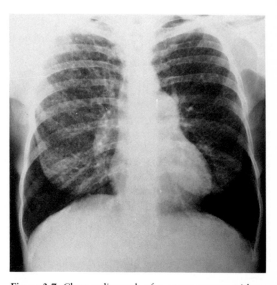

Figure 3.7. Chest radiograph of a young woman with tuberous sclerosis and the reticulated or "honeycomb" appearance of the lungs.

females with TS and in particular of prospective mothers at risk for TS.

Computed Tomography

Our present experience indicates that head CT scanning is the best method for the diagnosis of cerebral TS. For the detection of TS in any form of expression, that is, regardless of what organ is involved, it is only second to examination of the skin. The head CT scan is abnormal in 89% of all individuals with TS while specific skin lesions are present in 96%.

Abnormal findings in the head CT may be present at birth or in the first months of life while radiographic examination may show nothing unusual before the patient is several years old. The earliest recognized CT findings may be the nonspecific areas of decreased attenuation near the cortex or the calcified nodular subependymal lesions in the paraventricular region and especially near the foramina of Monro. The horizontal and coronal planes used in CT scans are preferable for detection of ventricular obstruction where following up these patients.

The type of abnormalities to be found in the head CT scan without contrast are

- Subependymal nodular calcifications.
- Intraventricular tumors.
- Ventricular dilatation with or without CSF obstruction.
- Cortical or subcortical areas of decreased attenuation.
- Widened gyri corresponding to tubers.
- Radial hypomyelinated tracts extending from the subependymal area to the cortex.
- Focal cerebral or cerebellar increased attenuation.
- Cortical atrophy.

The subependymal calcifications are the abnormalities most often recognized in head CT scans of TS patients (Figure 3.8). They do not correlate with the severity of the seizures and mental retardation. On the other hand, abundant and large-sized areas of decreased attenuation may parallel the severity and early development of seizures and the delay in psychomotor development (Figure 3.8). Although in two recent publications [65,66] low-attenuation lesions of the brain seen in sequential CT scans of young infants were attributed to cerebral embolism from an intracardiac tumor or from a cardiogenic thrombus, neither one of these two possible mechanisms has yet been confirmed pathologically. It is unlikely that fragments from a rhabdomyoma break

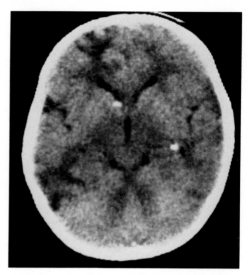

Figure 3.8. Computed tomography scan of the head without contrast showing the subependymal calcifications and areas of hypomyelination in subcortical regions adjacent to tubers and in centrum semiovale.

off from an intracavitary tumor but it is not unreasonable to propose that a thrombus is formed in the turbulence caused by intracavitary tumors and is the source of emboli.

The use of contrast material is of great help when an intraventricular tumor is suspected since these vascularized tumors may be "isodense" and not easily differentiated within the enlarged ventricle(s) (Figures 3.9A,B). They may form a cast within the ventricle. With aid of contrasting material the size and extent of the lesion may be shown. The low-attenuation intraventricular tumors calcify with aging. The cortical tubers do not enhance but, similar to giant cell astrocytomas, they calcify and may be detected in the head CT scan.

Dilated ventricles or hydrocephalus may or may not be associated with obstruction. A tumor obstructing the foramina of Monro will be accompanied by symptoms and signs of increased intracranial pressure but obstruction may be found when the symptoms are still subtle or lacking. Ventricular dilatation in the absence of obstruction and cortical atrophy may be found in patients who have had frequent and severe generalized seizures and are mentally subnormal.

Head CT scan is now a well-established method for the detection of asymptomatic cases of TS. Parents who have an affected child and who are seeking genetic counseling should have head CT scans.

The CT scan is also used to examine the kidneys,

Figure 3.9. Computed tomography scans of patients with tuberous sclerosis before *(A)* and after *(B)* injection of contrast material showing a large intraventricular uncalcified tumor and several small subependymal calcifications.

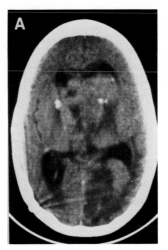
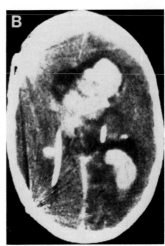

liver, and lungs. Examination of the kidneys may show multiple renal cysts. The angiomyolipomas in the kidneys or in the liver are revealed by areas of decreased attenuation within the parenchyma (Figure 3.10A). Examination of the lungs will reveal the increased attenuation of the fibrous trabeculae of the lung (Figure 3.10B).

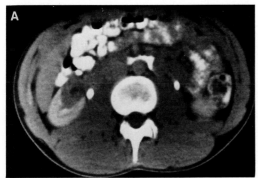
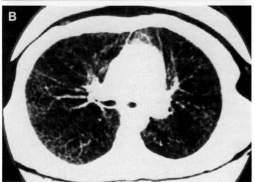

Figure 3.10. *(A)* Head CT scan showing the kidneys and a very large tumor with fat in the left kidney. *(B)* Computed tomography scan of the lung showing the reticulated pattern of the lungs in a patient with tuberous sclerosis and lung hyperinflation.

Magnetic Resonance Imaging

Magnetic resonance imaging has in a short time become a very useful tool for the diagnosis of specific lesions in the brains of patients with TS. Its advantages over the head CT scan are that it can give images of the brain in saggital sections, that the lesions not yet calcified may be visualized, and that areas of hypomyelination are easily demonstrated (Figures 3.11A,B). In patients suspected of having cerebral TS whose head CT scan was normal with MRI, cortical tubers or areas of subcortical hypomyelination have been displayed. A diagnosis of cerebral TS in an adult can probably be discarded if both CT and MRI are negative for cerebral lesions. Magnetic resonance imaging is also useful in discriminating between calcifications, and in evaluating fresh or clotted blood associated with cerebral angiomas.

Positron Emission Tomography

Although this is still an investigational tool, the value of positron emission tomographic scanning for the recognition of epileptogenic cortical lesions in TS has already been shown [67]. These lesions show a decreased uptake of [18F]-2-fluoro-2-deoxyglucose in the interictal state, a finding that may be helpful in conjunction with clinical and electroencephalographic data when considering surgery, an option for intractable seizures of focal origin.

Figure 3.11. Magnetic resonance imaging of a patient with multiple cerebral tubers.

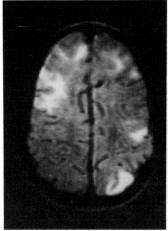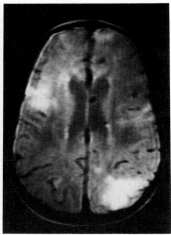

Ultrasound

Ultrasound is a radiation-free and economical imaging method for the detection of cystic and solid renal lesions. It is preferable to plain radiography and to intravenous pyelography (excretory urogram). CT scanning has the advantages over ultrasound that it can show the different degrees of x-ray attenuation between cystic lesions and fat-containing angiomyolipomas.

Pathology and Pathogenesis of Central Nervous System Lesions

The characteristic lesions found in the CNS of patients with TS are cortical tubers, subependymal nodules, and giant cell tumors. All CNS lesions are found within the cranium. The spinal cord, roots, nerves, and the rest of the peripheral nervous system to our knowledge are never involved.

Cortical Tubers

The focal cerebral dysplasias in the gyri are known as "tubers" or "tuberosities" (Figure 3.12) and are pathognomonic of the disease. The cerebral circumvolutions with the tubers are widened, pale, and hardened. The contrast between cortical tubers and the adjacent normal cortex is enhanced by illumination with ultraviolet light [62]. The number of cortical tubers varies from none to as many as 40, and their size ranges from a few millimeters to several centimeters. Their distribution over the two hemispheres is random and roughly symmetric or asymmetric. Close inspection of a tuber may reveal

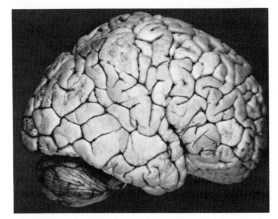

Figure 3.12. Brain of a patient with tuberous sclerosis showing multiple cerebral tubers.

a granular surface slightly raised above adjacent gyri and occasionally dimpled due to degeneration and retraction of the deeper regions within the gyrus [68]. Sectioning the brain reveals that the cortical tubers are pale and have indistinct borders. On microscopic examination they are characterized by disruption of the normal cortical lamination, reduction of the number of neurons that are replaced by giant cells of bizarre shape, and an increased number of astrocytic nuclei. The giant cells often contain several peripherally placed nuclei with prominent nucleoli. Some cells in the tuber show degenerative changes like shrinking, chromatolysis, or neurofibrillary tangles and contain an excessive amount of lipofuscin, glycogen, granulovacular bodies, and argentofilic globules [69]. The stroma of the tubers is abundant in glial fibers and poor in myelin (Figures 3.13A,B). With aging the gliosis increases, the neurons diminish in number, and calcium is deposited, although in

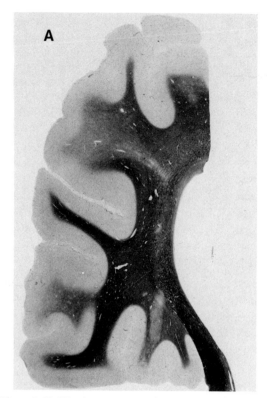 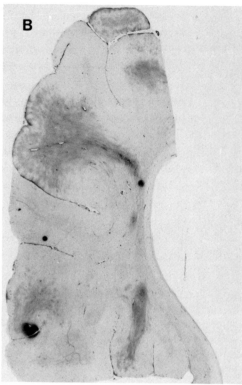

Figure 3.13. Histologic sections of two cortical tubers: *(A)* stained with luxol fast blue-cresyl violet to show subjacent area of hypomyelination; and *(B)* Holzer stain shows fibrillary gliosis. (Courtesy of Dr. Magda Erdohazi, Hospital for Sick Children, Great Ormond Street, London.)

smaller amount than in the subependymal lesions. Cystic degeneration of the central region of the tubers may occur [68]. Beneath the tubers, in the subcortical white matter, there are enlarged or bizarre neurons either in clumps or aligned in irregular rows, extending all the way from the ventricular wall to the cortex. These neurons, which have failed to migrate completely from the periventricular germinal matrix to the cortex, form a radial heterotopia visible in cut sections under the microscope, and, if large, are detectable in the head CT scan as areas of diminished attenuation. Tubers are seldom found in the cerebellum but heterotopic clusters of giant cells are not uncommon [70]. Abnormally large Purkinje cells are rare.

There is much controversy about the nature of the cellular elements forming the cortical tubers. Findings from the Golgi impregnation method and immunohistochemical and electron microscopy studies have given support to various interpretations. Huttenlocher and Heydemann [71], using the Golgi–Cox method, found that the neurons in cortical tubers are primitive and often lack a discernible axon but have well-developed dendrites with sparse spines. Neurons and glial cells are unevenly distributed within the tuber and tend to occur in clumps, which may explain discrepancies in different reports of EM studies. The neuronal population is predominantly made up of stellate neurons in contrast to the predominance of pyramidal neurons in a normal mammalian isocortex. The neuronal cell bodies are misaligned and disoriented, their dendritic spines are sparse or absent, and the dendrites have a beaded or varicose appearance. This type of neuron, uncommon in the mature brain, has led investigators to speculate that a cortical dysplasia occurs prenatally, perhaps as a result of localized disturbances in the embryonic or fetal environment, or that both neurons and glia in the tubers may be genetically defective cells that lack the capacity to differentiate into normal neocortical structures. A predominance of the stellate cell type of neurons, which fail to differentiate into mammalian neocortical cells and have a tendency to aggregate in clumps apart from the normal cortical neurons, suggested to Huttenlocher and Heydemann an alteration of cell surface properties;

cells lacking the necessary ingredients on their surface would move past the normal cellular elements and assume a superficial position during embryogenesis. An alternate hypothesis is that primitive cells in tubers retain mitotic potential, migrate to the cortical plate surface, and multiply in situ forming the characteristic cell nests. Other authors [72] also using the Golgi method have found a predominance of stellate cells in the intermediate and deep regions of the tubers, and based on the abnormal shape and aberrant orientation of the pyramidal cells, postulated a "focally accentuated disorder of cell migration and neuronal organization."

Ultrastructural studies of the cortical tubers have brought about further conflict of opinions on the origin of their giant cells. Arseni et al. [73] concluded they are large-sized neurons comparable to normal neurons, and that along with the glial cells and numerous neuronal and glial processes in the neuropil, the giant cells exhibit signs of early necrobiosis that suggest a metabolic factor in the etiopathogenesis of the disease. On the other hand, Ribadeau Dumas et al. [74] proposed that the abnormal cells they found in the cortical biopsy of a child with TS were of astrocytic origin and were very similar to those that they saw in a tumor of the caudate nucleus of another child with the same disease. Probst and Ohnacker [54] found astrocytic and ependymal differentiation in the cortical lesions of a premature infant with TS.

According to Trombley and Mirra [75] the majority of giant cells of a cortical tuber that they have seen resembled giant astrocytes similar to those seen in subependymal tumors. Also seen were abundant glial filaments with varying amounts of rough endoplastic reticulum, dense bodies, and mitochondria. Some astrocytes contained abundant fibers, and others were distended and filled with glycogen. The neuropil distant to the cortical tuber had abundant neurites and well-formed synapses. Intermediate zones closer to the tuber had a mixture of fibrillary glial processes and neurites while the center of the tuber contained relatively few neuronal processes or synapses and instead glial processes formed junctions with both astrocytic cell bodies and their processes [75].

Immunocytochemistry has been applied to the cerebral lesions of TS. Glial fibrillary acidic protein (GFAP) is a marker for both protoplasmic and fibrous astrocytes [76] never detected in oligodendrocytes, neurons, microglia, or cells from choroid plexus, endothelium, or meninges. Glial fibrillary acidic protein is present in cells that look like astrocytes in cortical tubers, in subependymal nodules,

and in retinal hamartomas. The giant cells in cortical tubers have no cytoplasmic GFAP staining. And although there are occasional giant cells that stain for GFAP their appearance is closer to the cells that do not take this stain than to conventional astrocytes [77]. What is found after staining with antiserum against GFAP is that a minority of giant cells in the cortical tubers are probably astrocytic [77].

Subependymal Nodules

The second, most striking, and also pathognomonic feature in the brain of patients with TS is the subependymal nodule (Figure 3.14). These are firm, tumor-like, and pea-size or larger excrescences on the ventricular wall of the ventricles that arise from under the ependyma and protrude into a ventricular cavity. Those in the lateral ventricles may be imbedded in the substance of the thalamus or caudate nucleus. They are seldom found in the third and fourth ventricles or are imbedded in the subcortical white matter of the cerebellum or brain stem. Their resemblance to the solidified wax that has dripped down the side of a candle has brought them the name "candle gutterings."

The subependymal nodules are composed almost entirely of large round or fusiform cells with nuclear

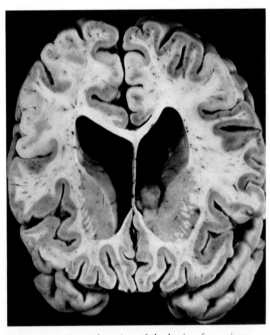

Figure 3.14. Coronal section of the brain of a patient with tuberous sclerosis showing a large nodule projecting into the ventricular cavity (candle guttering).

pleomorphism or multiple nuclei and glial fibers covered by a layer of ependyma. In the central parts of the nodules there are blood vessels with thickened walls and calcospherules with concentric layers. The subependymal nodules are benign or behave as a low-grade neoplasm but may obstruct the ventricles, usually at the foramina of Monro, to cause hydrocephalus. There is a unanimous belief that the giant cells in the subependymal nodules are astrocytic in origin. Electron microscopic examination as well as immunohistochemical studies have shown that they contain GFAP, the marker for astrocytes [77].

Subependymal Giant Cell Tumors

These lesions develop in the same region in which the subependymal nodules appear and may grow sufficiently to obstruct the foramina of Monro, or may even grow into one or both ventricles, forming a cast attached to the wall only by a small base. Since the subependymal nodules can also be considered tumors, the difference between subependymal nodules and subependymal "tumors" appears to be only that the latter can cause obstruction or grow inside the ventricle, producing progressive dilatation and symptoms of increased intracranial pressure. These tumors are not common and probably affect less than 2% of TS patients. Selected series of patients from neurosurgical sources may give the impression that these tumors are more frequent [78,79]. They rarely, if ever, become malignant and apparently originate from subependymal giant astrocytes, growing particularly when patients with TS are between 5 and 18 years old. They rarely bleed spontaneously. Histologically they consist of giant cells with abundant eosinophilic cytoplasm that resembles gemistocytic astrocytes. Ultrastructural examination shows an intact ependymal cell layer overlying glial cells and processes, most of which are packed with filaments [75]. The tumors are well vascularized, a feature that makes them distinct in contrasted CT scans. The giant cells have astrocytic features [54] and also contain large mitochondria. Immunohistochemical examination, however, has demonstrated that these cells lack GFAP, a fact not consistent with the opinion that they are astrocytes [77], but this finding has not been completely confirmed. Some authors [80] have found that in certain tumor areas the cells are totally negative when stained for GFAP while in other areas they show strong staining. Other authors have found a mosaic pattern of positive and negative cells [81]. The presence of a neuron-specific enolase in the giant cells has further reinforced the concept of neuronal

origin [82]. Recently it has been found [83] that in approximately 60% of TS patients who harbor a subependymal giant cell astrocytoma, the giant cells do not stain but that in the remaining 40% of patients the giant cells do stain for GFAP. This observation has led to the speculation that a mutational change in the astrocytes of TS patients results in the development of a phenomenon characteristic of neuronal cells, the inability to express GFAP. The demonstration of neuron-specific protein in some patients with subependymal astrocytoma remains unexplained.

Genetics

In 1913 Berg [17] described a family whose members in three generations had TS, and earlier Balzer and Menetrier [11] reported a mother and daughter with facial angiofibroma, unaware of the relationship of this disease with TS. Since then there have been reports of many families with affected members in up to five generations [32] with vertical transmission from father or mother to son or daughter. An autosomal-dominant type of inheritance with variable expressivity is well established. We have observed less variability in intrafamilial than in interfamilial expressivity. For instance, in one family all the affected members in three generations have periungual fibroma and facial angiofibroma but in all but one member normal intelligence prevails and white spots or seizures are rare or absent. Families have been described in which renal angiomyolipomas, pulmonary lesions, or just facial angiofibroma predominant among other clinical–pathologic features.

There are abundant reports of sporadic TS patients, that is, those having no known affected parent or sibling. It is exceptional, however, to find no affected member in a generation between two generations with affected members, that is, a "skipped" or "bracketed" generation. These two facts speak for a high mutation rate and high penetrance. In a large proportion of affected individuals, TS is believed to result from a new mutation of the gene responsible for the disease that may have occurred in the gonadal tissue of one of the direct ancestors either just before or during meiosis or after fertilization. Case history studies of sporadic cases looking for a predisposing factor toward a mutation have been fruitless [84–88].

It should be stressed that the "sporadic" cases reported in the past could have been in many instances patients born to an asymptomatic TS parent who today could be diagnosed with more effective methods of examination (ultraviolet light, head CT scan, renal ultrasound, and careful indirect ophthalmoscopy after mydriasis). Cassidy et al. [89] reported on 13 patients with TS and their apparently "unaffected" parents; when all 26 parents were properly examined, 4 were found to have TS.

Although reports of bona fide unaffected individuals "bracketed" between affected parents and children are missing, there are now on record two families, each with two affected siblings or half siblings and unaffected parents [90,91]. In the first family two severely affected children had unaffected parents and in the second two half siblings had a common father whose examination and ancillary tests, including intravenous pyelogram, pneumoencephalogram, head radiograph, and kidney ultrasound, were negative. A head CT scan was not done. The two obvious possibilities are that (a) two new mutations occurred in each family, and (b) the two apparently unaffected parents in the first family and the father of the two children in the second family had no signs of TS although they were affected. Another report discusses a set of twins with TS whose parents and other siblings were unaffected [92]; we suspect the twins were monozygotic, as were many other TS twins in the literature [93]. The reported monozygotic twins with TS appear to have resulted from a new mutation in the gonadal cells or before the first division of the fertilized egg [93].

Finally, it should be mentioned that when a family history of TS patients is obtained for genetic counseling, cases of fetal and early infant deaths should be noted. The increased incidence of stillbirths and neonatal deaths in affected families is due to cardiac rhabdomyoma, which causes hydrops fetalis [94] or neonatal heart failure.

In summary, genetic counseling in TS is simple when one of the proband's parents is affected. When, after a thorough examination of the skin and ocular fundi, and imaging of the head and kidneys, neither parent has been found to be affected, it can be assumed that the patient is the result of a new mutation. The possibilities of a second mutation are indeed small, probably on the order of 1 in 10,000, and the odds of a second new mutation occurring in a single generation of the same family is negligible.

Biochemical Markers

Several possible biochemical markers for TS have been investigated. Rundle et al. [95] screened propositi for changes in several serum proteins and found that 80% of 55 patients had one or more of the following: increased alpha-2 macroglobulin, increased IgM, and decreased transferrin, and 62% had the abnormality in all three of these markers. Other authors have failed to confirm these findings and have unsuccessfully searched for other markers, measuring serum amino acids and a series of polymorphic genetic markers (adenylate kinase, adenosine deaminase, sterase D, phosphoglucomutase I, acid phosphatase, glutamate pyruvate transaminase, glyoxylase I, phosphoglycolate phosphatase, glucose-6-phosphate dehydrogenase, 6-phosphogluconate dehydrogenase, and carbonic anhydrase II) [Draiger SP, Beaudet AL: unpublished data]. Tanaka et al. [96] measured serum levels of proline and hydroxyproline by high-performance liquid chromatography in 30 patients with TS and found that in the age group of patients 9 to 18 years a significantly higher mean free proline level compared to control subjects exists.

Most promising is the use of polymorphic DNA segments as linkage markers, which is now possible with the new recombinant DNA technology. This approach could be applied to mapping and characterization of the chromosomal defect causing TS. Such a DNA marker link to TS would allow the identification of individuals with TS who are nonexpressing or who have reduced expressivity phenotypes. Furthermore, the marker could permit antenatal recognition of this disease in families at risk for having affected children. Up to now the antenatal diagnosis of TS has been made only when a fetus at risk has been studied with ultrasound of the brain [97] or 2-D echocardiogram of the heart [97,98,99].

Course and Prognosis

The course of TS depends on the affected organ(s). In the medical literature the terms forme fruste and severely affected are often found but it is not quite clear what they mean. One's impression is that severely affected patients are those whose phenotype consists of signs or symptoms of CNS involvement, epilepsy, and mental retardation while the forme fruste refers to those who have either no or few and mild symptoms and no signs of CNS involvement. Forme fruste may refer only to involvement of the skin, the retina, or both, but with very few or no seizures. It should be noted that a patient with only mild signs of skin involvement may have asymptomatic kidney lesions or pulmonary TS leading to an early death. The course of the disease cannot be predicted from the clinical expression, whether severe or fruste, and it is therefore necessary to assess the involvement of each affected organ and in particular the kidneys, lungs, heart, and brain.

Judging only by postmortem findings in patients with TS, renal involvement is of greatest importance since it is always found and in a great majority of patients was the cause of death [48].

Treatment

Treatment also depends on what organs are affected. It is not our purpose to discuss this in detail in this chapter. There is obviously no treatment for the disease itself but many forms of treatment are available for CNS, cardiac, renal, pulmonary, and dermic symptoms or lesions of TS; this is often symptomatic or palliative, or may be surgical excision:

Symptoms	Treatment
CNS involvement	
Seizures	
Infantile spasms	Valproate, adrenocorticotropic hormone (ACTH)
Myoclonic	Clonazepam, ACTH
Atonic	Ethosuximide
Tonic-clonic	Phenobarbital Phenytoin
Partial seizures	Carbamazepine
Intracranial tumors	
Obstructive of CSF pathways	Shunting
Nonobstructive lesions	Tumor removal Need no treatment
Cardiac rhabdomyoma	
With obstruction	Surgical removal
With arrhythmia	Antiarrhythmic drugs
Renal angiomyolipomas, with no symptoms	Need no treatment
Persistent hematuria	Partial or total nephrectomy
With uremia	Dialysis
Large obstructive renal cysts	Surgical removal
Hypertension	Antihypertensive drugs
Pulmonary tuberous sclerosis	
Spontaneous pneumothorax	Reexpansion if recurrent
Pulmonary hyperinflation	Palliative
Retinal harmatomas	Need no treatment
Dermatologic lesions	
Facial angiofibromas	Dermabrasion, laser
Shagreen plaques	Rarely plastic surgery
Other skin lesions	Need no treatment

Detailed explanation of the appropriate treatments above can be found in general medical and specialty books.

Finally, it should be mentioned that the physician treating a patient with TS has a great responsibility to this individual and the family; many hours must often be spent explaining the nature of the disease, answering questions, and comforting the patient and immediate relatives.

References

1. Hunt A, Lindenbaum RH. Tuberous sclerosis: a new estimate of prevalence within the Oxford region. J Med Genet 1984;21:272–277.

2. Wiederholt WC, Gomez MR, Kurland LT. Incidence and prevalence of tuberous sclerosis in Rochester, Minnesota, 1950 through 1982. Neurology 1985;35:600–602.

3. D'Agostino AN, Kernohan JW. Tuberous sclerosis complex: report of a case in an 18-month-old child. J Neuropathol Exp Neurol 1962;21:79–84.

4. Tsukada Y, Pickren JW. Carcinoma of breast and asymptomatic tuberous sclerosis. NY State J Med 1967;67:593–597.

5. Gomez MR. Clinical experience at Mayo Clinic. In: Gomez MR, ed. Tuberous sclerosis. New York: Raven Press, 1979:11–26.

6. Von Recklinghausen F. Ein Herz von einem Neugeborenen welches mehrere Theils nach aussen, Theils nach den hohlen prominirende Tumoren (Myomen) trug. Verh Ges Geburtsh 25 Marz. Monatsschr Geburtskd 1862;20:1–2.

7. Bourneville DM. Sclérose tubéreuse des circonvolutions cérébrales: idiotie et épilepsie hémiplégique. Arch Neurol (Paris) 1880;1:81–91.

8. Hartdegen A. Ein Fall von multipler Verhärtung des Grosshirns nebst histologisch eigenartigen harten Geschwülsten der Seitenventrikel (Glioma gangliocellulare) bei einem Neugeborenen. Arch Psychiatr Nervenkr 1881;11:117–131.

9. Bourneville DM, Brissaud E. Encéphalite ou sclérose tubéreuse des circonvolutions cérébrales. Arch Neurol (Paris) 1881;1:390–412.

10. Bourneville, DM, Brissaud E. Idiotie et épilepsie symptomatiques de sclérose tubéreuse ou hypertrophique. Arch Neurol (Paris) 1900;10:29–39.

11. Balzer F, Menetrier P. Étude sur un cas d'adénomes sébacés de la face et du cuir chevelu. Arch Physiol Norm Pathol (série III) 1885;6:564–576.

12. Pringle JJ. A case of congenital adenoma sebaceum. Br J Dermatol 1890;2:1–14.

13. Rayer PFO. Traité théorique et pratique des maladies de la peau. 2nd ed. Paris: J B Baillière, 1835.

14. Perusini G. Über einen Fall von Sclerosis tuberosa hypertrophica. Monatsschr Psychiatr Neurol 1905;17:69–255.

15. Vogt H. Zur Diagnostik der tuberösen Sklerose. Z Erforsch Behandl Jugendl Schwachsinns 1908;2:1–12.

16. Schuster P. Beiträge zur Klinik der tuberösen Sklerose des Gehirns. Dtsch Z Nervenheilkd 1914;50:96–133.

17. Berg H. Vererbung der tuberösen Sklerose durch zwei bzw. drei Generationen. Z Ges Neurol Psychiatr 1913;19:528–539.

18. Campbell AW. Cerebral sclerosis. Brain 1905;28:382–396.

19. Critchley M, Earl CJC. Tuberous sclerosis and allied conditions. Brain 1932;55:311–346.

20. Sherlock FB. The feeble-minded. London: Macmillan, 1911.

21. Bielschowsky M. Über tuberöse Sklerose und ihre Beziehungen zur Recklinghausenschen Krankheit. Z Ges Neurol Psychiatr 1914;26:133–155.

22. Dalsgaard-Nielsen T. Tuberous sclerosis with unusual roentgen picture. Nord Med 1935;10:1541–1548.

23. Dickerson WW. Characteristic roentgenographic changes associated with tuberous sclerosis. Arch Neurol Psychiatr (Chi) 1945;53:199–204.

24. Yakolev PI, Corwin W. Roentgenographic sign in cases of tuberous sclerosis of the brain (multiple "brain stones"). Arch Neurol Psychiatr 1939;40:1030–1037.

25. Berg G, Vejlens G. Maladie kystique du poumon et sclérose tubéreuse du cerveau. Acta Paediatr (Uppsala) 1939;26:16–30.

26. Gold AP, Freeman JM. Depigmented nevi: the earliest sign of tuberous sclerosis. Pediatrics 1965;35:1003–1005.

27. Harris R, Moynahan EJ. Tuberous sclerosis with vitiligo. Br J Dermatol 1966;78:419–420.

28. Fitzpatrick TB, Szabó G, Hori Y, et al. White leaf-shaped macules: earliest visible sign of tuberous sclerosis. Arch Dermatol 1968;98:1–6.

29. Gastaut H, Roger J, Soulayrol R, et al. Encéphalopathie myoclonique infantile avec hypsarythmie (syndrome de West) et sclérose tubéreuse de Bourneville. J Neurol Sci 1965;2:140–160.

30. Della Rovere M, Hoare RD, Pampiglione G. Tuberous sclerosis in children: an EEG study. Dev Med Child Neurol 1964;6:149–157.

31. Pampiglione G, Moynahan EJ. The tuberous sclerosis syndrome: clinical and EEG studies in 100 children. J Neurol Neurosurg Psychiatry 1976;39:666–673.

32. Lagos JC, Gomez MR. Tuberous sclerosis: reappraisal of a clinical entity. Mayo Clin Proc 1967;42:26–49.

33. Zaremba J. Tuberous sclerosis: a clinical and genetic investigation. J Ment Defic Res 1968;12:63–80.

34. Donegani G, Gratarolla FR, Wildi E. Tuberous sclerosis. In: Vinken PJ, Bruyn GW, eds. Handbook of clinical neurology. The phakomatoses. Amsterdam: North–Holland; New York: American Elsevier, 1972;14:340–389.

35. Oppenheimer EY, Rosman NP, Dooling EC. The late appearance of hypopigmented maculae in tuberous sclerosis. Am J Dis Child 1985;139:408–409.

36. Rogers RS. Dermatologic Manifestations. In: Gomez MR, ed. Tuberous sclerosis. New York: Raven Press, 1979:95–119.

37. Blume RS, Wolff SM. The Chediak–Higashi syndrome: studies in four patients and review of the literature. Medicine 1972;51:240–280.

38. Awan KJ. Leaf-shaped lesions of ocular fundus and white eyelashes in tuberous sclerosis. South Med J 1982;75:227–228.

39. Alper JC, Holmes LB. The incidence and significance of birthmarks in a cohort of 4,641 newborns. J Pediatr Dermatol 1983;1:58–68.

40. Sishiba T, Shimozuma T. A case of tuberous sclerosis with subcutaneous nodules. J Dermatol 1983;10:391–394.

41. Gastaut H, Gastaut JL, Zifkin B, et al. Tuberous sclerosis. Summary of a clinical study of heredity, prognosis and associated epilepsies (abstr). Presented at the Tuberous Sclerosis Research Workshop, April 13, 1984, Harvard-MIT, Cambridge, MA.

42. Gomez MR. Neurologic and psychiatric symptoms. In: Gomez MR, ed. Tuberous sclerosis. New York: Raven Press, 1979:85–93.

43. Evans BK, Jankovic JJ. Tuberous sclerosis and chorea. Ann Neurol 1983;13:106–107.

44. Holanda FJCS, Holanda GMP. Tuberous sclerosis—neurosurgical indications in intraventricular tumors. Neurosurg Rev 1980;3:139–150.

45. Robertson DM. Ophthalmic findings. In: Gomez MR, ed. Tuberous sclerosis. New York: Raven Press, 1979:121–142.

46. Gutman I, Dunn D, Behrens M, et al. Hypopigmented iris spot, an early sign of tuberous sclerosis. Ophthalmology 1982;89:1155–1159.

47. Robbins TO, Bernstein J. Renal involvement. In: Gomez MR, ed. Tuberous sclerosis. New York: Raven Press, 1979:143–154.

48. Stillwell TJ, Gomez, MR, Kelalis PP. Renal lesions in tuberous sclerosis. J Urol (accepted for publication).

49. Wenzl JE, Lagos JC, Albers DD. Tuberous sclerosis presenting as polycystic kidneys and seizures in an infant. J Pediatr 1970;77:673–676.

50. Bender BL, Yunis EJ. The pathology of tuberous sclerosis. Pathol Annu 1982;17:339–382.

51. Alboliras ET, Hagler DJ, Gomez MR, et al. Cardiac involvement in tuberous sclerosis: an echocardiographic diagnosis (abstr). Presented at the American Heart Association 58th Scientific Sessions, November 11–14, 1985, Washington, DC.

52. Mair DD. Cardiac manifestations. In: Gomez MR, ed. Tuberous sclerosis. New York: Raven Press, 1979:155–169.

53. Ostor AG, Fortune DW. Tuberous sclerosis initially seen as hydrops fetalis. Arch Pathol Lab Med 1978;102:34–39.

54. Probst A, Ohnacker H. Sclérose tubéreuse de Bourneville chez un prématuré. Acta Neuropathol (Berl) 1977;40:157–161.

55. Sharp D, Robertson DM. Tuberous sclerosis in an infant of 28 weeks gestational age. Can J Neurol Sci 1983;10:59–62.

56. Crawford DC, Garrett C, Tynan M, et al. Cardiac rhabdomyomata as a marker for the antenatal detec-

tion of tuberous sclerosis. J Med Genet 1983;20:303–304.

57. Painter MJ, Pang D, Ahdab-Barmada M, et al. Connatal brain tumors in patients with tuberous sclerosis. Neurosurgery 1984;14:570–573.

58. Lie JT, Miller RD, Williams DE. Cystic disease of the lungs in tuberous sclerosis. Mayo Clin Proc 1980;55:547–553.

59. Liberman BA, Chamberlain DW, Goldstein RS. Tuberous sclerosis with pulmonary involvement. Can Med Assoc J 1984;36:287–289.

60. Gomez MR. Other visceral, vascular and osseus lesions. In: Gomez MR, ed. Tuberous sclerosis. New York: Raven Press, 1979:171–192.

61. Perou ML, Gray PT. Mesenchymal tumors of the kidney. J Urol 1960;83:240–261.

62. Cares RM. Tuberous sclerosis complex. J Neuropathol Exp Neurol 1958;17:247–254.

63. Westmoreland BF. Electroencephalographic experience at Mayo Clinic. In: Gomez MR, ed. Tuberous sclerosis. New York: Raven Press, 1979:55–68.

64. Ganji S, Hellmann CD. Tuberous sclerosis: long-term follow-up and longitudinal electroencephalographic study. Clin Electroencephalogr 1985;16:219–224.

65. Kandt RS, Gebarski SS, Goetting MR. Tuberous sclerosis with cardiogenic embolism: magnetic resonance imaging. Neurology 1985;35:1223–1225.

66. Konkol RJ, Walsh EP, Tower T, et al. Cerebral embolism resulting from an intracardiac tumor in tuberous sclerosis. Pediatr Neurol 1986;2:108–10.

67. Szelies B, Herholz K, Heiss W-D, et al. Hypometabolic cortical lesions in tuberous sclerosis with epilepsy: demonstration by position emission tomography. J Comput Assist Tomogr 1983;7:946–953.

68. Reagan TJ. Neuropathology. In: Gomez MR, ed. Tuberous sclerosis. New York: Raven Press, 1979:69–83.

69. Hirano A, Tuazon R, Zimmerman HM. Neurofibrillary changes, granulovacuolar bodies and argentophilic globules observed in tuberous sclerosis. Acta Neuropathol (Berl) 1968;11:257–261.

70. Norman RM. Malformations of the nervous system, birth injury and diseases of early life. In: Blackwood W, McMenemey WH, Meyer A, et al., eds. Greenfield's neuropathology. Baltimore: Williams & Wilkins, 1963:324–440.

71. Huttenlocher PR, Heydemann RT. Fine structure of cortical tubers in tuberous sclerosis. Ann Neurol 1984;16:595–602.

72. Ferrer I, Fabregues I, Coll J, et al. Tuberous sclerosis: a Golgi study of cortical tuber. Clin Neuropathol 1984;3:47–51.

73. Arseni C, Alexianu M, Horvat L, et al. Fine structure of atypical cells in tuberous sclerosis. Acta Neuropathol (Berl) 1972;21:185–193.

74. Ribadeau Dumas JL, Poirier J, Escourelle R. Étude ultrastructurale des lésions cérébrales de la sclérose tubéreuse de Bourneville. Acta Neuropathol (Berl) 1973;25:259–270.

75. Trombley IK, Mirra SS. Ultrastructure of tuberous sclerosis: cortical tuber and subependymal tumor. Ann Neurol 1981;9:174–181.

76. Eng LF, Rubinstein LJ. Contribution of immunohistochemistry to diagnostic problems of human cerebral tumors. J Histochem Cytochem 1978;26:513–522.

77. Stefansson K, Wollmann K. Distribution of glial fibrillary acidic protein in central nervous system lesions of tuberous sclerosis. Acta Neuropathol (Berl) 1980;52:135–140.

78. Kapp JP, Paulson GW, Odom Gl. Brain tumors with tuberous sclerosis. J Neurosurg 1967;26:191–202.

79. Holanda FJCS, Holanda GMP. Tuberous sclerosis—neurosurgical indications in intraventricular tumors. Neurosurg Rev 1980;3:139–150.

80. Velasco ME, Dahl D, Roessmann U, et al. Immunohistochemical localization of glial fibrillary acidic protein in human glial neoplasms. Cancer 1980;45:484–494.

81. Nakamura Y, Becker LE. Subependymal giant-cell tumor: astrocytic or neuronal? Acta Neuropathol (Berl) 1983;60:271–277.

82. Stefansson K, Wollmann R. Distribution of the neuronal specific protein 14-3-2 in central nervous system lesions of tuberous sclerosis. Acta Neuropathol (Berl) 1981;53:113–117.

83. Bonnin JM, Rubinstein LJ, Papasozomenos SCH, et al. Subependymal giant-cell astrocytoma. Acta Neuropathol (Berl) 1984;62:185–193.

84. Borberg A. Clinical and genetic investigations into tuberous sclerosis and Recklinghausen's neurofibromatosis. Contribution to elucidation of interrelationship and eugenics of the syndromes. Acta Psychiatr Scand 1951;(suppl)71:11–239.

85. Bundy S, Evans K. Tuberous sclerosis, a genetic study. J Neurol Neurosurg Psychiatry 1969;32:591–603.

86. Gunther M, Penrose LS. The genetics of epiloia. J Genet 1935;31:413–430.

87. Nevin NC, Pearce WG. Diagnostic and genetical aspects of tuberous sclerosis. J Med Genet 1968;5:273–280.

88. Zaremba J. Tuberous sclerosis: a clinical and genetical investigation. J Ment Defic Res 1968;12:63–80.

89. Cassidy SB, Pagon RA, Pepin M, et al. Family studies in tuberous sclerosis. Evaluation of apparently unaffected parents. JAMA 1983;249:1302–1304.

90. Wilson J, Carter C. Genetics of tuberous sclerosis. Lancet 1978;1:340.

91. Michel JM, Diggle JH, Brice J, et al. Two half-siblings with tuberous sclerosis, polycystic kidneys and hypertension. Dev Med Child Neurol 1983;25:239–244.

92. Primrose DA. Epiloia in twins: a problem in diagnosis and counselling. J Ment Defic Res 1975;19:195–203.

93. Gomez MR, Kuntz NL, Westmoreland BF. Tuberous sclerosis, early onset of seizures and mental subnormality: study of discordant monozygous twins. Neurology 1982;32:604–611.

94. Kuntz NL, Gomez MR. Genetics population studies and pathogenesis. In: Gomez MR, ed. Tuberous sclerosis. New York: Raven Press, 1979:207–220.

95. Rundle AT, Fannin CV, Bartlett K. Serum proteins and

serum enzymes in tuberous sclerosis. J Ment Defic Res 1967;11:85–96.

96. Tanaka H, Nakazawa K, Arima M, et al. Tuberous sclerosis: proline and hydroxyproline contents in serum. Brain Devel 1983;5:450–456.

97. Muller G, DeJong C, Falck V, et al. Antenatal ultrasonographic findings in tuberous sclerosis. South African Medical J 1986;69:633–638.

98. Crawford DC, Garrett C, Tynan M, Neville BG, Allan LD. Cardiac rhabdomyomata as a marker for the antenatal detection of tuberous sclerosis. J Med Genetics 1983;20:303–312.

99. Plais MH, Baril JY, Lebret M. Diagnostic anténatal d'une tumeur cardiaque évocatrice d'une sclérose tubéreuse de Bourneville. J Gynecol Obstet Biol Reprod 1985;14:759–762.

Chapter 4
Von Hippel–Lindau Disease

VIRGINIA V. MICHELS

Although von Hippel–Lindau (VHL) disease does not affect the skin as do all other diseases discussed in this book, there are enough similarities from clinical, pathologic, and genetic points of view to justify its inclusion.

Von Hippel–Lindau disease is a single gene disorder characterized by retinal and cerebellar hemangioblastomas; cysts of the kidneys, pancreas, and epididymis; and renal cancers. Other manifestations include hemangioblastomas of the medulla oblongata and spinal cord, cysts and hemangiomas of other visceral organs, and, in some families, pheochromocytomas (Table 4.1). The inheritance pattern is autosomal dominant with variable expression, so that not all patients have all the possible manifestations of the disease. Because of this variable expression, and because new mutation disease may occur, a negative family history does not exclude this diagnosis.

The diagnosis should be made in any person with a central nervous system or retinal hemangioblastoma plus one of the other characteristic physical abnormalities or a family history of VHL disease. In some cases, the diagnosis may be warranted in a patient with a positive family history who has no evidence of a CNS or retinal lesion, but who has one or more of the less specific findings (Table 4.2). It is important to make the diagnosis of VHL disease to ensure proper monitoring and early treatment of the patient and family members, as well as for genetic counseling purposes.

History

Panas and Remy described a retinal hemangioblastoma in 1879, although they did not recognize it as such. An earlier stage of the eye lesion was recognized and described further by Fuchs in 1882, who mistakenly considered the lesion to be an arteriovenous malformation [1]. In 1894, Collins, after examining autopsy material, suspected that the lesions originated in the capillaries and recognized their hereditary nature [1]. von Hippel in 1904 outlined the progressive nature of the retinal lesion; in 1911 he concluded that the lesion was a hemangioblastoma and called it "angiomatosis retinae" [1]. Hughlings Jackson reported a cerebellar hemangioblastoma in 1872 [2]. In 1884, Pye–Smith reported the autopsy findings of a cystic hemangioblastoma of the cerebellum in a patient with renal and pancreatic cysts that he dismissed as coincidental [3]. Another case later recognized as VHL disease was reported by Turner in 1887 [2]. In 1911, one of von Hippel's original two patients, whose retinal lesions had been serially examined, came to autopsy; he had a cerebellar tumor, hypernephromas, and renal, pancreatic and epididymal cysts [1]. He mistakenly thought the renal lesions were benign [4]. Tresling, in 1920, reported for the first time a family with both retinal and cerebellar tumors [2].

Finally in 1926, the Swedish pathologist, Arvid Lindau [5], published a monograph based on the findings in 40 patients, including 16 of his own, thus establishing the clinical–pathologic constellation of this unique disorder. He also recognized the histologic similarities of the retinal and cerebellar hemangioblastomas [2] and noted they may be found in the medulla and cord in association with syringomyelia. Ten percent of patients had multiple CNS tumors, and in his own cases 50% had pancreatic cysts, 62% renal cysts, 38% "benign renal hypernephroid tumors," and some had adrenal and liver adenomas and epididymal tumors [1,6]. Schubach first used the

Table 4.1. Major Organ Involvement in von Hippel–Lindau Disease

Organ	Lesion	Patients Affected[a] (%)
Eye	Hemangioblastoma; retina, optic disc	24–73 [21, 4]
Central nervous system	Hemangioblastoma; cerebellum, medulla oblongata, cord	22–66 [10, 8]
Kidney	Cysts, cancer, hemangiomas, adenomas	56–83 [7, 39]
Pancreas	Cysts, cancer, hemangioblastomas, hemangiomas	9–72 [48, 8]
Adrenal	Pheochromocytoma, adenomas, cysts, cortical hyperplasia	7–17 [8, 53]
Epididymis	Cysts, hemangiomas, adenomas	7–27 [8, 9]
Liver	Cysts, adenomas, hemangiomas	17 [8]

[a]Numbers indicate range in published series; reference numbers in brackets.

Table 4.2. Diagnostic Criteria for von Hippel–Lindau Disease

CNS and retinal hemangioblastoma
  or
CNS or retinal hemangioblastoma plus one of the
    following:
  Renal, pancreatic, hepatic, or epididymal cysts
  Pheochromocytoma
  Renal cancer
  or
Definite family history plus
  CNS or retinal hemangioblastoma
  Renal, pancreatic, or epididymal cysts
  Pheochromocytoma
  Renal cancer

term "von Hippel–Lindau complex" to refer to this syndrome in 1927, and in 1929 Möller recognized the inheritance pattern as autosomal dominant [1,2].

Since this early important work, there have been numerous case reports and studies addressing selected aspects of this disease in over 400 patients [7]. Of much value are the contributions by Melmon in 1964 [1] and in the past 10 years those by Horton [8], Fill [9], Blight [10], and Go [7], which provide information on the frequency of specific lesions and the clinical course of the disease. Still remaining unknown are the basic molecular defect, the location of the abnormal gene within the genome, the mechanism by which the single genetic defect results in multiple pathologic manifestations, the difference of expression in individuals of same families and between families, and the frequency of each lesion within the affected population. With greater awareness of this disease and improved medical technology, significant advances have been made in the early detection and treatment of probands and their relatives. In spite of these advances, the morbidity and mortality remain high.

Von Hippel–Lindau disease occurs in virtually all ethnic groups including people of European, African, Oriental, and Middle Eastern ancestry [7,11,12]. The disease is thought to be rare, but the exact incidence and prevalence are unknown. The mutation rate has been estimated to be 1.8×10^{-7} in the German population [13].

Clinical Symptoms and Signs

Eye

The typical ocular lesion of VHL disease is the retinal hemangioblastoma, sometimes referred to as a retinal angioma, hemangioma, or "angiomatosis retinae." This tumor, recognized as a benign hemangioblastoma since Lindau's time [2], is one of the earliest manifestations of VHL disease. The mean age at diagnosis is 25 or 28 years [8,14] for symptomatic and asymptomatic patients ascertained through family screening.

Retinal hemangioblastomas have been detected in 8-year-old children [15]. It is not unusual to find small lesions in teenagers from affected families [16]. New lesions have developed in retinas previously examined and found to be normal. Therefore, it is unlikely that the lesion is congenital, but this does not preclude the possibility that the lesions arise from the proliferation of vascular epithelium vestiges [17].

The earliest clinically detectable retinal lesion is a small red dot resembling an aneurysmal dilatation of retinal capillaries [17,18] that could be mistaken for a diabetic microaneurysm [18]. As it grows, the lesion may appear as a flat or slightly elevated gray disc and later as a globular, orange-red tumor (Figure 4.1) [17]. The hallmark of this mature tumor is a pair of dilated tortuous vessels running between the lesion and the disc. The dilated afferent arteriole and efferent venule reflect significant arteriovenous shunting [17,18]. The diameter of the lesions range between 0.5 and more than 10 mm [17].

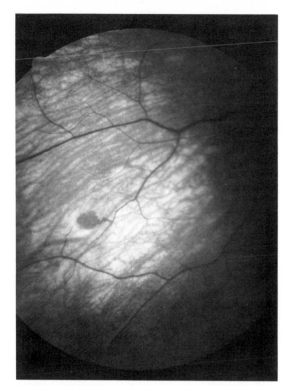

Figure 4.1. Retinal hemangioblastoma in patient with von Hippel–Lindau disease. (Courtesy of Dr. H. Gordon.)

As the retinal hemangioblastomas frequently are located in the periphery, a careful search by indirect opthalmoscopy may be needed to find the small ones [19]. Fluorescein angiography also is helpful [20], particularly in demonstrating the typical early filling and late leakage of small or atypical lesions. Without this technique, large lesions may be obscured by accumulated exudate on their surface and around their edges, resulting in gliosis [17]. Occasionally the lesions are associated with a cyst or may calcify [1].

The lesions progress at a variable rate, either rapidly over a period of 2 to 4 years, slowly over many years [8], or not at all [17]. If multiple, the lesions may be at different stages.

The lesions leak and fluid accumulates within or beneath the retina, between the lesion and the optic disc, or in the macular area. In the macula, this leakage may form an "exudative mound," that is, an exaggerated macular exudate next to an exudate-free area between lesion and macula [17]. Localized retinal detachment is a feature of all but the smallest tumors [16].

Retinal exudate and hemorrhage may result in reactive retinal inflammation and more extensive exudative retinal detachment, causing decreased visual acuity or blurred vision progressing to blindness [1].

Secondary neovascular glaucoma, cataracts, and uveitis may occur, ultimately resulting in pthisis requiring enucleation because of pain. Some of these secondary changes may mask the underlying lesions and result in the misdiagnosis, for example, of Coat's exudative retinitis [1]. Exophytic lesions that project into the vitreous may hemorrhage [17] and may also result in decreased vision.

Of patients known to have VHL, the frequency of those found to have at least one retinal lesion varied between series: 24% [21], 42% [10], 45% [9], 54% [7], 58% [8], and 73% [4]. This variability reflects, in part, the intrinsic variability of the disease as well as the selection of the subjects by age, clinical presentation, and method of study. Of those with VHL and eye lesions, 33 to 58% [1,22] had multiple lesions within one eye and 30 to 57% [16,22] had bilateral lesions.

Although small peripheral retinal hemangioblastomas frequently are asymptomatic, the eye tumor is one of the most frequently symptomatic lesions in VHL. In a large family studied by Horton, 16% of patients had symptoms. These included decreased visual acuity, progressive and painless visual loss, blurred vision, "floaters," and blindness [19]. There are numerous literature reports of blindness (unilateral or bilateral) in young patients in their twenties, and several reports of 8- and 9-year-old children with blindness due to retinal hemangioblastoma [15,23,24]. At the other end of the spectrum, patients with retinal lesions have remained asymptomatic past the age of 50 [16]. In one series of ophthalmologic patients with retinal involvement, 47% had normal vision and 36% had vision diminished to less than 20/200 [22]. Leukocoria and strabismus in children are rare manifestations [17]. Secondary changes resulted in painful glaucoma or phthisis necessitating enucleation in 11% of patients in one selected series [22].

Because retinal lesions are asymptomatic prior to significant retinal detachment and because early diagnosis increases the likelihood of successful treatment, all persons known to have VHL or to be at significant risk by virtue of family history should have annual ophthalmologic examinations beginning at age 6 years [18].

Hemangioblastomas of the optic disc also may occur in VHL. As of 1975, only 55 cases of this rare lesion had been reported [25]; 24% of the patients were considered to have VHL. In some instances an incorrect initial diagnosis of papilledema had been made; papilledema may occur in VHL in association with a posterior fossa tumor. Most patients with VHL and hemangioblastoma of the optic disc also have multiple retinal hemangioblastomas. The disc lesions appear as well-circumscribed, reddish-orange, round or oval elevated lesions obscuring part of the optic disc, usually temporally. Less commonly the lesion is flatter and grayish with poorly defined margins extending from the disc into the retina. Fluroscein angiography reveals that the mass consists of small-caliber vessels that fill early during the retinal arterial phase and leak. The most common symptom is visual loss resulting from chronic macular edema, with or without serous retinal detachment. In other cases visual loss results from repeated virtreous hemorrhages. Intraorbital optic nerve hemangioblastoma is even more rare, having been reported in only five patients [26].

What proportion of patients presenting with hemangioblastoma of the retina have VHL is unknown, since no unbiased study of such patients and their families looking for other extraretinal signs of VHL has been done. A rough estimate of the proportion of patients with retinal hemangioblastoma who have VHL can be made based on the fact that 10 to 20% of such patients have brain tumors [1,14]. All patients with retinal hemangioblastoma should be evaluated for other signs of VHL.

Central Nervous System

Central nervous system hemangioblastomas, when associated with VHL disease, occur most frequently in the cerebellum but also occur in the medulla oblongata, spinal cord, and rarely in the cerebrum.

Cerebellar hemangioblastoma, one of the most frequent manifestations of VHL, occurs in 66% of autopsy-confirmed cases [8]. In four different clinical series, this benign tumor was reported to occur in 22% [10], 35% [27], 36% [8], and 44% [7]. Although the cerebellar lesions have been detected in some cases only by computed tomography (CT) of the head in asymptomatic relatives of von Hippel–Lindau patients, many of these individuals later become symptomatic. When large families are studied, it is found to be the chief source (40%) of the first symptom [28], and the greatest cause of morbidity and mortality in VHL patients, resulting in more than 50% of disease-related deaths [8,9].

The average age of onset of symptoms from cerebellar hemangioblastoma is approximately 30 years [2,8] with an age range of 10 to 52 years [8,22]. The lesion is said to be rare before puberty [29], but there have been reports of 10- [22] and 11-year-old [30] children with VHL who were found to have papilledema when examined as part of a family study. The mean age of diagnosis is 8 to 12 years younger

than in patients in non-selected neurosurgical series with cerebellar hemangioblastoma [2]. The incidence of CNS hemangioblastoma in the general population is approximately 1/20,000 [5], accounting for 1 to 2.5% of all brain tumors [23] and 7 to 12% of all posterior fossa tumors in neurosurgical series [31]. In these general series, composed mainly of sporadic cases not known to have VHL disease, the male/female ratio is 1.5 or 2:1 [29], but in patients with VHL the sex ratio is closer to 1 [8]. Nevertheless, the signs and symptoms are similar in patients with or without VHL disease. The majority of patients (76%) present with symptoms of increased intracranial pressure [5].

Headache, the most common initial symptom, occurs in 53 to 90% of patients [19,31,32]. The headache may be frontal or occipital in location. Between 12% and 60% of patients have associated vertigo and dizziness [1,19,31]; a significant number of patients also present with nausea or vomiting (20 to 50%) [1,19]. Gait ataxia as a presenting symptom varies between 17% and 80% in frequency in reported series [2,19,31]. Visual disturbances also are frequent presenting symptoms: double vision in 24 to 32% of patients and decreased visual acuity in 11 to 26% [2,31]. The symptoms of cerebellar hemangioblastoma and their frequency and references are listed in Table 4.3. The duration of symptoms before hospitalization for surgery ranged from 3 weeks to 7 years [19], with an average of 7.5 months [2] to

Table 4.3. Symptoms of Cerebellar Hemangioblastoma

	Patients Affected[a] (%)
Headache	53–90 [19,32]
Gait imbalance	17–80 [19,31]
Vomiting	20–70 [1,32]
Double vision	24–32 [2,31]
Vertigo	28 [32]
Decreased visual acuity	11–26 [2,31]
Neck pain/stiffness	9–26 [19,32]
Mental changes[b]	12–18 [2,32]
Tinnitus	4–8 [2,32]
Anorexia	7 [2]
Lethargy	6 [2]
Sphincter disturbance	5 [32]
Limb weakness	4 [2]
Speech difficulty	4 [2]
Eye pain	4 [32]
Syncope	3 [1]

[a]Numbers indicate range in published series; reference numbers in brackets.
[b]Dementia, personality changes, irritability.

13.6 months, in different series [19]. The symptoms are those of a slowly growing lesion that gradually worsens, but occasionally there is sudden onset of symptoms due to bleeding into the tumor and rapid increase of intracranial pressure. In general, symptoms and signs of this benign tumor relate to the space-occupying effect of the tumor or the accompanying cyst. Subarachnoid hemorrhage, an infrequent complication [29], was suspected in some patients presenting with sudden onset of neck pain and stiffness [32].

The signs of cerebellar hemangioblastoma are listed in Table 4.4. Approximately 60 to 75% [5] of patients have cerebellar signs, while 20% of patients have signs of both cerebellar dysfunction and increased intracranial pressure [2]. The cerebellar signs are unilateral in half of these patients [32]. In addition to gait ataxia, dysarthria, and nystagmus, patients may have limb ataxia or hypotonia [32]. The abducens or the oculomotor nerves may be involved.

Between 3 and 10% of patients reported in non-selected neurosurgical series have multiple tumors [2,19]; however, it is sometimes difficult to differentiate between a second tumor and recurrence of an incompletely removed tumor [19]. Between 4 and 20% [31,32] of patients in these series have retinal hemangioblastomas, and 4 to 23% [5,31] have a positive family history of hemangioblastoma. The thoroughness of the history taking and ophthalmologic examinations in these various series was not uniform. In fact, there is no study of cerebellar hemangioblastoma in which all patients were fully investigated for signs of VLH disease. In a retrospective study of consecutive patients presenting with CNS hemangioblastoma, 30% were found to have VHL, even though most of them had not been fully evaluated [33].

Table 4.4. Signs of Cerebellar Hemangioblastoma

	Patients Affected[a] (%)
Papilledema	68–90 [19,31]
Ataxia/broad-based gait	44–76 [2,19]
Nystagmus	41–62 [2,31]
Cranial nerve palsies	30 [2]
Motor paresis	25 [19]
Corticospinal tract involvement	22 [32]
Facial paresis	18–21 [2,32]
Limb paresis	9 [2]
Decreased consciousness	9 [2]
Slurred speech	5 [2]
Seizures	2 [32]

[a]Numbers indicate range in published series; reference numbers in brackets.

The hemangioblastomas of VHL disease also may be located in the spinal cord or in the medulla. In nonselected neurosurgical series of CNS hemangioblastomas, 3 [32] to 8% [22] were spinal lesions, and in several instances a patient had both cerebellar and spinal lesions, suggesting that some of these patients may have had VHL disease. In series of VHL patients, the incidence of spinal hemangioblastomas was 10 [10] to 14% [4]. The methods by which these patients were ascertained and investigated are not clear. In one large family, spinal cord hemangioblastomas were found in 28% of deceased family members who had an autopsy, but most of these lesions had been asymptomatic and only 4% had a spinal hemangioblastoma that resulted in clinical symptoms.

The mean age of diagnosis in patients whose cord lesions were detected during life was 25 years (range 20 to 29 years) [8]. The cord lesions are associated with syringomyelia in most cases [8]. They may be located in any spinal segment [23] including the conus medullaris [28], although they are most common in the lower cervical and lower thoracic sites [1]. Initial symptoms may include loss of sensation and impaired proprioception. As cord compression progresses, weakness, muscle wasting, anesthesia, sphincter disturbances, and ultimately spasticity and paraplegia may develop [1]. There has been at least one report of paraplegia of sudden onset due to a "ruptured" cervical cord hemangioblastoma [34].

Hemangioblastomas of the medulla oblongata also may first be detected at autopsy in VHL patients (14%) or may be symptomatic (approximately 4%), but the mean age of diagnosis is greater (36 years; range 30 to 43 years) than for spinal lesions [8]. In some families this lesion is less common and occurs in only 2.5% [9,10] of family members. These lesions usually are associated with syringobulbia. In nonselected series of CNS hemangioblastomas, 4 [32] to 11% [22] are bulbar lesions, but in other series no such lesions are reported [2].

Supratentorial hemangioblastomas are very rare lesions in the general population and also are rare in VHL disease, accounting for less than 5% of CNS hemangioblastomas in nonselected neurosurgical series [2,19]. In a review published in 1981 [20], there were 62 case reports of supratentorial hemangioblastoma collected from the literature, and 14.5% of these were known to have VHL disease. These tumors were located in the pituitary [3]; the lateral wall and choroid plexus of the third ventricle; and in the parietal, occipitoparietal, temporal, or frontal lobes [20,35]. Care must be taken to exclude the diagnosis of metastatic renal carcinoma when supratentorial lesions are detected, since the histology can be confusing, even to very experienced pathologists [36]. It is possible that the correct diagnosis in some of the reported cases was metastatic renal carcinoma, which also is a feature of VHL disease, or that some lesions represented angioblastic meningiomas, particularly in those patients not known to have VHL.

There have been sporadic reports of other CNS tumors in VHL disease: meningioma [1], ependymoma [37], intraventricular neuroblastoma [37], and cerebellar astrocytoma [40].

Kidney

The renal lesions of VHL disease include cysts [1], hemangiomas [4], benign adenomas [8], and most importantly, malignant hypernephromas. In clinical and autopsy series, 56 [7] to 83% [38] of patients have some type of renal lesion [1].

The renal cysts are usually simple cysts [36] and are rarely symptomatic. Horton [8] reported finding at autopsy that 59% of patients with VHL have renal cysts. In one clinical survey, 22% [10] of VHL patients had cysts, but it is not clear how these persons were investigated. In a study of 17 affected persons who were screened by abdominal CT, 76% had cysts [21]; none were symptomatic.

The cysts vary in size from a few millimeters to more than 2 cm [38]; they frequently are bilateral and multiple. In contrast, the incidence of simple cysts in general autopsy patients is approximately 3 to 5% [40], being rare in children and adults under age 30 years [41], and increasing with age so that in adults over 50, more than 50% may have a cyst [42]. Newer imaging techniques such as CT and ultrasound have revealed that single renal cysts are even more common in the general population than had been expected from autopsy studies, and are of little or no clinical significance.

Rarely, the renal cysts of VHL disease may be so extensive as to mimic polycystic kidney disease. At least two VHL patients were misdiagnosed as having autosomal dominant ("adult-type") polycystic kidney disease because of hundreds of cysts that resulted in renal failure and the need for dialysis [10,43]. Although this presentation of VHL disease is rare, the diagnosis should be considered in any patient presenting with renal cysts.

Renal hemangiomas occur in approximately 7% of VHL patients [8] at autopsy and are virtually always incidental findings that had caused no symptoms. In one clinical series, only 2% of patients could be shown to have a renal angioma when screened with abdominal CT and ultrasound. Similarly, benign adenomas are asymptomatic with an incidence of 14% at autopsy in VHL patients.

Renal clear cell cancer (hypernephroma) is a common problem in patients with VHL and a major cause of morbidity and mortality. It is the most commonly symptomatic lesion of VHL disease, after cerebellar and retinal lesions.

Family studies reveal that 28% [8] of VHL patients develop symptoms due to hypernephroma that results in death in almost one-third [8]. In autopsy series of VHL patients, 45% had hypernephroma and sometimes it had been asymptomatic. The lesions are bilateral in 15 [40] to 75% [9] and multiple in 87% [9]; one 29-year-old patient had 15 tumors [44].

The frequency of malignant hypernephroma in clinical series of VHL patients reported in the literature is quite consistent, ranging between 25 [4,10] and 38% [9,21]. Renal cancer tends to be one of the later clinical manifestations of VHL, being detected on average 6 years after the disease is diagnosed [44]. As cerebellar hemangioblastomas are detected earlier and treated more effectively, allowing for more prolonged survival, renal cancer may pose an increasing burden for patients with VHL disease. The mean age of diagnosis of renal cancer was 41 years with a range of 20 to 61 years [8], and the average age of death from renal cancer was 44.5 years [44]. This is in contrast to renal cancer in the general population, in which the disease is rare before 40 years and peaks between the ages of 50 and 70 years. In sporadic cases, the male/female ratio is 2 or 3:1, but in VHL disease the sex ratio is close to 1 [40].

Initially, the cancer may be asymptomatic and may even be the first sign of the disease, as it was in two of four reported patients with renal cancer detected by family screening [21]. Patients may present with painless gross hematuria [36], but the absence of microscopic hematuria does not exclude the presence of large and multiple renal cancers [33].

Although previously thought to be benign, these lesions are definitely malignant and can metastasize. In a literature review, 40% of patients with renal cancer had metastases, the tumor being as aggressive as sporadic renal cancer in the general population [44]. The tumors often can be diagnosed by CT even if less than 3 cm in size, when they are unlikely to be invasive. Therefore, it can be anticipated that increased awareness of this lesion in VHL patients, with earlier detection, can result in successful removal before metastases occur.

The diagnosis of VHL disease must be considered in patients who present with renal cancer, particularly those who present at a young age or with a positive family history. If the patient also has a cerebellar lesion, it must be appreciated that this may be a removable hemangioblastoma rather than metastatic renal cancer with a poor prognosis [45]. Conversely, patients have presented with a cerebellar tumor misdiagnosed as a hemangioblastoma and were screened for renal lesions of VHL disease only to find that the primary lesion was sporadic renal cancer that had metastasized.

Pancreas

The pancreatic lesions of VHL disease may include cysts, and less frequently adenomas, hemangioblastomas, and malignancies.

Congenital cysts of the pancreas are rare in the general population [46], but simple cysts are common in VHL disease, being detected in 72% at autopsy [2]. The great majority of these cysts are asymptomatic. During life, between 9 [47] and 29% [21] have pancreatic cysts detectable by CT. The cysts frequently are multiple and rarely replace most of the pancreas leading to diabetes mellitus [48] or steatorrhea [49]. In these severe cases, the size of the cysts may be up to 10 cm in diameter and may cause displacement of the duodenum or abdominal distention [50]. Pancreatic disease is rarely the first manifestation of VHL disease [9]. It has been noted that symptomatic pancreatic disease tends to cluster within certain VHL families. For example, in one three-generation family, a man presented with pancreatic compression of the stomach and steatorrhea due to cystic pancreas; his mother's pancreas had been filled with cysts and cystadenomas, and his 28-year-old daughter presented with an epigastric mass found to be due to cystic and cystadenomatous replacement of the pancreas.

Benign angiomas and cystadenomas are found at autopsy in 7% of VHL patients [8]. These cystadenomas may be multilocular and asymptomatic; they rarely present as a palpable abdominal mass or cause abdominal pain. At least one VHL patient had a cystadenoma obstructing the common bile duct, causing jaundice.

Pancreatic hemangioblastomas, reported to occur in VHL disease [9], are very rare [49]. Other pancreatic tumors are also rare in most VHL families, but they tend to cluster within certain VHL disease families. In two families, 7.5 to 10% had pancreatic cancer [9,10] and in another family, two siblings had asymptomatic islet cell cancer detected at autopsy. Metastatic islet cell tumor [52] also has been reported. There have been occasional reports of VHL

patients with pancreatic "apudomas" that produced vasoactive intestinal peptide and that were associated with hypercalcemia [51].

Adrenal

Pheochromocytomas and, less frequently, medullary cysts, cortical hyperplasia, or adenomas, can occur in patients with VHL disease. The cysts and adenomas are benign and asymptomatic and are found in 3% of cases at autopsy [8]. Adrenal cortical hyperplasia has been found in 7% of autopsy cases [8]. Like significant pancreatic disease, the pheochromocytomas tend to cluster within certain VHL families, so that in three large families involving more than 85 affected members, none had a pheochromocytoma [9,7,47]. However, in other families 17 to 92% of patients were found to have pheochromocytomas [8,15]; more than one-third were not associated with high blood pressure when detected through family screening [15]. In reviews of VHL patients described in the literature, 3.5 [53] to 17% [21,44] had pheochromocytomas. Seventeen [15] to 34% [54] were bilateral, although not always detected simultaneously. The average age of diagnosis is 34 years [8] with a range of 10 to 56 years [8,15]. Rarely, pheochromocytoma is the first manifestation of VHL disease. Metastatic pheochromocytoma is extremely rare [44].

Benign adenomas and paragangliomas of the sympathetic chain are infrequently seen in VHL disease. In some families, no such lesions are found [9], while in other families 7% had lesions incidentally detected at autopsy [8]. For these lesions to be functional [54] or to metastasize is extremely rare [48].

Since surgery or renal arteriography can trigger hypertensive crises in patients with pheochromocytomas, it is important to screen VHL patients prior to these procedures, particularly when a positive family history of pheochromocytoma is present. In the general population, up to 10% of pheochromocytomas may be familial [40]; the diagnosis of VHL should be considered in these families.

Epididymis

Many males with VHL disease have benign and usually asymptomatic epididymal lesions. Simple cysts were reported in 7% of patients in one family autopsy series [8], but in another family studied clinically, 27% of males had cysts [9]. It has been said that most patients with bilateral cysts have VHL disease, whereas most who have a unilateral cyst do not [23]. The size of the cysts ranges from 0.5 to 2.0 cm [10], and they may be detected as a painless mass.

Hemangiomas of the epididymis are rare [4]. Benign adenomas were seen in 3% of cases in the previously mentioned autopsy series [8]. Papillary cystadenomas may feel cystic or firm and frequently are asymptomatic, although they occasionally cause slight discomfort or pain. In one series of patients with bilateral lesions, the age of detection was from 18 to 28 years [55]. The lesions sometimes had been noted to be present for many years before coming to medical attention, and lesions were sometimes not detected on the opposite side for up to 3 years later [55]. In one series of patients with papillary cystadenomas, there were no further genital lesions or complications 1 to 15 years later, regardless of whether or not the patient had VHL disease. There was no difference in the sporadic cases versus those who had VHL except for the tendency to bilaterality. Therefore, patients with bilateral cysts or adenomas should be evaluated for VHL disease.

Other Organs

There are many other organs that have the characteristic lesions of VHL disease. Cysts have been seen in the liver in 17% of VHL patients in one autopsy series; none had been symptomatic [8]. These liver cysts can be detected by CT and may be helpful in making the diagnosis in a family member when other signs of the disease are not present. Liver adenomas are less frequent (3%) and also are asymptomatic [8], as are liver hemangiomas (7%) [8,9].

Asymptomatic spleen angiomas and cysts occur in 3 to 7% of autopsied patients [8]. Lung cysts and angiomas [8], omentum cysts [8], parametrial cysts [1], ovarian angiomas [8], broad ligament papillary cystadenomas [23], bone cysts and hemangiomas [1,8], bladder hemangioblastomas [1], and skin hemangiomas have all been reported in patients with VHL disease. These lesions are uncommon and asymptomatic, and many were detected at autopsy. Bladder papillomas were present in von Hippel's original patient and have been noted subsequently [1]. There have been single case reports of VHL patients with a variety of other lesions such as adenocarcinoma of the ampulla of Vater [9], CNS neuroblastoma [56], and thyroid cancer [57], but these lesions may be coincidental.

In 1932, Van der Hoeve suggested categorizing VHL disease as one of the phakomatoses and cited a few patients and families that appeared to have features of VHL plus either Sturge–Weber, tuberous sclerosis, or neurofibromatosis [1]. The concept of phakomatosis has lost its initial appeal (see Preface). Furthermore, in spite of those interesting reports, VHL disease is a very distinct syndrome. It should not present diagnostic confusion with any of the other neurocutaneous diseases, particularly because the skin is not affected.

Laboratory Findings

The basic genetic defect in VHL disease is unknown, and there are no recognized biochemical markers for the disease. Therefore the diagnosis must be based on the clinical and radiographic findings, family history, and histopathologic examination of tissue specimens.

The organs or tissues involved in VHL disease lesions are mesodermal in origin [19]. It has been speculated that during the third month of fetal development, rests of benign mesoderm remain incompletely integrated and later enlarge to become manifest as cysts or hemangioblastomas [35,55].

The red blood cell count may be elevated in VHL patients who have cerebellar hemangioblastoma or renal cancer [1] because of erythropoetin activity in cyst fluid [23]. The frequency of polycythemia has ranged from 0 [7,9] to 49% [19] in reported series, with many reporting a mid-range value of 10 to 20% [2,5]. Polycythemia is less commonly attributable to renal cancer than to a cerebellar lesion [1]. A normal red blood cell count never excludes the diagnosis of a significant tumor and should not replace more sensitive roentgenographic investigations as a method of screening VHL patients or their family members.

Patients with CNS tumors, particularly those involving the medulla and cord, may have elevated cerebrospinal fluid protein [1,58].

Some patients with renal cancer have gross or microscopic hematuria, while others with extensive cancer have a normal urinalysis. Therefore, although patients with VHL should have a urinalysis as part of their annual evaluation, the absence of hematuria does not preclude the need for renal ultrasound or, preferably, CT of the abdomen.

Twenty-four-hour urine collections for epinephrine, norepinephrine, metanephrine, and vanillylmandelic acid also have been recommended on an annual basis [41,45] to screen for pheochromocytoma. This is particularly important for patients from families in which other members have had pheochromocytomas and for patients scheduled to have renal arteriography or surgery.

Radiography is the most important investigative tool for monitoring VHL disease patients and screening family members. All patients who have or who are suspected to have VHL disease should have CT of the head to search for intracranial hemangioblastomas. Early detection of tumors is important so that they may be surgically removed before secondary changes such as dilatation of the ventricles occur. Furthermore, surgical removal may be more difficult in some cases when the tumor or cyst is very large.

Cerebellar hemangioblastomas occur in the hemispheres or vermis and have a typical appearance by CT; they are round, hypodense, cystic nodules sometimes surrounded by a hyperdense ring-like shadow after contrast injection [59] (Figure 4.2). The less frequent, completely solid tumors are homogeneously isodense or hyperdense and enhance after contrast. These solid lesions are more apt to be located in the inferior vermis. A mass effect causing obliteration of the fourth ventricle and hydrocephalus may

be present. Computed tomography with contrast is helpful in defining the intensely enhancing mural nodule within the cystic component, which facilitates its complete removal by the surgeon [29]. Angiograms are helpful to better define the blood vessels connected to the lesion prior to surgical removal. Computed tomography is also helpful in detecting cerebral, medullary, and cord lesions.

Visceral cysts may be evident by abdominal ultrasound or CT examination; the latter may be more sensitive [48] and is probably the method of choice. Most cysts are asymptomatic and their detection is important for diagnostic purposes. Furthermore, since renal cancer can remain undetected after intravenous pyelography with tomography [6], CT is useful for annual screening [45]. In general, renal cancers can be detected when less than 3 cm in size, when they usually are noninvasive [21]. Angiography may be helpful for further definition of the lesions, but the risks make it impractical for routine screening [21].

Fluorescein angiography of retinal lesions may be

Figure 4.2. Cerebellar hemangioblastomas in patient with von Hippel–Lindau disease visualized by computed tomography with intravenous contrast injection. (Courtesy of Dr. H. Gordon.)

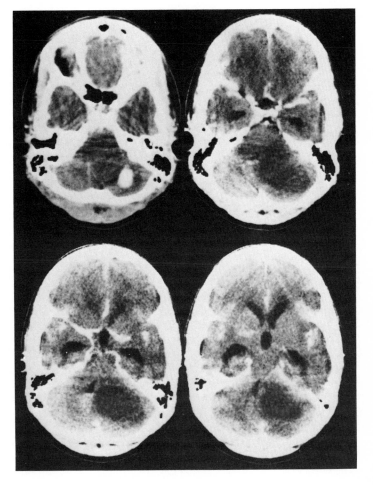

helpful in the diagnosis of tiny, incipient lesions or atypical lesions that are masked by secondary changes.

Course

Patients with VHL disease usually present with CNS or visual symptoms [1]. However, as physicians become more aware of the value of family screening and as diagnostic technology advances, a greater number of asymptomatic patients will be detected. In clinical series the age of onset of symptoms has ranged from 11 [9] to 65 years [1] with a mean age of 26 [7] to 33 years [1]. Although the onset of symptoms is rare before puberty, a few children have presented with significant visual loss due to retinal lesions or with CNS tumors. In one large family, the mean age of death of affected members was 41 years, with a range of 25 to 54 years. However, deaths directly related to VHL disease have been reported as young as 15 years (after neurosurgery) [4] and as late as 69 years (of metastatic renal cancer). In another family the average age of the affected members, all still living, was 43 years [38].

The importance of detecting retinal and CNS hemangioblastomas and renal carcinomas early, when more amenable to treatment, cannot be overemphasized.

Pathology

Central Nervous System

Cerebellar hemangioblastomas are benign, usually cystic, and filled with xanthochromic fluid. A highly vascular nodule, sometimes very small, can usually be identified in the wall of the cyst. This nodule is usually in contact with the pia-arachnoid near the surface of the cerebellum [31]. Approximately 20 to 32% [32] of lesions are solid [1]. The lesions are sharply demarcated and generally are not locally invasive and do not metastasize. Case reports of lesions thought to show malignant spread have been reported [60], but it is difficult to definitely exclude multiple primary lesions or metastatic renal carcinoma, which histologically can be confused with hemangioblastoma in these cases. Approximately 80% of tumors are located in the hemispheres, 13% in the vermis, and 7% in the fourth ventricle as they arise from the posterior medullary velum or occasionally from the floor or lateral margins [31]. Solid

lesions are more likely to be located at the inferior vermis [61]. The lesions have hypertrophied afferent and efferent cortical vessels [1].

Microscopically, the solid areas are composed of numerous thin-walled vascular channels [3] lined by plump endothelial cells that are separated by reticular and interstitial cells filled with abundant, vacuolated, lipid-rich cytoplasm. The lesions do not contain nerve cells or glial tissue [1]. There appear to be three cell types: endothelial cells, pericytes, and stromal cells, which may originate from primitive vasoformative elements [23].

The hemangioblastomas located elsewhere in the CNS have a similar pathologic appearance; they are more likely to be solid, although small cysts may be associated. Medulla and cord lesions are usually located posteriorly and are associated with syringobulbia or syringomyelia in up to 80% of cases [1]. Lesions in the sacral region and cauda equina are histologically different and may appear gelatinous or myxomatous [1].

Retina

The eye lesions are thought to be true hemangioblastomas derived from the anlage of capillary endothelium [14]. Although sometimes they still are referred to as hamartomatous hemangiomas, this probably is not the case [17]. The lesions are composed of relatively well-formed capillary-like structures and contain the same three cell types as do cerebellar tumors [23]. The vascular channels leak fluid into the subretinal space, which results in lipid accumulation and retinal detachment [18]. The lesion may involve part of the retina or its full thickness [14]. Small lesions may be entirely intraretinal, but large lesions can project into the vitreous or subretinal space [17].

Kidney

Grossly, the renal cysts are grayish, translucent, and filled with clear fluid. They range in size from a few millimeters to over 1.5 cm [44]. The cysts are lined by a single layer of atypical [23] cuboidal epithelium that is similar to that seen in solid tumors [10].

The solid tumors grossly are yellowish in color with a well-defined capsule [44]. The nodules may be solid or cystic and are surrounded by a fibrous pseudocapsule [23]. Some nodules are composed of loose fibrous tissue with occasional areas of myxoid

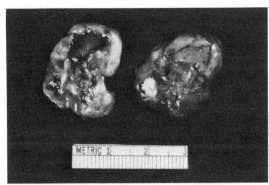

Figure 4.3. Cancerous kidney from patient with von Hippel–Lindau disease. (Courtesy of Dr. H. Gordon.)

degeneration [44] or foci of calcification [23]. The small (<3 cm) cortical tumors are sometimes classified as adenomas, but this distinction based on size is somewhat arbitrary, and they probably represent the early stage of the malignant lesions [40]. This is supported by the finding that some of these nodules have a clear cell pattern typical of malignant hypernephroma [23] and occasionally appear to be locally invading the pseudocapsule [10]. The clear cell renal tumors can invade veins and metastasize to the adrenal glands, spinal cord, and other distinct sites in the CNS [28]. Some of these solid tumors contain small cystic spaces, and it has been suggested that large cysts may be an exaggeration of this phenomenon [44]. Some large cysts appear to contain a nest of tumor cells within their walls.

Epididymis

Cysts and cystadenomas frequently are associated with the head of the epididymis but also can occur in the spermatic cord. Both the simple cysts and the cystadenomas are well circumscribed, and the cut surface of the latter appear spongy or multicystic, occasionally with a mural nodule. The cystadenomas appear to have three components: papillary processes surfaced by epithelial cells, ectatic ducts and microcysts lined by epithelial cells, and fibrous stroma [55].

Other Organs

The pheochromocytomas of VHL disease are histologically similar to sporadic lesions. Pancreatic cysts are lined by columnar epithelium consistent with ductal origin [3], while the pancreatic cystadenomas

are typical of the microcystic form of sporadic cystadenoma [62]. The cysts in other visceral organs are not distinctive and are lined by epithelium [23].

Treatment and Prognosis

The lesions of VHL disease that most commonly require treatment are retinal and CNS hemangioblastomas and malignant hypernephroma. Pheochromocytomas should be removed when detected. It is rarely necessary to treat pancreatic lesions. The lesions of other visceral organs, including the epididymis, should not be treated if asymptomatic.

Cerebellar hemangioblastomas generally are surgically removed with good success. Some patients with secondary hydrocephalus may require ventricular decompression by drainage before the posterior fossa is opened. Very rarely it is necessary to place a permanent shunt [2]. The surgeon should carefully inspect the cyst walls to ensure that the mural nodule also has been removed. Surgical treatment is successful in approximately 85 to 90% of patients, but mortality tends to be slightly greater in patients with solid lesions compared to those with cystic lesions [2]. Between 8 and 15% [2,5] of lesions recur, and recurrences are more frequent for solid tumors. However, it sometimes is difficult to distinguish between true recurrence and a second primary tumor, since the latter is particularly frequent in VHL patients. Such "recurrences" may occur up to 24 years later, but the average time interval is 5 years [32]. Tumors in the fourth ventricle, medulla, and spinal cord are more difficult to remove completely.

Radiotherapy seems to be of little if any benefit; however, it has been suggested that radiation may result in a decreased tumor volume [58]. In one case of bulbar hemangioblastoma not amenable to surgical treatment, radiation resulted in amelioration of symptoms and was said to have resulted in the appearance of dissection planes that facilitated surgery [58].

Since surgical outcome can be improved by early detection of CNS tumors, before surrounding edema and secondary effects become severe, it is hoped that increased awareness of the diagnosis and screening of family members will lead to improved outcome. It is recommended that patients and family members at risk have a head CT at the time of initial diagnosis and perhaps biannually thereafter.

Retinal lesions may be observed if small, peripheral, and stable in size. Careful serial observations are warranted to watch for retinal detachment and progressive visual impairment [9]. Some authors recommend obliteration of all lesions unless they are in or near the macula or disc [17]. The latter lesions also may require treatment if they cause significant visual impairment. In general, small lesions (<0.5 disc diameter in size) respond well to therapy; lesions of 1 to 1.5 disc diameter in size respond satisfactorily but may require repeated treatments; and large lesions (> 2 disc diameters in size) respond poorly, and treatment may result in further tractional detachment of the retina [16]. Lesions may be treated with cryocoagulation or photocoagulation [16]. It is hoped that earlier detection will lead to improved visual outcome over that in the series in which 36% of patients had visual acuity <20/200 and 11% had enucleation [22]. In one recent study of 12 patients, all retinal lesions were treated; over a 1- to 10-year period of observation (mean 4.5 years), visual acuity was the same or better in 16 eyes and worse in only one eye [63]. It has been recommended that annual ophthalmologic examinations be performed in patients and persons at-risk beginning at age 6 years [18].

It is probably safe not to treat small renal cysts [1]. However, it has been stressed that unroofing and gross examination of larger, apparently simple cysts are not adequate to exclude microscopic foci of cancer [44]. Both cysts and solid tumors, particularly if detected when small, usually are surrounded by a pseudocapsule of compressed parenchyma and can be shelled out [34]. It probably is safe to monitor tiny lesions (<1 cm in diameter) for rapid growth [28]. It is important to spare renal tissue, since bilateral and multiple lesions are apt to be present or to be detected subsequently. This conservative approach has led to prolonged survival that compares favorably to the alternative of nephrectomy requiring dialysis [34]. In the few cases that present with extensive polycystic disease and renal failure requiring dialysis, nephrectomy should be performed since cancer may still develop [10]. In any case in which renal transplant is contemplated, great care must be taken to avoid an affected but undiagnosed relative as donor [10]. As in other lesions of VHL disease, early diagnosis and treatment improves outcome, and annual screening of kidneys by CT in patients and individuals at risk should begin at 18 to 20 years [21]. It is hoped that this approach will lead to diminution of mortality and morbidity.

Pancreatic lesions require no treatment [1] except in the unusual case of malignancy or when large cysts cause symptoms. Aspiration of a cyst resulted in relief of abdominal swelling in one patient [50]. In more extensive polycystic disease with diabetes mellitus and steatorrhea, partial or complete pancreatectomy may be warranted [49].

Genetics and Counseling

The autosomal dominant inheritance of VHL disease is firmly established, and the risk of inheriting the gene for any child born to an affected person is 50%. There is no documented instance of nonpenetrance in families that have been evaluated using modern techniques and in which all pertinent family members had reached an age at which signs would have been expected [7].

An appropriate age at which to begin screening family members has been delineated, but it is not known at what age one can discontinue screening for at-risk members and assume they do not have the disease. Therefore, at the present time, screening must be continued indefinitely until further information becomes available.

The proportion of cases in which VHL disease arises by new mutation is not known. Males and females are affected equally.

Any patient with a CNS or retinal hemangioblastoma should have a complete family history investigation and should be screened by CT of the head or ophthalmologic examination and by CT of the abdomen to look for other signs of VHL disease. If the family history is positive or a second characteristic lesion is identified, the diagnosis should be made. Such screening should be done in patients who present with bilateral epididymal cysts or polycystic pancreas, and should be considered in patients presenting with pheochromocytomas, polycystic kidneys, or renal cancer, particularly when there is a suspicious family history or when the lesions are bilateral, multifocal, occur at an unusually young age, or are atypical in some other way.

Patients diagnosed as having VHL disease need an annual physical and ophthalmologic examination, a peripheral blood cell count, urinalysis, and CT of the abdomen. Annual evaluation of urinary catecholamines is reasonable, particularly if the patient is hypertensive or has a positive family history of pheochromocytoma. Initial CT of the head is essential. However, the necessity or frequency of subsequent monitoring is not clear, since small asymptomatic lesions may not require immediate removal. Until further information is available, biannual CT of the head in asymptomatic patients may be reasonable. All affected patients should have genetic counseling, and all first-degree relatives (parents, siblings, children) should have physical and ophthalmologic examinations and CT of head and abdomen. The need for further family investigation will be determined by the results of this initial family screening. Any at-risk person should be rescreened and should seek genetic counseling prior to reproduction. Prenatal diagnosis is not possible at this time.

In summary, the important elements of genetic counseling are (a) to inform the patients of the nature of their disease and to coordinate evaluation and treatment by other specialists; (b) to ensure adequate subsequent evaluations; (c) to document the family history and to arrange for investigations of other family members; and (d) to explain the inheritance pattern and discuss options for family planning (taking the 50% chance of having an affected child, remaining childless, adopting a child, or for affected males, artificial insemination of the wife with donor semen). In vitro fertilization of a donor egg implanted in an affected woman may be an increasingly available option in the future, since there are no known adverse effect of pregnancy on the disease.

References

1. Melmon KL, Rosen SW. Lindau's disease: review of the literature and study of a large kindred. Am J Med 1964;36:595–617.
2. Jeffreys R. Clinical and surgical aspects of posterior fossa haemangioblastomata. J Neurol Neurosurg Psychiatry 1975;38:105–111.
3. Dan NG, Smith DE. Pituitary hemangioblastoma in a patient with von Hippel–Lindau disease. J Neurosurg 1975;42:232–235.
4. Malek RS, Greene LF. Urologic aspects of Hippel–Lindau syndrome. J Urol 1971;106:800–801.
5. Obrador S, Martin-Rodriguez JG. Biological factors involved in the clinical features and surgical management of cerebellar hemangioblastomas. Surg Neurol 1977;7:79–85.
6. Campbell DR, Mason WF, Standen JR. Renal arteriography in von Hippel–Lindau disease. J Can Assoc Radiol 1978;29:243–246.
7. Go RCP, Lamiell JM, Hsia YE, et al. Segregation and linkage analyses of von Hippel–Lindau disease among 220 descendants from one kindred. Am J Hum Genet 1984;36:131–142.
8. Horton WA, Wong V, Eldridge R. Von Hippel–Lindau disease: clinical and pathological manifestations in nine families with 50 affected members. Arch Intern Med 1976;136:769–777.
9. Fill WL, Lamiell JM, Polk NO. The radiographic manifestations of von Hippel–Lindau disease. Diagm Radiol 1979;133:289–295.
10. Blight EM Jr, Biggers RD, Soderdahl DW, et al. Bilateral renal masses. J Urol 1980;124:695–700.
11. Yimoyines DJ, Topilow HW, Abedin S, et al. Bilateral peripapillary exophytic retinal hemangioblastomas. Ophthalmology 1982;89:1388–1392.
12. Bickler S, Wile AG, Melicharek M, et al. Pancreatic involvement in Hippel–Lindau disease. West J Med 1984;140:280–282.
13. Vogel F, Motulsky AG. Human genetics: problems and approaches. New York: Springer–Verlag, 1979.
14. Wing GL, Weiter JJ, Kelly PJ, et al. Von Hippel–Lindau disease: angiomatosis of the retina and central nervous system. Ophthalmology 1981;88:1311–1314.
15. Atuk NO, McDonald T, Wood T, et al. Familial pheochromocytoma, hypercalcemia, and von Hippel–Lindau disease: a ten year study of a large family. Medicine 1979;58:209–218.
16. Peyman GA, Rednam KRV, Mottow-Lippa L, et al. Treatment of large von Hippel tumors by eye wall resection. Ophthalmology 1983;90:840–847.
17. Augsburger JJ, Shields JA, Goldberg RE. Classification and management of hereditary retinal angiomas. Int Ophthalmol 1981;4:1–2, 93–106.
18. Greenwald MJ, Weiss A. Ocular manifestations of the neurocutaneous syndromes. Pediatr Dermatol 1984;2:98–117.
19. Palmer JJ. Haemangioblastomas: a review of 81 cases. Acta Neurochir 1972;27:125–148.
20. Diehl PR, Symon L. Supratentorial intraventricular hemangioblastoma: case report and review of literature. Surg Neurol 1981;15:435–443.
21. Levine E, Weigel JW, Collins DL. Diagnosis and management of asymptomatic renal cell carcinomas in von Hippel–Lindau syndrome. Urology 1983;21:1946–2150.
22. Hardwig P, Robertson DM. Von Hippel–Lindau disease: a familial, often lethal multi-system phakomatosis. Ophthalmology 1984;91:263–270.
23. Scully RE, Galdabini JJ, McNeely BU. Case records of the Massachusetts General Hospital. N Engl J Med 1978;95:101.
24. Kupersmith MJ, Berenstein A. Visual disturbances in von Hippel–Lindau disease. Ann Opthhalmol 1981;13:195–197.
25. Schindler RF, Sarin LK, MacDonald PR. Hemangiomas of the optic disc. Can J Ophthalmol 1975;10:305–318.
26. Seich I, Miyagi J, Kojho N, et al. Intraorbital optic nerve hemangioblastoma with von Hippel–Lindau disease. J Neurosurg 1982;56:426–429.
27. Levine E, Collins DL, Horton WA, et al. CT screening of the abdomen in von Hippel–Lindau disease. AJR 1982;139:505–510.
28. Kadir S, Kerr WS Jr, Athanasoulis CA. The role of arteriography in the management of renal cell carcinoma associated with von Hippel–Lindau disease. J Urol 1981;126:316–319.
29. Hellams SE, Cohen RJ, Young HF. Cerebellar hemangioblastomas and von Hippel–Lindau syndrome. Virginia Med 1981;108:42–45.
30. Sharif HS, Furneaux C, Srivatsa SR. Unusual uro-

graphic findings in a case of von Hippel–Lindau disease. Br J Radiol 1983;56:132–136.

31. Olivecrona H. The cerebellar angioreticulomas. J Neurosurg 1952;9:317–330.

32. Mondkar VP, McKissock W, Russell RWR. Cerebellar haemangioblastomas. Br J Surg 1967;54:45–49.

33. Michels VV, Gordon H. Investigative studies in von Hippel–Lindau disease. Proceedings, March of Dimes 1982 Birth Defects Conference. Birmingham Ala.

34. Pearson JC, Weiss J, Tanagho. A plea for conservation of kidney in renal adenocarcinoma associated with von Hippel–Lindau disease. J Urol 1980;124:910–912.

35. Ishwar S, Taniguchi RM, Vogel FS. Multiple supratentorial hemangioblastomas: case study and ultrastructural characteristics. J Neurosurg 1971;35:396–405.

36. Richards RD, Mebust WK, Schimke RN. A prospective study on von Hippel–Lindau disease. J Urol 1973;110:27–30.

37. Ho K-L. Von Hippel–Lindau disease and neurogenous tumors (letter to the editor). Arch Pathol Lab Med 1983;107:48.

38. Lee KR, Wulfsberg E, Kepes JJ. Some important radiological aspects of the kidney in von Hippel–Lindau syndrome: the value of prospective study in an affected family. Diagm Radiol 1977;122:649–653.

39. Hull MT, Roth LM, Glover JL, et al. Metastatic carotid body paraganglioma in von Hippel–Lindau disease: an electron microscopic study. Arch Pathol Lab Med 1982;106:235–239.

40. Ludmerer KM, Kissane JH. Renal mass in a man with von Hippel–Lindau disease. Am J Med 1981;71:287–297.

41. Kramer SA, Hoffman AD, Aydin G, et al. Simple renal cysts in children. J Urol 1982;128:1259–1261.

42. Witten DM, Myers GH, Utz DC, eds. Emmett's Clinical Urography. Philadelphia: WB Saunders, 1977;3:1371.

43. Lamiell JM, Stor RA, Hsia YE. Von Hippel–Lindau disease simulating polycystic kidney disease. Urology 1980;15:287–290.

44. Christenson PJ, Craig JP, Bibro MC, et al. Cysts containing renal cell carcinoma in von Hippel–Lindau disease. J Urol 1982;798–800.

45. Boker DK, Wassmann H, Solymosi L. Multiple spinal hemangioblastomas in a case of Lindau's disease. Surg Neurol 1984;22:439–443.

46. Barkin JS, Goldberg H, Bradley EL. Cysts and pseudocysts of the pancreas. In: Haubrick WS, Kalser MH, Roth JLA, et al., eds. Gastroenterology. Philadelphia: WB Saunders, 1985;6:4145.

47. Phytinen J, Suramo I, Lohela P, et al. Abdominal ultrasonography and computed tomography in von Hippel–Lindau disease. Ann Clin Res 1982;14:172–176.

48. Hull MT, Warfel KA, Muller J, et al. Familial islet cell tumors in von Hippel–Lindau's disease. Cancer 1979;44:1523–1526.

49. Fishman RS, Bartholomew LG. Severe pancreatic involvement in three generations in von Hippel–Lindau disease. Mayo Clin Proc 1979;54:329–331.

50. Jackaman FR. Polycystic pancreas: Lindau's disease. J R Coll Surg Edinb 1984;29:121–122.

51. Mulshine JL, Tubbs R, Sheeler LR, et al. Case report: clinical significance of the association of the von Hippel–Lindau disease with pheochromocytoma and pancreatic apudoma. Am J Med Sci 1984;288:212–216.

52. Cornish D, Pont A, Minor D, et al. Metastatic islet cell tumor in von Hippel–Lindau disease. Am J Med 1984;77:147–150.

53. Sybert VP. Pheochromocytomas in von Hippel–Lindau disease (letters). AJR 1978;131:736.

54. Hoffman RW, Gardner DW, Mitchell FL. Intrathoracic and multiple abdominal pheochromocytomas in von Hippel–Lindau disease. Arch Intern Med 1982;142:1962–1964.

55. Price EB Jr. Papillary cystadenoma of the epididymis: a clinicopathologic analysis of 20 cases. Arch Pathol 1971;91:456–470.

56. Pearl GS, Takei Y, Stefanis GS, et al. Intraventricular neuroblastoma in a patient with von Hippel–Lindau's disease. Light microscopic study. Acta Neuropathol (Berl) 1981;53:253–256.

57. Reyes CV. Thyroid carcinoma in von Hippel–Lindau disease (letter to the editor). Arch Intern Med 1984;144:413.

58. Helle TL, Conley FK, Britt RH. Effect of radiation therapy on hemangioblastoma: a case report and review of the literature. Neurosurgery 1980;6:82–86.

59. Baleriaux-Waha D, Retif J, Noterman J, et al. CT scanning for the diagnosis of the cerebellar and spinal lesions of von Hippel–Lindau disease. Neuroradiology 1978;14:241–244.

60. Mohan J, Brownell B, Oppenheimer DR. Malignant spread of hemangioblastoma: report on two cases. J Neurol Neurosurg Psychiatry 1976;39:515–525.

61. Gardeur D, Palmieri A, Mashaly R. Cranial computed tomography in the phakomatoses. Neuroradiology 1983;25:293–304.

62. Beerman MH, Fromkes JJ, Carey LC, et al. Pancreatic cystadenoma in von Hippel–Lindau disease: an unusual cause of pancreatic and common bile duct obstruction. J Clin Gastroenterol 1982;4:537–540.

63. Bonnet M, Garmier G. Treatment of retinal angiomatosis (von Hippel's disease). J Fr Ophthalmol 1984;7:545–555.

Chapter 5
Nevoid Basal Cell Carcinoma Syndrome

ROBERT J. GORLIN

The name of the syndrome is misleading since only about 50% of patients 20 years of age or older manifest the basal cell carcinomas and only the rare lesion becomes aggressive. Other names have been employed: Gorlin–Goltz syndrome, Gorlin's syndrome, basal cell nevi syndrome, and so forth. I am personally opposed to eponyms since they say nothing about the disorder and often give rise to argument regarding priority of discovery. The difficulty with the name we have employed is that it unjustly emphasizes only one aspect of a syndrome that has myriad manifestations.

History

There is remarkably good evidence to suggest that the nevoid basal cell carcinoma syndrome dates from at least the eleventh dynasty during Egyptian times. Satinoff and Wells [1] found Egyptian mummies exhibiting jaw cysts, bifid ribs, and short fourth metacarpal bones. However, the first reported case of the syndrome was probably that reported by Jarisch [2] in 1894. One cannot be certain since he emphasized the cutaneous lesions, considering them to be a variant of basal cell carcinoma. In the same year, White [3] described a patient who appears to me to have the syndrome. In 1932, Nomland [4] distinguished nevoid basal cell carcinomas as an entity. The inherited association of basal cell carcinomas and cysts of the jaws was probably first reported by Straith [5] in 1939, but his report was overlooked. In 1951, Binkley and Johnson [6] described a woman with multiple basal cell cancers and dental cysts. The jaw lesions were treated with radiotherapy over 7 years. A fibrosarcoma subsequently arose in the area and metastasized, causing her death. On autopsy, ovar-

ian fibroma, bifid rib, and agenesis of the corpus callosum were found. Her 6-year-old daughter had skin cancers but no jaw cysts. Again, this report went largely unnoticed. In 1958, Boyer and Martin [7] reported the syndrome under the mistaken diagnosis of Marfan's syndrome. Howell and Caro [8], in 1959, presented four patients with the syndrome, recognized the hereditary nature of nevoid basal cell carcinomas, and first brought this to the attention of the dermatologist. In 1960, Gorlin and Goltz [9] tabulated and analyzed all known cases, bringing the syndrome to the general attention of the readers of medical and dental books and pointing out its autosomal dominant inheritance pattern. Gorlin et al. [10] in 1963, Cernéa et al. [11] in 1969, Gorlin and Sedano [12] in 1971, and Gorlin [13] in 1987 updated all known associations in the syndrome.

Various components of the syndrome were discovered at various times by various investigators. For example, Jarisch [2] probably first reported the skin tumors. Palmar–plantar pits were first noted to be associated with basal cell carcinomas by Pollitzer [14] in 1905, although they were rediscovered by Calnan [15] in 1953 and by Ward [16] in 1960. Straith [5] appears to be the first observer to have linked skin tumors and jaw cysts and to mention ectopic calcification and epidermoid cysts of the skin. Herzberg and Wiskemann [17], in 1963, apparently first noted the association of medulloblastoma with the syndrome. In the same year, Block and Clendenning [18] suggested that ovarian fibromas and lymphomesenteric cysts were other components of the syndrome, although ovarian fibroma was noted by Binkley and Johnson [6] in 1951. Sprengel's deformity as part of the syndrome appears to have been first described by Swanson and Jacks [19] in 1961. Shortened fourth metacarpals possibly were first noted by Gorlin et al. [10] in 1963. Minor cortical defects of long bones probably were first documented by Cairns [20] in 1965 although Cernéa et al. [11] believed that they initially reported them. Bridging of the sella and medial hooking of the lower scapulae possibly were initially commented on by Pollard and New [21] in 1964. Kirsch [22] may well have been the first to have reported cleft lip or palate as a component. Agenesis of the corpus callosum was initially documented by Binkley and Johnson [6]. Excellent historical reviews are those of Howell [23] and Howell and Anderson [24].

Clinical Symptoms

Skin

The syndrome is characterized by basal cell carcinomas that generally appear between puberty and 35 years of age. Although they have been reported to occur as early as 2 years of age [25], I have seen patients whose skin lesions were present at birth. Only about 15% of patients manifest the nevoid basal cell carcinomas before puberty, and about 10% of individuals over the age of 30 years have none [26]. Patients may have from a few to literally thousands of basal cell carcinomas that may arise in any region of the skin but especially on the face, neck, and upper trunk [27,28]. The periorbital areas, eyelids, nose, malar region, and upper lip are the facial sites most often affected. Rarely are the abdomen, lower trunk, and extremities involved. The lesions may be pearly to flesh-colored to reddish-brown and isolated or grouped.

Small groups may resemble moles, skin tags, nevi, or hemangiomas. They range in size from 1 to 10 mm. There is some relationship to sunlight exposure, with affected blacks having fewer skin cancers which appear later in life. The basal cell cancers may grow rapidly for a few days to a few weeks, but most remain static. Rarely, a few spontaneously regress. Prior to puberty the lesions are harmless even when huge numbers are present. Only a few become malignant, and then only after adolescence, when they may be locally invasive, behaving like ordinary basal cell carcinomas. Dilated blood vessels that pervade the lesions may occasionally give rise to spontaneous hemorrhage following slight trauma. Evidence of malignant transformation is heralded by an individual lesion increasing in size, ulcerating, bleeding, and crusting [27]. Death has resulted in a few instances from invasion of the brain, lung, or peritoneum. Only

in the rare case has metastasis been documented [29,30].

Jaw Cysts

Cysts of the jaws, aptly named odontogenic keratocysts, develop during the first decade of life (usually after the seventh year) to peak during the second or third decades [26,31], which is approximately a decade earlier than the much more common isolated odontogenic keratocyst, not associated with the syndrome. The cysts are continuous in their development. They almost never cause symptoms unless secondarily infected following surgery. Rarely do they cause pathologic fracture [32,33]. Although rare, both ameloblastoma and squamous cell carcinoma have arisen in these jaw cysts (see Neoplasia, below). In my experience, only 15% of patients do not have radiographically demonstrable cysts at age 40. There are reports of individuals having their first jaw cysts in their sixth decade [26]. The cysts tend to occur mainly in the canine to premolar area, in the mandibular retromolar–ramus area, and in the region of the maxillary second molar [34].

Central Nervous System

Medulloblastoma developing within the first two years of life has been described in several patients, in their sibs, in their offspring, or in more distant relatives (see below). These tumors may lead to the death of the patient before the other, more usual, features of this syndrome have been elaborated. The tumor seems to appear earlier and to be less lethal than medulloblastoma not associated with the syndrome [35].

Mental retardation has been reported in about 3% of patients, but there are indications that the incidence is much higher [36,37].

Neoplasia

The syndrome has been associated with an increased tendency to various other neoplastic lesions: medulloblastoma [12,16,18,26,32–36,38–44], ovarian fibroma [6,17,18,28,32,36,45–50], ovarian fibrosarcoma [36,43,51–53], various other ovarian tumors [53,54], fibrosarcoma of the maxilla [6,47,55], cardiac fibroma [28,56–59], isolated neurofibroma [60], meningioma [32,55,61,62], ameloblastoma

[11,63–66], leiomyoma [48,67,68], craniopharyngioma [55], adrenal cortical adenoma [48], lymphangiomyoma [68], rhabdomyosarcoma [69,70], fetal rhabdomyoma [71], seminoma [72], and melanoma [73–75]. Lymphatic or chylous cysts of the mesentery, some of which are calcified, have been reported in several cases [12,20,27,32,47,63,68,76,77]. Gastric hamartomatous polyps [32], squamous cell carcinoma [44], and hamartomatous lung cyst [78] have been documented. A host of other tumors that may be adventitious have been reviewed by Gundlach and Kiehn [79], and I keep a current file.

Other Symptoms

In males, the syndrome may be associated with hypogonadotrophic hypogonadism, anosmia, cryptorchism, female pubic escutcheon, gynecomastia, or scanty facial or body hair [7,11,26,37,80,81]. Probably 75% of females referred to gynecologists have ovarian fibromas but they are often not discovered unless they become twisted on their pedicles. They do not seem to reduce fertility.

Congenital blindness due to corneal opacity, congenital cataract, glaucoma, or coloboma of the iris, choroid, and optic nerve coupled with convergent or divergent strabismus, have been reported in several patients [12,26,28,36,63,82,83].

Cleft lip or palate occurs in about 5% of patients. Seventeen cases were tabulated by van Dijk and Neering [83] in 1980. Additional examples have been noted [57,75,79,85–87,88–92].

Physical Findings

Musculoskeletal Abnormalities

A characteristic facies is present in about 70% of patients (Figure 5.1). This is due in part to increased size of the calvaria due to frontal and biparietal bulging (60 cm or more in adults), well-developed supraorbital ridges, heavy and often fused eyebrows, broadened nasal root, low position of the occiput, increased interorbital distance, exotropia, and exaggerated length of the mandible associated with pouting of the lower lip [12,36,50,58,93]. While congenital communicating hydrocephalus has been reported on several occasions, it is difficult to know how many examples merely represented abnormalities of head form.

Patients may be very tall, some exhibiting a marfanoid build. Kyphoscoliosis is found in about 40%.

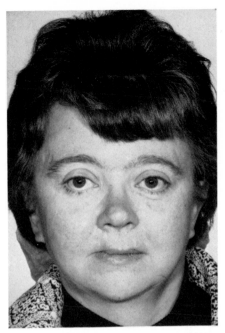

Figure 5.1. Typical facies. Macrocephaly, mild hypertelorism, and pouting of lower lip.

Several patients had inguinal hernia. A shortened metacarpal may be found, especially the fourth. Occasional anomalies include pre- or postaxial polydactyly, hallux valgus, pectus excavatum or carinatum, pes planus, syndactyly of second and third fingers, unusual clavicular form, Sprengel's deformity, and medial hooking or dysplasia of scapulae [12,32,36,72,94].

Skin Abnormalities

About 65% of patients present with small (1 to 2 mm) asymmetric palmar or plantar pits. They rarely occur on the sides or dorsa of the fingers or toes and are more common on the hands than on the feet. There is some suggestion that they are age related. Rarely are they seen in children. If the patient's occupation involves manual labor, the pits are usually more obvious due to ingrained dirt or grease. There are several cases in which basal cell carcinomas have arisen in the base of these pits [32,95–100].

The basal cell carcinomas are usually first noted in childhood. They are pink or pale brown papules, 1 to 10 mm in diameter. In my experience, the earliest manifestation is on the nape. From there, they become evident on the torso, face, and upper extremities [36].

Jaw and Skin Cysts

The jaw cysts usually do not cause symptoms and most often are detected on routine dental checkups. They are often very large before they effect expansion of the bony cortex. They may, however, perforate the cortex and extend to soft tissues where they cause swelling. Adjacent teeth may occasionally be loosened. The cysts are not painful unless secondarily infected.

Milia, that is, small keratin-filled cysts, are frequently found intermixed with the basal cell carcinomas on the face. They have been noted in at least 30% of patients [12,33,34,38]. Larger, often multiple epidermoid cysts (1 to 2 cm) occur on the limbs and trunk in over 50% of cases [32]. Several authors have described associated chalazion and comedones [25,50,101,102].

Radiologic Studies

Skeletal anomalies are common. There is usually a large calvaria with parietal and biparietal bossing, low occiput, and mildly increased interorbital distance [93]. Platybasia is relatively frequent. Lamellar calcification of the falx cerebri (Figure 5.2), which appears relatively early in life, is seen in at least 85% of patients (5% is normal). Calcification of the tentorium cerebelli (40%), petroclinoid ligament (20%), dura, pia, and choroid plexus, is common [35,103]. The frontal sinuses are enlarged in 60% [93]. Bridg-

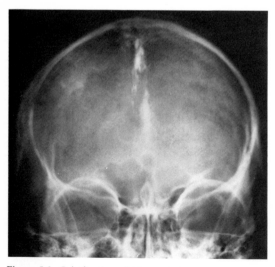

Figure 5.2. Calcification of falx cerebri.

ing of the sella turcica (calcification of the diaphragma sellae) is seen in at least 60 to 80%, a finding noted in only about 4% of the normal population [76,103]. Agenesis of the corpus callosum has been found in a few patients [6,12,37,104]. Cysts of the septum pellucidum have occasionally been noted [13].

About 60% of patients have anteriorly splayed, fused, partially missing, hypoplastic, or bifid ribs. Cervical ribs are frequent. Kyphoscoliosis with or without associated pectus excavatum or carinatum is present to some degree in about 30 to 40% of patients, and spina bifida occulta of the cervical or thoracic vertebrae is found in 60%. Cervical or upper thoracic vertebral fusion or lack of segmentation has been documented in about 40% [58]. Lumbarization of the sacrum occurs in about 40%. Sprengel's deformity is found in 5 to 10% of patients and in as high as 25% in some surveys [26]. Medial hooking or dysplasia of the lower scapular borders has been noted in several patients. Pes planus and defective medial portion of the clavicle have been documented [12].

Small pseudocystic lytic bone lesions are noted in at least 35%. Although they have been identified most often in the phalanges and in the metapodial, carpal, and tarsal bones, the long bones, pelvis, and calvaria may also be affected [79,103,105,106]. It is not inconceivable that some cases of "metastatic medulloblastoma" really represent these hamartomatous changes [107]. Spotted sclerotic osteopoikolytic lesions have also been reported [106]. Subcutaneous calcification of fingers and scalp has been documented by several authors [83,108].

The fourth metacarpal is short in perhaps 20% of patients but I view this "metacarpal sign" as poor diagnostic help since several studies have shown that about 10% of the normal population have either one or both fourth metacarpal bones.

Odontogenic keratocysts (Figure 5.3) are found in over 80% of patients, about three times as often in the mandible as in the maxilla [105,109]. They may be relatively small, single or multiple, but more often are large, bilateral, unilocular or multilocular, asymmetric, and involve both jaws. In young patients they can cause displacement of developing permanent teeth. Cysts in the molar–ramus area may extend into the coronoid process while those in the maxilla may involve the maxillary antra. Computed tomography has been employed in estimating the size of jaw cysts [110].

Ovarian fibromas are often bilateral and calcified. They may overlap medially as a single calcified mass, simulating a centrally located calcified uterine fi-

Figure 5.3. Multiple odontogenic keratocysts of maxilla and mandible. Note
extension of cyst in both coronoid processes.

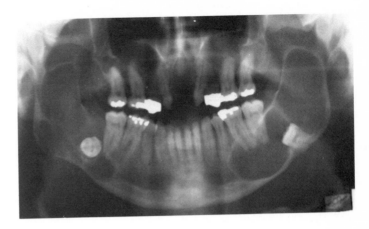

broid. Calcified lymphomesenteric cysts have also
been described.

Laboratory Studies

Happle and Hoehn [111] found an increased frequency of spontaneous chromosome breaks in fibroblasts from uninvolved skin. In our laboratory, we
have not been able to sustain this finding, nor have
we found an increased number of sister chromatid
exchanges. Römke et al. [112] reported no increase
in chromosome breaks.

Elejalde [113] noted increased transformation of
cells from patients with the syndrome when cultured
fibroblasts were exposed to N-acetylaminofluorine.
Ringborg et al. [114] found a 25% decreased level
of maximum DNA repair synthesis of ultraviolet
light-damaged leukocytes.

Featherstone et al. [115] found that fibroblasts
from patients with the syndrome were not unusually
sensitive to ionizing radiation, although lymphocytes
were. On the other hand, Nagasawa et al. [116]
studying survival curves of fibroblasts exposed to x-
rays, ultraviolet light, and mitomycin C found that
strains of fibroblasts from nevoid basal cell carcinoma patients were slightly hypersensitive to all three
of these DNA-damaging agents.

Biochemistry

Initially it was believed that since there were calcium
deposits in skin, cyst walls, ovarian fibromas, falx
cerebri, and so on, and because there were short
fourth metacarpals in some patients, a relationship
to pseudohypoparathyroidism might exist. Several
investigators found that there was hyporesponsiveness to parathormone, that is, absence of significant
phosphorus diuresis following intravenous injection
of parathormone (Ellsworth–Howard test [11,18,54,
117]. However, this finding has not been supported
by others [36,108,118,119].

The odontogenic keratocysts contain a remarkably low content of protein (less than 4 g/dl) and numerous keratinized squamous cells in the cyst fluid
in contrast to other dental cysts [120,121]. Histochemical studies have not been very informative.
Magnusson [122] found oxidative enzymes to be elevated and high acid phosphatase activity. Ultrastructural studies of the epithelium have suggested a
collagenolytic activity [123], which may reflect the
high leucine aminopeptidase activity noted in the cyst
capsule [122].

Pathology

The histopathology of nevoid basal cell carcinomas
cannot be differentiated from ordinary basal cell carcinoma [124]. They are composed of nests, islands,
or sheets of cells with large deeply staining nuclei
with indistinct cell membranes and variable number
of mitotic figures. At the periphery of each lesion,
the epithelial cells are large and well polarized,
suggestive of cutaneous basal cells. In view of the
pluripotentiality of the basal cells, a full spectrum of
basal cell carcinoma may develop in a patient, including morphea-like (1 to 2%), solid (50 to 70%),
superficial (9 to 10%), cystic (5 to 7%), adenoid (1
to 8%), and fibroepithelial (2 to 9%) carcinomas
[27,125]. Maddox et al. [66] and Mason et al. [27]
noted that about one-third of the patients had two
or more types of basal cell carcinoma patterns. Melanin pigmentation may be evident in many lesions

along with foci of calcification within the basal cell carcinomas [27,126]. In fact, calcified foci (rarely bone or osteoid), may occur in *normal-appearing* skin of patients with the syndrome [108,119].

Light microscopy of the palmar and plantar pits (Figure 5.4) show focal absence of the stratum corneum, thinning of the stratum granulosum, vacuolization of the spinous layer, and irregular rete ridges. Ultrastructurally, there are poorly developed tonofibrils, small keratohyaline granules, decreased desmosomal attachments, an increase in discharged cementosomes, and premature desquamation of horny cells [12,100,102,127]. Basal cell carcinomas have occasionally occurred on the palms and soles, developing at the base of the pits [97–100].

Odontogenic keratocysts present as multilocular or invaginated cysts (along with microdaughter cysts or epithelial rests in 25 to 50% of the cases), with a parakeratinized or rarely, an orthokeratinized (4%) stratified squamous epithelium consisting of five to eight rows of cells with a regularly oriented, well-defined basal epithelial cell layer with palisaded nuclei but without rete ridges (Figure 5.5). In some cases, the epithelial rests proliferate to produce a picture like that of squamous odontogenic tumor [128]. The mitotic index is comparable to that of the dental lamina. Budding of the epithelium into the connective tissue and suprabasilar splitting are noted in at least 50% of patients [129,130]. Inflammatory cells are rarely found in the underlying connective tissue. The cyst capsule is thin. Some cysts exhibit foci of calcification in the walls [87].

Bone radiolucencies, studied by Miller and Cooper [131], represent hamartomas composed of fibrous connective tissue, nerves, and vessels.

The ovarian fibromas do not differ microscopically from nonsyndromal ovarian fibromas but they are bilateral in about 75% of cases. In this syndrome, the ovarian fibromas are nearly always calcified and multinodular. The nonsyndromal ovarian fibroma is a single mass, unilateral, and calcified in only 10% of cases [132].

Pathogenesis

The pathogenesis of the nevoid basal cell carcinoma syndrome is unknown but is under the control of a single autosomal dominant gene that has complete penetrance and variable expressivity [50]. Many large pedigrees of the disorder involving several generations exist. About 40% of the patients do not have an affected parent. A paternal age effect has been demonstrated in cases of such new mutations [133]. Anderson [134] failed to find linkage with the common blood groups. However, Linss et al. [135] suggested that there might be loose linkage. Bale et al. [136] found loose linkage with a marker on 1p21.

The origin of the odontogenic keratocyst is not known but most authors now believe that they arise from the epithelial rests of the dental lamina [120,137].

The predilection of the odontogenic keratocysts for the ramus of the mandible suggests that they are primordial, that is, they originate from the distal extension of the dental lamina. Daughter or satellite cysts arise from epithelial rests. This probably accounts for the 50% postsurgical recurrence rate of the cysts [138].

The nevoid basal cell carcinomas are basically the

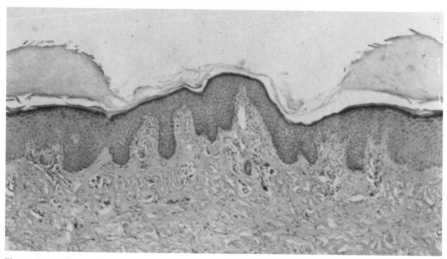

Figure 5.4. Palmar pit.

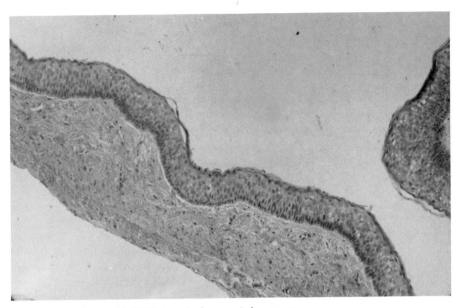

Figure 5.5. Uniform epithelial lining of odontogenic keratocyst.

same in origin as ordinary basal cell cancers but they differ in their early onset of appearance and are less related to sun exposure than are ordinary basal cell cancers. The tumors arise in the epidermis and in the upper part of the hair follicle.

Several authors have suggested that nevoid basal cell carcinoma seems to fit the Knudson two-hit hypothesis. The first hit represents the presence of the autosomal dominant gene, the second the radiation damage [52,139].

Rayner et al. [26] pointed out the increased susceptibility of the skin of patients with the syndrome to the oncogenic influence of tissue-damaging physical agents and stressed that radiotherapy is contraindicated as a form of therapy. Sunlight may play some role in the syndrome. The lesions are more often found on the head, neck, and other sun-exposed areas. In addition, blacks with the syndrome manifest skin tumors less than whites [52,87].

Among the patients with medulloblastoma treated with radiation, multiple basal cell carcinomas have developed within 6 months to 3 years of radiotherapy. This is distinctly earlier and in a distribution different from other family members with the syndrome [42,52]. The outline of the skin lesions often corresponds to the scalp and paraspinal area exposed to the radiation portal [20,43,97,140,141]. Cases of fibrosarcoma of the jaws appear to be secondary to radiation [6,55]. Ovarian fibrosarcoma has also developed in patients who received radiation to the spine [43,52].

The palmar and plantar pits represent a local re-tardation in the maturation process of the basal cells of the skin. The poorly developed tonofibrils, the small keratohyaline granules, and the cementosomes lacking intercellular cement, all make for focal premature desquamation of horny cells [100].

Differential Diagnosis

Unilateral linear nevoid basal cell carcinomas with comedones may well represent clonal manifestation of the syndrome [142,143]. Bazex's syndrome consists of multiple basal cell carcinomas (especially of the face), follicular atrophoderma (especially of tissue of hands and feet and elbows), hypotrichosis, and generalized hypohidrosis or anhidrosis of the face and head [144–146]. It has X-linked dominant inheritance. The so-called autosomal dominant Rombo's syndrome [147] has many features of Bazex's syndrome but the skin is normal until late in childhood. The basal cell carcinomas appear later and sweating is normal. Rasmussen [148] described a syndrome of trichoepitheliomas, milia, and cylindromas. There is superficial resemblance to multiple seborrheic keratoses of the trunk and extremities that may arise in a patient with adenocarcinoma (Leser–Trélat sign) [149].

The jaw cysts, if few in number, may be mistaken for conventional dentigerous cysts or isolated keratocysts. The calcification of several organs (falx cerebri, skin, ovaries) and short fourth metacarpals may suggest pseudohypoparathyroidism.

Course and Prognosis

The course of the syndrome is extremely variable. The basal cell carcinomas usually are not present in large numbers until adolescence. While some patients have only a few lesions during their entire lives, others have been estimated to have 10,000 lesions. Which ones will transform into aggressive basal cell carcinomas cannot be determined, hence the need for constant surveillance and early removal, especially of those situated around the eyelids, nose, or ears. Periodic total body inspection is necessary. For example, while the tumors occur less often below the waist, they have been found on the labia majora.

This disorder is seldom lethal but often leads to depression because of the continued appearance of one or more of its components. While patients may have hundreds of nevoid basal cell carcinomas, only a few of which become aggressive, the tumors or the scars resulting from treatment may be quite disfiguring, especially about the face.

As noted above, there is good evidence to suggest that radiation therapy causes the nevoid basal cell carcinomas to become aggressive or for new crops of lesions to appear on irradiated, otherwise normal skin.

The jaw cysts seldom are found earlier than the eighth year of life and then only accidentally at dental checkups. However, in most cases, increased number of cysts arise after puberty and into the fourth decade. They seldom cause symptoms since they characteristically extend throughout the bone, displacing developing teeth, even extending to the mandibular condyle and coronoid process. The cysts cross the midline but rarely cause dissolution of the cortex. However, when the cortex is perforated, the soft tissues may be involved in the cystic process. Only rarely does pathologic fracture of the mandible occur. In the maxilla, the maxillary sinuses may be invaded. Development of ameloblastoma or squamous cell carcinoma in an odontogenic keratocyst has been documented on several occasions. The cysts are especially annoying because of the high recurrence risk, which has been estimated in various series from 30 to 60% [150].

Medulloblastoma is lethal but survival of those with the syndrome is better than for those with the isolated tumor. There are a host of other neoplasms, as noted above, that do not appear to be adventitious. Ovarian fibroma does not appear to reduce fertility.

If one considers the number of individuals who have died from complication of the syndrome, one would say that prognosis is excellent. However, the progress of the disease appears inexorable.

Only a small number succumb to medulloblastoma during childhood. The nevi continue to appear from early childhood throughout life. Their appearance and the results of the modalities of treatment of the more aggressive basal cell cancers often result in severe cosmetic disfigurement. While jaw cysts seldom result in spontaneous jaw fracture, their frequent recurrence and their extensive growth throughout the jaws eventuate in what appears to the patient to be never-ending visits to the oral surgeon.

What the clinician considers to be of minor concern may be thought of as major in the mind of the patient. I have seen about 50 patients with the disorder. Some are truly depressed about the "hopelessness" of their case. Others seem fixated on their unilateral blindness due to coloboma of the optic nerve or feel that people are staring at their large head or at their kyphosis, or they simply feel they are "different" in some way. Some need psychiatric support. Because of the large number of systems involved and the numerous medical specialty disciplines required for their case, many patients resent their being treated as a "case of a very rare disorder rather than as a patient." Unfortunately this is often true. They often are presented at grand rounds by several departments in a single institution and feel less like a patient than a specimen. I cannot emphasize strongly enough that one must respect the rights of each individual.

Treatment

We will consider here only the treatment of the nevoid basal cell carcinomas and jaw cysts.

In view of the neoplastic skin changes, constant review of the patient is indicated, particularly between puberty and 35 years of age. Periodic 3- to 6-month follow-up visits are warranted. Total body cutaneous examinations should be performed. Special attention should be given to lesions that are located near orifices (eyelids, nostrils, ears) even if they do not appear active. Scalp lesions usually require special care at an early age due to their invasive destructive course [151]. Surgical or chemosurgical (Mohs' technique) removal of the basal cell carcinomas is the treatment of choice [152], but other modalities have been used with variable success [32]. Early reports recommended full-thickness skin grafts [153]. No attempt need be made to remove all the skin tumors since literally thousands may be present. Those that show growth, ulceration, or hemorrhage should be removed. The smaller ones can be electrodessicated and curetted. Cryotherapy can be skill-fully employed. Topical immunotherapy [154] and topical 5-fluorouracil [155–157] have been used with success. Oral ethretinoate may possibly be effective in preventing new lesions from appearing and ar-resting the growth of older lesions [158,159]. Radio-therapy is contraindicated since new lesions appear to be stimulated by radiation exposure.

From the beginning, the patient should be told about the high recurrence rate of the cysts and the marked proclivity toward the development of new cysts. The small odontogenic keratocysts should be completely enucleated surgically. Mucoperiosteal flaps are raised, the cystic cavity unroofed with a dental handpiece and bur, and the cyst enucleated [30,112,117,125,159–161]. Forssell [162] showed that recurrence was considerably lower for cysts that were enucleated intact, compared with those in which the lining was removed piecemeal. If possible, im-pacted canines should be preserved and brought into position orthodontically to preserve facial contour and arch form. The bony walls of the cavity should be curetted and planed. Cryosurgery, chemocautery, and electrocautery are contraindicated.

In the case of extensive cysts, one may consider the preoperative placement of arch bars to prevent fracture. Marsupialization, that is, cutting an ade-quate window in the outer wall of the cyst to remove its contents, may be performed. This is followed later by enucleation when the cyst cavity size has been adequately reduced, and appears to result in a slower recurrence rate [159]. Some surgeons prefer to leave the unerupted permanent teeth in situ and pack the cavity with iliac bone chips. Forssell [162] further showed that marsupialized cysts with a large open-ing have smaller recurrence than cysts enucleated in several pieces and packed open. Stoelinga et al. [163] and Voorsmit et al. [164] advocated removal of the oral mucosa overlying the cyst to reduce the number of satellite epithelial islands or cysts from which recurrence is thought to occur. This needs substantiation.

One should not neglect to provide emotional sup-port and encouragement to these patients. The dis-order seems never ending. Therapy by whatever modality is disfiguring and often causes the patient to become depressed and even reclusive. One cannot tell which basal cell nevoid lesion will become ag-gressive, and careful surveillance cannot be over-emphasized. Periodic examination can keep ahead of this seemingly inexorable disease.

Finally, genetic counseling should be carried out. The disorder has autosomal-dominant inheritance with probably complete penetrance. About 60% of cases represent new mutations. Hence, affected in-dividuals have a 50% chance for transmitting the disorder, and thus periodic examination of their progeny should be carried out.

References

1. Satinoff MI, Wells C. Multiple basal cell naevus syn-drome in ancient Egypt. Med Hist 1969;13:294–297.
2. Jarisch W. Zur Lehre von den Hautgeschwülsten. Arch Dermatol Syph (Berl) 1894;28:162–222.
3. White JC. Multiple benign cystic epitheliomas. J Cu-tan Genitourin Dis 1894;12:477–484.
4. Nomland R. Multiple basal cell epitheliomas origi-nating from congenital pigmented basal cell nevi. Arch Dermatol Syph (Chi) 1932;25:1002–1008.
5. Straith FE. Hereditary epidermoid cysts of the jaws. Am J Orthodont 1939;25:673–691.
6. Binkley GW, Johnson HH. Epithelioma adenoides cysticum: basal cell nevi, agenesis of corpus callosum and dental cysts. Arch Dermatol Syph 1951;63:73–84.
7. Boyer BE, Martin MM. Marfan's syndrome: report of a case manifesting a giant bone cyst of the man-dible and multiple (110) basal cell carcinomas. Plast Reconstr Surg 1958;22:257–263.
8. Howell JB, Caro MR. Basal cell nevus: its relation-ship to multiple cutaneous cancers and associated an-omalies of development. Arch Dermatol 1959;79:67–80.
9. Gorlin RJ, Goltz RW. Multiple nevoid basal-cell ep-ithelioma, jaw cysts and bifid rib syndrome. N Engl J Med 1960;262:908–912.
10. Gorlin RJ, Yunis JJ, Tuna N. Multiple nevoid basal-cell carcinoma, odontogenic keratocysts and skeletal anomalies syndrome. Acta Dermatol Venereol (Stockh) 1963;43:39–55.
11. Cernéa P, Kuffer R, Baumont M, et al. Naevomatose baso-cellulaire. Rev Stomatol (Paris) 1969;70:181–226.
12. Gorlin RJ, Sedano HO. The multiple nevoid basal cell carcinoma syndrome revisited. Birth Defects 1971; 7(8):140–148.
13. Gorlin RJ. Nevoid basal cell carcinoma syndrome. Medicine 1987;66:98–113.
14. Pollitzer J. Eine eigentümliche Karzinose der Haut (Carcinoderma pigmentosum Lang) nebenher: Punkt-und strichförmige Defekte im Hornstratum der Pal-mae und Plantae. Arch Dermatol Syph (Berl) 1905;76:323–345.
15. Calnan CD. Two cases of multiple naevoid basal cell epitheliomata? Porokeratosis of Mantoux. Br J Der-matol 1953;65:219–221.
16. Ward WH. Naevoid basal celled carcinoma associ-ated with dyskeratosis of palms and soles: new entity. Aust J Dermatol 1960;5:204–208.
17. Herzberg JJ, Wiskemann A. Die fünfte Phakomatose. Basalzellnaevus mit familiärer Belastung und Me-dulloblastom. Dermatologica 1963;126:106–123.
18. Block JB, Clendenning WE. Parathyroid hormone hy-

poresponsiveness in patients with basal-cell nevi and bone defects. N Engl J Med 1963;268:1157–1162.

19. Swanson AE, Jacks QD. An unusual propensity for odontogenic cyst formation. J Can Dent Assoc 1961;27:723–731.

20. Cairns RJ. Commenting on case of G.A. Caron: basal cell naevi with a neurological syndrome. Proc R Soc Med 1965;58:621–622.

21. Pollard JJ, New PFJ. Hereditary cutaneomandibular polyoncosis. A syndrome of myriad basal cell nevi of the skin, mandibular cysts, and inconstant skeletal anomalies. Radiology 1964;82:840–849.

22. Kirsch T. Pathologenetische Beziehungen zwischen Kieferzysten und Hautveränderungen unter besonderer Berücksichtigung der Hautkarzinomatose. Schweiz Monatsschr Zahnheilkd 1956;66:687–701.

23. Howell JB. The roots of naevoid basal cell carcinoma syndrome. Clin Exp Dermatol 1980;5:339–348.

24. Howell JB, Anderson DE. Transformation of epithelioma adenoides cysticum into multiple rodent ulcers: fact or fallacy. Br J Dermatol 1976;95:233–242.

25. Gilhuus-Moe O, Haugen LK, Dee PM. The syndrome of multiple cysts of the jaws, basal cell carcinomata and skeletal anomalies. Br J Oral Surg 1968;5:211–222.

26. Rayner CRW, Towers JF, Wilson JSP. What is Gorlin's syndrome? The diagnosis and management of basal cell naevus syndrome based on a study of thirty-seven patients. Br J Plast Surg 1977;30:62–67.

27. Mason JK, Helwig EG, Graham JH. Pathology of the nevoid basal cell carcinoma syndrome. Arch Pathol 1965;79:401–408.

28. Anderson DE, Cook WA. Jaw cysts and the basal cell nevus syndrome. J Oral Surg 1966;24:15–26.

29. Murphy KJ. Metastatic basal cell carcinoma with squamous appearance in the nevoid basal cell carcinoma syndrome. Br J Plast Surg 1975;28:331–334.

30. Goldberg HM, Pratt-Thomas HR, Harvin HS. Metastasizing basal cell carcinoma. Plast Reconstr Surg 1977;59:750–753.

31. McClatchey K, Batsakis JG, Hybels R, et al. Odontogenic keratocysts and nevoid basal cell carcinoma syndrome. Arch Otolaryngol 1975;101:613–616.

32. Southwick GJ, Schwartz RA. The basal cell nevus syndrome. Disasters occurring among a series of 36 patients. Cancer 1979;44:2294–2305.

33. Leppard BJ. Skin cysts in the basal cell naevus syndrome. Clin Exp Dermatol 1983;8:603–612.

34. Graham JK, McJimsey BA, Hardin JC. Nevoid basal cell carcinoma syndrome. Arch Otolaryngol 1968;87:72–77.

35. Neblett CR, Waltz TA, Anderson DE. Neurological involvement in the nevoid basal cell carcinoma syndrome. J Neurosurg 1971;35:577–584.

36. Jackson R, Gardere S. Nevoid basal cell carcinoma syndrome. Can Med Assoc J 1971;105:850–859.

37. Tasanen A, Lamberg MA, Nordling S. Skeletal anomalies and keratocysts in the basal cell nevus syndrome. Int J Oral Surg 1975;4:225–235.

38. Hermans EH, Grosfeld JCM, Spaas JAJ. The fifth phacomatosis. Dermatologica 1965;130:446–476.

39. Amin R. Basal cell naevus syndrome. Br J Radiol 1975;48:402–407.

40. Telle B. Multiple Basaliome bei einem jungen Mann. Dermatol Wochenschr 1965;151:1425–1431.

41. Esser R, Bohnert B. Neurologic symptoms of basal cell nevus syndrome. Eur Neurol 1980;19:335–338.

42. Cutler TP, Holden CA, MacDonald DM. Multiple naevoid basal cell carcinoma syndrome (Gorlin's syndrome). Clin Exp Dermatol 1979;4:373–379 [same case as ref. 19].

43. Kraemer BB, Silver EG, Sneige N. Fibrosarcoma of the ovary: a new component in the nevoid basal cell carcinoma syndrome. Am J Surg Pathol 1984;8:231–236.

44. Ramsden RT, Barrett A. Gorlin's syndrome. J Laryngol Otol 1978;89:615–621.

45. Burket RL, Rauh JL. Gorlin's syndrome: ovarian fibromas at adolescence. Obstet Gynecol 1976;47:43s–46s.

46. Raggio M, Kaplan AL, Harberg JF. Recurrent ovarian fibromas with basal cell nevus syndrome (Gorlin syndrome). Obstet Gynecol 1983;61:95s–96s.

47. Reed JC. Nevoid basal cell carcinoma syndrome with associated fibrosarcoma of the maxilla. Arch Dermatol 1968;97:304–306.

48. Taylor WB, Anderson DE, Howell JB, et al. The nevoid basal cell carcinoma syndrome. Arch Dermatol 1968;98:612–614.

49. McEvoy BF, Gatzek H. Multiple nevoid basal cell carcinoma syndrome: radiological manifestations. Br J Radiol 1969;42:24–28.

50. Anderson DE, Taylor WB, Falls HF, et al. The nevoid basal cell carcinoma syndrome. Am J Hum Genet 1967;19:12–22.

51. Ryan DE, Burkes EJ. The multiple basal cell nevus syndrome in a Negro family. Oral Surg 1973;36:831–840.

52. Strong LC. Genetic and environmental interactions. Cancer 1977;40:1861–1866.

53. Rittersma J. Het basocellulaire nevus syndroom. Master's Thesis. U. Gröningen, 1972.

54. Berlin NI, Van Scott EJ, Clendenning WE, et al. Basal cell nevus syndrome. Ann Intern Med 1966;64:403–421.

55. Tamoney HJ Jr. Basal cell nevoid syndrome. Am Surg 1969;35:279–283.

56. Hess J, Bink-Boelkens MTE. Fibroma cordis bij een zuilgeling met het basocellulaire naevussyndrom. Ned Tijdschr Geneeskd 1976;120:1796–1799.

57. Bunting PD, Remensnyder JP. Basal cell nevus syndrome. Plast Reconstr Surg 1977;60:895–901.

58. Littler BO. Gorlin's syndrome and the heart. Br J Oral Surg 1979;17:135–146.

59. Harris SA, Large DM. Gorlin's syndrome with a cardiac lesion and jaw cysts with some unusual histological features: a case report and review of the literature. Int J Oral Surg 1984;13:59–64.

60. Happle R, Mehrle G, Sander LZ, et al. Basalzellnä-vus-Syndrom mit Retinopathia pigmentosa, rezidivierender Glaskörperblutung und Chromosomenveränderungen. Arch Dermatol Forsch 1971;241:96–114.

61. Stoelinga PJW, Peters JH, van de Staak WJB, et al. Some new findings in the basal cell carcinoma syndrome. Oral Surg 1973;36:686–692.

62. Mortimer PS, Geaney DP, Liddell K, et al. Basal cell naevus syndrome and intracranial meningioma. J Neurol Neurosurg Psychiatry 1984;47:210–212.

63. Clendenning WE, Block JB, Radde IC. Basal cell nevus syndrome. Arch Dermatol 1964;90:38–53.

64. Happle R. Naevobasalom und Ameloblastom. Hautarzt 1973;24:290–294.

65. Jeanmougin M, Zeller J, Wechsler J, et al. Naevomatose basocellulaire et améloblastome. Ann Dermatol Venereol (Paris) 1979;106:691–693.

66. Maddox WD, Winkelmann RK, Harrison EG, et al. Multiple nevoid basal cell epitheliomas, jaw cysts and skeletal defects. JAMA 1964;188:106–111.

67. Kahn LB, Gordon W. Basal cell naevus syndrome. S Afr Med J 1967;41:832–835.

68. Rossi R, Libertino JA, Dowd JB, Braasch JW. Neurocutaneous syndromes and retroperitoneal tumors. Urology 1979;13:292–294.

69. Schweisguth O, Gerard-Marchant R, Lemerle J. Naevomatose baso-cellulaire; association à un rhabdomyosarcome congénital. Arch Fr Pediatr 1968;25:1083–1093.

70. Beddis IR, Mott MG, Bullimore J. Nasopharyngeal rhabdomyosarcoma and Gorlin's nevoid basal cell carcinoma syndrome. Med Pédiatr Oncol 1983;11:178–179.

71. Dahl I, Angervall L, Säve-Söderbergh J. Foetal rhabdomyoma. Acta Pathol Microbiol Scand (Sect A) 1976;84:107–112.

72. Zaun H. Basalzellnävussyndrom mit ungewöhnlicher Begleitsymptomatik. Hautarzt 1981;32:455–458.

73. Bansal MP, Sengupta SR, Krishnan EC. Basal cell nevus syndrome. Ind J Cancer 1975;12:214–218.

74. Kedem A, Even-Paz Z, Freund M. Basal cell nevus syndrome associated with malignant melanoma of the iris. Dermatologica 1970;140:99–106.

75. Summerly R, Hale AJ. Basal cell naevus syndrome. St Johns Hospital Dermatol Soc 1965;51:77–79.

76. Mills JJ, Foulkes J. Gorlin's syndrome: a radiological and cytogenetic study of 9 cases. Br J Radiol 1967;40:366–371.

77. Batschwarov B, Minkov D. Naevobasalioma, Mesenterialzysten und Malignom. Dermatol Wochenschr 1967;153:1294–1302.

78. Totten JR. The multiple nevoid basal cell carcinoma syndrome: report of its occurrence in four generations of a family. Cancer 1980;46:1456–1462.

79. Gundlach KKH, Kiehn M. Multiple basal cell carcinomas and keratocysts—the Gorlin and Goltz syndrome. J Maxillofac Surg 1979;7:299–307.

80. Davidson F. Multiple nevoid basal cell carcinomata

81. Oatis GW Jr, Burch MS, Samuels HS. Marfan's syndrome with multiple maxillary and mandibular cysts. J Oral Surg 1971;29:515–519.

82. Cawson RA, Kerr GA. The syndrome of jaw cysts and basal cell tumours. Proc R Soc Med 1964;57:799–801.

83. Wallace DC, Murphy KJ, Kelly L, et al. Report of a family with anosmia and a case of hypogonadotrophic hypopituitarism. J Med Genet 1973;10:30–33.

84. van Dijk E, Neering H. The association of cleft lip and palate with basal cell nevus syndrome. Oral Surg 1980;50:214–216.

85. Olson RAJ, Stroneck GG, Scully JR, et al. Nevoid basal cell carcinoma syndrome. J Oral Surg 1981;39:308–312.

86. Lahti A, Rintala A, Salo H. Polycystic jaws in patients with cleft lip and palate. Ann Chir Gynecol Fenn 1973;62:161–165.

87. Cotten S, Super S, SunderRay M, et al. Nevoid basal cell carcinoma syndrome. J Oral Med 1982;37:69–73.

88. Kamiya Y, Nareta H, Yamamoto T, et al. Familial odontogenic cysts: report of 3 cases and review of the Japanese dental literature. Int J Oral Surg 1985;14:73–80.

89. Lindberg H, Halaburt H, Larsen PO. The naevoid basal cell carcinoma syndrome. J Maxillofac Surg 1982;10:246–249.

90. Owens SC, Gillespie CA, Cole TB, et al. Gorlin's basal cell nevus syndrome. Arch Otolaryngol 1986;112:773–775.

91. Pritchard LJ, Delfino JJ, Ivey DM, et al. Variable expressivity of the multiple nevoid basal cell carcinoma syndrome. J Oral Maxillofac Surg 1982;40:261–269.

92. Southwick GJ, Schwartz RA. The basal cell nevus syndrome: disasters occurring among a series of 36 patients. Cancer 1979;44:2294–2305.

93. Dahl E, Kreiborg S, Jensen BL. Craniofacial morphology in the nevoid basal cell carcinoma syndrome. Int J Oral Surg 1976;5:300–310.

94. Lorenz R, Fuhrmann W. Familial basal cell nevus syndrome. Hum Genet 1978;44:153–163.

95. Howell JB, Mehregan A. Story of the pits. A historic vignette. Arch Dermatol 1970;102:583–585.

96. Howell JB, Mehregan A. Pursuit of the pits in the nevoid basal cell carcinoma syndrome. Arch Dermatol 1970;102:586–597.

97. Howell JB, Freeman RG. Structure and significance of the pits with their tumors in the nevoid basal cell carcinoma syndrome. J Am Acad Dermatol 1980;2:224–238.

98. Holubar K, Matros H, Smalik AV. Multiple basal cell epitheliomas in basal cell nevus syndrome. Arch Dermatol 1970;101:679–682.

99. Taylor WB, Wilkins JW. Nevoid basal cell carcinomas of the palm. Arch Dermatol 1970;102:654–655.

100. Hashimoto K, Howell JB, Yamanishi Y, et al. Electron microscopic studies of palmar and plantar pits of nevoid basal cell epithelioma. J Invest Dermatol 1972;59:380–393.

101. Howell JB, Anderson DE, McClendon JL. Multiple cutaneous cancers in children: the nevoid basal cell carcinoma syndrome. J Pediatr 1966;69:97–103.

102. Zackheim HS, Howell JB, Loud AV. Basal cell carcinoma syndrome. Arch Dermatol 1966;93:317–323.

103. Dunnick NR, Head GL, Peck GL, et al. Nevoid basal carcinoma syndrome: radiographic manifestations including cystlike lesions of the phalanges. Radiology 1978;127:331–334.

104. Naguib MG, Sung JH, Erickson DL, et al. Central nervous system involvement in the nevoid basal cell carcinoma syndrome: case report and review of the literature. Neurosurgery 1982;11:52–56.

105. Novak KD, Bloss N. Röntgenologische Aspekte des Basalzell-Naevus Syndroms (Gorlin-Goltz Syndrom). Roefo 1976;124:11–16.

106. Blinder G, Barke Y, Petz M, et al. Widespread osteolytic lesions of the long bones in basal cell nevus syndrome. Skel Radiol 1984;12:195–198.

107. Hawkins JC, Hoffman HJ, Becker LE. Multiple nevoid basal cell carcinoma syndrome (Gorlin's syndrome): possible confusion with metastatic medulloblastoma. J Neurosurg 1979;50:100–102.

108. Murphy KJ. Subcutaneous calcification in the naevoid basal-cell carcinoma syndrome. Response to parathyroid hormone and relationship to pseudo-hypoparathyroidism. Clin Radiol 1969;20:287–293.

109. Brannon RG. The odontogenic keratocyst: a clinicopathologic study of 312 cases. Part I. Clinical features. Oral Surg 1976;42:54–72.

110. MacKenzie GD, Oates GW, Mullen MP, et al. Computerized tomography in the diagnosis of an odontogenic keratocyst. Oral Surg 1985;59:302–305.

111. Happle R, Hoehn H. Cytogenetic studies on cultured fibroblast-like cells derived from basal cell carcinoma tissue. Clin Genet 1973;4:17–24.

112. Römke C, Gödde–Salz E, Grote W. Investigations of chromosomal stability in the Gorlin-Goltz syndrome. Arch Dermatol Res 1985;277:370–372.

113. Elejalde BR. In-vitro transformation of cells from patients with naevoid basal-cell carcinoma syndrome. Lancet 1976;2:1199–1200.

114. Ringborg V, Lambert B, Landegren J, et al. Decreased UV-induced DNA repair synthesis in peripheral leukocytes from patients with the nevoid basal cell carcinoma syndrome. J Invest Dermatol 1981;76:268–270.

115. Featherstone T, Taylor AMR, Harnden DG. Studies on the radiosensitivity of cells from patients with basal cell naevus syndrome. Am J Hum Genet 1983;35:58–66.

116. Nagasawa H, Little FF, Burke MJ, et al. Study of basal cell nevus syndrome fibroblasts after treatment with DNA damaging agents. Basic Life Sci 1984;29B:775–785.

117. Hickory JE, Gilliland RF, Wade WM, et al. Conservative treatment of cysts of the jaws in nevoid basal cell carcinoma syndrome. J Oral Surg 1975;33:693–697.

118. Kaufman R, Chase LR. Basal cell nevus syndrome: normal responsiveness to parathyroid hormone. Birth Defects 1972;7(8):149–155.

119. Murphy KJ. Subcutaneous bone formation in the naevoid basal cell carcinoma syndrome: normal urinary cyclic AMP response to parathyroid hormone infusion. Clin Radiol 1974;26:37–39.

120. Browne RM. The odontogenic keratocyst. Clinical aspects. Br Dent J 1970;128:225–231.

121. Kramer IRH, Toller PA. The use of exfoliative cytology and protein estimations in preoperative diagnosis of odontogenic keratocysts. Int J Oral Surg 1973;2:143–151.

122. Magnusson BC. Odontogenic keratocysts: a clinical and histochemical study with special reference to enzyme histochemistry. J Oral Pathol 1978;7:8–18.

123. Philipsen HP, Fejerskov O, Donatsky O, et al. Ultrastructure of epithelial lining of keratocysts in nevoid basal cell carcinoma syndrome. Int J Oral Surg 1973;5:71–81.

124. Gorlin RJ, Vickers RA, Kelln E, et al. The multiple basal-cell nevi syndrome. An analysis of a syndrome consisting of multiple nevoid basal cell carcinoma, jaw cysts, skeletal anomalies, medulloblastoma and hyporesponsiveness to parathormone. Cancer 1965; 18:89–104.

125. Lindeberg H, Jepsen FL. The nevoid basal cell carcinoma syndrome: histopathology of the tumors. J Cutan Pathol 1983;10:68–73.

126. Graham JH, Mason JK, Gray HR, et al. Differentiation of nevoid basal cell carcinoma from epithelioma adenoides cysticum. J Invest Dermatol 1965;44:197–200.

127. Ullman S, Sondergaard J, Kobayasi T. Ultrastructure of palmar and plantar pits in basal cell nevus syndrome. Acta Derm Venereol (Stockh) 1972;52:329–336.

128. Hodgkinson DJ, Woods JE, Dahlin DC, et al. Keratocysts of the jaw: clinicopathologic study of 79 patients. Cancer 1978;41:803–813.

129. Brannon RB. The odontogenic keratocyst: a clinicopathological study of 312 cases. Part II. Histologic features. Oral Surg 1977;43:233–255.

130. Ahlfors E, Larsson Å, Sjögren S. The odontogenic keratocyst: a benign cystic tumor. J Oral Maxillofac Surg 1984;42:10–19.

131. Miller RF, Cooper RR. Nevoid basal cell carcinoma syndrome. Histogenesis of skeletal lesions. Clin Orthop Rel Res 1972;89:246–252.

132. Scully RE, Galdabini JJ, McNeely BV. Case records of the Massachusetts General Hosp. N Engl J Med 1976;294:772–777.

133. Jones KL, Smith DW, Harvey MAS, et al. Older paternal age and fresh gene mutation: data on additional disorders. J Pediatr 1975;86:84–88.

134. Anderson DE. Linkage analysis of the nevoid basal cell carcinoma syndrome. Ann Hum Genet 1968;32:113–117.

135. Linss G, Scheibe E, Schielinksy C. Blutgruppen und eine Familie mit Nävobasaliomatose (Gorlin-Goltz Syndrom). Dermatol Monatsschr 1980;166:616–621.

136. Bale AE, Bale SJ, Mulvihill JJ. Linkage between the nevoid basal cell carcinoma syndrome (NBCCS) gene and chromosome 1 markers. Am J Hum Genet 1985;37:A44.

137. Stoelinga PJW, Cohen MM Jr, Morgan AF. The origin of keratocysts in the basal cell nevus syndrome. J Oral Surg 1975;33:659–663.

138. Donatsky O, Hjørting-Hansen E, Philipsen HP, et al. Clinical, radiologic and histopathologic aspects of 13 cases of nevoid basal cell carcinoma syndrome. Int J Oral Surg 1976;5:19–28.

139. Howell JB. Nevoid basal cell carcinoma syndrome: profile of genetic and environmental factors in oncogenesis. J Am Acad Dermatol 1984;11:98–104.

140. Scharnagel IM, Pack GT. Multiple basal cell epitheliomas in a 5 year old child. Am J Dis Child 1949; 77:647–651.

141. Golitz LE, Norris DA, Luekens CA, et al. Multiple basal cell carcinomas of the palms after radiation therapy. Arch Dermatol 1980;116:1159–1163.

142. Carney RG. Linear unilateral basal-cell nevus with comedones. Arch Dermatol 1952;65:471–476.

143. Wirth H, Tilgen W. Linearer unilateraler Basalzellnävus. Hautarzt 1983;34:620–624.

144. Gould DJ, Barker DJ. Follicular atrophoderma and multiple basal cell carcinomas (Bazex). Br J Dermatol 1978;99:431–435.

145. Plosila M et al. The Bazex syndrome: follicular atrophoderma with multiple basal cell carcinomas, hypotrichosis and hypohidrosis. Clin Exp Dermatol 1981;6:31–41.

146. Viknins P, Berlin A. Follicular atrophoderma and basal cell carcinoma: the Bazex syndrome. Arch Dermatol 1977;113:948–951.

147. Michaëlson G, Olsson E, Westermark P. The Rombo syndrome: a familial disorder with vermiculate atrophoderma, milia, hypotrichosis, trichoepitheliomas, basal cell carcinomas and peripheral vasodilation with cyanosis. Acta Dermato Vener (Stockh) 1981;61:497–503.

148. Rasmussen JE. A syndrome of trichoepitheliomas, milia and cylindromas. Arch Dermatol 1971;111:610–614.

149. Venencie PY, Perry HO. Sign of Leser-Trélat: report of two cases and review of the literature. J Am Acad Dermatol 1984;10:83–88.

150. Donatsky O, Hjørting-Hansen E. Recurrence of the odontogenic keratocyst in 13 patients with the nevoid basal cell carcinoma syndrome—a 6-year follow-up. Int J Oral Surg 1980;9:173–179.

151. Howell JB, Anderson DE. The nevoid basal cell carcinoma syndrome. Arch Dermatol 1982;118:824–825.

152. Mohs FE, Jones DL, Koranda FC. Microscopically controlled surgery for carcinomas in patients with nevoid basal cell carcinoma syndrome. Arch Dermatol 1980;116:777–779.

153. Thorne FL, Miller F, Garrett WS. The surgical approach to trichoepithelioma and the basal cell nevus syndrome. Plast Reconstr Surg 1966;38:438–443.

154. Klein E, Holtermann O, Milgrom H, et al. Immunotherapy for accessible tumors utilizing delayed hypersensitivity reactions and separated components of the immune system. Med Clin North Am 1976;60: 389–418.

155. Klein E, Stoll HL Jr, Milgrom H, et al. Topical 5-fluorouracil for epidermal neoplasms. J Surg Oncol 1971;3:331–349.

156. Moynahan EJ. Multiple nevoid basal cell naevus syndrome—successful treatment of basal cell tumors with 5-fluorouracil. Proc R Soc Med 1973;66:627–628.

157. Amon RB, Goodkin PE. Topical 5-fluorouracil and the basal cell nevus syndrome. N Engl J Med 1976;295:677–678.

158. Peck GL, Gross EG, Butkus D, et al. Chemoprevention of basal cell carcinoma with isotretinoin. J Am Acad Dermatol 1982;6:815–823.

159. Christofolini M, Zumiani G, Scappini P, et al. Aromatic retinoid in the chemoprevention of the progression of nevoid basal cell carcinoma syndrome. J Dermatol Surg 1984;10:778–781.

160. Howell JB, Byrd L, McClendon JL, et al. Identification and treatment of jaw cysts in the nevoid basal cell carcinoma syndrome. J Oral Surg 1967;25:129–138.

161. Totten JR. Multiple basal cell naevi syndrome: management of the young patient. Br J Oral Surg 1979;17:147–156.

162. Forssell K. The primordial cyst, a clinical and radiographic study. Proc Finn Dent Soc 1980;76:129–174.

163. Stoelinga PJW, Cohen MM Jr., Morgan AF. The origin of keratocysts on the basal cell nevus syndrome. J Oral Surg 1975;33:659–663.

164. Voorsmit RA, Stoelinga PJ, van Hoelst VJ. The management of keratocysts. J Maxillofac Surg 1981; 9:228–236.

Chapter 6
Lentiginosis-Deafness-Cardiopathy Syndrome

DONALD J. HAGLER

Lentiginosis, or multiple lentigines, is the hallmark of this familial syndrome, which is appropriately considered a neuroectodermal defect. Similar to other neurocutaneous syndromes, multiple lentigines are inherited in an autosomal dominant fashion and have variable expression or manifestations. Sporadic cases that are possibly due to heterogeneity of expression or to a new mutation also have been recognized.

The inclusion of multiple lentigines as a cardiocutaneous syndrome is also appropriate because another clinically very important aspect of this syndrome has been an associated hypertrophic obstructive cardiomyopathy. In some cases, this feature has been progressive and responsible for a patient's demise.

Progressive generalized lentigines were reported in 1936 by Zeisler and Becker [1]. However, the associated syndrome with cardiac abnormalities and short stature was reported by Moynahan in 1962 [2]. Walther et al. [3] described a family with lentiginosis and cardiac abnormalities in 1966. Moynahan and Polani [4] reported the association of lentiginosis in hypertrophic obstructive cardiomyopathy in 1968. A similar syndrome of multiple lentigines, electrocardiographic conduction abnormalities, ocular hypertelorism, abnormalities of genitalia, growth retardation, sensory neural deafness, and pulmonary stenosis with an autosomal dominant hereditary pattern was reported by Gorlin et al. in 1969 [5].

The progressive nature and a more complete description of the associated hypertrophic obstructive cardiomyopathy were reported by Polani and Moynahan [6] in 1972. They also postulated a neuroectodermal defect with "extensive dysfunction of pigmentary and other elements of neural crest origin." Because of the apparent association of progressive lentigines and progressive obstructive cardiomyopathy, the neural crest origin hypothesis was expanded by Somerville and Bonham-Carter [7] in 1972 to include a possible metabolic or enzyme defect resulting in excessive pigmentation and excessive cardiac muscle hypertrophy. They also pointed out that the progressive nature of the cardiac abnormality may explain the apparent discrepancies in earlier cardiac diagnoses. Thus, mild pulmonary stenosis may have been recognized in some cases as an early feature before the later development and appearance of the typical hypertrophic obstructive features involving the left heart.

The association of hypertrophic obstructive cardiomyopathy and other neurocutaneous syndromes—neurofibromatosis, tuberous sclerosis, and pheochromocytoma—has also been reported [8] and seems consistent with a neuroectodermal defect. The report of experimental production of ultrastructural myocardial changes, similar to those observed in hypertrophic obstructive cardiomyopathy, by daily injections of nerve growth factor in puppies lends further support to a suspected neuroectodermal defect [9].

Diagnosis

Table 6.1 lists the primary and associated abnormalities that constitute the syndrome of multiple lentigines (Figure 6.1). Skin biopsies of the lesions have demonstrated moderate hyperactivity of the melanocytes, pigment accumulation in the dermis, and a generalized tendency to hyperpigmentation. An equal male to female sex ratio has been reported [1–7,10]. The electrocardiographic abnormalities described seem most consistent with variable degrees of right or left ventricular hypertrophy with associated inter-

Table 6.1. Primary and Associated Abnormalities of the Syndrome of Multiple Lentigines

Lentigines
Hypertrophic obstructive cardiomyopathy
Electrocardiographic abnormalities
    Left axis deviation
    Ventricular conduction delay
    Right or left ventricular hypertrophy
Genital abnormalities
Growth retardation, short stature
Psychomotor retardation
Poor skeletal muscle development associated with
    scoliosis or winging of the scapula
Sensorineural deafness
Ocular hypertelorism

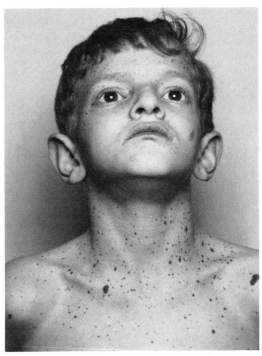

Figure 6.1. Nine-year-old boy with multiple lentigines, psychomotor retardation, growth retardation, and hypertrophic obstructive cardiomyopathy. He did not have genital abnormalities or sensorineural deafness.

ventricular conduction delays and usually with left axis deviation (Figure 6.2). Several case reports suggest early death during the second decade of life because of progressive obstructive hypertrophic cardiomyopathy or sudden death because of associated apparent serious dysrhythmia [6,7,10]. In this context, the importance of the associated progression of both lentigines and cardiomyopathy has been recognized. Some patients present in infancy without lentigines, but throughout childhood and adolescence the lentigines and cardiomyopathy become progressively more evident.

Cardiac evaluation in suspected cases should include complete two-dimensional and Doppler echocardiographic study in addition to routine clinical cardiac examination. During infancy, the clinical features may be characterized by failure to thrive and symptoms suggestive of cardiac failure. During childhood and adolescence, the clinical cardiac findings may be relatively nonspecific. A somewhat prominent ventricular impulse may be noted with a variable-intensity systolic ejection murmur at the left sternal border. In addition to the previously described electrocardiographic abnormalities, the chest radiograph frequently demonstrates some cardiomegaly. Echocardiographic study demonstrates the presence of asymmetric septal hypertrophy and systolic anterior motion of the mitral valve leaflets or chordae as pathognomonic features of hypertrophic obstructive cardiomyopathy. Doppler echocardiographic examination may demonstrate the presence of a resting right or left ventricular outflow tract obstruction. In addition, mitral regurgitation and left atrial enlargement may be evident. In the absence of resting outflow tract gradients, provocative measures such as amyl nitrite inhalation may allow their demonstration. The assessment of more fixed or

severe right or left ventricular outflow tract obstruction and the response to provocative isoproterenol infusion, or the therapeutic response to propranolol or verapamil, may require detailed cardiac catheterization or angiographic study [7,8]. Right ventricular angiocardiography may demonstrate infundibular hypertrophy and right ventricular obstruction (Figure 6.3). Left ventricular angiocardiography demonstrates ventricular hypertrophy, systolic cavity obliteration, and subvalvular outflow obstruction (Figure 6.4). Simultaneous right and left ventriculograms in a long axial oblique projection will allow demonstration of the asymmetric ventricular septal hypertrophy. In addition, variable degrees of mitral regurgitation may be evident secondary to systolic anterior motion of the mitral valve leaflets.

In addition, patients should be studied for the possible presence of serious dysrhythmia such as ventricular ectopy or supraventricular tachycardia, which may be responsible for sudden death in patients with hypertrophic obstructive cardiomyopathy. Such examinations should include 24-hour ambulatory electrocardiographic monitoring and exercise stress testing.

Short stature, psychomotor retardation, and de-

Figure 6.2. Twelve-lead electrocardiogram *(A)* and vectorcardiogram *(B)* of 10-year-old patient with lentigines and documented hypertrophic obstructive cardiomyopathy. Note mild ventricular conduction delay, left axis deviation, and left ventricular hypertrophy.

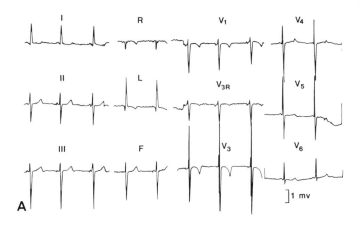

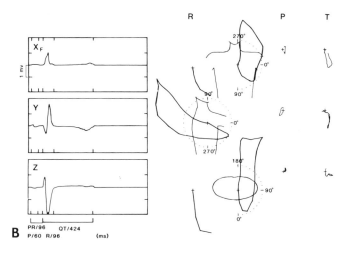

layed sexual maturation are frequently described as associated features of this syndrome. Genital abnormalities have included cryptorchidism, hypospadias, and ovarian disorders and may also be related to an abnormality of melanocytes.

Treatment

Genetic counseling should be used for prevention after examination of other family members. Treatment of the cardiac abnormalities may include restriction from participation in strenuous competitive athletics in the presence of outflow tract obstruction or significant dysrhythmia. Surgery is necessary to relieve severe

degrees of outflow tract obstruction until medical treatment is available for less significant obstruction. Therapeutic regimens include β-adrenergic receptor (propranolol) or calcium channel blocking (verapamil) agents to reduce outflow tract obstruction and adrenergic responsiveness. These agents may be clinically efficacious by other mechanisms such as their beneficial effects on ventricular relaxation and diastolic filling [11–13]. Recently, life-threatening ventricular ectopy prompted treatment with amiodarone [13,14]. Surgical treatment may also be necessary for other associated defects such as cryptorchidism or hypospadias, when present. Other supportive measures may be indicated for disabilities such as psychomotor retardation and sensorineural deafness.

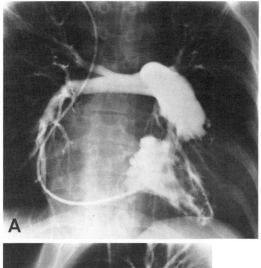

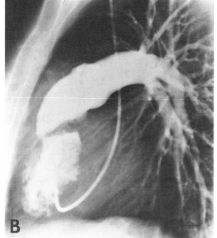

Figure 6.3. Anteroposterior *(A)* and lateral *(B)* biplane right ventricular angiograms of patient with hypertrophic obstructive cardiomyopathy demonstrate severe subvalvular pulmonary stenosis.

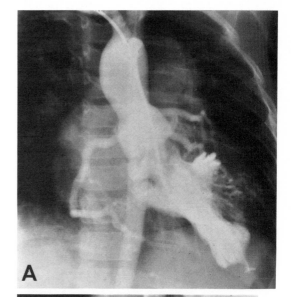

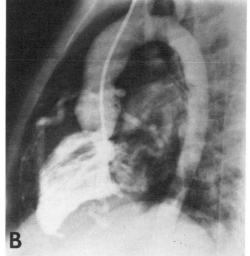

Figure 6.4. Anteroposterior *(A)* and lateral *(B)* biplane left ventricular angiograms of patient shown in Figure 6.1 demonstrate severe hypertrophic obstructive cardiomyopathy with typical subaortic obstruction. Resting left ventricular outflow tract gradient was 63 mm Hg.

References

1. Zeisler EP, Becker SW. Generalized lentigo: its relation to systemic nonelevated nevi. Arch Dermatol Syph 1936;33:109–125.
2. Moynahan EJ. Multiple symmetrical moles, with psychic and somatic infantilism and genital hypoplasia: first male case of a new syndrome. Proc R Soc Med 1962;55:959–960.
3. Walther RJ, Polansky BJ, Grots IA. Electrocardiographic abnormalities in a family with generalized lentigo. N Engl J Med 1966;275:1220–1225.
4. Moynahan EJ, Polani P. Progressive profuse lentiginosis, progressive cardiomyopathy, short stature with delayed puberty, mental retardation or psychic infantilism, and other developmental anomalies: a new familial syndrome. In: Jadassohn W, Schirren CG, eds. XIII. Congressus internationalis dermatologiae. Berlin: Springer–Verlag, 1968;2:1543.
5. Gorlin RJ, Anderson RC, Blaw M. Multiple lentigenes syndrome: complex comprising multiple lentigenes, electrocardiographic conduction abnormalities, ocular hypertelorism, pulmonary stenosis, abnormalities of genitalia, retardation of growth, sensorineural deaf-

ness, and autosomal dominant hereditary pattern. Am J Dis Child 1969;117:652–662.

6. Polani PE, Moynahan EJ. Progressive cardiomyopathic lentiginosis. Q J Med 1972;41:205–239.

7. Somerville J, Bonham-Carter RE. The heart in lentiginosis. Br Heart J 1972;34:58–66.

8. Elliott CM, Tajik AJ, Giuliani ER, et al. Idiopathic hypertrophic subaortic stenosis associated with cutaneous neurofibromatosis: report of a case. Am Heart J 1976;92:368–372.

9. Witzke DJ, Kaye MP. Myocardial ultrastructural changes induced by administration of nerve growth factor. Surg Forum 1976;27:295–297.

10. Voron DA, Hatfield HH, Kalkhoff RK. Multiple lentigines syndrome: case report and review of the literature. Am J Med 1976;60:447–456.

11. Bonow RO, Rosing DR, Bacharach SL, et al. Effects of verapamil on left ventricular systolic function and diastolic filling in patients with hypertrophic cardiomyopathy. Circulation 1981;64:787–796.

12. Canedo MI, Frank MJ. Therapy of hypertrophic cardiomyopathy: medical or surgical? Clinical and pathophysiologic considerations. Am J Cardiol 1981;48:383–388.

13. Criley JM, Siegel RJ. Has 'obstruction' hindered our understanding of hypertrophic cardiomyopathy? Circulation 1985;72:1148–1154.

14. McKenna WJ, Oakley CM, Krikler DM, et al. Improved survival with amiodarone in patients with hypertrophic cardiomyopathy and ventricular tachycardia. Br Heart J 1985;53:412–416.

Chapter 7

Hypomelanosis of Ito

IGNACIO PASCUAL-CASTROVEIJO

Ito in 1952 [1] described a new neurocutaneous entity under the name incontinentia pigmenti achromians, which was subsequently also known by the names systematized achromic nevus or hypomelanosis of Ito (HI).

The number of patients with this disorder reported to date is a very small proportion of the existing cases. In our experience HI is one of the most common neurocutaneous disorders associated with melanin disturbance—the 30 patients we have collected to date represent 1 of every 8,000 to 10,000 patients referred to our hospital.

Clinical Symptoms

The skin lesions consist of linear, vorticose, or irregular areas of hypopigmentation, well defined from the normally pigmented surrounding skin and varying in size and location. In addition to the skin, other organs may be affected, in particular the CNS, peripheral nervous system (PNS), eyes, blood vessels, thorax, and musculoskeletal system. It is estimated that the CNS is affected in at least 50% of patients and that altogether noncutaneous signs occur in 76.4% [2]. In our experience CNS involvement occurs in 76% of patients in the first decade of life.

By definition the skin manifestation is found in 100% of patients. It consists of hypopigmented lesions on any part of the trunk, head, or extremities, on one or both sides of the body, and near or away from the midline. The shape of the spots varies from a fine line following a dermatome distribution to a large or small whorl or a spot with irregular borders. The normally pigmented skin stands out better than the affected hypochromic spot (Figure 7.1). Hypomelanotic spots in zigzag are particularly evident on the back and are common. It is easier to detect this hypomelanosis when the normal surrounding skin is

rich in pigment as occurs in blacks and others with dark skin. Ultraviolet light helps to find the lesions in individuals of Nordic descent and others with pale skin. There is no known racial predominance of HI although recently a large number of nonwhite individuals were reported [3]. We suspect this was due to a high prevalence of black individuals in the population studied. The disorder is said to be more prevalent in females than males. Our experience with 30 patients, 16 male and 14 female, does not support this contention.

The skin lesions are of the congenital type and although they seem to be the result of an embryopathy are seldom detected in the newborn period. In most instances the hypopigmented lesions are discovered within the first months of life. Conceivably they may remain unrecognized by the patient's parents until some neurologic symptoms appear. In our experience, the skin lesions are found in the first year of life in 70% of patients. Other skin lesions, mongolian spots [4] and café-au-lait spots, are associated with the hypomelanosis in these patients. One of our patients had, in addition to hypomelanotic spots, large mongolian spots covering both gluteal areas and spreading to cover the back almost entirely, a facial venous angioma on one cheek, and a nevus fuscoceruleus of Ota on both sclerae.

The hair arising from a hypomelanotic skin lesion on the scalp is white or gray-white, mottled and hirsute, or trichorrhexic. Sometimes the hair appears late on these hypomelanotic areas of the scalp. Individuals with these dermic signs on the head usually have other associated facial disturbances such as hemihypertrophy or, less frequently, hemihypotrophy or dental/ocular alterations. The hypomelanosis may affect the iris [5].

In a review of 38 patients Hamada et al. [2] found that 76% had associated noncutaneous anomalies, 50% had CNS involvement, the musculoskeletal sys-

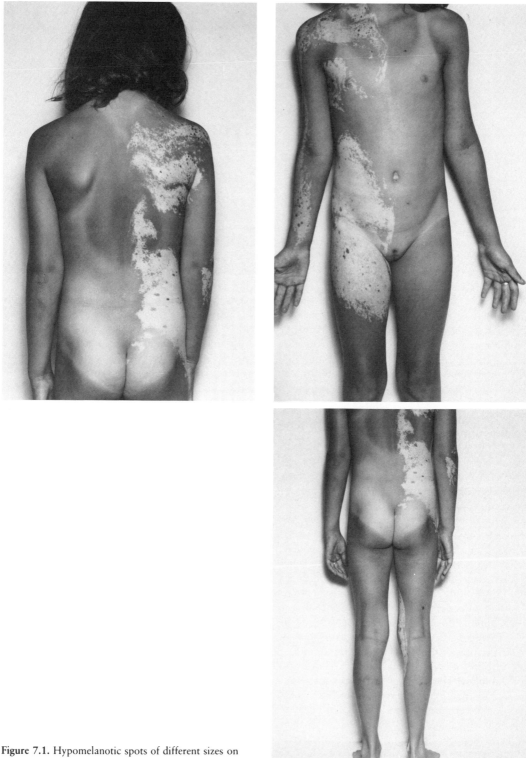

Figure 7.1. Hypomelanotic spots of different sizes on right side of neck, trunk, and right upper and lower limbs. (Courtesy of Dr. Manuel R. Gomez.)

tem was affected in 36%, and the eyes were affected in 31%. Mental retardation and seizures are the most frequent neurologic symptoms. Mental deficit occurred in 76% of our patients and was the most common presenting symptom. Some patients exhibited autistic behavior. The majority of patients with mental retardation had suffered seizures early in life, particularly infantile spasms or myoclonic seizures. Mental retardation may also occur in patients who have never had epilepsy. Patients with seizures in the first year of life are likely to be mentally defective, particularly those who had a poor response to anticonvulsant medication. About half of our patients presented with seizures, and in almost all cases they began in the first year of life. Two patients had West's syndrome, one of whom progressed toward Lennox–Gastaut syndrome. Another one with Lennox–Gastaut syndrome had begun having partial seizures. Nine of our 14 patients experienced seizures of focal onset. Regardless of the seizure type, control with anticonvulsants was unsatisfactory.

Eye signs, although frequently described, are not specific. Among them are strabismus, esotropia, optic nerve atrophy, microphthalmus, hypertelorism, and nystagmus [2,6,7]. More important, but rarely described, are choroidal atrophy [8] and corneal opacity [6].

As has been previously recognized [7,9,10], macrocephaly is one of the most frequent findings: 7 of our 30 patients, or 23%, had it. The brain of a 22-month-old patient who came to autopsy weighed 1,435 gm [9].

Cardiac anomalies are seldom mentioned. One patient had a septal defect [4], and one of our patients had tetralogy of Fallot and global hemihypertrophy. The genitalia are rarely involved. One patient had microgenitosomia and another just microphallus (Figure 7.2).

Hypotonia is frequently described in association with normal deep reflexes, hip dislocation, and kyphoscoliosis which seems to be secondary to hemihypertrophy [11], since constitutional vertebral anomalies have not been detected.

Reported oral anomalies are irregularly spaced teeth [12,13], dental hypoplasia, partial anodontia, defective dental implantation and conic teeth [14], enamel defects, dysplasias, and hamartomatous cuspids protruding from the dental crowns or the permanent teeth [5,15], which are histologically reminiscent of an odontoma. Gothic palate, hairlip [16], bifid uvula, and submucosal cleft palate [7] have been reported rarely.

In the extremities ectrodactyly has been reported as part of a complex group of anomalies [16]. Mal-

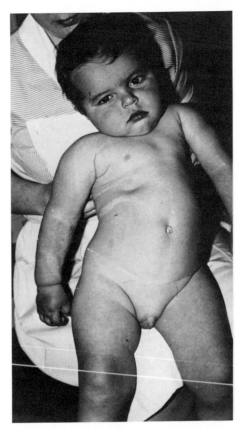

Figure 7.2. Boy with hypomelanotic spots in the hemithorax and right superior extremity. Also note macrocephaly and microphallus. The patient also has severe hypotonia and mental retardation.

formations of the nails are described with greater frequency [6,13]. Anisomelia is frequent and may involve a fragment of a limb, usually a foot or hand, and, in most instances, the lower legs [7]. Hemihypertrophy, which may affect any part of the body or its entirety, is found on the side where there is hypomelanosis of the skin. We have found it, partial or total, in 20% of our patients. Half of these patients appear to have a bilateral distribution of hypertrophy. These anomalies, which are in our opinion nonspecific, can be found in many of the neurocutaneous syndromes, such as neurofibromatosis, urge–Weber disease, nevus unis lateris, cutis marmorata telangiectatica congenita, and tuberous sclerosis.

Diagnostic Studies

Biochemical analyses are of no assistance for making the diagnosis. The blood, urine, and CSF examinations are negative. Nerve conduction velocity studies have demonstrated slowed sensory nerves [17].

Imaging

Skeletal radiographs clearly demonstrate asymmetric limbs kyphoscoliosis, microcephaly, hip subluxation, and other alterations. The dental anomalies as well as deformities of the facial bones can also be demonstrated.

There are few neuroradiologic studies. Up to 1974, when only pneumoencephalography was available, usually normal images were obtained in patients whose neurologic symptoms had been recognized after the age of 2 or 3 years [7,14,17]. When the seizures and psychomotor deterioration have been present earlier, either general or focal cortico-subcortical cerebral atrophy exists [1], which can be interpreted as primary and concomitant with the neurocutaneous disorder or acquired and related to the seizures. The same applies to CT, which can demonstrate either generalized or focal cerebral atrophy in patients with significant neurologic deficit [2,4,18,19]. In addition, this investigation can also demonstrate changes in the attenuation coefficient of the white matter and in particular low attenuation [3], giving images similar to those seen in some types of leukodystrophy. In patients more recently studied we have not seen any abnormality of this type either in the head CT scan or in magnetic resonance imaging (MRI). To our knowledge, no angiographic findings have been reported in this disorder.

Chromosomal Studies

The association of HI with chromosomal abnormalities has been reported in only two articles. Miller and Parker [19] described a 6-month-old girl who had generalized seizures and who had been treated for the Wolff–Parkinson–White syndrome. The karyotype with high-resolution prophases demonstrated a balanced translocation between chromosomes 2 and 8 with the formula 46,XX t(2,8) (q37.2;p21.1). Her parents had normal karyograms. The girl had a right hemiparesis, and her CT scan showed atrophy of her left hemisphere with enlargement of the left ventricle and the cerebral sulci. An EEG demonstrated poorly developed background activity over the left hemisphere and epileptiform activity emanating from the right mid and posterior temporal regions. The seizures were poorly controlled with anticonvulsant medications. Ishikawa et al. [17] reported a Japanese boy with seizures, mental retardation, sensory neuropathy, an epidermoid lesion in the parietal bone dipole, a mediastinal cystic teratoma, and a ventricular septal defect in addition to the cutaneous lesions. His karyogram demonstrated a mosaicism of 45,XY, – 14, – 21, + t(14q,21q) and 46,XY, – 14, – 21, + t(14q,21q) + mar in a 1:2 proportion. Both parents had normal karyotypes.

Pathology

The histopathologic examination of the hypopigmented areas of the skin demonstrates diminished number, size, and pigment content of the melanocytes in the basal layer of the epidermis [20]. Ultrastructural studies show incomplete melanization and a diminished number of melanosomes [21]. These findings are similar to those of the hypomelanotic macules of tuberous sclerosis [22] (see Chapter 3).

The macroscopic and microscopic changes in the brain explain the generalized seizures and severe psychomotor retardation. The patient studied by Ross et al. [9] had paquigyria, caudal displacement of the brain stem, bilateral uncal herniation, multiple heterotopias of gray matter, multiple whitish areas with an irregular configuration and random distribution through the basal ganglia, cerebellar atrophy, and corticospinal tract hypoplasia in the brain stem. The cerebral cortex looked pale and was ill defined. Histologic examination of the widened gyri showed incomplete cortical lamination and gliosis. The glial cells were of fibrous and gemistocytic type, and the latter were often of gigantic size and with more than one nucleus. The neuronal population was clearly diminished and many neurons looked abnormal. There were Rosenthal fibers. The heterotopic gray matter showed neurons and multiple gemistocytic astrocytes similar to those observed in the widened gyri. In the cerebellum there was diminution of the Purkinje cells and an increment of Bergmann's glia. Both the cerebellum and the brain stem were hypoplastic. The corticospinal tracts were poorly myelinated.

The above-described alterations are reminiscent of those found in some neurocutaneous syndromes such as tuberous sclerosis, neurofibromatosis, and incontinentia pigmenti [23,24] and are considered the nonspecific result of a dysplasia or embryopathy affecting the CNS and the skin. The skin and CNS defects should be chronologically related during embryogenesis.

Between the gestational ages of 2 and 4 months there is a great proliferation of nervous tissue, which if defective or absent leads to microcephaly. Between 3 and 6 months of gestation there is neuronal migration, which when altered gives origin to such pathologies as agyria, lissencephaly, pachygyria, and polymicrogyria. At this same time or more exactly at about 3.5 months of gestation the melanoblasts migrate from the neural crest toward their different destinations in the skin where they mature and are transformed into melanocytes. Interference with this migration may give origin to depigmentation in the form of whorls. From the sixth month of gestation to term there is a period of cerebral organization which continues until cortical lamination is complete. In the sixth month the hair anlage is present. Thus, interference with development in the sixth month may affect both cerebral cortex and hair.

Genetics

The hereditary nature of HI is as yet unclear. It appears that in some families there is an autosomal dominant transmission [6,8,14,21,25]. In other cases the hereditary nature is obscure and could be explained if one admits the existence of minisymptomatic forms or formes frustes and "asymptomatic carriers," that is, a clinically unaffected descendant of a patient passing it on to a subsequent descendant. This could have occurred in case 2 of Schwartz et al. [7] and in one of our patients who had severe psychomotor retardation, West's syndrome, macrocephaly, and an extensive hypomelanosis, while her grandmother had a hypomelanotic spot more than 25 cm^2 on the left side of the face but no neurologic findings. The patient's mother was free of skin or organ involvement. Case 1 of Schwartz et al. [7] is very similar to one of our patients who had a brother with a hypomelanotic spot similar to those observed in tuberous sclerosis. For other cases recently reported in the literature [4,26] an autosomal-recessive form of inheritance cannot be ruled out.

Treatment and Prognosis

There is no treatment for the hypomelanosis of the skin. The differences in intensity of pigmentation between the nevus and the normal skin surrounding it is more noticeable in individuals with dark skin and increases with exposure to sunlight.

The seizures, whatever their type, often respond poorly to anticonvulsant medication and have a tendency to recur after temporary remission. The seizures of children with West's syndrome and those with early-onset myoclonic seizures are particularly resistant to all types of anticonvulsant drugs and tend to progress to a Lennox–Gastaut syndrome.

The mental retardation remains stable through the years. Only in patients with poorly controlled seizures can one observe a tendency to regression; that is, lowering of their intellectual ability. Those with autistic behavior do not seem to change.

Finally, patients with musculoskeletal deformities such as scoliosis, hip dislocation, and asymmetry of the extremities have no other option than orthopedic management when feasible.

References

1. Ito M. Studies of melanin XI. Incontinentia pigmenti achromians. A singular case of nevus depigmentosus systematicus bilateralis. Tohoku J Exp Med 1952;(suppl)55:57–59.
2. Hamada K, Tanaka T, Ohdo S, et al. Incontinentia pigmenti achromians as part of a neurocutaneous syndrome. A case report. Brain Dev 1979;1:313–317.
3. Rosenberg S, Arita FN, Campos C, et al. Hypomelanosis of Ito. Case report with involvement of the central nervous system and review of the literature. Neuropediatrics 1984;15:52–55.
4. David TJ. Hypomelanosis of Ito: a neurocutaneous syndrome. Arch Dis Child 1981;56:798–800.
5. Happle R, Vakilzadeh F. Hamartomatous dental cusps in hypomelanosis of Ito. Clin Genet 1982;21:65–68.
6. Jelinek JC, Bart RS, Schiff GM. Hypomelanosis of Ito ("incontinentia pigmenti achromians"). Arch Dermatol 1973;107:596–601.
7. Schwartz MF Jr, Esterly NB, Fretzin DF, et al. Hypomelanosis of Ito (incontinentia pigmenti achromians): a neurocutaneous syndrome. J Pediatr 1977;90:236–240.
8. Pinol J, Mascaro JM, Romaguera C, et al. Considérations sur l'incontinentia pigmenti achromians de Ito. Bull Dermatol 1969;76:553–555.
9. Ross DL, Liwnicz BH, Chun RWM, et al. Hypomelanosis of Ito (incontinentia pigmenti achromians). A clinicopathologic study: macrocephaly and gray matter heterotopias. Neurology 1982;32:1013–1016.
10. Pena L, Ruiz-Maldonado R, Tamayo L, et al. A. Incontinentia pigmenti achromians (Ito's hypomelanosis). Int J Dermatol 1977;16:194–202.
11. Pascual–Castroviejo I. Cuadros neurológicos que cursan con alteraciones en la piel. In: Neurologia Infantil. Barcelona: Editorial Científico Médica, 1983:649–712.
12. Sacrez R, Gigonnet J-M, Stoll C, Grosshans E, et al. Quatre cas de maladie d'Ito familiale (encéphalopathie congénitale et dyschromie). Discussion nosologique. Rev Int Pediatr 1970;7:5–23.
13. Maize JC, Headington JT, Lynch PJ. Systematized hypochromic nevus. Incontinentia pigmenti achromians of Ito. Arch Dermatol 1972;106:884–885.

14. Grosshans EM, Stoebner P, Bergoend H, et al. Incontinentia pigmenti achromians (Ito). Étude clinique et histopathologique. Dermatologica 1971;142:65–78.

15. Brown RM, Byrne JPH. Dental dysplasia in incontinentia pigmenti achromians (Ito). An unusual form. Br Dent J 1976;140:211–214.

16. Stewart RE, Funderburk S, Setoguchi Y. A malformation complex of ectrodactyly, clefting and hypomelanosis of Ito (incontinentia pigmenti achromians). Cleft Palate J 1979;16:358–362.

17. Ishikawa T, Kanayama M, Sugiyama K, et al. Hypomelanosis of Ito associated with benign tumors and chromosomal abnormalities: a neurocutaneous syndrome. Brain Dev 1985;7:45–49.

18. Donat JF, Walsworth DM, Turk LL. Focal cerebral atrophy in incontinentia pigmenti achromians. Am J Dis Child 1980;134:709–710.

19. Miller CA, Parker WD Jr. Hypomelanosis of Ito: association with a chromosomal abnormality. Neurology 1985;35:607–610.

20. Hamada T, Saito T, Sugai T, et al. Incontinentia pigmenti achromians (Ito). Arch Dermatol 1967;96:673–676.

21. Cram DL, Fukuyama K. Proceedings of the San Francisco Dermatological Society, March 31, 1973: unilateral systematized hypochromic nevus. Arch Dermatol 1974;109:416.

22. Jimbow K, Fitzpatrick TB, Szabo G, et al. Congenital circumscribed hypomelanosis: a characterization based on electron microscopic study of tuberous sclerosis, nevus depigmentosus and piebaldism. J Invest Dermatol 1975;64:50–62.

23. Pearce J. The central nervous system pathology in multiple neurofibromatosis. Neurology (Minneap) 1967;17:691–697.

24. O'Doherty NJ, Norman RM. Incontinentia pigmenti (Bloch–Sulzberger syndrome) with cerebral malformation. Dev Med Child Neurol 1968;10:168–174.

25. Rubin MB. Incontinentia pigmenti achromians. Multiple cases within a family. Arch Dermatol 1972;105:424–425.

26. Griffiths A, Payne C. Incontinentia pigmenti achromians. Arch Dermatol 1975;111:751–752.

Chapter 8
Other Autosomal Dominant Diseases

MANUEL R. GOMEZ

Waardenberg Syndrome I

The clinical features of this autosomal dominant disorder are frontal white forelock, heterochromia iridis, white eyelashes, lateral displacement of the inner canthus (dystopia canthorum) with or without cochlear deafness, leukoderma, premature graying of hair, and partially or completely albinotic fundi [1]. The deafness is probably related to inability to control endolymphatic fluid production. There are no neurologic deficits in these patients.

Waardenberg Syndrome II

This syndrome, separated from the Waardenberg syndrome by Arias [2], is characterized by the same features as Type I except that there is no dystopia canthorum. On the other hand, deafness is more frequent in Type II, and some patients may have vestibular symptoms. No other neurologic or neurosensory disturbances have been reported.

Dominant Piebald Trait with Neurologic Impairment

The clinical features of this syndrome are similar to the two forms of Waardenberg syndrome except for the lack of deafness and dystopia canthorum. Characteristically there is depigmentation of the skin on the medial portion of the forehead, chin, anterior chest, abdomen, and extremities, and white forelock and eyebrows. There is hyperpigmentation on the borders of the depigmented areas, sensorineural

hearing loss, cerebellar ataxia, impaired motor coordination, and mental retardation of variable severity [3].

Klein–Waardenberg Syndrome

Before Waardenberg reported the syndrome now under his name, Klein [4] reported the association of congenital anomalies of the upper limbs: hypoplasia of the muscles, flexion contractures, fusion of carpal bones, and syndactyly. In addition, the patients also exhibit other features of the Waardenberg syndrome.

Type VII Oculocerebral Albinism

This is described in Chapter 34 under Albinism.

References

1. Waardenberg PJ. A new syndrome combining developmental anomalies of the eyelids, eyebrows and nose root with pigmentary defects of the iris and head hair and with congenital deafness. Am J Human Genet 1951;3:195–253.
2. Arias S. Genetic heterogeneity in the Waardenberg syndrome. Birth Defects 1971;7:87–101.
3. Telfer MA, Sugar M, Jaeger EA, et al. Dominant piebald trait (white forelock and leukoderma) with neurological impairment. Am J Hum Genet 1971;23:383–389.
4. Klein D. Albinisme partiel (leucisme) accompagné de surdimutité, d'ostéomyodysplasie, de raideurs articulaires congénitales multiples et d'autres malformations congénitales. Arch Julius Klaus Stift 1947;22:336–342.

PART TWO

DISEASES WITH AUTOSOMAL RECESSIVE INHERITANCE

Chapter 9
Ataxia-Telangiectasia

ELENA BODER

Although ataxia-telangiectasia (A-T) can usually be diagnosed on purely clinical grounds, and often on inspection, it was peculiarly elusive until 1957 when it was first delineated clinicopathologically [1,2], establishing it as a disease entity, and given its name. Although it was clearly a familial syndrome, its three major components, all of them progressive—cerebellar ataxia, oculocutaneous telangiectasia, and sinopulmonary infection—were seemingly unrelated. After more than 25 years of diverse and exciting research developments, which have revealed A-T to be an increasingly complex multisystem disease, many of its facets are still seemingly unrelated.

Ataxia-telangiectasia* can now be defined as an autosomal recessive multisystem disorder comprising progressive cerebellar ataxia with onset in infancy, progressive oculocutaneous telangiectasia, and unusual susceptibility to progressive bronchopulmonary disease and to lymphoreticular neoplasia. Its multiple facets also include characteristic facies and posture; progressive apraxia of eye movements, simulating ophthalmoplegia; choreoathetosis; progeric changes of hair and skin; growth retardation; endocrine abnormalities, including ovarian dysgenesis and insulin-resistant diabetes; an abnormal immune mechanism with hypoplasia and occasional absence of the thymus gland; clinical and cellular radiosensitivity; chromosomal instability; and a DNA-repair/

In using the pronouns "we" and "our" in this chapter, I am referring to the work that Dr. Robert P. Sedgwick and I, longtime collaborators, have done, and to the patients we have followed. Special thanks are due to my husband, Dr. Nathaniel Levien, for his helpful criticism of the manuscript and his enduring interest in my study of A-T, to Sylvia Jarrico for her skillful editorial contributions, and to the newly established Ataxia-Telangiectasia Medical Research Foundation.

*The term ataxia-telangiectasia [1,2] is used predominantly in the literature. Synonyms include the eponyms Louis–Bar syndrome [3,4] and Boder–Sedgwick syndrome [4].

processing defect. Mental retardation, though it may occur, is not typical.

Reported in all races and regions of the world, A-T occurs equally among males and females and is transmitted as an autosomal recessive trait. In our experience its incidence is at least that of Friedreich's ataxia. In 1970, we were able to make a preliminary analysis of the prevalence of A-T in Los Angeles by relating the number of children and adolescents with A-T in the Schools for the Physically Handicapped to the total enrollment in the Los Angeles City School District. We arrived at an estimated prevalence of about 1 in 40,000 [5]. Based on their epidemiologic studies of A-T, Swift [7] recently estimated that the probable incidence of A-T is about 1 in 100,000 births.

Historical Review

The first description of patients with A-T was published by Syllaba and Henner [8] in 1926. They reported three adolescent Czech siblings with progressive choreoathetosis and striking ocular telangiectasia as having a variant of Ramsay Hunt's familial double athetosis. There was no postmortem examination.

In 1941, after a gap of 15 years, a second clinical description was published by Louis-Bar [9]. It was another clinical report without pathologic study: a 9-year-old Belgian boy with progressive cerebellar ataxia and extensive cutaneous telangiectasia distributed in nevoid patches but no family history. The author identified the syndrome as a previously undescribed entity belonging among the phakomatoses, either as a variant of the Sturge–Weber syndrome or as a separate new entity. Until Martin's paper [10] in 1964 called attention to the report by Syllaba and Henner, Louis-Bar's report was believed to be the first clinical description, and A–T was sometimes referred to as the Louis-Bar syndrome.

Both of these early case reports were lost in the literature, and the syndrome remained unknown until 1957 when two independent clinicopathologic reports appeared in two widely separated areas of the world. The first clinicopathologic report, based on eight cases, six of them familial, was by Boder and Sedgwick [1,2], who named the syndrome ataxia-telangiectasia. It included a report on the first autopsy of an A-T patient that noted the absence of the thymus and the ovaries. The second, by Biemond, was based on four familial cases and two autopsies, without reference to the thymus or the ovaries [11]. His report emphasized the occurrence of extrapyramidal manifestations in the absence of histopathologic findings in the basal ganglia. Both of the initial clinicopathologic reports [1,11] emphasized the heredofamilial nature of the syndrome and called attention to severe recurrent sinopulmonary infection as a third major component of the syndrome and as the main cause of death.

Wells and Shy [12] also published a report in 1957, this one on two sisters without an autopsy entitled "Progressive choreoathetosis with cutaneous telangiectasia." Like Syllaba and Henner, Wells and Shy classified the syndrome as a basal ganglia disorder rather than a cerebellar syndrome. This points out that the choreoathetotic component of A-T, now known to occur in about 85% of cases [13], may be severe enough in older children to overshadow the cerebellar ataxia.

In 1958, in a paper based on two nonfamilial cases, Centerwall and Miller [3] provided a fourth autopsy. Our second and third papers on the syndrome [2,14], in 1958 and 1960, differentiated A-T clinically and pathologically from Friedreich's ataxia and identified A-T as the only predominantly cerebellar degeneration of infancy and childhood.

With the rapid proliferation of reports in the world literature after 1958, within 4 years it was possible for us to develop a tabular analysis of 101 known cases that definitively confirmed the syndrome's stereotypical clinical symptomatology. It also identified lymphoreticular malignancy as the second most frequent cause of death [14], a finding definitively corroborated in 1964 [15].

The identification of susceptibility to sinopulmonary infection, in 1957, as a cardinal feature stimulated early immunologic studies of A-T. However, the results of serum electrophoresis were inconsistent [2,3,5]. Ataxia-telangiectasia was not established as an immunodeficiency disease until 1963, although the absence of the thymus was noted in our first autopsy report in 1957 and selective deficiency of serum IgA was first reported by Thieffry et al. [16] in 1961.

Peterson et al. [17] confirmed the inconstant hypogammaglobulinemia and the selective deficiency of serum IgA in 1963. In addition, they reported that their A-T patients had abnormal delayed hypersensitivity responses, were unresponsive to a variety of antigenic stimuli, and showed delayed and impaired skin homograft rejection. They postulated that a fundamental immunologic defect of A-T lies in the thymus gland and suggested that A-T patients may represent human counterparts of animals rendered immunologically incompetent by thymectomy at birth. This initial hypothesis was further supported by the findings of Peterson et al. [15] and others [5], both on autopsy and biopsy, that the thymus in A-T, although sometimes absent, was usually hypoplastic and so lacking in normal architecture as to resemble an embryonic thymus [1,2,15].

Independent concurrent studies further documented the immunologic defect in A-T in 1964 and emphasized dysgammaglobulinemia as a specific diagnostic feature [18,19]. In 1965 Eisen et al. [20] observed decreased peripheral lymphoid tissue, including tonsils and adenoids, and called attention to lymphopenia as an early sign. In contrast, in studies of patients with Friedreich's ataxia, Eisen et al. reported delayed hypersensitivity responses to be normal and Young et al. [19] demonstrated normal IgA levels. Lymphoid tissue abnormalities were extensively studied as an integral aspect of A-T in 1966 by Peterson et al. [21], who confirmed the presence of general lymphoid hypoplasia and found frequent structural abnormality of lymph nodes and tonsils.

In the first patient–family study of the immunologic aspects of A-T, reported by Epstein et al. [22] in 1966, depressed or absent delayed hypersensitivity responses were found in almost half of the parents and normal siblings as well as in all of the 19 patients. This is especially significant in light of the unusual family history of malignant neoplasms and leukemia among the parents and immediate relatives of A-T patients, first noted by Reed et al. in 1966 [23]. Through systematic epidemiologic genetic studies of A-T in 1976, Swift et al. [24] definitively established the increased predisposition among the parents and immediate families of A-T patients to cancer and diabetes and identified the types of cancer most frequently found.

Decreased in vitro blast cell transformation of A-T lymphocytes in response to phytohemagglutinin (PHA) was first reported in 1966 [25]. Having also found increased chromosomal breakage (20 to 30%)

in the cultured lymphocytes, Hecht et al. [26] suggested that chromosomal breakage may predispose A-T patients to lymphocytic leukemia and lymphoma. Their cytogenetic findings were soon confirmed by others [27], giving further support to the hypothesis that there is an inherent genetic defect in the lymphocytes of A-T patients.

A comprehensive historical review of the early immunologic, genetic, cytogenetic, endocrine, and neuropathologic aspects of A-T is available elsewhere [5,28–30]. There has been a rapid proliferation of research reports in the literature in the last decade, increasingly by laboratory scientists [29, 31–33]. In pursuit of A-T's pathogenesis, most of the studies focus on the cellular and molecular basis of the neurologic, immunologic, cytogenetic, radiobiological, and oncological aspects of A-T. It has become clear that immune dysfunction is only one of many defects in A-T patients. Among other established dysfunctions are a striking cellular radiosensitivity, with increased chromosomal instability following exposure of A-T cell cultures to ionizing radiation, and abnormality in DNA-repair/processing. Another emphasis in current research is on heterozygote detection in A-T families and prenatal diagnosis. The most significant research developments of the past decade are discussed in detail in two recently published books [29,30].

Clinical Observations

The clinical features of A-T, based on our review of 101 cases, are summarized elsewhere [14]. Since the classic clinical picture of A-T is now well known, I shall emphasize here the more subtle and variable signs that I have found to be helpful in making an early diagnosis and in diagnosing mild cases. Familiarity with the subtle signs and with the evolution of the clinical features of A-T from the early to the later stages is important in order to avoid the pitfalls in making a diagnosis. Our comprehensive discussions of all known clinical features of A-T, including variant features, appear elsewhere [5,28].

Neurologic Features

Ataxia is always the first and presenting symptom, having its onset in infancy and typically becoming apparent when the child begins to walk, usually between 12 and 14 months. Predominantly a truncal ataxia, it is first manifested in a swaying of the head and trunk when the child stands and even on sitting.

Both ataxia of gait and truncal ataxia are slowly and steadily progressive. However, the normal development of motor skills between the ages of 2 and 5 years tends to mask the progression of ataxia, so that an actual improvement in gait may be reported by the parents. At this point a diagnosis of cerebral palsy, ataxic or athetoid, is frequently made.

Beyond the age of 5 years, the progression of the ataxia becomes increasingly apparent and a misdiagnosis of Friedreich's ataxia may be made, particularly if the telangiectasia has not yet appeared. At the typical rate of progression, the child requires a wheelchair by the age of 10 or 11 years, even when muscular strength continues to be good.

Dyssynergia and intention tremor of the extremities become prominent features later. Myoclonic jerks of the trunk and extremities, particularly on intention, occur in an occasional A-T patient, but not before the age of 9 or 10. The myoclonus may result in sudden and frequent falling and, in itself, make the child nonambulatory. Romberg's sign is negative, but it is often reported to be positive from the failure to observe that swaying of the trunk is equally marked with the eyes open or closed. Slow initiation and performance of all voluntary activity and muscular hypotonia are characteristic and are also manifestations of cerebellar symptomatology. Deep reflexes may be normal in the younger child but are usually diminished or absent after the age of 7 or 8; the plantar responses are flexor or equivocal. All modalities of sensation are intact, although vibratory and position sense are usually impaired in older patients.

Intact sensation and a negative Romberg's sign are helpful in differentiating the cerebellar ataxia of A-T from Friedreich's ataxia, in which the ataxia is predominantly spinal, or sensory, and Romberg's sign is positive. The early absence of spinal signs in younger A-T patients is consistent with histopathologic findings that significant spinal cord involvement occurs much later than the devastating early cerebellar degeneration.

Choreoathetosis is the most prominent extrapyramidal feature in A-T [11,14]. In some patients it may be severe enough to mask the presence of ataxia [7,12]. In general, the choreoathetotic component is more prominent in older than in younger children, in whom the purely cerebellar picture predominates.

Characteristic facies and postural attitudes, observed in all of the children, are part of the cerebellar hypotonia and ataxia [2,5]. The facies is usually relaxed, dull, sad, and seemingly inattentive, which is in sharp contrast to the cheerful, alert appearance when the patient is smiling. The hypotonic cerebellar facies, though often described in the literature as mask-like, appears so only in older A-T patients, in whom the facial skin has become atrophic and inelastic. Stooping, with the shoulders drooped and the head sunk forward and usually tilted to one side, becomes the characteristic posture, and gives an impression of muscular weakness and fatigue that contributes to an appearance of premature aging. Dystonic posturing of the fingers is characteristic. In fact, a 10-year-old A-T patient with severe progressive dystonia has recently been described [34]. One patient I have followed developed a torsion dystonia at age 15; two other patients, aged 27 and 41, had, when last seen, in addition to signs of progressive spinal muscular atrophy of the extremities, a marked torticollis with dystonic posturing of the fingers and secondary contractures (Figure 9.1).

Oculomotor signs are present in virtually all A-T patients and are diagnostically important, particularly since they frequently precede the appearance of the ocular telangiectasia. Like the ataxia, the disorder of eye movements is steadily progressive.

Voluntary eye movements are slowly initiated and then interrupted. The eyes halt midway on lateral and upward gaze. Rapid, almost spasmodic blinking and head thrusts occur with the halting, apparently in an effort to overcome the interruption of movement. Coarse nystagmoid oscillations, or fixation nystagmus, occurs on the return to forward gaze. In contrast to ophthalmoplegia, the movements can be completed given sufficient time. When conjugate gaze is attempted, the head tends to turn before the eyes do. The lag in eye movements is especially apparent

when the head turns suddenly to the side toward a target; the eyes first deviate tonically in the opposite direction and then slowly follow the head toward the target. The abnormalities of conjugate gaze are seen only on voluntary movement; the eye movements appear smooth and full in range on involuntary movement, as when the head is moved passively from side to side. Conjugate convergence is incomplete, although full convergence of each eye separately is possible [2,5].

The complex oculomotor signs in A-T, initially described as a "peculiarity of eye movements" [1,2], have been extensively studied. Smith and Cogan [35] reported optokinetic nystagmus to be absent and concluded that the oculomotor disorder in A-T closely resembles congenital oculomotor apraxia. Thieffry et al. [16] identified the disorder with the "viscosity" of eye movements described in certain cerebellar and spinocerebellar degenerations.

More recently, electro-oculographic studies by Baloh et al. [36] have demonstrated the difficulty in initiating voluntary and involuntary saccades, and the increased reaction time of voluntary saccades. The authors emphasized that the oculomotor signs of A-T differ from those of other cerebellar degenerations, in that they combine features of both cerebellar and extrapyramidal disorders. A later electro-oculographic study indicated that the oculomotor abnormality of A-T is sufficiently different from that of Friedreich's ataxia to be valuable in their differential diagnosis. [37].

Non-neurologic Cardinal Features

Telangiectasia usually has a later onset than the ataxia, typically first noticed between the ages of 3 and 6 years. Steadily progressive, like the ataxia, it spreads in a characteristic symmetrical pattern. It is first noticed in the angles of the eyes and spreads horizontally across the exposed portion of the bulbar conjuctivae as fine, bright red, symmetrical horizontal streaks (Figure 9.2). By the age of 5 or 6 years the ocular telangiectasia usually spreads sufficiently to the rest of the conjunctiva to simulate conjunctivitis but characteristically fades out at the border of the cornea (Figure 9.2).

Subtle telangiectasia may also involve the internal ear, the eyelids, the butterfly area of the face, the creases and V of the neck, the antecubital and popliteal spaces, in which they may be mistaken for fine petechiae, and less frequently, the dorsum of the hands and feet and the hard and soft palate. These are essentially the areas most exposed to the sun and wind or subject to irritation.

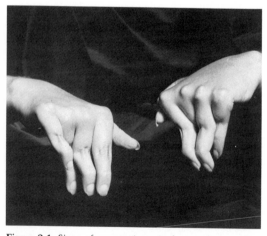

Figure 9.1. Signs of progressive spinal muscular atrophy in a 27-year-old female with ataxia-telangiectasia. Note interosseous atrophy with striking combined flexion-extension contractures of fingers, suggestive of early dystonic posturing.

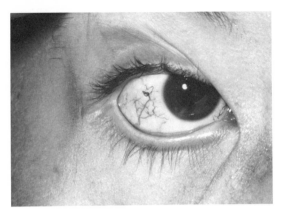

Figure 9.2. Patient at 9 years of age, showing advanced telangiectasia of the bulbar conjunctiva with characteristic fading out at the border of the cornea. Note telangiectasia on the bridge of the nose.

It is very rare for the telangiectatic vessels of A-T to hemorrhage [38–40]. The telangiectases of A-T were originally thought to be arterial in origin, but capillary microscopy indicates that they are of predominantly venous origin and are not arteriovenous fistulas [23,41,42]. Long-term observation suggests that they are progeric changes, since in location and appearance they resemble those found in the aged.

Progeric changes of hair and skin are a cardinal feature of A-T (Figure 9.3). Some gray hairs are usually found even in young children if carefully looked for; diffuse graying of the hair may continue to increase slightly through adolescence, but is no more than normally progressive thereafter. The facial skin tends to become atrophic and sclerodermoid in adolescence; atrophic areas resembling large varicella scars may appear. The ears tend to become inelastic. The wasted face, the scattered gray hairs, the oculocutaneous telangiectasia, and the stooped posture give the older children an appearance of premature aging. Chronic seborrheic blepharitis is frequent, simulating in association with the ocular telangiectasia a blepharoconjunctivitis [2].

In a dermatologic study of 22 of our patients, Reed et al. [23] and Epstein et al. [42] reported a variety of lesions. Pigmentary changes were frequent, occurring in a mottled pattern of hyper- and hypopigmentation with cutaneous atrophy and telangiectasia, similar to the poikiloderma seen in scleroderma, advanced actinodermatitis, or radiodermatitis as well as in premature aging. Other skin changes included café-au-lait spots, usually single rather than multiple; frequent hyperpigmented macules, resembling large freckles; and occasional vitiligo. Seborrheic dermatitis, keratosis pilaris, common warts, and in female patients hirsutism of the arms and legs are

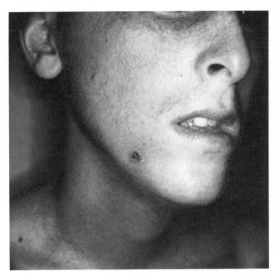

Figure 9.3. Progeric skin changes in a 21-year-old male, showing pronounced facial telangiectases with cutaneous hyperpigmentation and atrophy. The deep scar on the right side of the chin resulted from the removal of a basal cell carcinoma.

also frequently found. Multiple senile keratoses [38] and basal cell carcinomas of the face have been reported in patients in their twenties [23,43] (Figure 9.3). A review of the common and uncommon cutaneous findings in A-T has recently been published [44].

Biopsy specimens have shown that the typical skin changes in A-T are similar to those seen in cumulative actinic damage and thus are suggestive of progeric changes [5,23,42]. The predilection of both the progeric skin changes and the oculocutaneous telangiectases for sun-exposed areas further suggests increased propensity to actinic damage.

Retardation of somatic growth with significant dwarfing is a prominent feature of A-T that is found in most patients [2,5,28]. The heights and weights of children between 4 and 7 years of age are typically at the tenth percentile and tend to fall below the third percentile by adolescence. Only an exceptional A-T patient achieves somatic growth at the fiftieth percentile or beyond. In my experience the A-T patients who develop normal puberty are the ones most likely to achieve somatic growth within the normal range [6,45].

The stunting of growth is not well understood. Chronic sinopulmonary disease may be a contributing factor, but stunting of growth also occurs in its absence. Other factors may include the hypogonadism typical of A-T [2,46,47] as well as the thymic dysplasia, as suggested by Peterson et al. [15,17]. Endocrine studies done on a number of our patients give no evidence of hypothyroidism or hypopituitarism.

Other Neurologic Features

The dysarthric speech noted in all A-T patients is of cerebellar type [2,5], slow, slurred, labored, and slowly initiated. A stereotypical inflection pattern develops as the ataxia progresses, and the speech may become somewhat explosive and indistinct. Drooling is frequent.

Mental retardation is not a characteristic feature of A-T. However, the results of psychometric testing show wide scatter, and IQ scores may drop below the normal range as the disease progresses. In fact, in our tabular analysis of 101 cases, mental deficiency was reported in one-third of the 22 patients on whom information was available [14].

Analysis of serial test results in the early decades of life gives no indication that cognitive function is lost. Rather, the drop in IQ scores that tends to occur as the disease progresses appears to reflect an increasing disparity between mental age and chronological age. It is a leveling off of mental function rather than an actual mental deterioration. Most of our A-T patients have been able to function well enough academically to complete high school. Two of them have completed college. Some older patients in their twenties and thirties, however, have shown a selective severe loss of short-term memory, suggestive of premature aging [5,43].

The equable disposition characteristic of patients with A-T helps them to make a good adjustment to their progressively severe handicap. They are generally socially responsive, appreciative, and undemanding. The parents comment on their being "easy to take care of " and having "a good sense of humor."

Pathologic Observations

The causes of death in A-T, based on the current total of 58 complete autopsies reported in the available literature [48–90] are summarized in Table 9.1. Despite the longer survival of A-T patients with the

Table 9.1. Causes of Death in Ataxia-Telangiectasia Based on a Review of the 58 Published Complete Autopsies

Year	Authors	Sex	Age	Cause of Death
1957–58	Boder and Sedgwick [1] (n = 1)	F	10½	Sinopulmonary infection with chronic progressive bronchiectasis, pulmonary fibrosis, and pneumonitis
1957–59	Biemond and van Bolhuis [11,48] (n = 2)	F	15	Chronic progressive bronchiectasis and pneumonitis
		M	15	Chronic progressive bronchiectasis and pneumonitis
1958	Centerwall and Miller [3] (n = 1)	M	12	Chronic progressive sinopulmonary disease with severe bronchiectasis and pneumonitis
1962–63	Bowden et al. [49] (n = 1)	F	15	Diffuse bronchiectasis with miliary tuberculosis
1963	Guttman and Lemli [50] (n = 1)	F	8	Staphylococcus pneumonia with multiple pulmonary abscesses, empyema, and fibrinous pericarditis
1964	Dunn et al. [51] (n = 1)	F	17	Bronchiectasis with pneumonia and ovarian dysgerminoma
1964	Osetowska and Traczynska [52] (n = 1)	F	7	Bronchiectasis with pneumonia and pulmonary cyst
1964	Peterson et al. [15] (n = 2)	F	8	Generalized small cell lymphosarcoma and chronic pulmonary infection
		M	5½	Pneumococcal meningitis and generalized reticuloendotheliosis of lymphoid tissue
1966	Centerwall and Centerwall [53] (n = 1)	M	23	Bronchopneumonia
		M	10	Acute leukemia with massive leukemic infiltration
1966	Shuster et al. [55] (n = 1)	F	13	Cerebellar medulloblastoma and acute pneumonitis
1966	Sourander et al. [56] (n = 1)	F	14	Acute purulent bronchopneumonia
1966	Strich [57]	M	15	Acute confluent bronchopneumonia

Table 9.1. *Continued*

Year	Authors	Sex	Age	Cause of Death
	(n = 3)	F	11	Chronic pulmonary infection and bilateral pneumothorax
		F	12	Pulmonary infection and collapse
1966	Thieffry et al. [58]	F	5	Giant cell pneumonia complicating measles
	(n = 1)			
1966–67	Harley et al. [54]	F	6	Chronic bronchitis and pneumonia
	(n = 3)	F	7	Malignant lymphoma and pseudomonas pneumonia
1967	Gotoff et al. [59]	M	10½	Lymphosarcoma, acute severe bronchopneumonia, and untoward effect of radiation; tuberous sclerosis
	(n = 1)			
1967	Hassler [60]	F	17	Acute purulent, confluent bronchopneumonia
	(n = 1)			
1967	Miller and Chatten [47]	F	11	Severe acute and chronic pulmonary infection
	(n = 1)			
1967	Solitare and Lopez [61]	F	14	Acute bronchopneumonia
	(n = 1)			
1968	Solitare [62]	F	22	Pulmonary fibrosis, bronchiectasis, and acute bronchopneumonia
	(n = 1)			
1968	Aguilar et al. [46][a]	M	21	Malignant lymphoma and chronic sinopulmonary disease with bronchiectasis and pneumonia
	(n = 5)	F	10	Reticulum cell lymphoma, bronchiectasis, and extensive pneumonitis
		M	19	Pulmonary fibrosis and bronchiectasis; severe acute and chronic pneumonitis
		M	10	Bronchiectasis and pulmonary fibrosis
1968	Dorantes et al. [39]	M	9	Complications of exploratory laparotomy for rectal hemorrhages
	(n = 1)			
1968	Morgan et al. [63]	M	9	Hodgkin's disease and lymphomatous pneumonitis; complications of radiation therapy
	(n = 1)			
1969	Castaigne et al. [64]	M	7	Diffuse histiocytosarcoma
	(n = 1)			
1969	Haerer et al. [65]	F	19	Mucinous adenocarcinoma of the stomach
	(n = 1)			
1969	Itatsu and Uno [66]	F	11	Complications of pneumoretrography for examination of thymus in presence of chronic pulmonary disease
	(n = 1)			
1969	Scott [67]	M	8 mos.	Acute pneumonia
	(n = 1)			
1969	Terplan and Krauss [68]	F	18	Bronchiectasis and pneumonia
	(n = 1)			
1969	Teleb et al. [69]	M	9	Acute lymphoblastic leukemia
	(n = 1)			
1970	Feigin et al. [70]	F	30 mos.	Reticulum cell sarcoma; granulocytopenia and oropharyngeal ulcerations; untoward reaction to chemotherapy
	(n = 1)			
1970	Cawley and Schenken [71]	F	9	IgM monoclonal gammopathy; diffuse plasmacytosis; necrotizing arteritis of kidney, liver, bone marrow, and lungs
	(n = 1)			
1970	Matsuo et al. [72]	F	14	Bronchiectasis, pulmonary fibrosis, and pneumonia; follicular adenoma of the thyroid gland; hypoplastic spleen
	(n = 1)			
1971	Grossi–Bianchi et al. [73]	F	6	Lymphatic leukemia
	(n = 1)			
1972	Hoerni et al. [74]	M	23	Acute lymphoblastic leukemia with generalized leukemic infiltrations
	(n = 1)			
1972	Navarro and Martin [75]	M	9	Lymphocytic lymphosarcoma
	(n = 1)			

Table 9.1. *Continued*

Year	Authors	Sex	Age	Cause of Death
1973	Hecht et al. [76] (n = 1)	M	23	Bronchiectasis and pulmonary fibrosis
1975	Goldsmith and Hart [77] (n = 1)	F	17	Ovarian gonadoblastoma with contralateral dysgerminoma; chronic bronchiectasis with pulmonary fibrosis
1975	Scully and McNealy [78] (n = 1)	M	23	Interstitial pneumonitis and bronchopneumonia; hyperplasia of lymphoid tissue of unknown cause
1976	Buyse et al. [79][b] (n = 1)	F	16	Ovarian gonadoblastoma with contralateral dysgerminoma; chronic bronchiectasis with pulmonary fibrosis and respiratory failure
1976	De Leon et al. [80] (n = 1)	M	17	Chronic pulmonary disease with recurrent spontaneous pneumothorax, bronchopneumonia, and pulmonary insufficiency
1977	Cameron et al. [81] (n = 1)	M	12	Acute lymphoblastic T-cell leukemia complicated by pneumonia following chemotherapy
1977–79	Amromin et al. [43,84] (n = 1)	F	32	Chronic T-cell leukemia, with uterine leiomyosarcoma, complicated by late-onset chronic bronchopulmonary disease with bilateral pulmonary infiltrates and pleural effusion; possible untoward reaction to chemotherapy
1978	Levitt et al. [82] (n = 1)	F	26	Atypical subacute T-cell leukemia complicated by terminal bronchopneumonia due to *Pneumocystis carinii* and *Candida albicans* following chemotherapy
1979	Agamanolis and Greenstein [83] (n = 1)	M	31	Unresolved bilateral bronchopneumonia with pleural effusion and pneumothorax
1979	Krishna Kumar et al. [85] (n = 1)	F	24	Hepatocellular carcinoma with terminal pneumonia and pleural effusion following laparotomy
1980	Yoshitomi et al. [86] (n = 1)	M	22	Renal cell carcinoma, hepatoma, and malignant hepatic mixed tumor with acute pulmonary insufficiency
1981	Pascual–Pascual et al. [87] (n = 1)	M	4½	Widespread lymphosarcoma, including infiltration of the cerebrum, basal ganglia, cerebellum, and meninges; chronic tracheobronchitis and pneumonia
1982	Casaril et al. [40] (n = 1)	M	26	Decompensated hepatic cirrhosis following hepatitis, with hemorrhage from ruptured esophageal varices; multiple cerebral hemorrhages
1982	Pritchard et al. [88] (n = 1)	F	3½	Stage 1A Hodgkin's disease; untoward reaction to radiation therapy, with terminal esophagitis and pneumonitis
1984	Perry et al. [89] (n = 1)	M	25	Repeated episodes of aspiration pneumonia in last year of life
1985	Weinstein et al. [90] (n = 1)	F	15	Hepatocellular carcinoma with metastases, ascitis, gastrointestinal hemorrhage, and terminal pneumonitis

Summary

Cause of Death	Number of Autopsies	Percent
Pulmonary disease alone	27	46
Malignancy alone	12	21
Both pulmonary and neoplastic disease	16	28
Other	3	5
	58	100

Source: modified from Boder [6].

[a]One of the autopsy reports by Aguilar et al. is a review of the autopsy reported by Boder and Sedgwick in 1957–58.

[b]The patient reported by Buyse et al. appears to be the same as the one reported by Goldsmith and Hart in 1975.

introduction of new antibiotics, pulmonary disease is still the most frequent cause of death and neoplasia the second most frequent. In fact, pulmonary disease and neoplasia, separately or combined, account for virtually all deaths among A-T patients on whom autopsy reports are available.

Malignant lymphomas, including small cell lymphosarcoma, reticulum cell sarcoma, or histiocytosarcoma, and Hodgkin's disease, markedly predominate among the reported neoplasias (Table 9.1). Among the other types of neoplasia reported in association with A-T are cerebellar medulloblastoma [55] and astrocytoma [6]; glioma of the frontal lobe [19]; ovarian dysgerminoma, gonadoblastoma [51,77,79], and cystadenofibroma [43]; uterine leiomyoma and leiomyosarcoma [43]; adenocarcinoma of the stomach [65]; basal cell carcinoma [23,43]; follicular adenoma of the thyroid gland [72]; hepatocellular carcinoma [85,90] and hepatoma with malignant hepatic mixed tumor and renal cell carcinoma [86]. A cyst of the adenohypophysis [51] and an intracranial angioma [5] have also been described. Monoclonal gammopathy with diffuse plasmocytosis has been reported in one patient [71]. Acute lymphocytic leukemia has been frequently reported as a cause of death in A-T [69,73,91]. T-cell lymphocytic leukemia has recently been reported in three female patients ranging in age from 26 to 50 years and in a 12-year-old boy [43,81,82,92]. Tabular analyses of the types of neoplasia in A-T appear elsewhere [5,93,94].

On the basis of their study of malignancy in immunodeficiency disease, Gatti and Good [93] have estimated the incidence of malignant neoplasms among A-T patients to be 10 to 15%.j Spector et al. [94] reported that in their ongoing study of malignant neoplasms A-T accounts for about one-third of all the cases of malignancy in 17 primary immunodeficiency diseases. In a recent review, based on 45 reported A-T patients, of the types of malignant neoplasms in A-T, Yoshitomi et al. [86] found that lymphoreticular neoplasms and leukemia predominate in patients under the age of 15 years and that epithelial tumors predominate in patients beyond 16 years. Since epithelial tumors are characteristic of older adults, the authors regard this observation as further evidence of the progeric changes that occur in A-T.

In the 58 complete autopsy reports that have been published (Table 9.1), 12 deaths (21%) were due to malignancy alone, 27 (46%) to pulmonary disease alone, and 16 (28%) to a combination of both. The 3 remaining deaths were attributable to other causes [39,40,66]. Three of the early autopsy reports called attention for the first time to untoward and ultimately fatal reactions to radiation and chemotherapy in conventional doses and suggested that these measures are contraindicated in the treatment of malignancies associated with A-T [59,63,70]. This hypersensitivity of A-T patients to radiation therapy and chemotherapy is corroborated in several other recent publications [81,88,91,95,96].

Neuropathologic Observations

A comprehensive historical review of the pathologic and neuropathologic findings in A-T appears elsewhere [5,28]. The discussion here emphasizes the most provocative pathologic findings in our own series of 11 autopsies [2,5,43,46] and the significant new findings in the 3 recent autopsy reports on older patients, reviewed in some detail in a recent publication [6].

The neuropathologic hallmark of the disease is diffuse cortical cerebellar degeneration, involving mainly the Purkinje and granular cells and to a much lesser extent the basket cells (Figure 9.4). Neuronal degeneration is usually more severe in the vermis than in the cerebellar hemispheres [11,48]. Degenerative changes in the dentate and olivary nuclei were noted in several of the early autopsies, and slight pallor of the fasciculus gracilis was observed in the first autopsy, but no other abnormalities were found in the cerebrum, brain stem, or spinal cord [1–3,48,49]. Except for some acute neuronal changes in the corpus striatum observed in one autopsy [52], no changes had been demonstrated in the basal ganglia until recently. The absence of changes in the basal ganglia was unexpected in view of the frequent choreoathetotic component in A-T.

With the increasing number of autopsies, it became apparent that the changes in the CNS were more diffuse, especially in older patients, than they were initially reported to be, although the striking degenerative changes were still seen predominantly in the cerebellum. The CNS lesions are of great variety, including often extensive changes in the spinal cord and spinal ganglia along with more subtle or inconstant changes in the cerebrum, basal ganglia, and brain stem. Significant changes have also been demonstrated in peripheral nerve and skeletal muscle [61,97–100].

The four most recent complete autopsy reports [40,43,80,83], which include the three oldest patients [40,43,83] on whom autopsies have been published, describe new findings as well as a more widespread degenerative process in the nervous system than has been previously encountered.

Among the findings in the cerebellum, in addition

Figure 9.4. Section through cerebellar folia showing diffuse absence of Purkinje cells with many empty baskets and marked attenuation of the granular layer. (Same 32 year old female patient as in Figures 9.5, 9.6, 9.7, and 9.8.) Bielschowsky's stain (original magnification × 110). (From Amromin et al. [43]; courtesy of J Neuropathol Exp Neurol.)

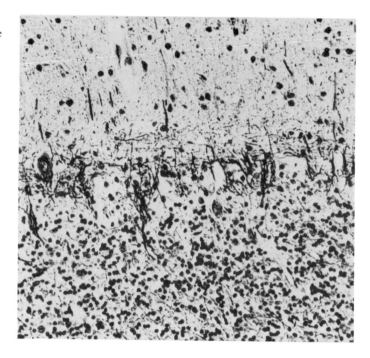

to the more extensive degenerative changes, are dystrophic changes involving the dendrites and axons of the Purkinje cells, including axonal torpedoes, and eosinophilic inclusion bodies in the cytoplasm and dendrites of some of the Purkinje cells [43,46,57,80,83]. Vinters et al. [101] reported the presence of ectopic Purkinje cells and interpreted this as evidence for the expression of the A-T genes in embryonic life.

The reported changes in the cerebrum and brain stem in the early autopsies were not uniform and were regarded as relatively minor. Frequently, no changes were noted [46,51,61]. In the four most recent autopsies [40,43,80,83], however, the findings in the cerebrum include moderate cortical gliosis of the central and parietal gyri, numerous neurofibrillary tangles in large neurons of the cerebral cortex and hippocampus, and lipofuscin-like pigment in the cortical neurons.

In addition to the neuronal degeneration in the dentate and olivary nuclei noted in the early autopsies, the changes in the brain stem later reported include neuroaxonal dystrophy in the tegmentum of the medulla [46], with axonal swellings, or Schollen, in the nuclei gracilis and cuneatus, similar to those seen in neuroaxonal dystrophy due to vitamin-E deficiency. All four of the most recent autopsy reports [40,43,80,83] described a more advanced involvement of the brain stem nuclei, especially the nuclei of the cranial nerves, and degenerative changes in the

substantia nigra, including both severe loss of pigment and loss of nerve cells with gliosis. Eosinophilic intracytoplasmic inclusions in the pigmented neurons of the substantia nigra, identified as Lewy bodies, were reported for the first time [83].

In addition to the neuronal changes in the corpus striatum noted in an earlier autopsy [52], the findings in the most recent autopsies are a small hamartomatous tumor in the thalamus [80], mild gliosis of the thalamic and caudate nuclei, occasional small vascular anomalies [83], and numerous neurofibrillary tangles throughout the basal ganglia, with many of the neurons containing lipofuscin granules [43]. However, the new findings in the basal ganglia in the autopsies on older patients still fail to explain the choreoathetotic component in A-T, which is an early and very frequent feature of the disease.

Of the 21 autopsies to date in which the spinal cord has been examined [6], only 2 demonstrated no abnormalities [49,66]. The reported changes include diffuse demyelination in the posterior columns, especially in the fasciculus gracilis (Figure 9.5), with the variable presence of microglial cells and loss of axons; glial nodules in the white matter of the spinal cord [57]; and partial demyelination of the spinocerebellar tracts [53,58] and, less frequently, of the corticospinal tracts [43,80,83]. Degenerative and dystrophic changes in the neurons of the anterior horns, first described by Aguilar et al. [46], have been noted frequently and are consistent with the

Figure 9.5. Section through lumbar cord, showing extensive demyelination of posterior columns and to a lesser degree of the lateral columns. Luxol fast blue–PAS stain (original magnification × 4). (From Amromin et al. [43]; courtesy of J Neuropathol Exp Neurol.)

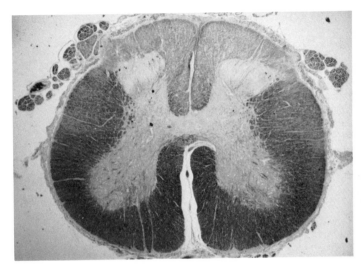

clinical picture of progressive spinal muscle atrophy that occurs in older patients and with the denervation atrophy of distal skeletal muscle demonstrated on autopsy as well as biopsy [61,99,100]. Another distinctive neuropathologic feature of A-T that is confirmed in the four most recent autopsies is bizarre dystrophic changes and nucleomegaly of satellite cells in the dorsal root and sympathetic ganglia and in the Schwann cells of peripheral nerves. A sural nerve biopsy specimen from a 38-year-old patient, studied by electron microscopy [99], showed no evidence of demyelination in the myelin sheaths, but revealed striking cytoplasmic lipid cytosomes, including so-called zebra bodies in Schwann cells, perineurial smooth muscle cells, and endothelial cells. This finding has been confirmed in other electron microscopic studies [100].

Early reports on vascular pathology in the CNS were inconsistent. Enlarged venules in the cerebellum and dentate nuclei, suggestive of telangiectases, were reported in only a few of the early autopsies [2,3,56,58]. Other autopsy reports emphasized the absence of vascular anomaly [46,48,49,57,60]. Sourander et al. [56] were the first to report vascular changes in the spinal cord suggestive of telangiectases. Terplan and Krauss [68] reported perivascular hemosiderotic glial scars in the pallium, concluding that they might be the result of stasis in the capillaries and veins within the cerebral white matter.

Distinctive vascular abnormalities, widely distributed in the cerebral white matter and to a lesser extent in the brain stem and spinal cord, have been found in the autopsies on all three of the oldest patients [40,43,83]. First described by Amromin and Boder [84], these gliovascular nodules consist of prominent dilated capillary loops, many with fibrin thrombi, with perivascular hemorrhages and hemosiderosis, surrounded by demyelinated white matter, reactive gliosis, and numerous atypical astrocytes (Figure 9.6), some of them containing eosinophilic cytoplasmic inclusions. The gliovascular abnormalities were only occasionally seen in the cerebral cortex and the basal ganglia [43,83]. Unexpectedly, none at all were seen in the cerebellum. It has been suggested that the gliovascular abnormalities are either hamartomatous in origin or, more likely, due to a progressive degenerative vascular process [43,83]. In addition, Casaril et al. [40] reported two macroscopic areas of hemorrhagic infarction in the cerebral white matter as well as multiple pinpoint hemorrhages. Vascular abnormality in the CNS can therefore be considered a feature of A-T in older patients. It is so variable and inconstant in younger patients, however, that it cannot account for the devastating early cerebellar degeneration or the later degenerative changes in the spinal cord. The interrelationship between the neurologic and vascular components of the disease remains obscure.

Nucleocytomegaly

Large, bizarre, hyperchromatic nuclei, often irregular in shape, were first described in the anterior pituitary by Bowden et al. [49] and in the spinal ganglia and peripheral nerves by Strich [57]. As first noted by Aguilar et al. [46] and confirmed in later autopsy reports [43,75,80,83], the nucleocytomegaly in A-T involves cells in virtually all organs and tissues of the body, including the CNS—the anterior pituitary, thymus, thyroid, and adrenal glands, liver, kidney,

Figure 9.6. Gliovascular nodule with partial occlusion of vessels by fibrin thrombi. *(Upper left)* Thrombus also distends large feeding vessel. There is pronounced gliosis around the vascular channels, and spongiosis and slight demyelination of adjoining white matter. Phosphotungstic acid hematoxylin stain (original magnification × 110). (From Amromin et al. [43]; courtesy of J Neuropathol Exp Neurol.)

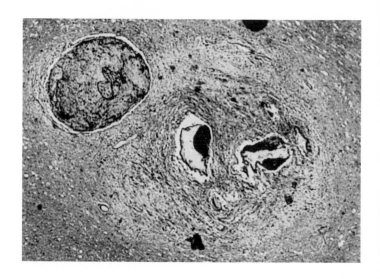

lung, heart, epididymis, smooth muscle, and capsular cells of the spinal ganglia, myenteric plexus, and peripheral nerves (Figures 9.7, 9.8).

Similar nucleomegalic changes have been found in association with progressive multifocal leukoencephalopathy (PML), which may develop under conditions of long-standing immunosuppression and in other virus-induced lesions. However, electron microscopy failed to demonstrate any virus particles in the autopsy of our oldest patient [43], and viral isolation studies performed on brain tissue obtained at autopsy from another of our A-T patients failed to detect a viral agent. Studies seeking evidence of C-type RNA tumor virus in dermal fibroblasts cultured from skin biopsy specimens from several of our A-T patients also gave negative results [102]. In addition, three species of primates were inoculated with brain tissue extracts obtained at autopsy from two of our patients, with negative results [Gajdusek DC, Gibbs C: personal communication, 1973]. Nucleocytomegaly has also been found in association with normal aging [46,103] and has been described in two recently autopsied cases of progeria [104].

Progeric Changes in the CNS

The progeric changes in the CNS reported by Amromin et al. [43] include occasional Alzheimer's plaques, neurofibrillary tangles in neurons of the cerebral cortex, hippocampus, basal ganglia, and spinal cord, with granules of lipofuscin in many of the neurons and in satellite cells of the dorsal root ganglia and Schwann cells. Other changes in the CNS that Kamoshita et al. [103] regarded as evidence of precocious aging include axonal dystrophy in Goll's nu-

clei, generalized nucleomegaly, notably in the spinal ganglia, and the Marinesco bodies that were observed in the pigmented neurons of the substantia nigra and locus ceruleus in a 21-year-old patient [46]. In addition, the gliovascular nodules in the cerebral white matter found in the autopsies on the three oldest patients (26 to 32 years of age) [40,43,83] are suggestive of progeric degenerative vascular changes (Figure 9.6).

In a recent neurochemical study of the autopsied brain of a 25-year-old A-T patient, Perry et al. [89] found glutamic acid and phosphoethanolamine content and gamma-aminobutyric acid (GABA) receptor binding to be markedly reduced in the cerebellar cortex, while GABA was greatly reduced in the dentate nucleus. Phosphoethanolamine was the only neurochemical compound found to be markedly deficient in both cerebellar and extracerebellar brain regions.

Course and Prognosis

Ataxia of gait and fatigability on walking have usually progressed by the age of 10 or 11 years to a point where the child is confined to a wheelchair, in spite of continuing good muscular strength. As has been noted, the purely cerebellar picture of A-T gradually evolves in the direction of Friedreich's ataxia [5,10] and progresses to include peripheral neuropathy [5,28,97] and, eventually, progressive spinal muscular atrophy [43,83,98], but usually not before age 25. Most patients surviving beyond adolescence develop denervation muscle atrophy and spinal signs such as loss of vibratory and position sense. This neurological progression is consistent with

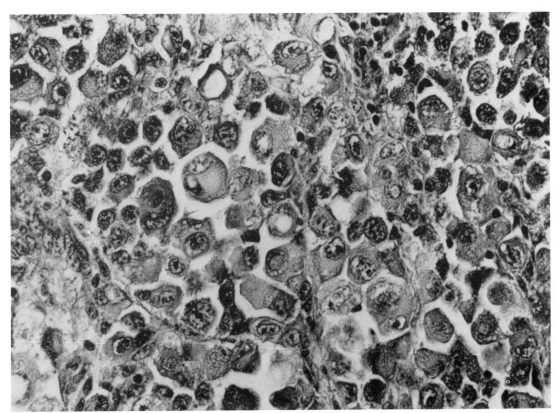

Figure 9.7. Representative portion of anterior pituitary showing marked cellular atypism with nucleocytomegaly and bilobed or multinucleated cells. Hematoxylin and eosin stain (original magnification × 400). (From Boder [6]; courtesy of Alan R. Liss.)

the degenerative changes in the anterior horn cells [46,58] and posterior columns [5,43,46,80,83] of the spinal cord found at autopsy and with changes in peripheral nerves found on both autopsy and biopsy [97,99,100].

The evolution of A-T to include progressive spinal muscular atrophy is clearly illustrated by the two oldest reported patients, aged 42 and 38, both of whom died at age 50 [92,98,99]. Both patients showed marked distal atrophy and gross fasciculations of muscle, with secondary flexion contractures of the fingers and bilateral foot drop. The electromyograms were consistent with denervation [98]. Muscle biopsy, though showing changes compatible with a myopathy, was also suggestive of denervation atrophy. Our oldest autopsied patient showed similar clinical and laboratory evidence of progressive spinal muscular atrophy [43]. Our two current oldest patients, aged 27 and 44 years, also show marked distal atrophy, with striking flexion contractures of the fingers and bilateral foot drop (Figure 9.1).

Until recently, death occurred typically in early or middle adolescence, usually from bronchopulmonary infection and less frequently from malignancy, or a combination of both (Table 9.1). In the absence of chronic bronchopulmonary disease and lymphoreticular malignancy, however, A-T is consistent with survival into the fifth and even into the sixth decade [43,92,98].

An insulin-resistant diabetes may also develop in the postadolescent period, sometimes in association with hepatic dysfunction [97], as is illustrated by our oldest autopsied patient [43].

The rate of disease progression and its severity vary considerably from one patient to another, and it has become evident that mild forms of the disease exist [6,45]. For example, two brothers, now 27 and 33 years old, whom I have been following have had an unusually benign course. Neither brother began to need a wheelchair until late adolescence. Both have normal sexual development and are above the fiftieth percentile in weight and height. Ocular telangiectasia did not become prominent in either brother before early adolescence. Both have had a normal

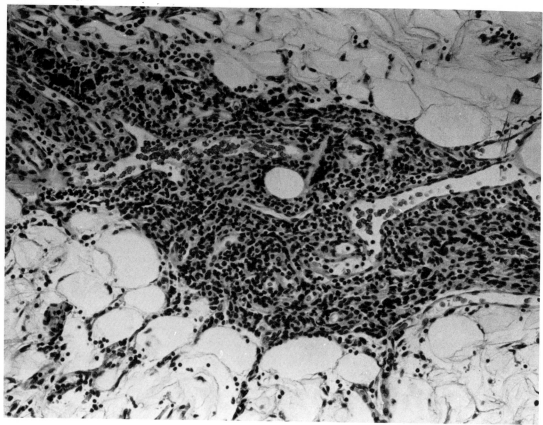

Figure 9.8. Dysplastic thymic fragment without Hassel's corpuscles found amidst predominantly fibroareolar tissue. Note numerous atypical nucleocytomegalic cells throughout the thymic fragment. Hematoxylin and eosin stain (original magnification × 200). (From Boder [6]; courtesy of Alan R. Liss.)

incidence of respiratory infections and show only minimal impairment of delayed hypersensitivity, mildly elevated alpha-fetoprotein, and normal levels of serum immunoglobulins, including IgA.

An observation on the female patients in our series appears to have prognostic significance. All six of our female patients who have come to autopsy had either absent or hypoplastic and dysplastic ovaries. The two who survived beyond the age of 30— one to age 32 [43] and the other to age 50 [92]— had well-developed secondary sexual characteristics, although menses were somewhat irregular; neither was unusually susceptible to pulmonary infections and both died of T-cell leukemia. Furthermore, all four of the postadolescent female patients, age 17 to 27, that Dr. Gatti and I are currently following also give clinical evidence of functional ovaries with irregular menses and are not prone to respiratory infections. It would appear, therefore, that the prognosis for long-term survival is notably improved for female A-T patients who undergo normal pu-

berty. More specifically, they appear to be less predisposed to chronic pulmonary disease and early-onset neoplasia. Our long-term observations indicate that this also may be true, though less consistently, of our older male patients who have reached normal puberty and who have achieved well-developed secondary sexual characteristics. These observations suggest a rationale for gonadal hormone therapy. To my knowledge it has not yet been tried.

Classification

Ataxia-telangiectasia can best be classified, according to its major clinical and pathologic features, as a predominantly cerebellar form of spinocerebellar degeneration, which is transmitted as an autosomal recessive trait [105] and evolves ultimately to include motor neuron disease, with spinal muscular atrophy and peripheral neuropathy. Ataxia-telangiectasia can also be classified among the neurocutaneous syndromes, though not among the phakomatoses as originally proposed [2,5], since the vascular and cutaneous lesions of A-T are not congenital nevi (phakomas), but develop in the course of the disease as a progeric manifestation.

In addition, for the purposes of differential diagnosis and research, it is important to consider A-T in the context of the entities with which it has features in common. For example, A-T should be considered among the immunodeficiency diseases, cancer-prone genetic disorders, chromosomal instability syndromes, disorders with abnormal radiosensitivity, syndromes with possible DNA-repair/processing defects, and, as is now evident, the progeroid syndromes. Both the similarities and the differences between A-T and the other diseases in each of these groups can be expected to offer valuable insights in the search for the pathogenesis of A-T as a unique entity.

Is A-T Genetically Heterogeneous?

Because of the variability in some of the clinical and laboratory features of A-T, there is a current trend to consider the possibility that A-T is genetically heterogeneous and may comprise more than one disease entity. A recently proposed tentative clinical classification of types of A-T is based on the presence or absence within sets of A-T siblings of such clinical features as pulmonary infection, mental retardation, and ovarian failure [106]. Our experience suggests, however, that genetic subtypes of A-T cannot be reliably based on clinical features alone; there is no clear concordance within the sets of A-T siblings in our series for any of the clinical features that have been proposed as possible criteria for subtypes of A-T. This is well illustrated by two sisters in our series, on whom a detailed clinicopathologic comparison is published elsewhere [6]. From the age of 3 years, the younger sister had chronic progressive bronchopulmonary disease that was the cause of her death at age 10½; the older sister did not have recurrent pulmonary infections until shortly before her death of T-cell leukemia and terminal bronchopneumonia at age 32. The younger sister had absent ovaries at autopsy, whereas the older sister gave clinical evidence of functional ovaries, including menses, although the ovaries were found to be dysplastic at autopsy, as is typical of all A-T patients in whom the ovaries are present.

In brief, our experience and that of others [107] indicate that the fundamental factors that allow the clinical and pathologic variability of A-T to be understood best are the severity of the disease, the rate of progression, and the age of the patient. In fact, over time, with long survival, the evolving clinical and pathologic picture is so stereotyped in most A-T patients as to be inconsistent with a concept of genetic heterogeneity. If A-T proves, nevertheless, to be genetically heterogeneous, it would appear that its subtypes will have to be established on systematic correlations between the clinical features of A-T and its distinctive laboratory markers rather than on clinical features alone. The only such correlation that has so far provided positive results is still the study by McFarlin et al. [97] who were able to classify A-T patients into three categories by correlating the kind and degree of immunodeficiency with the frequency and severity of pulmonary infection. The authors did not suggest, however, that the three categories might indicate that A-T is genetically heterogeneous.

Recent genetic complementation studies of A-T, based on cell-fusion techniques, have demonstrated the existence of several distinct complementation groups in A-T fibroblast strains [108], and have thereby given impetus to the concept that A-T may be genetically heterogeneous. However, to what extent there may be correlations between such complementation groups and the clinical features of A-T has not been studied.

Pathogenesis

The continuing proliferation of research on A-T in the last decade has been done increasingly by laboratory scientists [29–33,109,110], who are focusing on its cellular and molecular basis in search of its pathogenesis and on heterozygote detection and prenatal diagnosis. However, the clinical observation of A-T is far from being a closed chapter. Systematic study of variant clinical features and long-term observation of A-T patients, especially older patients, and their families may continue to reveal new clinical and pathologic features and perhaps formes frustes of the disease.

Autopsies on older patients have shown that the progeric manifestations are not limited to the cutaneous changes and to oculocutaneous telangiectasia, but that they also occur in the CNS. The most impressive new evidence of premature aging in the CNS includes the neurofibrillary tangles and lipofuscin granules found in the neurons of the cerebrum, basal ganglia, and spinal cord of our oldest autopsied patient [43], and the multiple gliovascular nodules with perivascular hemorrhages in the cerebral white matter, found in all three of the oldest autopsied patients [40,43,83]. In addition, the widespread visceral nucleocytomegaly reported in many autopsies on A-T patients is similar to the nucleocytomegaly described in two autopsied cases of progeria [103,104]. More autopsies on older patients with careful clinicopathologic correlations are needed to establish the full range of pathologic changes in A-T. Only 3 of the 58 published autopsy reports are on adult A-T patients over the age of 25 years.

Although the basic enzymatic defect in A-T still eludes us, we have come a long way in our knowledge of this complex disease through the exciting research developments of the last 20 years. Beyond its neurologic importance as the only chronic, predominantly cerebellar degeneration of infancy and childhood, A-T has become a unique model for the study of cancer-proneness, immunodeficiency, endocrine abnormality, radiosensitivity, and abnormality in DNA-repair/processing. It now appears, from our long-term clinical observation and the autopsy findings in older patients, that A-T can also serve as a model for the study of the multisystem processes of aging. Each of the cardinal clinical components that come together in A-T represents a major field of contemporary medical research, and we can anticipate that A-T will continue to provide keys to each of its multisystem components and to the links between them. The frontier for A-T research in the foreseeable future [111] appears to be the close collaboration of the clinician and the laboratory scientist in search of the pathogenesis of A-T and, ultimately, its prevention and specific treatment.

Diagnosis

The two diagnostic hallmarks are early-onset cerebellar ataxia and the oculocutaneous telangiectasia that appears somewhat later. The association of these hallmarks with the characteristic cerebellar hypotonic facies and posture is so striking that the diagnosis can usually be made on purely clinical grounds and often on inspection.

Before the appearance of ocular telangiectasia, however, a purely clinical diagnosis may not be possible unless the patient already manifests either the characteristic oculomotor apraxia or recurrent sinopulmonary infection, or has an affected sibling with typical A-T. The most common misdiagnosis in early childhood, when the progression of ataxia may be masked by the normal development of motor skills, is cerebral palsy, usually ataxic or athetoid. In later childhood, when the progression of the ataxia becomes obvious, the most common misdiagnosis is Friedreich's ataxia. It is important, therefore, to consider a diagnosis of A-T in the differential diagnosis of any chronic ataxia of early onset.

Laboratory Markers

The diagnosis of A-T in the pretelangiectatic stage can be facilitated by a number of specific laboratory tests. The most constant biochemical markers of A-T are elevated serum levels of alpha-fetoprotein (AFP) [112] and carcinoembryonic antigen (CEA) [113]. In a study of 12 of our patients, AFP was elevated in 9 [114]. In a more recent study of fetal proteins in 7 of our patients, all 7 had elevated levels of CEA and all but one had elevated AFP levels; the levels of all the other fetal proteins were within normal range [115].

The demonstration of humoral or cellular immunologic defect also permits a diagnosis of A-T in the pretelangiectatic stage. In current practice it usually is demonstrated through absent or low serum levels of IgA, diminished responses to skin test antigens, and peripheral lymphopenia. The dysgammaglobulinemia of A-T may also include normal or low levels of IgG, deficiency of IgG_2 and IgE, and normal or elevated IgM. In spite of the fact that the immunologic findings vary from one patient to another and may be normal in an occasional patient, A-T remains the only progressive ataxia that typically is associated with immunodeficiency.

Spontaneous chromosomal breaks and rearrangements in lymphocytes in vitro and in cultured skin fibroblasts are also an important laboratory marker of A-T [26,27,116], although not invariably present. When chromosomal breakage is present, it helps, in uncertain cases, to make the diagnosis of A-T. Moreover, rearrangements of chromosomes 2, 7, and 14 [116–118] in peripheral blood lymphocytes, and especially a 14:14 translocation, may presage the development of lymphoreticular neoplasia or leukemia. Among the 12 A-T patients in our series who were studied cytogenetically with cultured lymphocytes by Teplitz, only 4 patients, all of them between 5 and 10 years of age, showed no chromosomal abnormalities [Teplitz RL, Boder E: unpublished data]. Of the remaining 8 patients, who showed a variety of chromosomal breaks and rearrangements, 6 ranged in age from 19 to 50 years and only 2 were younger than 10 years. The 2 oldest patients, both females, showed 14:14 translocations for several years before they died of T-cell leukemia, one at age 32 and the other at 50 [43,92].

Increased chromosomal breakage after exposure to ionizing radiation in cell cultures is of rapidly increasing diagnostic importance, although it is primarily a research procedure and is not routinely available to the clinician. In addition to its value in diagnosing atypical cases, it holds promise for prenatal diagnosis [109] and as a means of identifying heterozygotes [33], who recently have been estimated to constitute between 0.1 and 5% of the general U.S. population [7].

In summary, elevated AFP and CEA, immunologic defect, and chromosomal abnormality are laboratory markers that may be crucial in the diagnosis of an atypical, uncertain, or early case of A-T. They can also serve to differentiate A-T from Friedreich's ataxia, in which none of them is present. Although the presence of these markers confirms the diagnosis in an obvious case of A-T, their absence does not rule it out. Ultimately, the clinical diagnosis still takes precedence [6,119].

Special Diagnostic Procedures

A number of special procedures can be helpful in the differential diagnosis of an early or uncertain case, but they should not be regarded as routine.

Radiologic findings of decreased or absent adenoidal tissue in the nasopharynx on lateral skull x-rays are so typical in A-T that they are of value in confirming the diagnosis. Sinus x-rays often show a pansinusitis. Chest x-rays may show a small or absent thymic shadow, decreased mediastinal lymphoid tissue, and pulmonary changes similar to those seen in cystic fibrosis. In fact, hypoplastic peripheral lymphoid tissue is such a consistent clinical finding in A-T [15,20] that the appearance of lymphadenopathy or even easily palpable lymph nodes has been, in my experience and that of others [120], highly suggestive of lymphoma.

Electro-oculography is valuable, as has been noted, in corroborating the characteristic oculomotor abnormality of A-T and in differentiating A-T from Friedreich's ataxia [36,37].

Electromyograms and nerve conduction velocities are usually normal in the early stages of A-T. Later, when the anterior horn cells are involved and peripheral neuropathy has occurred, the electromyograms will show signs of denervation [43,97,98], and the nerve conduction studies will show slightly reduced velocity in motor fibers and markedly reduced velocity in sensory fibers [121]. The nerve conduction findings in A-T and Friedreich's ataxia are so similar as to be of limited value in their differentiation.

Only a few reports of computerized tomography (CT) in A-T have appeared in the literature [119,122], but in each of them CT scans have been found to be of definite diagnostic value in demonstrating cerebellar atrophy. All three of our patients on whom CT scans have been done show enlargement of the fourth ventricle, with variable widening of the cerebellar sulci, indicative of cerebellar atrophy [Boder E, Gatti RA, Shields D: unpublished data]. Magnetic resonance imaging (MRI) promises to be of even greater diagnostic value in A-T, particularly because of its superior ability to visualize structures in the posterior fossa. A further advantage of MRI for the A-T patient, in addition to its being completely noninvasive, is that it does not use ionizing radiation. A recent MRI study of two of our patients, sisters age 17 and 12, clearly demonstrated cerebellar atrophy with widened cerebellar sulci in both patients and enlargement of the fourth ventricle in the older [6] (Figure 9.9).

Diagnosis of Atypical Cases

A current emphasis in the literature is that a diagnosis of A-T can be made in the absence of pulmonary infection and regardless of the immunologic findings [123,124]. This is a practical emphasis, especially for the clinician whose experience with the disease is limited and who may be reluctant to make a diagnosis of A-T unless the full range of its clinical features is present. It was clear from our original

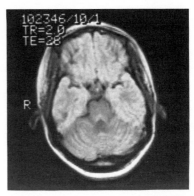

Figure 9.9. Magnetic resonance imaging showing cerebellar atrophy in a 17-year-old female. Note the prominent cerebellar folia and enlarged fourth ventricle.

series of eight patients that although pulmonary disease was sufficiently frequent to constitute a triad with ataxia and telangiectasia, it was not an invariable component of the syndrome; it was also apparent that the severity of the neurologic features of A-T was not directly related to the severity of the pulmonary infection [2,5,28]. Granted that elevated AFP levels and chromosomal abnormality permit a confident diagnosis of A-T in the absence of pulmonary disease or immunodeficiency, pulmonary disease is still the most frequent cause of death in A-T, and immunodeficiency, in spite of its variable manifestations, is still one of the most consistent components of the disease.

With increasing awareness of A-T, there is an increased tendency to report patients who manifest some of its features as "benign variants" or "presumed A-T" [125–128]. However, in some of these case reports, the diagnosis of A-T seems dubious, since neither ataxia nor ocular telangiectasia is present. For example, one patient had an elevated AFP, but the predominant picture was one of late-onset peripheral neuropathy rather than of early-onset cerebellar ataxia [126]. In another case report there was recurrent infection and low IgA but no ataxia [125]. Ocular telangiectasia was absent in both of these cases and in three recently reported siblings [128].

No matter how mild or atypical the clinical picture may be, the main diagnostic hallmark of the disease and its first presenting sign is progressive cerebellar ataxia. Ataxia-telangiectasia evolves only with long survival to include spinocerebellar signs, progressive spinal muscular atrophy, and peripheral neuropathy. Although the association of cerebellar ataxia with oculocutaneous telangiectasia is a unique diagnostic key, A-T could conceivably exist without telangiectasia, but the more likely possibility in any given case is that telangiectasia will appear later on, or is so subtle that it has been overlooked. It is not conceivable, however, that a variant of A-T might exist without ataxia.

Differential diagnosis presents no problems in a typical case of A-T. In early, mild, or uncertain cases, however, A-T will have to be differentiated systematically from other ataxic diseases of childhood. The differential diagnosis is discussed in some detail in two of our earlier publications [5,28].

Management

No specific treatment has been found to halt the progression of A-T. All treatment is symptomatic and must be highly individualized because of the variable multisystem manifestations and the occasional occurrence of mild forms. General supportive and rehabilitative measures are therefore of paramount importance. Early diagnosis makes unnecessary such invasive and potentially hazardous diagnostic procedures as angiography and posterior fossa exploration for cerebellar neoplasms; it also alerts the physician to the child's unusual susceptibility to bronchiectasis so that an appropriate program of antibiotic therapy can be instituted promptly to combat recurrent sinopulmonary infection [129]. In addition to an appropriate regimen of antibiotic therapy with adequate hydration, a cystic fibrosis regimen, including aerosol inhalation therapy and chest percussion with postural drainage, is essential for patients with chronic bronchiectasis.

Immunotherapy

The results of immunotherapy have usually been inconclusive, although an improvement in immunologic reactivity and a decrease in the frequency and severity of sinopulmonary infection have been reported with a variety of therapies. Exploratory trials of immunotherapy have included gammaglobulin injections, plasmapheresis, fetal thymus transplants, and the use of transfer factor, levamisole, thymosin, and, more recently, synthetic serum thymic factor (FTS). Few of these therapies have been tried with sufficient numbers of patients to be certain of their clinical value. The most promising results have been obtained from the following:

Gamma globulin (0.6 to 0.8 ml per kg of body weight) given intramuscularly or intravenously at 3- to 4-week intervals may prove useful in combating sinopulmonary infections when hypogammaglobulinemia is marked (i.e., less than 200 mg/100 ml), or when only moderate but in association with selective deficiencies of IgA and IgG_2.

Fetal thymus transplants aimed at reconstituting the immune system were tried on eight patients by Lopukhin et al. [130] with reported clinical improvement and increased immunologic reactivity, but the results in other trials of thymic transplants have been inconclusive [131]. Trials of thymosin in a few A-T patients have had variable effects on immunologic reactivity, without clinical improvement at the dosages used [131]. More recently, treatment of two A-T patients with synthetic serum thymic factor (FTS) by Bordigoni et al. [132] resulted in decreased frequency and severity of infections and significant immunologic improvement, including IgA synthesis. However, the improvement lasted only for the period of treatment.

Initial trials of levamisole by Medici et al. [133] on four A-T children, administered orally twice a week for two 6-month periods, resulted in improved immunologic reactivity. T-cell levels increased to the normal range and were still normal 5 years after discontinuance of therapy.

Bone marrow transplants merit therapeutic trial, but to my knowledge have not been tried yet [Good RA, Stiehm R: personal communication, 1985].

Other Medical Treatment

Because of the predilection of progeric skin changes and oculocutaneous telangiectases for sun-exposed areas, the avoidance of undue exposure to sunlight is recommended.

Strabismus is often transient in A-T and should be treated conservatively.

The insulin-resistant diabetes mellitus that develops primarily in postadolescent A-T patients requires no specific treatment; it does not appear to be progressive, glycosuria occurs rarely, and there is no ketosis [97].

Steroid therapy cannot be recommended, since it has been tried with inconclusive results and some untoward reactions.

Vitamin E therapy, which is increasingly used in a variety of neurologic conditions, has been tried in several of our patients because the neuroaxonal dystrophy in the brain stem observed in autopsies of our patients is similar to the neuroaxonal dystrophy associated with vitamin E deficiency [46]. Definite improvement was reported by the parents of several patients, but the results as a whole were inconclusive at the dosage used (alpha-tocopherol, 800 mg once or twice daily).

Propranolol has been found to be useful in improving the fine motor coordination of some A-T patients. In our initial trial of propranolol in six A-T patients, with a dosage of 10 to 20 mg tid, all showed noticeable improvement in their handwriting and in their ability to feed themselves [129]. Although the results of subsequent trials have been variable, propranolol merits a routine trial in A-T patients with severe functional impairment of the upper limbs.

The use of radiation therapy and chemotherapy in conventional doses is contraindicated in the treatment of the malignancies associated with A-T be-cause of reported untoward and ultimately fatal reactions [59,63,70,88,96]. Recent reports suggest, however, that when there is no adequate alternative treatment, and especially when the neoplasm is localized, reduced-dose radiotherapy and chemotherapy may result in better control of the malignancy and even prolonged remission [91,95]. The precautions that have been emphasized include the following: in chemotherapy, the use of a small enough dose of cytotoxic drugs to prevent immunosuppression and the avoidance of radiomimetic drugs, including bleomycin, actinomycin D, and cyclophosphamide [70,95,96]; in radiation therapy, a dose not to exceed 1,200 to 2,000 rad, administered in fractions not greater than 100 rad, and termination of radiation at the first sign of sensitivity [88,95,96]; and in treating A-T patients with leukemia (ALL), avoidance of both CNS irradiation and chemotherapy with Vinca alkaloids, because of their neurotoxic effects [91].

Rehabilitative Measures

Physical therapy is useful in maintaining good muscular strength, preventing limb contractures, and learning techniques of falling to avoid injury. Occupational therapy helps to develop functional adaptations in the activities of daily living. Speech therapy may be useful in improving articulation and increasing voice volume. In addition, daily participation to tolerance in a structured physical fitness program, which may include swimming, use of a special bicycle, and graduated weight lifting, is useful in maintaining function and muscle strength and in preventing contractures. My long-term observations confirm that keeping A-T patients physically active can offset the progression of their motor handicap sufficiently to prolong ambulation by several years and thus postpone confinement to a wheelchair.

Good educational progress is possible in either special classes or regular classes in schools that have safety provisions for children with physical handicaps. The school program will need to be adapted to the slow initiation and incoordination of all voluntary activity characteristic of A-T patients, especially their labored speech, slow reading, and poor writing. Since IQ scores tend to drop below normal range as the disease progresses, the educational program should be adapted accordingly.

Parent counseling is of paramount importance and should include tactful genetic counseling that avoids aggravating parental guilt feelings; explanation of the multisystem nature of the disease, its variable severity and course, the existence of mild forms, and the possibility of long-term survival; early setting of realistic goals, emphasizing the child's assets, such as the equable disposition, relatively good intelligence, and good muscle strength typical of most A-T patients; calling attention to the susceptibility of adult members of A-T families to malignant neoplasms and to the importance of regular examinations for early cancer detection; and emphasizing that A-T is the focus of interdisciplinary research by clinicians and laboratory scientists that may well lead to breakthroughs in specific therapy in the foreseeable future that would halt the progression of the disease, ameliorate its symptoms, and point the way to its ultimate prevention and possible cure.

References

1. Boder E, Sedgwick RP. Ataxia-telangiectasia: a familial syndrome of progressive cerebellar ataxia, oculocutaneous telangiectasia and frequent pulmonary infection. A preliminary report on 7 children, an autopsy, and a case history. Univ South Calif Med Bull 1957;9:15–28.

2. Boder E, Sedgwick RP. Ataxia-telangiectasia. A familial syndrome of progressive cerebellar ataxia, oculocutaneous telangiectasia and frequent pulmonary infection. Pediatrics 1958;21:526–554.

3. Centerwall WR, Miller MM. Ataxia, telangiectasia, and sinopulmonary infections. A syndrome of slowly progressive deterioration in childhood. Am J Dis Child 1958;95:385–396.

4. Jablonski S. Illustrated dictionary of eponymic syndromes and diseases and their synonyms. Philadelphia: Saunders, 1969:35, 191.

5. Sedgwick RP, Boder E. Ataxia-telangiectasia. In: Vinken PJ, Bruyn GW, eds. Handbook of clinical neurology. Amsterdam: North–Holland, 1972;14:267–339.

6. Boder E. Ataxia-telangiectasia: an overview. In: Gatti RA, Swift M, eds. Ataxia-telangiectasia: genetics, neuropathology, and immunology of a degenerative disease of childhood. New York: Alan R. Liss, 1985:1–63.

7. Swift, M. Genetics and epidemiology of ataxia-telangiectasia. In: Gatti RA, Swift M, eds. Ataxia-telangiectasia: genetics, neuropathology, and immunology of a degenerative disease of childhood. New York: Alan R. Liss, 1985:133–144.

8. Syllaba L, Henner K. Contribution à l'indépendance de l'athétose double idiopathique et congénitale. Rev Neurol (Paris) 1926;1:541–562.

9. Louis-Bar D. Sur un syndrome progressif comprenant des télangiectasies capillaires cutanées et conjonctivales symétriques, à disposition naevoïde et de troubles cérébelleux. Confin Neurol (Basel) 1941;4:32–42.

10. Martin L. Aspect choréoathétosique du syndrome d'ataxie-télangiectasie. Acta Neurol Belg 1964; 64:802–819.

11. Biemond A. Palaeocerebellar atrophy with extrapyramidal manifestations in association with bronchiectasis and telangiectasis of the conjunctiva bulbi as a familial syndrome. In: van Bogaert L, Radermecker J, eds. Proceedings of the First International Congress of Neurological Sciences, Brussels, July 1957. London: Pergamon Press, 1957:206.

12. Wells CE, Shy GM. Progressive familial choreoathetosis with cutaneous telangiectasia. J Neurol Neurosurg Psychiatry 1957;20:98–104.

13. Boder E, Sedgwick RP. Ataxia-telangiectasia: a review of 101 cases. In: Walsh G, ed. Little Club Clinics in Develop. Med., no. 8. London: Heinemann Medical Books, 1963:110–118.

14. Sedgwick RP, Boder E. Progressive ataxia in childhood with particular reference to ataxia-telangiectasia. Neurology 1960;10:705–715.

15. Peterson RD, Kelly WD, Good RA. Ataxia-telangiectasia: its association with a defective thymus, immunological-deficiency disease, and malignancy. Lancet 1964;1:1189–1193.

16. Thieffry S, Arthuis M, Aicardi J, et al. L'ataxie-télangiectasie. Rev Neurol (Paris) 1961;105:390–405.

17. Peterson RD, Blaw M, Good RA. Ataxia-telangiectasia: a possible clinical counterpart of the animals rendered immunologically incompetent by thymectomy. J Pediatr 1963;63:701–703.

18. Fireman P, Boesman M, Gitlin D. Ataxia-telangiectasia. A dysgammaglobulinaemia with deficient gamma 1A (B2A)-globulin. Lancet 1964;1:1193–1195.

19. Young RR, Austen KF, Moser HW. Abnormalities of serum gamma 1A globulin and ataxia telangiectasia. Medicine 1964;43:423–433.

20. Eisen AH, Karpati G, Laszlo T, et al. Immunologic deficiency in ataxia-telangiectasia. N Engl J Med 1965;272:18–22.

21. Peterson RD, Cooper MD, Good RA. Lymphoid tissue abnormalities associated with ataxia-telangiectasia. Am J Med 1966;41:342–359.

22. Epstein WL, Fudenberg HH, Reed WB, et al. Immunologic studies in ataxia-telangiectasia. I. Delayed hypersensitivity and serum immune globulin levels in probands and first-degree relatives. Int Arch Allergy 1966;30:15–29.

23. Reed WB, Epstein WL, Boder E, et al. Cutaneous manifestations of ataxia-telangiectasia. JAMA 1966;195:746–753.

24. Swift M, Sholman L, Perry M, et al. Malignant neoplasms in the families of patients with ataxia-telangiectasia. Cancer Res 1976;36:209–215.

25. Oppenheim JJ, Barlow M, Waldmann TA, et al. Impaired in vitro lymphocyte transformation in patients with ataxia-telangiectasia. Br Med J 1966;2:330–333.

26. Hecht F, Koler RD, Rigas DA, et al. Leukemia and lymphocytes in ataxia-telangiectasia. Lancet 1966; 2:1993.

27. Gropp A, Flatz C. Chromosome breakage and blastic transformation of lymphocytes in ataxia-telangiectasia. Humangenetik 1967;5:77–79.

28. Boder E, Sedgwick RP. Ataxia-telangiectasia. In: Goldensohn ES, Appel SH, eds. Scientific approaches to clinical neurology. Philadelphia: Lea & Febiger, 1977:926–952.

29. Bridges BA, Harnden DG, [eds]. Ataxia-telangiectasia: a cellular and molecular link between cancer, neuropathology, and immune deficiency. New York: John Wiley & Sons, 1982.

30. Gatti RA, Swift M, eds. Ataxia-telangiectasia: genetics, neuropathology, and immunology of a degenerative disease of childhood. New York: Alan R. Liss, 1985.

31. Paterson MC, Smith BP, Knight PA, et al. Ataxia-telangiectasia: an inherited human disease involving radiosensitivity, malignancy and defective DNA repair. In: Castellani A, ed. Research in photobiology. New York: Plenum, 1977.

32. Taylor AM, Harnden DG, Arlett CF, et al. Ataxia-telangiectasia: a human mutation with abnormal radiation sensitivity. Nature 1975;258:427–429.

33. Arlett CF, Priestley A. An assessment of the radiosensitivity of ataxia-telangiectasia heterozygotes. In: Gatti RA, Swift M, eds. Ataxia-telangiectasia: genetics, neuropathology, and immunology of a degenerative disease of childhood. New York: Alan R. Liss, 1985:101–109.

34. Bodensteiner JB, Goldblum RM, Goldblum AS. Progressive dystonia masking ataxia in ataxia-telangiectasia. Arch Neurol 1980;37:464–465.

35. Smith JL, Cogan DG. Ataxia-telangiectasia. Arch Ophthalmol 1959;62:364–369.

36. Baloh R, Yee RD, Boder E. Eye-movements in ataxia-telangiectasia. Neurology 1978;28:1099–1104.

37. Furman JM, Perlman S, Baloh RW. Eye-movements in Friedreich's ataxia. Arch Neurol 1983;40:343–346.

38. Reye C. Ataxia telangiectasia. Am J Dis Child 1960; 99:238–241.

39. Dorantes S, Perez-Pena C, Molina B, et al. Sangrado en ataxia-telangiectasia. Un aspecto de la enfermedad previamente no estudiado. Bol Med Hosp Infant (Mexico) 1968;25:161–172.

40. Casaril M, Gabrielli GB, Capra F, et al. Atassia-telangiectasia: descrizione di un caso con emorragie cerebrali multiple e cirrosi epatica. Minerva Med 1982;73:2183–2188.

41. Williams HE, Demis DJ, Higdon RS. Ataxia-telangiectasia: a syndrome with characteristic cutaneous manifestations. Arch Dermatol 1960;82:937–942.

42. Epstein WL, Reed WB, Boder E, et al. Dermatologic aspects of ataxia-telangiectasia. Cutis 1968;4:1324–1332.

43. Amromin GD, Boder E, Teplitz R. Ataxia-telangiectasia with a 32 year survival: a clinicopathological report. J Neuropathol Exp Neurol 1979;38:621–643.

44. Cohen LE, Tanner DJ, Schaeffer HG, et al. Common and uncommon cutaneous findings in patients with ataxia-telangiectasia. J Am Acad Dermatol 1984; 10:431–438.

45. Boder E. Ataxia-telangiectasia: some historic, clinical and pathologic observations. In: Bergsma D, ed. Birth defects: original article series. New York: Alan R. Liss, 1975;11:255–270.

46. Aguilar MJ, Kamoshita S, Landing BH, et al. Pathological observations in ataxia-telangiectasia: a report on 5 cases. J Neuropathol Exp Neurol 1968;27:659–676.

47. Miller ME, Chatten J. Ovarian changes in ataxia-telangiectasia. Acta Paediatr Scand 1967;56:559–561.

48. Biemond A, van Bolhuis JH. Atrophia cerebelli met oculocutane telangiectasieen en bronchiectasieen als familial syndroom. Ned T Geneeskd 1959;103:2253–2258.

49. Bowden D, Danis PG, Sommers SC. Ataxia-telangiectasia: a case with lesions of ovaries and adenohypophysis. J Neuropathol Exp Neurol 1963;22:549–554.

50. Gutmann L, Lemli L. Ataxia-telangiectasia associated with hypogammaglobulinemia. Arch Neurol 1963;8: 318–327.

51. Dunn HG, Meuwissen H, Livingstone CS, et al. Ataxia-telangiectasia. Can Med Assoc J 1964;91: 1106–1118.

52. Osetowska E, Traczynska H. Sur l'ataxie avec télangiectasie, une observation anatomoclinique. Acta Neuropathol (Berlin) 1964;3:319–325.

53. Centerwall SA, Centerwall WR. Ataxia-telangiectasia: A familial degenerative disease leading to mental retardation—a case report. Am J Ment Defic 1966;71:185–190.

54. Harley RD, Baird HW, Craven EM. Ataxia telangiectasia: report of 7 cases. Arch Ophthalmol 1967;77:582–592.

55. Shuster J, Hart Z, Stimson CW, et al. Ataxia telangiectasia with cerebellar tumor. Pediatrics 1966; 37:776–786.

56. Sourander P, Bonnevier JO, Olsson Y. A case of ataxia-telangiectasia with lesions in the spinal cord. Acta Neurol Scand 1966;42:354–366.

57. Strich S. Pathological findings in 3 cases of ataxia-telangiectasia. J Neurol Neurosurg Psychiatry 1966;29:489–499.

58. Thieffry S, Arthuis M, Farkas–Barceton E, et al. L'ataxie-télangiectasie: une observation anatomoclinique familiale. Ann Pediatr 1966;13:749–762.

59. Gotoff SP, Amirokri E, Liebner EJ. Ataxia-telangiectasia: neoplasia, untoward response to X-irradiation, and tuberous sclerosis. Am J Dis Child 1967;114:617–625.

60. Hassler O. Ataxia-telangiectasia (Louis-Bar's syndrome): a case examined by micro-angiography with no telangiectases in the central nervous system. Acta Neurol Scand 1967;43:464–471.

61. Solitare GB, Lopez VF. Louis-Bar's syndrome (ataxia-telangiectasia): neuropathologic observations. Neurology 1967;17:23–31.

62. Solitare GB. Louis–Bar's syndrome (ataxia-telangiectasia): anatomic considerations with emphasis on neuropathologic observations. Neurology 1968;18:1180–1186.

63. Morgan JL, Holcomb TM, Morrissey RW. Radiation reaction in ataxia telangiectasia. Am J Dis Child 1968;116:557–558.

64. Castaigne P, Cambier J, Brunet P. Ataxie-télangiectasie, désordres immunitaires, lymphosarcomatose terminale chez deux frères. Presse Med 1969;77:347–348.

65. Haerer AF, Jackson JF, Evers CG. Ataxia-telangiectasia with gastric adenocarcinoma. JAMA 1969;210:1884–1887.

66. Itatsu Y, Uno Y. An autopsy case of ataxia-telangiectasia. Acta Pathol Jpn 1969;19:229–239.

67. Scott RE. Ataxia-telangiectasia. Arch Pathol 1969;88:78–84.

68. Terplan KL, Krauss RF. Histopathologic brain changes in association with ataxia-telangiectasia. Neurology 1969;19:446–454.

69. Taleb N, Thome S, Chostine S, et al. Association d'une ataxie-télangiectasie avec une leucémie aiguë lymphoblastique. Presse Med 1969;77:345–347.

70. Feigin RD, Vietti TJ, Wyatt RG, et al. Ataxia telangiectasia with granulocytopenia. J Pediatr 1970;77:431–438.

71. Cawley LP, Schenken JR. Monoclonal hypergammaglobulinemia of the M type in a nine-year-old girl with ataxia-telangiectasia. Am J Clin Pathol 1970;54:790–801.

72. Matsuo T, Muto Y, Tsuchiyama H. Ataxia-telangiectasia. Acta Pathol Jpn 1970;20:379–385.

73. Grossi–Bianchi ML, Moscatelli P, Tassara A. Atassia-telangiectasia: 3 casi clinici con studio immunologico ed un reperto autoptico. Minerva Pediatr 1971;23:1350–1358.

74. Hoerni B, Vital C, Bonnaud E. Leucémie aiguë lymphoblastique chez un sujet atteint d'ataxie-télangiectasie. Acta Haematol 1972;47:250.

75. Navarro C, Martin JJ. Particularités lésionnelles dans l'ataxie-télangiectasie de Louis–Bar. J Neurol Sci 1972;17:219.

76. Hecht F, McCaw BK, Koler RD. Ataxia-telangiectasia: clonal growth of translocation lymphocytes. N Engl J Med 1973;289:286.

77. Goldsmith CI, Hart WR. Ataxia-telangiectasia with ovarian gonadoblastoma and contralateral dysgerminoma. Cancer 1975;36:1838–1842.

78. Scully RE, McNeely BU. Case records of the Massachusetts General Hospital weekly clinicopathological exercises: Case 22–1975. N Engl J Med 1975;292:1231–1237.

79. Buyse M, Hartman CT, Wilson MG. Gonadoblastoma and dysgerminoma with ataxia-telangiectasia. In: Bergsma D, ed. Birth defects: original article series. New York: Alan R. Liss, 1976;12:165–169.

80. De Leon GA, Grover WE, Huff DS. Neuropathologic changes in ataxia-telangiectasia. Neurology 1976;26:947–951.

81. Cameron E, Seshadri RS, Pai KR, et al. Heat stable E-receptors on leukemic lymphoblasts in ataxia-telangiectasia. J Pediatr 1977;91:269–271.

82. Levitt R, Pierre RV, White WL, et al. Atypical lymphoid leukemia in ataxia-telangiectasia. Blood 1978;52:1003–1011.

83. Agamanolis DP, Greenstein JL. Ataxia-telangiectasia: report of a case with Lewy bodies and vascular abnormalities within cerebral tissue. J Neuropathol Exp Neurol 1979;38:475–488.

84. Amromin GD, Boder E. Autopsy findings in a 32 year old woman. Presented at the 53rd Annual Meeting of the American Association of Neuropathologists. Chicago, June 1977. J Neuropath Exp Neurol 1977;(abstr)36:591.

85. Krishna Kumar G, Al Saadi A, Yang S-S, et al. Ataxia-telangiectasia and hepatocellular carcinoma. Am J Med Sci 1979;278:157–160.

86. Yoshitomi F, Zaitsu Y, Tanaka K. Ataxia-telangiectasia with renal cell carcinoma and hepatoma. Virchows Arch A [Path Anat Histol] 1980;389:119–125.

87. Pascual-Pascual SI, Pascual-Castroviejo I, Fontan G, et al. Ataxia-telangiectasia (A-T): contribution with eighteen personal cases. Brain Dev 1981;3:289–296.

88. Pritchard J, Sandland MR, Breatnach FB, et al. The effects of radiation therapy for Hodgkin's disease in a child with ataxia telangiectasia. Cancer 1982;50:877–886.

89. Perry TL, Kish SJ, Hinton D, et al. Neurochemical abnormalities in a patient with ataxia-telangiectasia. Neurology 1984;34:187–191.

90. Weinstein S, Scottolini AG, Loo SY, et al. Ataxia-telangiectasia with hepatocellular carcinoma in a 15-year-old girl and studies of her kindred. Arch Pathol Lab Med 1985;109:1000–1004.

91. Toledano SR, Lange BJ. Ataxia-telangiectasia and acute lymphoblastic leukemia. Cancer 1980;45:1675–1678.

92. Saxon A, Stevens RH, Golde DW. Helper and suppressor T-lymphocyte leukemia in ataxia-telangiectasia. N Engl J Med 1979;300:700–704.

93. Gatti RA, Good RA. Occurrence of malignancy in immunodeficiency diseases. Cancer 1971;28:89–98.

94. Spector BD, Filipovich AH, Perry GS, et al. Epidemiology of cancer in ataxia-telangiectasia. In: Bridges BA, Harnden DG, eds. Ataxia-telangiectasia. New York: John Wiley & Sons, 1982:103–138.

95. Abadir R, Hakami N. Ataxia telangiectasia with cancer: an indication for reduced radiotherapy and chemotherapy doses. Br J Radiol 1983;56:343–345.

96. Cunliffe PN, Mann JR, Cameron AH, et al. Radiosensitivity in ataxia-telangiectasia. J Pediatr 1977;91:269–271.

97. McFarlin DE, Strober W, Waldmann TA. Ataxia-telangiectasia. Medicine 1972;51:281–314.

98. Goodman WN, Cooper WC, Kessler GB, et al. Ataxia-telangiectasia: a report of 2 cases in siblings present-

ing a picture of progressive spinal muscular atrophy. Bull Los Angeles Neurol Soc 1969;34:1–22.

99. Gardner MB, Goodman WN. Ataxia-telangiectasia. Electronmicroscopic study of a nerve biopsy. Bull Los Angeles Neurol Soc 1969;34:23–38.

100. Jerusalem F, Bischoff A. Ataxia telangiectasia: electron microscopic study of two nerve biopsies. Z Neurol 1972;202:128.

101. Vinters HV, Gatti RA, Rakic P. Sequence of cellular events in cerebellar ontogeny relevant to expression of neuronal abnormalities in ataxia-telangiectasia. In: Gatti RA, Swift M, eds. Ataxia-telangiectasia. New York: Alan R. Liss, 1985:233–255.

102. Gardner MB, Rasheed S, Shimizu S, et al. Search for RNA tumor virus in humans. In: Hiatt HH, Watson JD, Winsten JA, eds. Origins of human cancer. Book B, mechanism of carcinogenesis. Cold Spring Harbor, NY: Cold Spring Harbor Laboratory, 1977:1235–1252.

103. Kamoshita S, Aguilar MJ, Landing BH. Precocious aging in ataxia-telangiectasia: pathological evidence in the central nervous system. Proceedings of the First International Congress of Child Neurology. Toronto, 1975.

104. Reichel W, Garcia–Bunuel R. Pathologic findings in progeria. Am J Clin Pathol 1970;53:243–253.

105. Ionasescu V, Zellweger H. Genetics in neurology. New York: Raven Press, 1983:145–149.

106. Hecht F, Kaiser-McCaw B. Ataxia-telangiectasia: genetics and heterogeneity. In: Bridges BA, Harnden DG, eds. Ataxia-telangiectasia. New York: John Wiley & Sons, 1982:197–201.

107. Olivares L, Gutierrez J, Boissin G. Caracterización neurológica de la ataxia-telangiectasia: revisión de la literatura y análisis de ocho nuevos casos. Rev Clin Esp 1974;135:359–366.

108. Jaspers NG, Bootsma D. Genetic heterogeneity in ataxia-telangiectasia studied by cell fusion. Proc Natl Acad Sci USA 1982;79:2641–2644.

109. Schwartz S, Flannery DB, Cohen MM. Tests appropriate for the prenatal diagnosis of ataxia-telangiectasia. Prenat Diagn 1985;5:9–14.

110. Shiloh Y, Tabor E, Becker Y. In vitro phenotype of ataxia-telangiectasia (AT) fibroblast strains: clues to the nature of the "AT DNA lesion" and the molecular defect in AT. In: Gatti RA, Swift M, eds. Ataxia-telangiectasia. New York: Alan R. Liss, 1985:111–121.

111. Miller RW. Highlights in clinical discoveries relating to ataxia-telangiectasia. In: Bridges BA, Harnden DG, eds. Ataxia-telangiectasia. New York: John Wiley & Sons, 1982:13–21.

112. Waldmann TA, McIntire KR. Serum-alpha-fetoprotein levels in patients with ataxia-telangiectasia. Lancet 1972;2:1112–1115.

113. Sugimoto T, Sawada T, Tozawa M, et al. Plasma levels of carcinoembryonic antigen in patients with ataxia-telangiectasia. J Pediatr 1978;92:436–439.

114. Gatti RA, Bick M, Tam CF, et al. Ataxia-telangiectasia: a multiparameter analysis of eight families. Clin Immunol Immunopathol 1982;23:501–516.

115. Richkind KE, Boder E, Teplitz RL. Fetal proteins in ataxia-telangiectasia. JAMA 1982;248:1346–1347.

116. McCaw BK, Hecht F, Harnden DG, et al. Somatic rearrangement of chromosome 14 in human lymphocytes. Proc Natl Acad Sci USA 1975;72:2071–2075.

117. Davis MM, Gatti RA, Sparkes RS. Neoplasia and chromosomal breakage in ataxia-telangiectasia: a 2:14 translocation. In: Gatti RA, Swift M, eds. Ataxia-telangiectasia. New York: Alan R. Liss, 1985:197–204.

118. Levin S, Gottfried E, Cohen M. Ataxia-telangiectasia: a review—with observations on 47 Israeli cases. Paediatrician 1977;6:135–146.

119. Sedgwick RP. Neurological abnormalities in ataxia-telangiectasia. In: Bridges BA, Harnden DG, eds. Ataxia-telangiectasia. New York: John Wiley & Sons, 1982:23–35.

120. Brown LR, Coulam CM, Reese DF. Ataxia-telangiectasia (Louis-Bar syndrome). Semin Roentgenol 1976; 11:67–70.

121. Dunn HG. Nerve conduction studies in children with Friedreich's ataxia and ataxia-telangiectasia. Dev Med Child Neurol 1973;15:324.

122. Assencio-Ferreira VJ, Bancovsky I, Diament AJ, et al. Computed tomography in ataxia telangiectasia. J Comput Assist Tomogr 1981;5:660–661.

123. Jason JM, Gelfand EW. Diagnostic considerations in ataxia-telangiectasia. Arch Dis Child 1979;54:682–686.

124. Hansen RL, Marx JJ, Ptacek LJ, et al. Immunological studies on an aberrant form of ataxia-telangiectasia. Am J Dis Child 1977;131:518–521.

125. Stankler L, Bennett FM. Ataxia-telangiectasia. Br J Dermatol 1973;88:187–189.

126. Terenty TA, Robson P, Walton JH. Presumed ataxia-telangiectasia in a man. Br Med J 1978;2:802.

127. Ying KL, Decoteau WE. Cytogenetic anomalies in a patient with ataxia, immune deficiency, and high alpha-fetoprotein in the absence of telangiectasia. Cancer Genet Cytogenet 1981:4:311–317.

128. Byrne E, Hallpike JF, Manson JI, et al. Ataxia-without-telangiectasia. J Neurol Sci, 1984:66:307–317.

129. Boder E. Neurocutaneous syndromes. In: Gillis SS, Kagan BM, eds. Current pediatric therapy. 7th ed. Philadelphia: Saunders, 1976:59–64.

130. Lopukhin Y, Morosov Y, Petrov R. Transplantation of neonate thymus-sternum complex in ataxia-telangiectasia. Transplant Proc 1973;5:823.

131. Wara DV, Ammann AJ. Thymosine treatment of children with primary immunodeficiency disease. Transplant Proc 1978;10:203–212.

132. Bordigoni P, Bene MC, Bach JF, et al. Improvement of cellular immunity and IgA production in immunodeficient children after treatment with synthetic serum thymic factor (FTS). Lancet 1982;2:293–297.

133. Medici MA, Bick M, Boder E, et al. Long-term treatment of ataxia-telangiectasia with levamisole. (Unpublished data.)

Chapter 10
Xeroderma Pigmentosum

JAY H. ROBBINS

Xeroderma pigmentosum (XP) is a neurocutaneous disease with autosomal recessive inheritance in which there is defective repair of damaged deoxyribonucleic acid (DNA) [1–4]. As a result of this defect in DNA repair, XP patients are afflicted by an accelerated aging of tissue exposed to sunlight and, in some cases, by a premature degeneration of nerve cells [1–4].

History and Epidemiology

In the 1860s and 1870s Kaposi [5,6] observed several patients who developed chronic solar cutaneous damage after minimal exposure to sunlight. He named the disease "xeroderma pigmentosum" because the skin of the patients was dry and atrophic and had numerous pigmentation abnormalities [5,6]. In 1883 Neisser [7] described the clinical features of XP together with neurodegeneration. This neurodegeneration was described in more detail in 1932 by De Sanctis and Cacchione [8] in clinical studies of three siblings and in autopsy studies of one of them. In 1968 Cleaver [9] found that cultures of skin fibroblasts from XP patients were unable to repair damage induced in their DNA by ultraviolet (UV) radiation. Epstein et al. [10] demonstrated in 1970 that this DNA nucleotide-excision repair process was defective in all types of the patients' skin cells in vivo. Two years later DeWeerd–Kastelein et al. [11] found genetic heterogeneity among excision-deficient XP patients by demonstrating complementation of the repair defect in cell fusion studies in vitro. In 1971 Burke et al. [12] described a form of XP, subsequently designated the "XP variant" form [13], in which DNA nucleotide-excision repair was normal. Lehmann et al. [14] subsequently showed that XP variant cells had a marked defect in the DNA-repair process known as postreplication repair. In 1974 Robbins et al. [1] described a patient with XP together with Cockayne's syndrome. The report in 1983 by Moshell et al. [15] of a second patient with both XP and Cockayne's syndrome established the combination of these two rare disorders as a distinct syndrome.

Large series of XP cases have been reported in the United States [1], Japan [16], England [17], Germany [18], Egypt [19], and Israel [4]. Xeroderma pigmentosum occurs in the United States [1] and Europe [20] with a frequency of 1 in 250,000 persons and has a higher frequency in Japan (1 in 30,000) [20] and Israel (1 in 100,000) [4]. Xeroderma pigmentosum occurs in all races and affects both sexes equally. As expected with an autosomal recessive disease, consanguinity is found in all series.

Clinical Features

Cutaneous Abnormalities

The cutaneous abnormalities of XP are listed in Table 10.1. Only areas of skin exposed to UV radiation (in sunlight) develop these abnormalities (Figure 10.1A). Areas receiving the most sun exposure typically include the face, neck, ears, dorsa of the hands and forearms, and the V-area of the chest. The cutaneous lesions can be classified into the following stages [2,4,21]: (a) erythematous, (b) pigmented, (c) telangiectatic and atrophic, and (d) neoplastic. With the exception of those XP infants seen at the time of an acute sunburn reaction, most XP patients when first evaluated have features of the last three stages. Fifty percent of XP patients have onset of symptoms by 8 months of age, 75% by 4 years, 95% by 15 years, and the remaining 5% after 15 years of age [4].

During infancy some XP patients suffer one or

Table 10.1. Cutaneous and Ocular Abnormalities in Xeroderma Pigmentosum

Cutaneous Abnormalities	
Erythema and bullae (acute sun sensitivity in infancy)	Neoplasms
Freckles, hypopigmentation	Actinic keratoses
Xerosis (dryness) and scaling	Basal and squamous cell carcinomas
Telangiectases	Malignant melanomas
Atrophy	Others (keratoacanthomas, angiomas, fibromas, sarcomas)

Ocular Abnormalities	
Lids	Symblepharon, inflammatory nodules
Blepharitis, erythema, pigmentation, keratoses	Neoplasms
Atrophy leading to entropion, ectropion, loss of cilia, and loss of lower lid	Intraepithelial epitheliomas
	Squamous cell carcinomas
Neoplasms	Cornea
Papillomas	Exposure keratitis with edema, cellular invasion, vascularization
Epitheliomas of free border of lid	Dryness, opacification, ulceration, scarring
Basal and squamous cell carcinomas	Neoplasms
Conjunctiva	Iris
Conjunctivitis with photophobia, lacrimation, edema	Iritis, synechiae, atrophy
Pigmentation, telangiectases, dryness	Neoplasms

Source: adapted from Robbins et al. [1].

more episodes of acute sun sensitivity, that is, a marked degree of erythema or blistering after minimal sun exposure [1]. After subsidence of the acute reaction, the involved skin gradually develops pigmentation abnormalities, which are manifested chiefly as colored macules. While these macules have certain clinical and histopathologic criteria distinguishing them from freckles [21,22], the term freckle has become a convenient and accepted clinical designation for the XP macule. In XP patients without an acute sunburn reaction the development of these freckles may not initially appear abnormal. Xeroderma pigmentosum freckles are irregularly shaped pigmented macules, ranging from pinpoint size to a centimeter or more in diameter (Figure 10.1A, B) [1]. While each freckle is usually all of one color [1], in any one patient the freckles will be of many shades of brown, gray, and black [1]. After several years the freckles enlarge and become so numerous that large areas of skin become pigmented [4]. Another distinctive feature of the pigmentation abnormalities of XP skin is the development of hypopigmented (achromic) areas, ranging from a millimeter to several centimeters in diameter.

The pigmented stage gradually merges with the ensuing stage of telangiectases and atrophy. Vascular dilatations give rise to numerous telangiectases. The skin becomes dry and scaly. There is clinical evidence of epidermal and dermal atrophy (Figure 10.1B). As the atrophic process continues, the skin becomes wrinkled and tight. Neoplastic changes,

which are occasionally apparent in the early pigmented stage, become most numerous in the late atrophic stage.

All types of cutaneous tumors can occur in XP patients (Figure 10.1 C, D) [1]. Benign lesions include keratoses, warty papillomatous growths (including keratoacanthomas), angiomas, fibromas, nevi, and senile and juvenile lentigos [1,4,22]. Among the neoplastic changes, actinic keratoses are the most frequent, followed in decreasing frequency by basal and squamous cell carcinomas, and, except in the Japanese [4,16], by malignant melanomas [1,4]. Sarcomas occasionally develop [1]. Xeroderma pigmentosum patients under 20 years of age have an approximately 5,000-fold increase in the frequency of basal and squamous cell carcinomas (in comparison with the general population), and their median age of skin cancer onset is 8 years (versus 58 years for the general population) [4].

Ocular Abnormalities

As shown in Table 10.1, the sun-exposed portions of the eye develop numerous abnormalities [1,2,4,23,24]. Almost all XP patients suffer from photophobia and conjunctivitis. The thin skin of the eyelids becomes damaged by the UV radiation in sunlight in the same manner as other exposed XP skin (Figure 10.1E, F). As the lids undergo atrophic changes, they turn in (entropion) or out (ectropion)

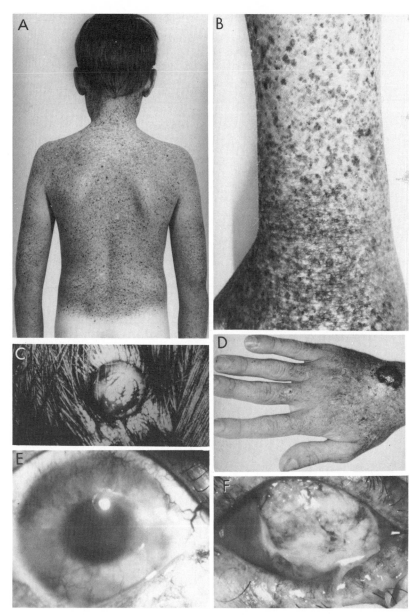

Figure 10.1. Effects of sunlight on xeroderma pigmentosum skin. *(A)* Sun-exposed skin of a 12-year-old patient shows numerous freckles. The buttocks, which had been protected from sunlight, show no clinical manifestations of xeroderma pigmentosum. A long hair style might have prevented damage to the upper neck. *(B)* Close-up view of the dorsum of the patient's arm and wrist. Differences in size, shape, and color intensity of the freckles are apparent. Achromic spots are prominent on the wrist. The exaggerated skin lines at the wrist are the result of elastotic changes in the underlying dermis. *(C)* Nodular malignant melanoma in the scalp of a young adult with xeroderma pigmentosum. This patient had a history of very short crew haircuts as a child, which exposed his scalp to sunlight. *(D)* Large fungating squamous cell carcinoma on dorsum of the patient's hand. *(E)* Eye of 28-year-old xeroderma pigmentosum patient. Many eyelashes have been lost from the lower lid, and the cornea is clouded and vascularized. *(F)* Five years later an invasive squamous cell carcinoma involved the anterior orbital tissues. *(E and F adapted from Gaasterland et al. [24].)*

and can no longer mechanically protect the cornea and conjunctiva; severe exposure keratitis can occur. The cornea is prone to ulceration and scarring and can become opacified (Figure 10.1E). The tissues of the outer eye are also damaged directly by the UV radiation, leading to inflammation as well as to benign and malignant neoplasms of the lid, conjunctiva, cornea, and iris (Figure 10.1F). The lens and retina are not damaged because the harmful UV radiation cannot reach them.

Neurologic Abnormalities

Worldwide, approximately 20% of XP patients develop neurologic abnormalities [4]. In Japan, however, approximately 90% of patients are so affected [16]. With the exception of microcephaly, the neurologic abnormalities affecting XP patients differ only in the time of their appearance and in the rate of their progression [1,7,25–29]. In the most severely affected patients sensorineural deafness and all the abnormalities originally described by De Sanctis and Cacchione [8] are present clinically before 7 years of age [25]. These abnormalities include retarded growth and sexual development, microcephaly, progressive mental deterioration, choreoathetosis, ataxia, spasticity, extensor plantar responses, Achilles-tendon shortening, hyporeflexia progressing to areflexia, and a neuropathic electromyogram and muscle biopsy. In less severely affected patients growth and sexual development are normal, and the neurologic abnormalities usually become clinically evident between 7 and 12 years of age [1,7,25–28]. In all cases the neurologic abnormalities are relentlessly progressive.

Patients with Both Xeroderma Pigmentosum and Cockayne's Syndrome

Cockayne's syndrome is an autosomal recessive disease characterized clinically by cachectic dwarfism, acute sun sensitivity, and ocular, skeletal, and neurologic abnormalities [30–32]. Among the latter are optic atrophy, pigmentary retinal degeneration, cataracts, sensorineural deafness, premature death of nerve cells, central and peripheral demyelination, cerebellar and extrapyramidal movement disturbances, hyperreflexia, microcephaly, and normal pressure hydrocephalus. The skin of typical Cockayne's syndrome patients does not develop the pigmentation abnormalities or the cutaneous malignancies of XP patients. However, the two patients who have both XP and Cockayne's syndrome have the cutaneous abnormalities of XP and the ocular, skeletal, and neurologic abnormalities of Cockayne's syndrome [1,15]. Although Cockayne's syndrome patients' cultured cells have defective repair of UV radiation-induced DNA damage, their defective DNA-repair process is different from that in XP [15,32–34]. The repair defects in the two patients who have both diseases have not yet been fully characterized.

Pathology

Dermatopathology

The following nonspecific histopathologic changes [21,22] are seen in the skin of a typical XP patient who clinically has only some erythema, scaling, and freckling: hyperkeratosis, irregular acanthosis alternating with areas of epidermal atrophy, a chronic inflammatory infiltrate in the upper dermis, and irregular accumulation of melanin in the basal cell layer. These changes accelerate as the clinical damage becomes severe. Figure 10.2 shows histopathologic features in sun-damaged skin from a 28-year-old XP patient who had been avoiding sun exposure of the biopsied area for at least the previous 15 years. Premalignant and malignant lesions occurring in XP skin have the same histopathology as those occurring in the skin of normal individuals [1,22]. All these changes in sun-exposed XP skin appear similar to chronic solar degeneration seen in normal individuals with excessive sun exposure [22].

Neuropathology

The neurologic abnormalities of XP are the result of a primary neuronal degeneration [1,8,35]: neurons of a particular type die without any histopathologic evidence of their pathogenesis. The progressiveness of the neurologic abnormalities of XP results from the extension of primary neuronal degeneration to increasingly larger numbers of neurons [35]. Neuronal loss occurs primarily in the pyramidal cells of the cerebral cortex, the Purkinje cells of the cerebellum, the deep nuclei of the basal ganglia and cerebellum, the locus ceruleus, and the zona compacta of the substantia nigra [1,35]. The spinal cord, with degeneration of the posterior columns, lateral and anterior corticospinal tracts, and dorsal roots and ganglia, eventually resembles that of Friedreich's ataxia [35]. Peripheral nerve conduction studies and electromyographic studies, together with nerve and

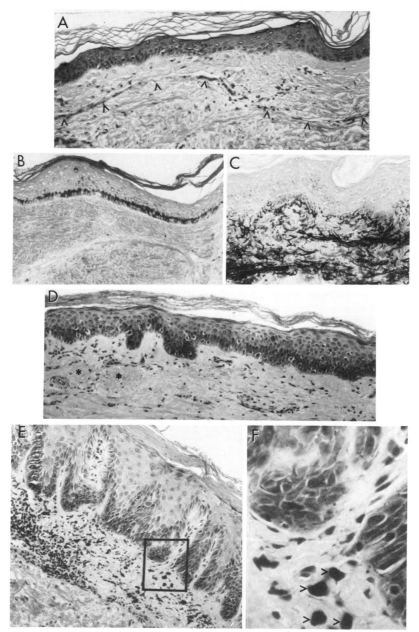

Figure 10.2. Histopathology of sunlight-damaged xeroderma pigmentosum skin. *(A–C)* Dermatome shaving from forearm. *(D)* Biopsy of pigmented macule on posterior calf. *(E and F)* Biopsy of a flat pigmented lesion (classified as a senile lentigo) on the inner aspect of the midthigh. *(A)* The epidermis is thin, shows no significant cellular atypia, and has no rete pegs. The dermis shows an elongated telangiectatic vessel *(arrowheads)*. Hematoxylin and eosin staining (original magnification × 40). *(B)* Fontana–Masson stain of section from same shaving showing irregular accumulations of melanin in the basal layer in the absence of any marked increase in the number of melanocytes (original magnification × 40). *(C)* Verhoeff–van Gieson elastic tissue stain showing elastotic changes in the dermis (original magnification × 40). *(D)* Hematoxylin and eosin stain of section showing a compact and parakeratotic stratum corneum, blunt rete ridges, numerous melanocytes (cells with clear cytoplasm) in basal layer, and basophilic (elastotic) degeneration in the dermis (areas surrounding asterisks). *(E)* The elongated and club-shaped rete pegs contain increased melanin. A nonspecific dermal infiltrate containing numerous melanophages is also present. Inset shown in *F*. Hematoxylin and eosin stain (original magnification × 40). *(F)* High-power magnification (original magnification × 160) of inset of *E* showing melanophages *(arrowheads)* in the dermis. *(A–F* adapted from Robbins and Moshell [22].)

muscle biopsy results, indicate that there is a chronic denervation atrophy of the muscles [1,36]. Sensorineural hearing loss is also progressive [26]. Degeneration of the eighth cranial nerve has been reported [35], and audiometric testing suggests damage to the hair cells of the cochlea [37].

Cellular Characteristics

Xeroderma pigmentosum cells in tissue culture are more readily killed by UV radiation than are normal cells [25–28]. Cultured cells from XP patients with a history of acute sun sensitivity and an early age of onset of neurological abnormalities are the most readily killed [25]. Cultured XP cells are more readily mutated [38] and transformed [39] than are normal cells by UV radiation. Certain UV-radiation-mimetic DNA-damaging chemicals, including certain carcinogens, produce essentially the same effects as UV radiation in these in vitro tests [4]. An abnormally increased frequency of chromosomal aberrations and sister chromatid exchanges is also found in XP cells treated with UV radiation or these DNA-damaging chemicals [3,4].

Biochemical Characteristics

Ultraviolet radiation in sunlight produces several types of DNA damage, the most important of which is the cyclobutane dimer that forms covalently between adjacent pyrimidine bases on the same DNA strand [1]. Normal cells are able to repair this damage by a series of enzymatic reactions comprising a nucleotide-excision DNA-repair process [1,3,4]. In this process the dimer-containing region of the DNA strand is removed from the DNA double helix, the resulting space is then filled in by a DNA polymerase, which inserts bases by using the opposing intact DNA strand as a template, and the newly synthesized portion is joined to the remainder by a polynucleotide ligase. The cells of most XP patients are excision deficient, since they are unable to make the initial incision required to begin removal of the dimer-containing DNA segments [40], and consequently retain dimers in their DNA longer than do normal cells [3,4]. There is a group of XP patients whose cells are excision proficient [1,12,13]; these XP variants have a severe defect in a different DNA repair process, known as postreplication repair [14]. Cells from XP variants [41] and from excision-deficient XP patients [42,43] are also unable to repair double-stranded DNA viruses that have been exposed to UV radiation before they infect the cells.

Such host-cell reactivation studies, in which the virus but not the XP cell is irradiated, confirm that XP cells have a primary defect in their ability to repair DNA damaged by UV radiation [3,4].

Somatic Cell Genetic Studies

By fusing tissue culture cells from one XP patient with those from another, multinucleated cells are obtained [1]. If, after cell fusion, DNA repair in the nuclei is restored to normal in both cell donors, the donors are considered to be in different complementation groups because they have different defective gene products, and each can supply a normal version of the product that is defective in the other [1,11]. When no complementation occurs in the fused cells, the cell donors are considered to be in the same complementation group, that is, they have the same defective gene product [1,11]. Nine complementation groups, referred to as groups A through I, have been identified among DNA excision-deficient XP patients [44]. Most neurologically affected XP patients are in complementation groups A and D [28]. Groups A, C, and D have numerous members, while the remaining groups comprise very few kindreds. Complementation groups B [1] and H [15] are composed of a single patient each; these two patients are the only ones known to have both XP and Cockayne's syndrome. The complementation between these two patients' cells in the cell-fusion tests indicates that the gene defects responsible for XP are different in each of these patients.

Pathogenesis

Sunlight-induced Damage

The consequences of the defective DNA-repair processes in XP patients explain many of their clinical and pathologic abnormalities. Tissue culture studies have shown that defective DNA repair makes UV-irradiated XP cells more readily mutable [38], transformable [39], and susceptible to death [25] than are normal cells. Freckles and achromic spots on the sun-exposed skin of normal people result from sunlight-induced mutations in melanocytes [1]. Consequently, the increase in such pigmentation abnormalities in XP and the increased frequency of skin cancers are the result of hypermutability. The atrophy of XP skin, as well as the acute sun sensitivity seen in some patients, is caused, at least in part, by the increased rate of cell death that results from defective DNA repair. Since the DNA-repair defect in

XP is present in all types of nucleated cells studied [1,10], including conjunctiva [45], the ocular abnormalities of XP can also be explained by defective DNA-repair processes.

Neurodegeneration

The ability of XP fibroblasts and lymphoblastoid cells to survive in tissue culture after treatment with UV radiation depends on the severity of the patient's DNA-repair defect [1,25–28,46]. From these postirradiation survival studies, it is known that XP patients whose neurologic abnormalities presented early have the most severe DNA-repair defects. Those with a later age of onset and a slower progression of neurologic abnormalities have a milder defect, while XP patients who do not develop neurologic abnormalities have the mildest of defects. Based upon these studies [25–28], it has been concluded that the death of XP neurons occurs because of their accumulation of unrepaired DNA damage. Since the UV radiation contained in sunlight is unable to reach the nervous system [1], the damage to neuronal DNA must be due to UV-mimetic intracellular metabolites or spontaneous hydrolysis of the DNA bases [28]. In the presence of normally functioning DNA-repair processes, this DNA damage would be repaired; however, in the presence of the severely defective DNA-repair processes of some XP patients, the damage remains unrepaired, accumulates, and eventually kills the nerve cells.

Clinical Management

Early Diagnosis

If XP is diagnosed early enough, measures can be instituted to protect the patient from the harmful UV radiation in sunlight. The diagnosis of XP should be considered in an infant or young child who has an acute sunburn reaction on minimal exposure to sunlight. Photophobia, conjunctivitis, and freckling are additional reasons for suspecting the presence of XP. The diagnosis of XP can be established only by performing the appropriate diagnostic tests for the XP DNA-repair defects on the patients' cultured fibroblasts or lymphocytes.

Protection from Ultraviolet Radiation

As reviewed in more detail elsewhere [2], UV radiation in sunlight is probably harmful up to a wave-

length of at least 340 nm even when reflected. This radiation is not filtered out by rain clouds but is completely blocked by window glass [2]. Xeroderma pigmentosum patients must, of course, avoid sunlamps. They should also avoid unshielded fluorescent light, since some commonly employed fluorescent light tubes emit wavelengths as low as approximately 313 nm [2]. Light from incandescent bulbs is not known to be harmful to XP patients [2].

Since no clinical abnormalities develop on XP skin that has been protected from sunlight (Figure 10.1A), the most important preventive measure for XP patients is the avoidance of harmful UV radiation. Five specific approaches for avoidance have been utilized [1,2,4,23]: (a) when traveling outdoors during daylight hours can not be avoided, it should be for as brief a time as possible and during the very early morning or late afternoon to avoid exposure to the sun's damaging UV radiation when it is at its highest intensity; (b) all skin surfaces, and particularly those not protected by clothing, should be treated daily with a chemical sunblocker (for example, a titanium dioxide compound) or sunscreen (for example, para-aminobenzoic acid in alcohol); (c) as much skin surface as possible should be covered by clothing (two layers of clothing where possible); (d) areas of the head and neck should be protected by a long hair style and a wide-brimmed hat; (e) the eyes should be protected by eyeglasses or sunglasses that are impenetrable to the harmful UV radiation in sunlight (that is, the lenses should be glass or specifically UV-impenetrable plastic). The glasses should have UV-impenetrable side shields to block radiation from the sides.

Protection from DNA-damaging Chemicals

It has been shown in cells cultured from XP patients that these cells cannot remove DNA damage induced by a certain type of carcinogen present in tobacco smoke [4]. Thus, XP patients should not smoke. Providing XP patients with a "protective" skin tan induced by photochemotherapy (orally administered methoxsalen followed by irradiation of the skin with long-wavelength UV-A radiation) is contraindicated, for XP cells cannot remove the DNA damage induced by this procedure [4].

Management of Lesions

Prompt Diagnosis

The prompt treatment of neoplastic lesions while they are small is particularly important for XP patients for the following reasons [1]: (a) since typical XP patients develop numerous lesions, each of which requires the removal or destruction of adjacent uninvolved skin, it is important to treat these lesions at the earliest possible stage; (b) since XP patients (other than the Japanese) have a greatly increased risk of developing malignant melanomas, it is important to diagnose melanomas as soon as possible in order to remove them before they metastasize.

Xeroderma pigmentosum patients should examine their eyes and all skin surfaces weekly [2]. "Unexposed, covered" areas (for example, the scalp and torso), as well as areas known to be exposed to sunlight, must be included in the examination, and any lesions that might be neoplastic should be reported to a dermatologist immediately. A careful examination by a dermatologist should be performed every 3 months, and most XP patients who have any active eye involvement should be examined by an ophthalmologist every 6 months.

Treatment

Treatment of the cutaneous neoplastic lesions in XP patients is essentially the same as that for normal individuals [1,2,4]. Liquid nitrogen cryotherapy is used for premalignant lesions such as actinic keratoses. As reviewed elsewhere [1,2,4], areas of XP skin with numerous premalignant lesions have been successfully treated with topical 5-fluorouracil, dermatome shaving, or dermabrasion. Cutaneous malignancies are treated with cryosurgery, electrodesiccation and curettage, surgical excision, and Mohs' chemosurgery. X-ray treatment can be employed for those malignant lesions not amenable to these modalities. Grafts of uninvolved skin from sun-protected areas are frequently required.

When the cornea and conjunctiva are subject to excessive dryness resulting from damaged eyelids, methylcellulose eye drops can be used [1,4,23,24]. A soft contact lens will help protect the cornea from mechanical damage [1,4,23]. Neoplasms of the conjunctiva and cornea are usually removed surgically [1,24], and a corneal transplant may restore sight in patients whose corneas have become scarred and opacified [24].

Prenatal Diagnosis

As reviewed elsewhere [4], prenatal diagnosis has been successfully accomplished by studying DNA-repair processes in fetal cells obtained by amniocentesis. No practical and reliable test for identifying XP heterozygotes has been reported.

Prognosis

Provided that the principles for avoiding sunlight and for treating lesions are rigorously adhered to, the prognosis is good for patients with XP who do not develop neurologic abnormalities. Increasingly, more XP patients are living well into adulthood, are completing their education, and are raising families. There is, however, no effective treatment for the progressive neurologic degeneration that affects some XP patients.

References

1. Robbins JH, Kraemer KH, Lutzner MA, et al. Xeroderma pigmentosum: an inherited disease with sun sensitivity, multiple cutaneous neoplasms and abnormal DNA repair. Ann Intern Med 1974;80:221–248.
2. Robbins JH. Xeroderma pigmentosum. In: Fitzpatrick TB, Eisen AZ, Wolff K, et al., eds. Dermatology in general medicine. New York: McGraw–Hill, 1979;2:390–394.
3. Cleaver JE. Xeroderma pigmentosum. In: Stanbury JB, Wyngaarden JB, Fredrickson DS, et al., eds. The metabolic basis of inherited disease. New York: McGraw–Hill, 1983;5:1227–1248.
4. Kraemer KK, Slor H. Xeroderma pigmentosum. In: Demis DJ, Dobson RL, McGuire J, eds. Clinics in dermatology. Hagerstown: Harper & Row, 1985;3:33–69.
5. Hebra F, Kaposi M. On diseases of the skin, including the exanthemata. Tay W, trans. and ed. London: The New Sydenham Society, 1874;3:252–258.
6. Kaposi M. Xeroderma pigmentosum. Med Jahrb Wien 1882;619–633. [French translation in Ann Dermatol Syph (Paris) 1883;4:29–38.]
7. Neisser A. Ueber das "Xeroderma pigmentosum" (Kaposi), Liodermia essentialis cum melanosi et telangiectasia. Vrtljschr Dermatol Wien 1883:47–62.
8. De Sanctis C, Cacchione A. L'idiozia xerodermica. Riv Sper Freniatr 1932;56:269–292.
9. Cleaver JE. Defective repair replication of DNA in xeroderma pigmentosum. Nature (Lond) 1968;218:652–656.
10. Epstein JH, Fukuyama K, Reed WB, et al. Defect in DNA synthesis in skin of patients with xeroderma pigmentosum demonstrated in vivo. Science 1970;168:1477–1478.
11. De Weerd–Kastelein EA, Keijzer W, Bootsma D. Genetic heterogeneity of xeroderma pigmentosum demonstrated by somatic cell hybridization. Nature New Biol 1972;238:80–83.
12. Burke PG, Lutzner MA, Clarke DD, et al. Ultraviolet stimulated thymidine incorporation in xeroderma pigmentosum lymphocytes. J Lab Clin Med 1971;77:759–767.
13. Cleaver JE. Xeroderma pigmentosum: variants with

normal DNA repair and normal sensitivity to ultraviolet light. J Invest Dermatol 1972;58:124–128.

14. Lehmann AR, Kirk–Bell S, Arlett CF, et al. Xeroderma pigmentosum cells with normal levels of excision repair have a defect in DNA synthesis after ultraviolet-irradiation. Proc Natl Acad Sci USA 1975;72:219–223.

15. Moshell AN, Ganges MB, Lutzner MA, et al. A new patient with both xeroderma pigmentosum and Cockayne syndrome comprises the new xeroderma pigmentosum complementation group H. In: Friedberg EC, Bridges BA, eds. Cellular responses to DNA damage. New York: Alan R. Liss, 1983:209–213.

16. Takebe H, Miki Y, Kozuka T, et al. DNA repair characteristics and skin cancers of xeroderma pigmentosum patients in Japan. Cancer Res 1977;37:490–495.

17. Pawsey SA, Magnus IA, Ramsay CA, et al. Clinical, genetic and DNA repair studies on a consecutive series of patients with xeroderma pigmentosum. Q J Med 1979;48:179–210.

18. Fischer E, Thielmann HW, Neundorfer B, et al. Xeroderma pigmentosum patients from Germany: clinical symptoms and DNA repair characteristics. Arch Dermatol Res 1982;274:229–247.

19. Hashem N, Bootsma D, Keijzer W, et al. Clinical characteristics, DNA repair, and complementation groups in xeroderma pigmentosum patients from Egypt. Cancer Res 1980;40:13–18.

20. Neel JV, Kodani M, Brewer R, et al. The incidence of consanguineous matings in Japan: with remarks on the estimation of comparative gene frequencies and the expected rate of appearance of induced recessive mutations. Am J Hum Genet 1949;1:156–178.

21. Lever WF, Schaumburg-Lever G. Histopathology of the skin. Philadelphia: Lippincott, 1975.

22. Robbins JH, Moshell AN. DNA repair processes protect human beings from premature solar skin damage: evidence from studies on xeroderma pigmentosum. J Invest Dermatol 1979;73:102–107.

23. Robbins JH. Xeroderma pigmentosum. In: Fraunfelder FT, Roy FH, eds. Current ocular therapy. Philadelphia: Saunders, 1980;136–138.

24. Gaasterland DE, Rodrigues MM, Moshell AN. Ocular involvement in xeroderma pigmentosum. Ophthalmology 1982;89:980–986.

25. Andrews AD, Barrett SF, Robbins JH. Xeroderma pigmentosum neurological abnormalities correlate with colony-forming ability after ultraviolet radiation. Proc Natl Acad Sci USA 1978;78:1984–1988.

26. Robbins JH, Polinsky RJ, Moshell AN. Evidence that lack of deoxyribonucleic acid repair causes death of neurons in xeroderma pigmentosum. Ann Neurol 1983;13:682–684.

27. Robbins JH. The significance of repair of human DNA: evidence from studies of xeroderma pigmentosum. J Natl Cancer Inst 1978;61:645–656.

28. Robbins JH, Brumback RA, Polinsky RG, et al. Hypersensitivity to DNA-damaging agents in abiotrophies: a new explanation for degeneration of neurons, photoreceptors, and muscle in Alzheimer, Parkinson and Huntington diseases, retinitis pigmentosa, and Duchenne muscular dystrophy. In: Woodhead AD, Blackett AD, Hollaender A, eds. Molecular biology of aging. New York: Plenum, 1985:315–344.

29. Mimaki T, Naoyuki I, Abe J, et al. Neurological manifestations in xeroderma pigmentosum. Ann Neurol 1986;20:70–75.

30. Guzzetta F. Cockayne–Neill–Dingwall syndrome. In: Vinken PH, Bruyn GW, eds. Handbook of clinical neurology. Amsterdam: North–Holland, 1972;13:431–440.

31. Brumback RA, Yoder FW, Andrews AD, et al. Normal pressure hydrocephalus: recognition and relationship to neurological abnormalities in Cockayne's syndrome. Arch Neurol 1978;35:337–345.

32. Otsuka F, Robbins JH. The Cockayne syndrome—an inherited multisystem disorder with cutaneous photosensitivity and defective repair of DNA. Comparison with xeroderma pigmentosum. Am J Dermatopathol 1985;7:387–392.

33. Schmickel RD, Chu EHY, Trosko JE, et al. Cockayne syndrome: a cellular sensitivity to ultraviolet light. Pediatrics 1977;60:135–139.

34. Andrews AD, Barrett SF, Yoder FW, et al. Cockayne's syndrome fibroblasts have increased sensitivity to ultraviolet light but normal rates of unscheduled DNA synthesis. J Invest Dermatol 1978;70:237–239.

35. Yano K. Xeroderma pigmentosa mit Störungen des Zentralnervensystems: eine histopathologische Untersuchung. Folia Psychiatr Neurol Jpn 1950;4:143–175.

36. Thrush DC, Holti G, Bradley WG. Neurological manifestations of xeroderma pigmentosum in two siblings. J Neurol Sci 1974;22:91–104.

37. Kenyon GS, Booth JB, Prasher DK, et al. Neuro-otological abnormalities in xeroderma pigmentosum with particular reference to deafness. Brain 1985;108:771–784.

38. Maher VM, Dorney DJ, Mendrala AL, et al. DNA excision-repair processes in human cells can eliminate the cytotoxic and mutagenic consequences of ultraviolet irradiation. Mutation Res 1979;62:311–323.

39. Maher VM, Rowan LA, Silinskas KC, et al. Frequency of UV-induced neoplastic transformation of diploid human fibroblasts is higher in xeroderma pigmentosum cells than in normal cells. Proc Natl Acad Sci USA 1982;79:2613–2617.

40. Fornace AJ, Kohn KW, Hann HE. DNA single-strand breaks during repair of UV damage in human fibroblasts and abnormalities of repair in xeroderma pigmentosum. Proc Natl Acad Sci USA 1976;73:39–43.

41. Day RS. Xeroderma pigmentosum variants have decreased repair of ultraviolet-damaged DNA. Nature (Lond) 1975;253:748–749.

42. Rabson AS, Tyrrell SA, Legallais FY. Growth of ultraviolet-damaged herpes-virus in xeroderma pigmentosum cells. Proc Soc Exp Biol Med 1969;132:802–806.

43. Day RS. Studies on repair of adenovirus 2 by human

fibroblasts using normal, xeroderma pigmentosum and xeroderma pigmentosum heterozygous strains. Cancer Res 1974;34:1965–1970.

44. Fischer E, Keijzer W, Thielmann HW, et al. A ninth complementation group in xeroderma pigmentosum, XP I. Mutation Res 1985;145:217–225.

45. Newsome DA, Kraemer KH, Robbins JH. Repair of DNA in xeroderma pigmentosum conjunctiva. Arch Ophthalmol 1975;94:660–662.

46. Moshell AN, Tarone RE, Newfield SA, et al. A simple and rapid method for evaluating the survival of xeroderma pigmentosum lymphoid lines after irradiation with ultraviolet light. In Vitro 1981;17:299–307.

Chapter 11
Cockayne's Syndrome

DONALD ZIMMERMAN

In 1936, Cockayne [1] described a 7-year 11-month-old girl and her 6-year 3-month-old brother who were affected with a condition characterized by dwarfism, pigmentary degeneration of the retina, optic atrophy, and deafness. Other features described in the initial report included microcephaly, enophthalmos, prominent maxillae, disproportionately long extremities in comparison with the size of the trunk (with particular enlargement of the hands and feet), mental subnormality, erythematous scaly photosensitive dermatitis, thick cranial vault, shallow pituitary fossa, carious dentition, and anorexia. Ten years later, Cockayne reported additional developments in his patients. These included cataracts, extreme inanition, secondary hypomenorrhea, spasticity of the lower extremities with flexion contractures, cardiac arrhythmias, proteinuria, and marked delay in pubertal development [2]. Approximately 70 cases of Cockayne's syndrome have been described [3]. Its pattern of inheritance and some aspects of its pathogenesis have been elucidated.

Clinical and Laboratory Features

Growth

At birth, patients have normal size, proportions, and facial appearance [4–9]. Not infrequently, feeding difficulties occur in the neonatal period [5–7,10,11]. Some of the neonates suck poorly [6,10] and some vomit frequently [6,11]. In nearly all cases neonatal feeding difficulties remit during infancy and growth normalizes. Some infants take as long as 6 months to establish a normal weight gain pattern [6]. However, poor feeding and poor growth recur.

Many patients manifest growth failure in height and weight by 12 months of age [6,7,8]. Some manifest poor growth by 6 to 7 months of age [5,11] and others by 2 to 3 years of age [2,12,13]. Growth in weight has declined prior to growth in height in our patients and in some reported in the literature [4]. Skeletal maturation as estimated by bone age is often normal [2,6,8,14] but may be delayed [15] or advanced [16–18]. In some instances, bone age becomes advanced, and there is premature fusion of phalangeal epiphyses at approximately 9 years of age [15,17,19].

As patients become progressively cachectic, they acquire a distinctive facial appearance characterized by a thin prominent nose and zygomatic processes, prognathism, enophthalmos, and absent fat [3]. This appearance is usually well developed by the age of 4 years [12] (Figure 11.1).

Skin

The most dramatic cutaneous feature observed in some patients with Cockayne's syndrome [1,5,6,7,11,12,20], though not in all [10,21], is a photosensitive dermatitis associated with erythema, bullae, and scarring.

Other abnormalities of the skin include general thinness of the skin with absence of subcutaneous tissue [6,9,10], cold and blue extremities (in our patients, these features have been indistinguishable from findings in other patients with undernutrition) [1,2,6,20], increased numbers of pigmented nevi (especially over the extremities, head, and neck) [2,8], anhydrosis [11,22], and decreased hair over the scalp and eyebrows [10–12,21]. In some patients, the nails are dystrophic [12]. Other ectodermal abnormalities include abnormally small [10] or carious [6,8,10,12] teeth.

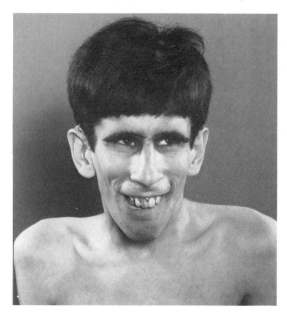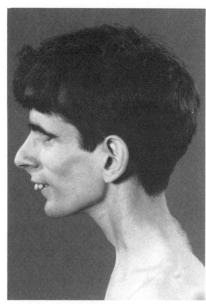

Figure 11.1. Facial appearance of a patient with Cockayne's syndrome. The nose and zygomatic processes are prominent. Enophthalmos is present, and fat is absent.

Central and Peripheral Nervous Systems

Among the neurologic abnormalities in patients with Cockayne's syndrome, progressive deterioration of mental function is particularly prominent [2,5–8,10–12,22–24]. The degree of psychomotor delay in patients with Cockayne's syndrome comprises a broad spectrum from severe retardation [11] to essentially normal intelligence [4]. Patients with Cockayne's syndrome manifest a higher level of social functioning than of general intellectual functioning [5,22]. Gradual mental deterioration may occur for a period of time. Later in childhood or early in adult life, psychomotor deterioration characteristically accelerates. This deterioration culminates, after a period of many months, in loss of ability to sit, walk, and talk as well as in fecal and urinary incontinence [5,12,24].

Psychomotor delay in Cockayne's syndrome is frequently associated with microcephaly and normal pressure hydrocephalus. Although microcephaly may be evident at birth [25], it is usually first noted in the second or third year of life [15,26]. In patients with Cockayne's syndrome the contrast between their intact social adaptation and their diminished intellectual functioning is similar to that observed in other patients with normal pressure hydrocephalus [5,22]. The same can be said for the progression of dementia to apathy, inertia, and decreased consciousness [5,27]

and for the enlargement of all cerebral ventricles despite normal intracranial pressure [5]. Ventricular enlargement and basal ganglia calcification are evident on head CT (Figure 11.2).

Like other patients with normal pressure hydrocephalus [27,28], patients with Cockayne's syndrome manifest a complex movement disorder associated with spasticity greater in the lower extremities, apraxia, ataxia, and extrapyramidal features including inertia and retropulsion. Choreoathetosis is frequently prominent as are intention tremor, dysdiadochokinesia, and myoclonic jerks. Peripheral sensorimotor neuropathy may contribute to the gait disturbance [11,25,29,30].

Seizures have been described [4,5,6,31,32] and have their onset as early as the age of 1 year [4] or as late as 21 years [31]. Optic atrophy has been reported in approximately 50% of reported patients [5]. Patients with optic atrophy have tended to be older than those without it, suggesting that, like many of the other neurologic abnormalities, optic atrophy may develop as a relatively late finding [33]. In addition to optic atrophy, approximately 70% of patients have atypical retinopigmentary degeneration [5]. Cockayne described this finding in his original report: "scattered all over the fundus but particularly aggregated towards the central areas, are a number of fine blackish dots like those seen in 'salt and pepper fundus,' but differing from the classical

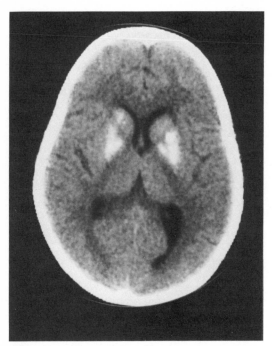

Figure 11.2. CT scan image of basal ganglia mineralization in a patient with Cockayne's syndrome.

Approximately 25% of patients with Cockayne's syndrome are resistant to pupillary dilatation by mydriatic agents [5]. Other ocular abnormalities described in these patients include cataracts [2,33], keratopathy [33], strabismus, and nystagmus [33].

Sensorineural deafness has been described in approximately 45% of patients with Cockayne's syndrome [5]. Like blindness and other neurologic abnormalities in patients with Cockayne's syndrome, sensorineural deafness tends to be progressive. Vestibular reflexes tend to remain intact in Cockayne's patients with deafness [34].

Kidneys

Other significant clinical findings in patients with Cockayne's syndrome include hypertension and kidney disease. The prevalence of these complications is unknown because many reports focus on other findings. Both hypertension and kidney disease have been found together in some patients with Cockayne's syndrome [13,17,20]. At least one patient with histologic evidence of kidney disease was initially normotensive; hypertension supervened over a period of 16 months [20]. While hypertension is mild to moderate [6,13,17] in some patients, in others it is more severe. In one instance, there was fatal malignant hypertension [20].

Decreased glomerular filtration rates [13,17,20] and trace proteinuria [17,20] have been described in patients with pathologically documented kidney disease. However, one rather severely affected patient had no proteinuria [13]. The urine sediment is gen-

picture in the distinct and symmetrically heavier involvement of the central areas. Nowhere does the pigmentary disturbance tend to follow the blood vessels." The combination of retinitis pigmentosa and optic atrophy ultimately contribute to progressive loss of vision [2,5,22,33]. As these abnormalities progress, the retinal vessels become progressively narrower [2,33] (Figure 11.3).

Figure 11.3. Photograph of the ocular fundus in a patient with Cockayne's syndrome. Optic atrophy is present, as is pigmentary degeneration and narrowing of the blood vessels.

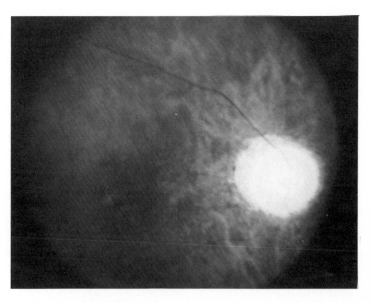

erally normal but occasionally red or white blood cells are present [13,17,20]. In one of our patients with progressive azotemia, the urinary sediment eventually showed granular casts with increasing proteinuria.

Pubertal Development

A number of abnormalities in sexual development have been described in patients with Cockayne's syndrome. Some degree of hypogonadism is often present, particularly in affected boys [22].

Some boys with Cockayne's syndrome have been reported to have normal genitalia [30], and others undescended testes [1,6,9,11]. Testes were found to be absent at autopsy in one patient [35]. Pubertal changes are frequently absent or subnormal [8,22]. A 19-year-old boy treated at the Mayo Clinic had small testes and laboratory evidence of partial primary testicular failure (normal serum testosterone levels but markedly elevated serum levels of luteinizing hormone and follicle stimulating hormone).

Girls with Cockayne's syndrome manifest pubertal development more frequently than do boys [22]: they have small breasts and, frequently, oligomenorrhea [2,22]. One patient was reported with pubertal precocity [24].

Skeleton

Skeletal radiographs are usually normal until sometime between 2 and 3 years of age. Thereafter, the skull fails to grow normally—the ocular orbits and sella turcica remain particularly small. The calvaria and skull base become dense. Vertebral bodies assume a pear shape with posterior tapering. Eventually, kyphosis and osteoporosis appear. The pelvis remains small (particularly the iliac crests), and the iliac angle becomes abnormally steep. Coxa valga may develop. The long bones develop slender diaphyses with thickened dense cortices and narrowed medullary canals. Long bone epiphyses, and, to a lesser extent, metaphyses, are disproportionately large and osteoporotic. Some epiphyses in the hands and feet become sclerotic. The carpal and tarsal bones become large and osteoporotic. Ribs and clavicles become slender [15,30].

Prognosis

Among a number of patients reported to have died from Cockayne's syndrome, the average age at death was 11.67 years. The shortest lived had unusually early symptoms and manifestations and died between 8 months and 6 years 5 months of age [23,35]. The remainder died between 11 and 31 years of age [10,12,20,24,31,36,37]. Approximately one-half of the patients died from pneumonia [12,24,35,36,37]. Other causes of death included status epilepticus, malignant hypertension, and renal and pulmonary dysfunction.

Genetics

Cockayne's syndrome is thought to be inherited in an autosomal recessive manner [3,22,33]. Among the 70 cases reported, there are more males than females [30]. Several reports have described two or more affected siblings with Cockayne's syndrome [1,2,5,7,10,12,20,23,29,30,33,35,36]. No parent and child have been affected in the same family. Some affected patients had consanguineous parents [17,33,36,38].

Pathology

Skin

Pathologic examination of the skin shows atrophy of the epidermis with hyalinization of dermal collagen. Hair follicles and sweat glands are abnormally small. Hair follicles show sebaceous transformation, a normal finding in fetal life [10].

Brain

Cerebral atrophy is a prominent pathologic finding in Cockayne's syndrome [10,23,24,35,36]. In large measure, the small brain size is related to loss of cerebral white matter [10,23,24,35,36,38]. The cerebellum has been described, in a number of reports, as more atrophic (specifically manifesting loss of white matter) than the cerebrum [23,31,36]. Frank atrophy of the brain stem was evident in some autopsied cases [24,36,37], and patchy demyelination with generalized nerve cell loss has been frequently noted [24,31,36,37]. The spinal cord also is characterized by patchy demyelination and gliosis [31,37].

Neuronal abnormalities are most prominent in the cerebellum. Focal sclerosis may be present in areas of Purkinje and granular cell loss [10,23,31,36,37]. Two reports describe abnormal dendritic morphology in the Purkinje cells [23,36]. Purkinje cell changes include axonal swelling ("torpedoes") [10,36], dendritic expansion ("cactus flowers") [36], and mineralization of soma and dendrites [24,36]. Nuclear abnormalities in cerebellar neurons include multinucleation [23,36], hyperchromia, and enlargement [23]. The dentate nucleus cell bodies of one patient contained large amounts of lipofuscin [37].

Neuronal abnormalities are less severe in the cerebrum than in the cerebellum. Neuronal loss [24,31,37] sometimes associated with gliosis [24,31], lipofuscin accumulation in cortical neurons [36,37], neurofibrillary tangles [36], and Hirano bodies [36] has been described. Some cortical neurons are calcified and appear as globular or stellate bodies [24]. Nuclear atypia has been described in cerebral neurons [23]. The basal ganglia neurons of one patient contained large amounts of lipofuscin [37], and in another patient there was a brown-black pigment, possibly melanin [36].

Vascular abnormalities are present in the CNS of some patients [10,24,31,36,37] and are most marked in the basal ganglia but also in the cerebral and cerebellar white matter and, to a smaller extent, in the gray matter [37]. The capillaries are most frequently affected with globules of PAS-positive material within their walls and over their outer surface [31]; these globules are frequently mineralized. The mineral in and around cortical capillaries is chiefly calcium while that in the basal ganglia and especially in the globus pallidus is predominantly iron [31,37]. In some areas pericapillary mineral deposits form large coalescent laminated "brain stones" [36]. Similar accumulations of mineralized PAS-positive material are found in the adventitia and media of arterioles [10,31,36,37]. Granular ependymitis and choroid plexus atrophy [22,24,31,32,37] are frequently present.

Peripheral Nerves and Eye

In addition to segmental demyelination [11,23,24, 25,30,31,32,36,37,39] peripheral nerves may show onion-bulb formation [25,30]. In one patient, granular lysosomal inclusions were observed in perineuronal cells and in Schwann cells on ultrastructural examination of peripheral nerve [25].

Pathologic examination of the eye reveals gliosis of the inner layers of the retina. The choroidal pigment layer is thickened and disrupted. The optic disc and optic nerve are gliotic, and the retinal arteries are thickened [24].

Kidney

Pathologic examination of the kidney has shown thickening of the glomerular basement membrane and mesangium along with some collapse and hyalinization of glomeruli. Tubular atrophy and interstitial fibrosis also have been observed [10,17,20]. Segmented granular deposits of IgG, IgM, IgA, and C3 have been found in portions of the glomerular basement membrane and mesangium, and C3 was found in the walls of small arterioles and in the tubular basement membrane [20].

Pathogenesis

Growth Deficiency

While one report suggests that poor growth in stature may be related to growth hormone deficiency [10], one of our patients and two recorded in the literature [13,14] had normal responses to growth hormone provocative tests. The possibility that poor growth in patients with Cockayne's syndrome results from cachexia-induced underproduction of somatomedin-c [39,40] has not been systemically studied. One of our patients had a normal somatomedin-c level, normal growth hormone secretion in response to exercise, normal thyroid function, and normal renal function. These findings suggest that growth deficiency in patients with Cockayne's syndrome may result from the inability of bone to respond to normal amounts of somatomedin-c.

Photosensitive Dermatitis

A number of experimental studies suggest that photosensitivity in Cockayne's syndrome may result from the increased susceptibility of skin cells to damage produced by ultraviolet radiation [7]. This susceptibility to ultraviolet radiation damage may be the result of a defect in the ability of Cockayne cells to repair ultraviolet radiation-induced damage in cellular DNA [41–45].

Neurologic Abnormalities

While psychomotor deterioration may be related in part to progressive cerebral atrophy, normal pressure hydrocephalus may also contribute [5].

The pathophysiologic substrate of the movement

abnormalities in patients with Cockayne's syndrome is complex. Normal pressure hydrocephalus may contribute to the abnormal gait as well as to spasticity [5]. Ataxia as well as intention tremor and dysdiadokinesia may be related to profound abnormalities in cerebellar myelin as well as in cerebellar neurons. Spasticity may be due in part to central demyelination. Finally, peripheral neuropathy may contribute to gait disturbance in these patients. Seizures have been described in patients with pathologic evidence of neuronal damage and gliosis. Neuronal injury may be the result of calcifying vasculopathy, a frequent finding in the brain of patients with Cockayne's syndrome [31].

Since vestibular reflexes remain intact in patients with Cockayne's syndrome, deafness has been attributed to degeneration of the organ of Corti [34].

Kidney Dysfunction

Deposits of immunoglobulin and complement in the glomerular basement membrane and mesangium raise the possibility that immunologic mechanisms may contribute to the problems of hypertension and renal dysfunction.

Etiologic Hypotheses

No single pathogenic mechanism has been demonstrated to be responsible for the diverse abnormalities present in patients with Cockayne's syndrome. Robbins [3,23] has presented evidence supporting the hypothesis that a central pathogenic mechanism in this syndrome is the inability to repair long-patch errors in DNA sequence (the type of error induced by ultraviolet radiation and a number of chemicals). As noted above, the sensitivity of skin fibroblasts to the effects of ultraviolet radiation [41–45] provide a particularly plausible explanation for the photosensitive dermatitis found in patients with Cockayne's syndrome. A similar hypersensitivity to ultraviolet radiation has been demonstrated in lymphoid cells in affected patients, raising the possibility that the inability to repair long-patch DNA damage may be pervasive or indeed ubiquitous among various tissues in affected patients.

Some of the neuropathologic changes in this disease are shared with other disorders in which there is defective repair of DNA errors [23]. For instance, abnormalities in the nuclei of certain CNS cells [23,36] in Cockayne's syndrome—including multi-

nucleation and nuclear hyperchromia of astrocytes, binucleation of Purkinje cells [23,36], and abnormally large Schwann cell nuclei [10]—are similar to those observed in ataxia-telangiectasia and in tuberous sclerosis (conditions in which DNA repair of the short-patch type error produced by ionizing radiation are defective). Similar cell nucleus abnormalities have also been demonstrated in mammalian fibroblasts exposed to supralethal doses of ionizing radiation [46]. Purkinje cells in Cockayne's syndrome may show two other pathologic changes found in ataxia-telangiectasia [47]—abnormal dendrites [23,36] and axonal swelling with "torpedo" formation [10,23,36].

It should be noted that direct evidence of abnormal DNA repair in nervous tissue from patients with Cockayne's syndrome has not yet been reported. Pathologic findings suggesting abnormal DNA repair in this tissue have only been observed in a small minority of patients. Thus, additional studies will be needed to investigate a possible role for defective DNA repair in the pathogenesis of CNS abnormalities in Cockayne's syndrome.

Other hypotheses have been proposed to explain the varied abnormalities in patients with Cockayne's syndrome. The presence of lipofuscin in the majority of neurons in the basal ganglia, pons, medulla, and dentate nucleus has raised the possibility that Cockayne's syndrome is a type of sudanophilic lipodystrophy, perhaps related to a specific abnormality in myelin regeneration [22,32].

Finally, an inflammatory hypothesis has been suggested by some investigators [20,37,48]. Thickening of the leptomeninges seen in patients with Cockayne's syndrome [5] has been observed in many patients with normal pressure hydrocephalus [48]. Ependymitis is present in patients with Cockayne's syndrome as well as in others with normal pressure hydrocephalus and has been thought to cause normal pressure hydrocephalus in these patients [48]. The presence of immune complexes in the kidneys and blood of some patients lends support to an inflammatory etiology [20].

Treatment

No specific treatment is available. Supportive measures consist of special education because of psychomotor delay, hearing aids for sensorineural deafness, and physical therapy to prevent limb contractures. Anticonvulsants have been effective in controlling seizures. Sun exposure should be avoided to prevent exacerbation of photosensitive dermatitis. It is uncertain whether vigorous avoidance of ultraviolet radiation would reduce or minimize the ocular abnormalities in this condition.

It is not known what might be the effect of treating the normal pressure hydrocephalus with a shunt. It is unlikely that this treatment would diminish the psychomotor regression of these patients but perhaps the gait abnormalities and the prominent headache of some patients would improve.

References

1. Cockayne EA. Dwarfism with retinal atrophy and deafness. Arch Dis Child 1936;11:1–8.
2. Cockayne EA. Case reports: dwarfism with retinal atrophy and deafness. Arch Dis Child 1946;21:52–54.
3. Otsuka F, Robbins JH. The Cockayne syndrome—an inherited multisystem disorder with cutaneous photosensitivity and defective repair of DNA. Am J Dermatopathol 1985;7:387–392.
4. Lanning M, Simila S. Cockayne's syndrome: report of a case with normal intelligence. Z Kinderheilkd 1970;109:70–75.
5. Brumbach RA, Yoder FW, Andrews AD, et al. Normal pressure hydrocephalus: recognition and relationship to neurological abnormalities in Cockayne's syndrome. Arch Neurol 1978;35:337–345.
6. Macdonald WB, Fitch KD, Lewis IC. Cockayne's syndrome: an heredo-familial disorder of growth and development. Pediatrics 1960;25:997–1007.
7. Schmickel RD, Chu EHY, Trosko JE, et al. Cockayne syndrome: a cellular sensitivity to ultraviolet light. Pediatrics 1977;60:135–139.
8. Neill CA, Dingwall MM. A syndrome resembling progeria: a review of two cases. Arch Dis Child 1950;25:213–221.
9. Pfeiffer RA, Bachmann KD. An atypical case of Cockayne's syndrome. Clin Genet 1973;4:28–32.
10. Sugarman GI, Landing BH, Reed WB. Cockayne syndrome: clinical study of two patients and neuropathologic findings in one. Clin Pediatr 1977;16:225–232.
11. Moosa A, Dubowitz V. Peripheral neuropathy in Cockayne's syndrome. Arch Dis Child 1970;45:674–677.
12. Proops R, Taylor AMR, Insley J. A clinical study of a family with Cockayne's syndrome. J Med Genet 1981;18:288–293.
13. Fujimoto WY, Greene ML, Seegmiller JE. Cockayne's syndrome: report of a case with hyperlipoproteinemia, hyperinsulinemia, renal disease, and normal growth hormone. J Pediatr 1969;75:881–884.
14. Cotton RB, Keats TE, McCoy EE. Abnormal blood glucose regulation in Cockayne's syndrome. Pediatrics 1970;46:54–60.
15. Riggs W Jr, Seibert J. Cockayne's syndrome: roentgen findings. AJR 1972;116:623–633.
16. Land VJ, Nogrady MB. Cockayne's syndrome. J Can Assoc Radiol 1969;20:194–203.
17. Ohno T, Hirooka M. Renal lesions in Cockayne's syndrome. Tohoku J Exp Med 1966;89:151–166.
18. Spark H. Cachectic dwarfism resembling Cockayne's–Neill type. J Pediatr 1965;66:41–47.
19. Alton DJ, McDonald P, Reilly BJ. Cockayne's syndrome: report of three cases. Radiology 1972;102:403–406.
20. Higginbottom MC, Griswold WR, Jones KL, et al. The Cockayne syndrome: an evaluation of hypertension and studies of renal pathology. Pediatrics 1979;64:929–934.
21. Pfeiffer RA, Bachmann KD. An atypical case of Cockayne's syndrome. Clin Genet 1973;4:28–32.
22. Guzzetta F. Cockayne–Neill–Dingwall syndrome in neuroretinal degenerations. In: Vinken PJ, Bruyn GW, eds. Handbook of clinical neurology. Amsterdam: Elsevier–North–Holland, 1972;13:431–440.
23. Leech RW, Brumback RA, Miller RH, et al. Cockayne syndrome: clinicopathologic and tissue culture studies of affected siblings. J Neuropathol Exp Neurol 1985;44:507–519.
24. Rowlatt U. Cockayne's syndrome: report of a case with necropsy findings. Acta Neuropathol (Berl) 1969;14:52–61.
25. Grunnet ML, Zimmerman AW, Lewis RA. Ultrastructure and electrodiagnosis of peripheral neuropathy in Cockayne's syndrome. Neurology 1983;33:1606–1609.
26. Bensman A, Faure C, Kaufman HJ. The spectrum of x-ray manifestations in Cockayne syndrome. Skel Radiol 1981;7:173–177.
27. Wood JH, Bartlet D, James AE Jr, et al. Normal pressure hydrocephalus: diagnosis and patient selection for surgery. Neurology 1974;24:517–526.
28. Chawla JC, Woodward J. Motor disorder in "normal pressure" hydrocephalus. Br Med J 1972;1:485–486.
29. Srivastava RN, Gupta PC, Mayekar G, et al. Case report: Cockayne's syndrome in two sisters. Acta Paediatr Scand 1964;63:461–464.
30. Smits MG, Gabreels FJM, Renier WO, et al. Peripheral and central myelinopathy in Cockayne's syndrome. Neuropediatrics 1982;13:161–167.
31. Crome L, Kanjilal GC. Cockayne's syndrome: case report. J Neurol Neurosurg Psychiatry 1971;34:171–179.
32. Norman RM, Tingey H. Syndrome of microcephaly, striocerebellar calcifications, and leucodystrophy. J Neurol Neurosurg Psychiatry 1966;29:157–163.
33. Pearce WG. Ocular and genetic features of Cockayne's syndrome. Can J Ophthalmol 1972;7:435–444.
34. Franceschetti A, Francois J, Babel J. Les Hérédo-Dégénérescenses Choriorétiennes. Paris: Masson, 1963:1153–1156.
35. Moyer DB, Marquis P, Shertzer ME, et al. Cockayne syndrome with early onset of manifestations. Am J Med Genet 1982;13:225–230.
36. Soffer D, Grotsky HW, Rapid IN, et al. Cockayne syndrome: unusual neuropathological findings and review of the literature. Ann Neurol 1979;6:340–348.

37. Moossy J. The neuropathology of Cockayne's syndrome. J Neuropathol Exp Neurol 1967;26:654–660.

38. Paddison RM, Moossy J, Derbes VJ, et al. Cockayne's syndrome: a report of five new cases with biochemical, chromosomal, dermatologic, genetic and neuropathologic observations. Dermatol Trop 1963;2:195–203.

39. Grant DB, Hambley J, Becker D, et al. Reduced sulfation factor in undernourished children. Arch Dis Child 1973;48:596–600.

40. Clemmons DR, Klibansky A, Underwood LE, et al. Reduction of plasma immunoreactive somatomedin-c during fasting in humans. J Clin Endocrinol Metab 1981;53:1247–1250.

41. Marshall RR, Arlett CF, Harcourt SA, et al. Increased sensitivity of cell strains from Cockayne's syndrome to sister-chromatid-exchange induction and cell killing by UV light. Mutat Res 1980;69:107–112.

42. Cheng WS, Tarone RE, Andrews AD, et al. Ultraviolet light-induced sister chromatid exchanges in xeroderma pigmentosum and in Cockayne's syndrome lymphocyte cell lines. Cancer Res 1978;38:1601–1609.

43. Day RS III, Ziolkowski CHJ, DiMattina M. Decreased host cell reactivation of UV-irradiated adenovirus 5 by fibroblasts from Cockayne's syndrome patients. Photochem Photobiol 1981;34:603–607.

44. Lytle CD, Tarone RE, Barrett SF, et al. Host cell reactivation by fibroblasts from patients with pigmentary degeneration of the retina. Photochem Photobiol 1983;37:503–508.

45. Watatani M, Ohtani H, Takai SI, et al. Host cell reactivation of ultraviolet light irradiated adenovirus 5 in fibroblasts from patients with Cockayne syndrome: a study with six Japanese cases. J Radiat Res 1984;25:150–159.

46. Scudiero DA, Moshell AN, Scarpinato RG, et al. Lymphoblastoid lines and skin fibroblasts from patients with tuberous sclerosis are abnormally sensitive to ionizing radiation and to a radiomimetic chemical. J Invest Dermatol 1982;78:234.

47. Strich SJ. Pathological findings in three cases of ataxia telangiectasia. J Neurol Neurosurg Psychiatry 1966;29:489–499.

48. Adams RD, Victor M. Principles of Neurology. New York: McGraw–Hill, 1985:461–473.

Chapter 12
Rothmund–Thomson Syndrome

ROBERTA A. PAGON

Rothmund–Thomson syndrome (poikiloderma con-genitale) is an autosomal recessive disorder in which obligatory and characteristic skin changes frequently are associated with ectodermal dysplasia and juve-nile-onset cataracts. Hypogonadism, short stature, and skeletal abnormalities are common. Character-istic facies may be present. Intelligence is normal. The metabolic basis of this rare disorder is unknown.

History

This disorder was first described by Rothmund, a German ophthalmologist, in 1868 [1], who noted cutaneous abnormalities in a child with cataracts. Upon hearing that there were affected relatives in an isolated Austrian valley, he visited it on holiday and discovered six more children from a total of three related families. Thomson, a British dermatologist, described two sisters in 1923 [2] and subsequently a third unrelated patient in 1936 [3]. None had cata-racts. Thomson, who was unaware of or disregarded Rothmund's report, introduced the term poikilo-derma congenitale [3]. Rothmund–Thomson syn-drome was proposed by Taylor in 1957 [4] and Rook et al. in 1959 [5], who recognized the similarity of the cutaneous changes of Rothmund syndrome and Thomson's poikiloderma congenitale. It is now com-monly accepted that the two disorders are identical. The acceptance of the designation Rothmund–Thomson syndrome indicates that the cutaneous finding "poikiloderma" is not pathognomonic and that this is a multisystem disorder.

Physical Findings

Cutaneous and Dental Changes

Skin manifestations are described in detail by Rook et al. [5]. The skin is usually normal at birth with the first lesions appearing typically between 3 and 6 months of age. Occasionally skin changes appear as early as 1 month of age [2] or as late as 18 months of age. The earliest lesions are discrete erythematous patches on the buttocks or cheeks. Simultaneously or shortly thereafter similar changes appear on the extensor surfaces of the limbs. The dorsum of the hands, the distal third of the forearms, and the ex-ternal aspect of the thighs, knees, and posterolateral aspects of the lower legs are typically affected (Fig-ure 12.1). The trunk is usually spared. The cheeks are often the first area affected, usually more se-verely than other parts of the face, although the chin, forehead, and ears may have milder changes.

Along with the diffuse, bright vermilion color, the skin takes on a swollen, tense, and shiny appearance. This stage usually is fully manifest by 12 to 18 months of age. In general, sun-exposed skin is more severely affected. The palms and soles are normal in this stage. There may be a follicular, papular rash with minute hyperkeratoses that impart a scratchy feel. Soon a capillary network becomes visible through this pink discoloration and develops into a macular, reticu-lated, net-like pattern. As the acute phase resolves, over months or years, the erythema fades and the chronic stage evolves. The patient is asymptomatic through the acute and chronic stages. The mucous membranes are not involved.

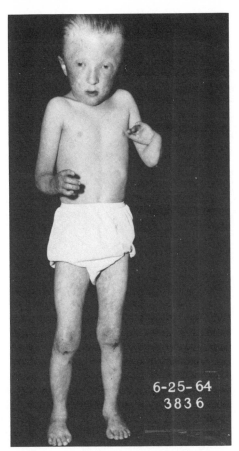

6-25-64
3836

Figure 12.1. A 5-year 11-month-old girl with Rothmund–Thomson syndrome exhibiting typical distribution of poikilodermatous changes on the face and extensor surfaces of the limbs with sparing of the trunk. She has absence of the thumbs with absence of the left radius and hypoplasia of the right radius. (Am J Dis Child 1980;134:165–169. Copyright 1980, American Medical Association. Used with permission.)

The mature cutaneous changes, or poikiloderma, include linear telangiectases and areas of dermal atrophy, depigmentation, and hyperpigmentation [6] (Figures 12.2, 12.3). The vascular changes suggest exaggerated cutis marmorata with mottled, dull red, confluent, and slightly depressed zones that blanch under pressure. These telangiectatic vessels constrict with the cold, causing the skin to look bluish, and dilate in the heat or sunlight, giving a reddish appearance. The atrophy may be either diffuse or limited to ill-defined islands within the reticulated telangiectatic vascular net. Scarring does not occur, but the overlying skin is soft, shiny, finely wrinkled, and transparent (Figure 12.3).

Dull brown pigmentation develops in the affected areas after the atrophy and telangiectasia. This hyperpigmentation may also extend onto otherwise normal skin, particularly on the neck and trunk. The hyperpigmented areas are irregularly macular or reticulate. Depigmented macules without atrophy may dapple the affected areas.

The chronic poikilodermatous stage has usually completely evolved by the third to fifth year, after which the lesions persist throughout life [3]. In this stage the telangiectatic changes may predominate on the face and the pigmentary disturbance on the limbs and trunk [5]. Affected areas are devoid of hair.

Photosensitivity is present in about one-third of cases and in early childhood may result in bullous formation on sun exposure. Photosensitivity is usually the most severe between the ages of 2 and 4, after which it may improve spontaneously. Although it may diminish, sun sensitivity may persist through adolescence and even indefinitely [5]. Except for one case in which skin lesions progressed in childhood despite avoidance of the sun and the use of topical sun screens [7], little has been reported about this type of therapy.

In adolescence and adulthood keratoses often appear in sun-exposed areas, especially in individuals with a history of sun sensitivity. In time, these increase in size and number. Warty keratoses also may appear on prominences such as elbows, knees, malleoli, heels, tips of toes, and the metacarpophalangeal and interphalangeal joints of the hands. At this stage the palms and soles may become involved, and the skin is generally dry, harsh, and atrophic [5,8].

A rare complication is atypical calcinosis cutis reported in a 15-year-old boy [9] and a 4-year-old girl [10].

Some degree of ectodermal dysplasia occurs in the majority of Rothmund–Thomson patients. Scalp hair, eyebrows, and eyelashes in any combination may be sparse or absent (Figure 12.2). Lanugo hair is always missing from poikilodermatous skin but may also be missing from apparently normal skin. Facial hair in males is either normal or soft and downy. Axillary and pubic hair may be sparse. Scalp hair, eyebrows, and eyelashes occasionally are lost suddenly; subsequent regrowth of hair varies [3,5,9,11]. Scalp hair may become prematurely gray [5]. Hypohydrosis and heat intolerance vary. In about 25% of patients, the nails are hypoplastic and rudimentary or rigid and overgrown.

Dental abnormalities include multiple unusual crown malformations, microdontia, delayed erup-

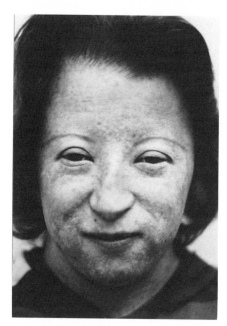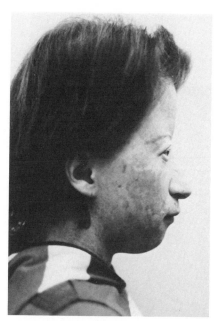

Figure 12.2. Same patient as in Figure 12.1 at 19 years of age. Characteristic facies includes high forehead, lack of supraorbital ridges, long slender nose, and absent eyebrows and eyelashes. Pigmentary changes involve the entire face and neck. (Am J Dis Child 1980;134:165–169. Copyright 1980, American Medical Association. Used with permission.)

Figure 12.3. Characteristic poikilodermatous changes are variegated pigment, fine wrinkling and atrophy of the skin, and absence of lanugo hair.

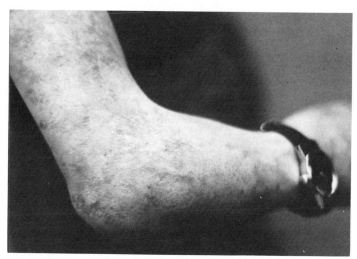

tion, ectopic eruption, and supernumerary and congenitally missing teeth [11,12,13].

Ocular Findings

The ophthalmologic findings and pertinent literature were reviewed in detail by Kirkham and Werner in 1975 [1]. Although they reported that cataracts occur in 75% of well-documented Rothmund–Thom-

son cases, prevalence in this review was closer to 40 to 50%. Lens changes usually appear suddenly between the ages of 18 months and 7 years and progress rapidly to total cataracts over several weeks. Occasionally they appear as early as 3 months, but rarely appear after 7 years. The cataracts are always bilateral and affect both eyes at the same time and to the same extent. Children with previously normal eye exams have been noted to develop spoke-like anterior and posterior subcapsular opacities that quickly evolve into total lens opacity [11,14,15]. Opacification of the lenses occasionally proceeds more slowly, in which case a prolonged stage of posterior subcapsular and radially oriented cortical snowflake opacities can occur [16]. Lens extraction is usually technically successful and results in satisfactory visual acuity. Strabismus and amblyopia, common complications of early lens extraction, are reported frequently [11].

Microcornea appears to be present in all cases described in sufficient detail, whether cataracts are present or not. Corneal diameter ranges from 7 to 9 mm [11]. Less common ocular findings are band keratopathy that may be mild or severe, keratoconus, absence of the anterior mesodermal leaf of the iris, and posterior staphylomas with tilted optic discs. Abnormalities of the chamber angle and glaucoma have not been reported.

Skeletal Changes

Skeletal changes include short stature, limb anomalies, and unusual radiographic appearance of the bones. Proportionate short stature occurs in the majority of cases and reflects both prenatal and postnatal growth deficiency. Low birth weight, present in the majority of cases, has been reported to be as low as 1,500 to 1,600 grams [17,18,19]. Severe short stature may occur [18].

Limb anomalies range from absence of the radii or tibiae to short, stubby fingers (Figure 12.1). Absence of the thumb with hypoplasia of the radius occurred in one of Thomson's original two cases and in about 5 to 10% of subsequently reported cases.

Involvement may be unilateral or bilateral. Bilateral absence of the tibiae rarely occurs [19]. Unilateral ulnar hemimelia has been reported in one case [20].

Very short stubby fingers with hypoplasia or absence of the terminal phalanges is the most commonly recognized skeletal abnormality [11,21,22,23]. Case 1 of Werder et al. [23] exhibited absent terminal phalanges with radiographic changes suggesting a peripheral dysostosis. Cupping and flaring of the proximal phalanges' metaphyses has also been reported [11]. Shortening of the middle phalanges occasionally accounts for the stubby appearance of the fingers [18,24] (Figure 12.4).

Other radiographic abnormalities include fibrous dysplasia-like cystic bone lesions and focal sclerotic areas in the metaphyses of major long bones [4, 21,24,25], hypotubulation of long bones, and a prominent trabecular pattern (Figure 12.4) as well as frank osteoporosis. Pathologic fractures have been described in cases where there is normal calcium metabolism [9,10,25]. Vertebral anomalies [16] have included rectangular shape with increased vertical height [11] and irregular and fused cervical vertebrae [18]. Significant idiopathic scoliosis has occurred [26]. Absent, abnormal, and congenitally dislocated patellae [11,18,26] have been reported, as has subluxation of the proximal tibiae [18].

In the earlier literature numerous patients were reported to have normal radiographic studies, and it is not clear if these patients had entirely normal studies or subtle changes that may have been overlooked. Kozlowski et al. [21] speculate that more patients with Rothmund–Thomson syndrome might manifest skeletal changes if radiographs were obtained at an older age when certain changes are more apparent.

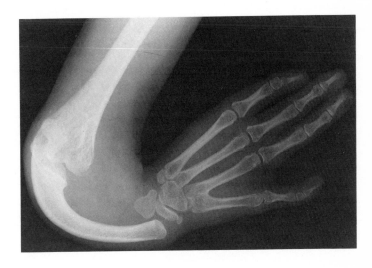

Figure 12.4. Radiograph from the same patient at 19 years of age showing absence of the first metacarpal and thumb, the left radius, and small second and fifth middle phalanges. Trabecular pattern is prominent. (Am J Dis Child 1980;134:165–169. Copyright 1980, American Medical Association. Used with permission.)

Hypogonadism

Hypogonadism and infertility appear to be exceedingly common in Rothmund–Thomson syndrome, although most reported cases lack sufficient detail to determine the incidence. At least one-third of the 60 cases reviewed by Rook et al. [5] had clinical hypogonadism. The cause of hypogonadism in this condition has not been well studied, and the few existing reports are contradictory. Werder et al. [23] evaluated two cases in detail and found normal FSH and LH but low estrogen levels in a 36-year-old woman with primary amenorrhea, and elevated FSH and LH in a 19-year-old male who had small testes but normal testosterone levels. Three siblings, ages 16, 17, and 18 years, reported by Kirkham and Werner [11] had hypogonadism with prepubertal levels of FSH, LH, and gonadal steroids. These meager data suggest that both hypogonadotrophic hypogonadism and end organ unresponsiveness can be causative. Micropenis (penile length less than 2.5 cm at birth), a common manifestation of hypogonadotrophic hypogonadism, has been reported in two young boys [27].

Facies

Although a characteristic facies (Figures 12.2, 12.3) with either a saddle nose reminiscent of congenital lues or delicate features with a bird-like nose are often observed, many patients have completely normal facies. Rook et al. [5] declared that there was no pathognomonic facies.

Central Nervous System Manifestations

Both a disproportionately large cranial vault [2] and microcephaly [27] have been reported. Asymmetric cortical atrophy on pneumoencephalography in a mentally retarded girl [25] and dilated ventricles on cranial CT in a 2-year-old boy with a disproportionately large head and normal psychomotor development [7] constitute the only reports of CNS imaging in this disorder. Intelligence is generally normal, although some patients with mental deficiency have been reported [5,23,25,28].

Malignancy

Development of squamous cell carcinoma in poikilodermatous areas of skin was recognized by the earliest investigators as a potential complication. It has been reported in patients in and beyond their fourth decade (30-year-old male [9], 32-year-old female [23], 32-year-old female [29], 91- and 92-year-old females [30]). Since most reported patients with this disorder are children on whom no follow-up data are available, the actual risk for this complication remains unknown. Of interest are four recent reports of osteosarcoma in patients ranging in age from 5 to 19 years [13,21,26,31] and of fibrosarcoma in a 32-year-old [9].

Other Findings

Other complications that have been reported in single cases are subendothelial arterial calcification causing hypertension [32], parathyroid adenoma [23], hypothyroidism [21], akinetic seizures [23], and epilepsy and myopathy [33].

Pathology and Pathogenesis

While histologic changes of the skin are consistent, they are not diagnostic. In early childhood there is edema of the basal layer and variable edema of the dermis with capillary dilatation and lymphocytic infiltration. Later the epidermis displays focal atrophy with flattened papillae and focal hyperkeratosis. The pilosebaceous follicles and sweat glands may be lost and pigment-laden chromatophores accumulate in the upper dermis.

Autosomal recessive inheritance of Rothmund–Thomson syndrome is accepted. In the only report alleging two-generation involvement [34], the mother appears to have a different cutaneous disorder. A previously reported abnormal sex ratio with a 2:1 female preponderance [5,13] was not confirmed in this review of over 90 published cases in which 48 were female and 43 male. The high incidence of consanguinity in reported cases suggests that the gene frequency in the general population is low. Prevalence rates for Rothmund–Thomson syndrome have not been calculated.

The biochemical basis of Rothmund–Thomson syndrome is unknown. A defect in DNA-repair mechanisms that would explain the sun sensitivity and the apparently increased risk for malignancy has been postulated [35] but is unproven [36].

Differential Diagnosis

Although earlier reports painstakingly differentiated Werner syndrome, an autosomal recessive disorder, from Rothmund–Thomson syndrome, the skin lesions in Werner syndrome are primarily sclerodermatous, and both the skin and ocular changes are of much later onset. Kindler syndrome, an autosomal recessive disorder, involves spontaneous or trauma-induced blistering of the hands and feet from birth. Early photosensitivity and erythema of the face diminish with age and are followed by poikilodermatous changes with marked atrophy involving most of the skin area. Cataracts do not occur. Hallermann–Streiff syndrome, dyskeratosis congenita, progeria, Cockayne's syndrome, ataxia-telangiectasia, and epidermolysis bullosa have all been considered to be in the differential diagnosis of Rothmund–Thomson syndrome, but can be distinguished easily by their characteristic clinical findings.

Treatment

Although it is hypothesized that avoidance of sun and protection of skin from ultraviolet radiation through the use of topical sunscreens may reduce the extent of the primary cutaneous involvement and the rate at which cutaneous malignancy develops, no data are available. Surveillance of affected skin for carcinomatous changes is advised. Routine ophthalmologic evaluations, especially during the first decade, and lens extraction when visual acuity is significantly reduced, are the major ophthalmic considerations.

References

1. Rothmund A. Uber cataracten in Verbindung mit einer eigentümlichen Hautdegeneration. Graefes Arch Ophthalmol 1868;14:159–182.
2. Thomson MS. An hitherto undescribed familial disease. Br J Dermatol Syph 1923;35:455–462.
3. Thomson MS. ? Poikiloderma congenitale: two cases for diagnosis. Proc R Soc Med 1936;29:453–455.
4. Taylor WB. Rothmund's syndrome—Thomson's syndrome. Congenital poikiloderma with or without juvenile cataracts: a review of the literature, report of a case, and discussion of the relationship of the two syndromes. Arch Dermatol 1957;75:236–244.
5. Rook A, Davis R, Stevanovic D. Poikiloderma congenitale: Rothmund–Thomson syndrome. Acta Dermatol Venereol 1959;39:392–420.
6. Gellis SS, Feingold M. Denoument and discussion: Rothmund–Thomson syndrome (poikiloderma congenital). Picture of the month. Am J Dis Child 1978;132:619–620.
7. Mitchell EA, Cairns LM, Hodge JLR. Rothmund–Thomson syndrome (poikiloderma congenitale) asso-

ciated with hydrocephalus. Aust Paediatr J 1980; 16:290–291.
8. Sexton GB. Thomson's syndrome (poikiloderma congenitale). Can Med Assoc J 1954;70:662–665.
9. Davies MG. Rothmund–Thomson syndrome and malignant disease. Clin Exp Dermatol 1982;7:455–457.
10. Cheesbrough MJ, Kinmont PDC. Poikiloderma congenitale (Thomson–Rothmund syndrome). Br J Dermatol 1978;(suppl)16:66–67.
11. Kirkham TH, Werner EB. The ophthalmic manifestations of Rothmund's syndrome. Can J Ophthalmol 1975;10:1–14.
12. Kraus BS, Gottlieb MA, Meliton HR. The dentition in Rothmund's syndrome. J Am Dent Assoc 1970;81:894–915.
13. Starr DG, McClure JP, Connor JM. Non-dermatological complications and genetic aspects of the Rothmund–Thomson syndrome. Clin Genet 1985;27:102–104.
14. Lepard CW. Poikiloderma congenitale (Rothmund's syndrome). Trans Am Ophthalmol Soc 1956;54:301–309.
15. Loftus BG, Meenan FOC, O'Loughlin S, et al. Rothmund–Thomson syndrome—a report of 2 cases. Irish J Med Sci 1985;154:83–86.
16. Merz EH, Tausk K, Dukes E. Meso-ectodermal dysplasia and its variants. Am J Ophthalmol 1963;55:488–504.
17. Wahl JW, Ellis PP. Rothmund–Thomson syndrome. Am J Ophthalmol 1965;60:722–726.
18. Hall JG, Pagon RA, Wilson KM. Rothmund–Thomson syndrome with severe dwarfism. Am J Dis Child 1980;134:165–169.
19. Bosch MIF, Aparicio AM, Garcia JC, et al. Poikilodermie congénitale type Thomson avec dysplasies osseuses majeures. Ann Dermatol Venereol 1984; 111:429–433.
20. Hailey H, Hailey H, Clemens H. Poikiloderma congenitale: report of a case in America. Arch Dermatol 1941;44:345–348.
21. Kozlowski K, Scougall JS, Oates RK. Osteosarcoma in a boy with Rothmund–Thomson syndrome. Pediatr Radiol 1980;10:42–45.
22. Maurer RM, Langford OL. Rothmund's syndrome: a cause of resorption of phalangeal tufts and dystrophic calcification. Radiology 1967;89:706–708.
23. Werder EA, Murset G, Illig R, et al. Hypogonadism and parathyroid adenoma in congenital poikiloderma (Rothmund–Thomson syndrome). Clin Endocrinol 1975;4:75–82.
24. Oates RK, Lewis MB, Walker–Smith JA. The Rothmund–Thomson syndrome: case report of an unusual syndrome. Aust Paediat J 1971;7:103–107.
25. Kassner EG, Qazi QH, Haller JO. Rothmund–Thomson syndrome (poikiloderma congenitale) associated with mental retardation, growth disturbance, and skeletal features. Skel Radiol 1977;2:99–103.
26. Tokunaga M, Sato K, Funayama K, et al. Rothmund Thomson syndrome associated with osteosarcoma. J Jpn Orthop Assoc 1976;50:287–293.

27. Silver HK. Rothmund–Thomson syndrome: an ocu-locutaneous disorder. Am J Dis Child 1966;111:182–190.

28. Cole HN, Driver JR, Giffen HK, et al. Ectodermal and mesodermal dysplasia with osseous involvement. Arch Dermatol Syph 1941;44:773–787.

29. Rook A, Whimster I. Congenital cutaneous dystrophy (Thomson's type). Br J Dermatol Syph 1949;61:197–205.

30. Sexton GB. Comment. Arch Dermatol 1960;82:116–117.

31. Dick DC, Morley WN, Watson JT. Rothmund–Thomson syndrome and osteogenic sarcoma. Clin Exp Dermatol 1982;7:119–123.

32. Dechenne CH, Chantraine JM, Davin JC. A Roth-mund–Thomson case with hypertension. Clin Genet 1983;24:266–272.

33. Lessem J, Bjerre I, Forslund M. Epilepsy and myopathy in a patient with Rothmund–Thomson's syndrome. Acta Med Scand 1980;207:237–239.

34. Hallman N, Patiala R. Congenital poikiloderma atrophicans vasculare in a mother and her son. Acta Dermatol Venereol 1951;31:401–406.

35. Smith PJ, Patterson MC. Enhanced radiosensitivity and defective DNA repair in cultured fibroblasts derived from Rothmund Thomson syndrome patients. Mutat Res 1982;94:213–228.

36. Cleaver JE. DNA damage and repair in light-sensitive human skin disease. J Invest Dermatol 1970;54:181–195.

Chapter 13
Fucosidosis

MICHEL PHILIPPART

Fucosidosis is an autosomal recessive lysosomal storage disorder in which an α-fucosidase deficiency causes a multisystem accumulation of a diverse array of oligosaccharides and sphingoglycolipids. Two clinical presentations have been delineated: Type I and Type II. In Type I a rapid psychomotor regression leads to death in the midst of the first decade. In Type II, dysmorphic facial and skeletal features suggest a mucopolysaccharide storage disorder (MPSD). Extensive angiokeratomas occur by the age of 6. The neurologic regression and clinical course are protracted, with survival until adulthood.

Clinical Presentation

Type I (Severe Form)

Sixteen cases (six males, nine females) have been reported [1–14] (Table 13.1). Seven have been subject to comprehensive reports; only abstracts and abbreviated descriptions are available for the nine others. Based on these reports, gestation, delivery, and development for the first 6 to 12 months were normal. Frequent pulmonary or upper respiratory tract infections started as early as the first month of life. Cystic fibrosis may be suspected. Excessive perspiration and increased sweat electrolytes have been reported in the first few years. Psychomotor retardation, which is constant, became apparent between 5 and 15 months of age. At this stage the children were hypotonic. No further developmental progress was achieved for the next few months. A slow neurologic regression then takes place with loss of previously acquired mental and motor skills. Progressive spasticity has been noted in patients from age 1 year 11 months to 3 years 9 months. In the two original patients dystonia of the axis and feet was evident [1]. Seizures were infrequent. Mild EEG abnormali-

ties included slowing, low voltage, and rarely, paroxysmal features. The head may be slightly enlarged. Full facial features, especially cheeks and lips, were reminiscent of a MPSD although the gross coarsening and distorted bone structure of the face and skull that are associated with these disorders were not found. The tongue may be large and the gingivae thickened, giving another touch of resemblance to MPSD. The skin may be thick. The heart may be slightly enlarged. The abdomen is protuberant but hepatomegaly is generally discrete, with the liver reaching 4 to 6 cm below the costal margin in only two cases [2,3]. A moderate thoracolumbar kyphosis is common. A peculiar livid red color due to microangiomata was observed under the distal ends of the fingers and toenails in a child aged 3 years [4]. Bone marrow aspiration was negative or showed foam cells or dark inclusions in histiocytes. Vacuolized lymphocytes were often present. Death occurred between about 2½ and 6 years of age after a period of progressive weight loss that was often complicated by infections and dehydration.

Type II (Chronic Form with Angiokeratoma)

Thirty-one cases (twenty-two males, nine females) have been reported [15–37] (Table 13.2). The patients ranged in age from 1½ to 33 years, ten being 14 years or older. Respiratory infections started as early as 2 months of age. Delayed psychomotor development appeared between 8 months and 3¾ years. Except for two children who had an IQ of 42 to 48 at 4 years [15,34], no other cases progressed beyond a mental age of 10 to 15 months. Neurologic regression was not well described but most patients became hypertonic. There was one case of dystonic posturing [15] and another of athetosis [16]. Regression was often insidious but ambulation was lost as

Table 13.1. Clinical Features of Patients with Type I Fucosidosis

Case Number	1	2	3	4	5	6	7	8	9	10	11	12	13	14	15	16
Age	45m	62m	39m	30m	42m	50m	58m	36m	6y	3y	2y	31m	4y	46m	28m	
Sex	M	F	M	F	M	F	M	F	F	F	F	M	?	F	F	M[b]
Siblings	⎯⎯⎯	⎯⎯⎯					⎯⎯⎯	⎯⎯⎯		⎯⎯⎯	⎯⎯⎯					
Ancestry	I	I	I	I	G	J	NE	NE	B	A	A	FC	FC	U	U	U (B)
Consanguinity	+		+	0	+	0			0	0			+			0
Infections[a]	3m	6m	16m		6m	8m	+					4m			1m	
Retardation	15m	12m	39m	30m	6m	12m	6m	12m	+	+	+	5m	14m	6m	14m	+
Hypotonia	15m	12m				50m	12m	3y				11m		20m		
Hypertonia	45m	30m			30m		58m		26m			29m			23m	
Seizures[a]	8m	0			4y							17m				
Head circumference		± ↑	↑		N		N					N	↑	↓		
Coarse facies	0	0	+	±	+	+	+	±	±			±				+
Enlarged tongue	0	0	+	±	+											
Kyphosis	+	+	+	+	±	+	+					+		0	0	
Thick skin	+	+		+		0	0	+								+
Hepatomegaly	0	0	±	±	+	+	+	+	±			+ +		0	0	
Sweating	↑					↑	N					↑				
Sweat electrolytes	↑	↑			±	↑	N					↑				
Vacuolized lymphocytes	+	+		+	+	+	0		+ +			0				
Brain weight	↑	885gm											1,305gm			
Death	45m	62m					60m		6y			31m	5y			
Source (reference number)	[1]	[1]	[4]	[8]	[2]	[5]	[6,7]	[6,7]	[8,9]	[10]	[10]	[3]	[11]	[12]	[13]	[14]

[a] age of onset

[b] Patient's brother died at age 3, possibly with fucosidosis, but no details are available.

⎯⎯⎯⎯⎯ The two patients are siblings.

m = month; y = year; N = normal; ↑ = increased; ↓ = decreased; + = present; 0 = absent; M = male; F = female;
A = Algeria; B = Belgium; FC = French Canada; G = Germany; I = Italy; J = Japan; NE = Netherlands; U = United States; U(B) = United States, black

early as the age of 2 [17]. Seizures were infrequent. The EEG may be slightly abnormal, exhibiting low voltage, slow waves, and rarely, spikes. Nerve conduction velocities generally have been normal but they have not been widely investigated. Two cases (Table 13.2, no. 5, 6) were normal except for decreased velocities in the median nerves suggesting possible carpal tunnel syndrome, a common complication in MPSD and which can also be anticipated in other storage disorders involving connective tissue. Sweat electrolytes are rarely increased. Perspiration is decreased. The skin is thickened. Angiokeratomas, which are the hallmark of Type II, were by definition present in all cases, shortly after birth in one [6], and by age 6½ years at the latest. Coarse facial features, often compared to MPSD, were frequent, especially in older patients. The neck was short, and bone age markedly delayed. Height fell below the third percentile by age 3, reaching 120 to 130 cm in young adults. Other features included a large head, kyphosis, scoliosis, and splenomegaly. Gingival telangiectases may be seen [17]. Corneal opacities were described in six cases, including the three oldest patients [18]. Tortuosity and aneurysmal dilations of the veins have been seen in the conjunctiva and retina. Pigmentary abnormalities of the retina with bull's eye retinopathy [19, case no. 3] and papilledema (case no. 4) were exceptional. Vacuolized lymphocytes were uncommon: 4 patients had none, 2 had 1%, and 1 had 10%.

Three patients, aged 13 to 25 years (see Table 13.2, cases no. 29–31), had a chronic course and findings entirely compatible with Type II but did not present any angiokeratoma. Because of the slower neurologic regression with spasticity seen in these patients (in one at around age 8, in another around 5 years, and never in a third patient [case no. 27] who was briefly reported when the diagnosis was made at age 17 years during a survey of atypical MPSD [20]) these cases cannot be classified as Type

I. This last patient never developed angiokeratomas and remained ambulatory until his death in his mid-twenties (personal examination). It would be meaningless at this stage to define a Type III just for such patients. It is likely, indeed, that many similar patients with a chronic neurodegenerative disorder have not been diagnosed in the absence of the distinctive angiokeratomas that provide a clue to the diagnosis.

Angiokeratoma

The angiokeratoma (Figures 13.1–13.3) is similar to that which has been the hallmark of Fabry–Anderson disease (FAD). Tending to occur earlier in fucosidosis, the angiokeratoma is also more diffuse and spreads more rapidly than it does in FAD. The first description [22] mentions "a mild skin rash about the age of 5 years," "small generalized capillary telangiectasis" at age 11 years, "an extensive maculopapular rash" and "dark red, soft papillomata" near

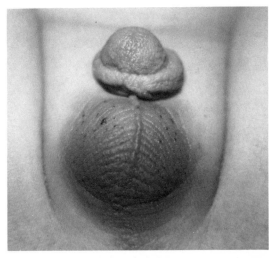

Figure 13.1. Pinhead-shaped, dark glistening angiokeratomas over the scrotum of a 3-year-old boy. Although these lesions are indistinguishable from those observed in FAD (see Figure 29.3), they occur in a much younger patient population. (Courtesy of Dr. Russell Snyder.)

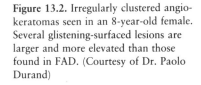
Figure 13.2. Irregularly clustered angiokeratomas seen in an 8-year-old female. Several glistening-surfaced lesions are larger and more elevated than those found in FAD. (Courtesy of Dr. Paolo Durand)

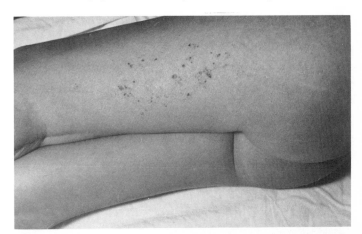

Figure 13.3. Innumerable small angiokeratomas over the thighs of a 10-year-old boy. The underlying skin has an irregularly erythematous appearance. (Courtesy of Dr. Paolo Durand.)

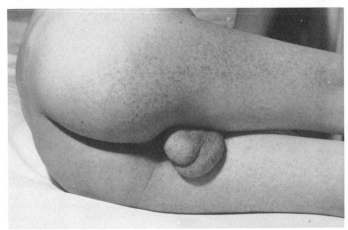

Table 13.2. Clinical Features of Patients with Type-II Fucosidosis

Case Number	1	2	3	4	5	6	7	8	9	10	11	12	13	14	15
Age (y)	20	24	17	5	10	5	12	14	6	1½	3	7	14	4	7
Sex	M	F	M	F	M	M	M	M	M	M	M	M	M	M	M
Siblings															
Ancestry	U	S	I	I	G	G	I	I	U (M)		U (S)		U (S)	I	I
Consanguinity	0	?	+		0		+		0					+	0
Infections[a]	2y				+	+	+	+	+	+	2m	+	+		+
Retardation[a]	14m	+	2m	1y	18m	18m			45m	0	2y	+	+	+	22m
Hypotonia	24m						+	?	0	0					
Hypertonia		+	+	+	+	±	±	+	+	0	+	+	+		+
Nerve velocity					N,↓	N,↓									
Seizures[a]	18y	0					12y						10y		
Bone age					6y	4y									
Head circumference		N			N	N									
Height (cm) [perc]	120	130	124	110							[3]		[3]		94
Coarse facies	+	+	+	+	+	+	+	+	+	±	+	+			+
Enlarged tongue	+	+	+				+	+	+		+		+		+
Kyphosis	+	(+)	+		+	+	+	±							+
Thick skin					+	+	+	+	+	0	+	+	+		
Angiokeratoma[a]	4y	5y	5y	5y	5y	5y	+	+	+	0	3y	+	infant		+
Hepatomegaly	0	0	0	+	0	0	0	0	0	0	0	0	0		0
Sweating	↓										↓	↓	↓		
Sweat electrolytes				N	N	N	N							N	N
Vacuolized lymphocytes		±		1%	10%	0	+	+	+						
Corneal opacity											+				+
Tortuous veins		+	+								+	+	+		
Source (reference number)	[21]	[19, 22, 23, 24]	[25, 17, 35]	[25, 17, 5]	[15, 36]	[15, 36]	[20, 36]	[20, 36]	[20]	[20]	[26, 27]	[26, 27]	[26, 27]	[28]	[29]

[a]age of onset

————The two patients are siblings.

m = month; y = year; N = normal; ↑ = increased; ↓ = decreased; perc = percentile; + = present; 0 = absent; M = male; F = female; FR = France; G = Germany; I = Italy; J = Japan; NE = Netherlands; NO = Norway; S = Scotland; U = United States; U (B) = United States, black; U (M) = United States, Mexican; U (S) = United States, Spanish

flexures at age 20 years. The small raised lesions on the scrotum and penis are certainly similar to those found in FAD. The increased subcutaneous markings on the chest, palms, and soles [15], which may correspond to the macular appearance described by Primrose et al. [22], are not a feature of FAD. A female with FAD and extensive angiokeratoma has never been reported.

Radiographic Features

Skull radiographs may show a slight diastasis of the sutures in Type I [1]. Vertebral bodies are slightly ovoid. Wedging of the first three lumbar vertebral bodies is the most common finding associated with the characteristic thoracolumbar kyphosis. These abnormalities may be quite discrete [13].

In Type II, vertebral beaking, odontoid hypoplasia, pelvic and femoral head deformities, widening of the shafts of the long bones, and sinus hypoaeration resemble the discrete dysostosis multiplex found in MPSD Type III [33,34]. Progressive diploic thickening of the skull develops; noted also are early synostosis of one or more sutures, flattening and hypoplasia of the cervical vertebral bodies, "phantom" lumbar discs, and esophageal and possibly small bowel mucosal thickening [35]. Cranial computed

16	17	18	19	20	21	22	23	24	25	26	27	28	29	30	31
20	6½	6½	4	17	4	6	4	7	5	28	31	33	17	25	13
M	F	M	M	M	F	M	M	F	F	F	F	F	M	M	M
NO	I	U	U	U	U	FR	FR	G	G	J	J	J	U (M)	NE	NE
0	+	0		0	0			0		+			?	0	
+		+						+	+	?			?	+	+
2y	12m	6m	2y			8m	12m	2y	9m	2–3y	2–3y	2–3y	19m	2y	18m
		6m				9m			9m					2y	18m
+		+		+		6y	4y		4y	+	+	+		8y	5y
						N	N			N	N	N			
	0		2y					0	+						
														8y	4y
														↑	↑
										124	124	124		dwarf	dwarf
±	+	+		+		+	+	+	0				+	+	+
0	+							+					+		
+	+	+		+	+	+	+			+	+	+	+	+	
												+	+		
(late?)	6½y	6½y		+		4y	2y	+		+	+	+	0	0	0
±	±					±	±	0	0	0	0	0	±		
								N	↑						
± ↑	↑												N		
0							0		0						
	+								+	+	+				
						+	+								
[16]	[30]	[31]	[23, 31]	[31]	[31]	[23, 31, 32]	[32, 33]	[23, 34]	[34]	[18]	[18]	[18]	[20, 37]	[35]	[35]

tomography [30] is normal at age 4, and in one case showed mild infiltrative changes two years later in the gray and white matter. In a 17-year-old considerable ventricular dilation with cerebral and cerebellar atrophy was exhibited. Another child had decreased white matter density at just under 4 years of age [12].

Pathology

In both types of fucosidosis skin biopsies show severe vacuolation in the sweat glands and endothelial cells of the capillaries [8,38]. Electron microscopy reveals clear and dense inclusions in histiocytes, fibroblasts, endothelial cells of the blood (Figure 13.2) and lymphatic capillaries, and perineural cells of the skin and conjunctiva [8,38]. Most clear inclusions contain fine granular material with a few concentric lamellar membranes that are often organized in half rings in contact with the limiting membranes. The dense inclusions, which have an almost homogeneous content, are less numerous and have not been reported in any other storage disease [8]. Storage in the vascular endothelium may vary in intensity from cell to cell in the same vessel and also from vessel to vessel [38]. Myoepithelial cells in eccrine sweat glands contain lamellated inclusions only [3]. Schwann cells may contain no inclusions [8], lamellated inclusions only [3], or the two types of inclusions (Figure 13.4). Unmyelinated axons occasionally exhibited large composite inclusions with few lamellar structures (Figures 13.5, 13.6).

A sural nerve biopsy in a Type-I case [39] showed large foam cells and nonspecific demyelination with axonal degeneration. A biopsy from another case with fucosidase activity in the heterozygous range showed a less severe, nonspecific neuropathy which, in the absence of acceptable clinical features, makes clear that the patient reported as case 3 [6] does not have

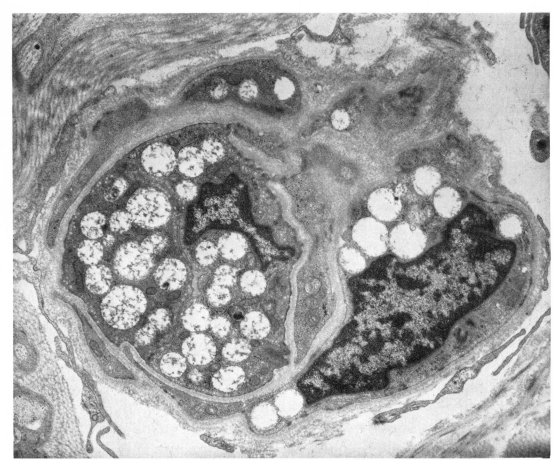

Figure 13.4. Skin biopsy. This electron micrograph of a skin biopsy reveals prominent inclusions that contain fine granuloreticular material in the endothelial cells of a blood capillary. The lumen is almost occluded. The perithelial cell on the right contains large inclusions optically almost empty (original magnification × 13,500). (Courtesy of Dr. W. Jann Brown.)

fucosidosis. Liver biopsies in Type I revealed widespread vacuolation of hepatocytes and Kupffer cells, with scattered foam cells [2]. The hepatocytes may have an empty appearance as they would in a glycogen storage disease [1]. Ultrastructural study of the liver revealed many dense granular or lamellar inclusions as well as large electron-lucent inclusions containing vesicles [1,4,39]. Massive storage in retinal ganglion cells was found at autopsy of a Type I case [9] (Table 13.1, no. 9).

The brain of the original patient (Table 13.1, no. 1) showed diffuse vacuolation in the cortical neurons, subcortical nuclei, and glia [40]. Most vacuoles were empty or contained homogeneous material that did not have an affinity for usual dyes. The globus pallidus had a rusty discoloration and fatty degeneration similar to cases of infantile Hallervorden–Spatz disease. Granular inclusions were found in the neurons of the basal ganglia and in the large motor neurons of the cortex and brain stem. A mild cellular and dense fibrous gliosis was present throughout. The white matter was almost completely depleted of oligodendroglia. Axons were generally preserved. There was no sign of active demyelination. Similar brain findings and storage in anterior horn cells were exhibited in case no. 12 of Type I [3].

Biochemistry

Enzyme

α-Fucosidase activity can be assayed with a fluorogenic substrate in the tissues, cells, or body fluids. Serum should not be used because a small number of normal individuals have very low enzymatic ac-

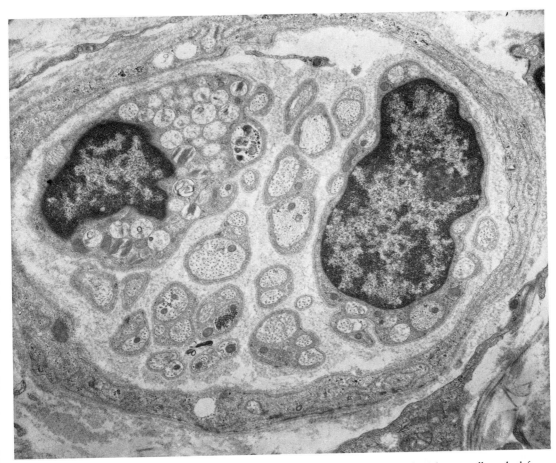

Figure 13.5. Skin biopsy. Electron micrograph of a small unmyelinated dermal nerve. The Schwann cell on the left contains multiple faintly granular inclusions and a few inclusions with stacks of lamellae. The larger inclusion containing larger coarser granules is probably an axon (original magnification × 13,500). (Courtesy of Dr. W. Jann Brown.)

tivity [41]. Cultured fibroblasts provide a reliable source of enzymatic activity, but unexplained inactivation has been reported [16]. The activity is also absent in HeLa cells and in animal fibroblasts transformed by oncogenic viruses [42]. An occasional homozygote may exhibit activity in the heterozygous range [13]. Leukocytes appear to be safe for the diagnosis of homozygotes but heterozygote detection requires the use of purified mononuclear cells [43,44]. Prenatal diagnosis is feasible [10] but affected twin fetuses were mistakenly thought to be heterozygous [45].

Natural Substrates

Fucose is a methylpentose found in small quantities in glycoproteins, glycolipids, and gangliosides. During cellular turnover proteases remove the protein moiety of the glycoproteins, leaving oligosaccharide chains of varying complexity that contain up to 27 carbohydrate residues [46]. Fucose is always attached to the periphery of these chains and needs to be removed by α-fucosidase to allow further degradation of the molecule. Such components probably account for the bulk of oligosaccharides that accumulate in the lysosomes and are excreted in the urine of patients with fucosidosis. Already more than 20 of these substances have been isolated from patients' urine [47,48].

Another group of fucose derivatives are sphingolipids, which are known as blood group substances A, B, H, Lewis a, Lewis b, and Lewis x [49]. They also accumulate in patients with fucosidosis [50,51] but the initial expectation that patient blood types might influence phenotypic expression of α-fucosidase deficiency has not yet been confirmed.

Fucosyl-gangliosides are the third group of sub-

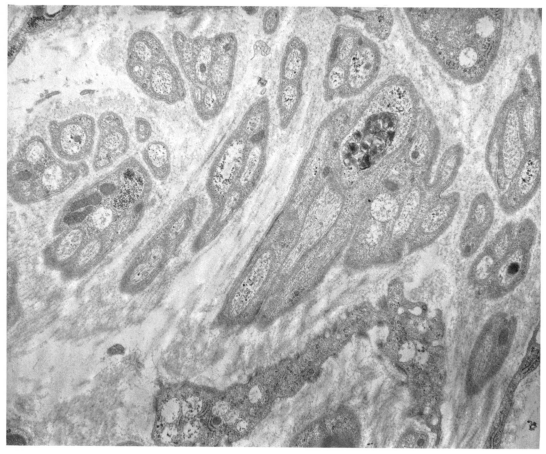

Figure 13.6. Electron micrograph of a skin biopsy reveals an unmyelinated dermal nerve. A large axon contains a composite granular inclusion with a few coarse lamellae (original magnification × 13,500). (Courtesy of Dr. W. Jann Brown.)

stances that are found in small amounts in a variety of tissues. Seven types have been isolated from human cataracts [52] and one type from the human brain [53]. Keratan sulfate is the only glycosaminoglycan that contains α-fucose, and was found to be increased as much as five- and tenfold in several patients [25,30,54]. There may be several dozens of complex fucosyl derivatives, many of which accumulate in relatively small amounts in patients with fucosidosis. The task of sorting them out represents a formidable technologic challenge.

Genetics

The disease is rare and possesses a high rate of consanguinity (8 of 30 families of both types). The excess number of Type I females is likely due to the small number of cases reported. However, the excess of Type II males cannot be explained. To differentiate the two types on the basis of angiokeratoma does not validate genetic heterogeneity for several reasons. First, two sets of siblings of both types have been identified in two Italian pedigrees [55]. Second, the enzyme deficiency is equally profound in both types. Third, the angiokeratoma does not express differences in the type of capillary storage but rather in the length of life span of the patient [15,56]. It can no longer be used to discriminate sibships that have the protracted form since a child with Type I (Table 13.1, no. 9) developed the lesion before dying at age 6 [9]. Moreover, three Type II families included a sibling who died at age 4 or 5 years [31,34]. Even though there is inadequate information on the deceased patients [31], that both types occurred in the same sibship negates the usefulness of angiokeratoma as a predictor of milder clinical outcome. Actually, patients who have experienced a mild protracted course [20,35] in the absence of angiokeratoma further contradict this point of view.

Phenotypic variability has become the rule in many recessive disorders. Genetic heterogeneity undoubtedly exists without easily detectable clinical correlates.

Pathophysiology

Rare disorders often shed light or bring attention to aspects of metabolism whose functional importance is not readily appreciated. Widespread neuronal storage of oligosaccharides leads to the early arrest of psychomotor development. Glycoprotein synthesis is intimately associated with higher mental functions such as learning [56]. The α-fucosidase deficiency impairs the turnover of the complex molecules synthesized and in some way interferes with brain function. Profound mental retardation is the rule in fucosidosis as it is in other disorders of oligosaccharide degradation. Yet to be understood are the metabolic steps involved in these important neuronal functions. The basic cellular activities do not seem seriously hindered by the lysosomal storage itself. This is especially true for the vessels in which the endothelial cells are markedly enlarged and thus might be expected to cause ischemia. That a similar vascular impairment prevails in FAD indicates that it takes several decades before ischemia becomes a significant factor, and thus requires a longer life span than has been reported in most cases of fucosidosis. Dwarfism is related mostly to delayed bone age and points to another functional consequence of deranged oligosaccharide metabolism. The frequent infections seen in early childhood may be secondary to thickened secretions [1], a problem also observed in several types of MPSD. The spasticity probably results from a combination of impaired myelination and low-grade demyelination, although active demyelination has not been reported [40]. On the basis of basal ganglia involvement, especially of the globus pallidus [40], one would expect more extrapyramidal signs, dystonia, for example, than have been reported so far.

Table 13.3. Differential Diagnosis of Lysosomal Storage Disorders

| | Lysosomal Inclusions | | | Deficient Enzyme | Urine | |
	Endothelial Cells	Schwann Cells	Fibroblasts		Oligosaccharide	GAG
Fucosidosis	Clear	Lamellar	Clear	α-Fucosidase	4 +	N, ±
GM₁ gangliosidosis	Clear	Lamellar	Clear	β-Galactosidase	4 +	N, ±
Fabry–Anderson disease	Lamellar	(Lamellar)	Lamellar	α-Galactosidase	N	N
Sandhoff disease	Lamellar	Lamellar	Clear, lamellar	β-Hexosaminidase (A + B)	+	N
Mannosidosis	Clear	Clear	Clear	α-Mannosidase	4 +	N
Sialidosis	?	?	?	Sialidase (+ β-galactosidase)	+	N
Aspartylglucosaminuria	?	?	?	Aspartyl-glucosaminidase	4 +	N
I-cell disease	Lamellar	Clear	Clear	Transferase	±	N
Mucolipidosis IV	Clear, lamellar	Clear, lamellar	Clear, lamellar	Uncertain	N	N
Multiple sulfatase deficiency	(Clear)	Lamellar	Clear	Arylsulfatase a,b,c	N	N,1 +
Hunter (MPSD II)	0	(Lamellar)	Clear	Iduronate sulfatase	0	N,2 +
Sanfilippo syndrome (MPSD III,A)	0	(Lamellar)	(Clear)	Heparan N-sulfatase	0	N,2 +
Morquio syndrome (MPSD IV)	0	0	0	Specific sulfatase	0	N,2 +

GAG = Glycosaminoglycans (mucopolysaccharide)
  ? = Not reported
  N = Normal
  0 = Absent
  ( ) = Inconstant

Table 13.4. Distinctive Clinical Features of Lysosomal Storage Disorders Which May Resemble Fucosidosis

	Mental Retardation	Angiokeratoma	Corneal Opacities
Fucosidosis	Severe to profound	Frequent after age 4 to 6 years	Rare
GM$_1$ gangliosidosis	Severe to profound	Exceptional	Slight
Fabry–Anderson disease	Exceptional	Rare before age 10 years; generally discrete	Requires slitlamp (whorls)
Sandhoff disease	Severe to profound	Absent	Absent
Mannosidosis	Severe to profound	Absent	Frequent
Sialidosis	Variable	Occasional	Occasional
Aspartylglucosaminuria	Moderate to severe	Absent	Absent
I-cell disease (mucolipidosis II, III)	Severe to profound	Absent	Rare
Mucolipidosis IV	Severe to profound	Absent	Dense, early
Multiple sulfatase deficiency	Severe to profound	Absent	Generally absent
Hunter syndrome (MPSD II)	May be absent	Absent	Absent
Sanfilippo syndrome (MPSD III)	Severe to profound	Absent	Requires slitlamp
Morquio syndrome (MPSD IV)	Generally absent	Absent	Requires slitlamp

Differential Diagnosis

Sorting out an inborn disorder of metabolism from the large still undifferentiated mass of apparently static encephalopathies is an increasingly difficult endeavor. Ultrastructural studies on skin or conjunctival biopsies provide the most informative technique to demonstrate the existence of lysosomal storage, its general nature—water soluble (oligosaccharides or glycosaminoglycans) or lipidic (membranous or lamellar)—and its distribution in the different cell types (Table 13.3). Enzyme studies are in some ways more convenient but are generally restricted to the most common disorders unless they can be better focused when the nature of the storage has been broadly identified. Clinical clues such as organomegaly, coarse facial features, or bony abnormalities may suggest a MPSD, which has been the first diagnostic consideration in the majority of fucosidosis cases. Coarsening of the facies is found in many other storage disorders as well, such as GM$_1$ gangliosidosis, Sandhoff disease, sialidosis, I-cell disease (mucolipidosis II and III), mucolipidosis IV, α-mannosidosis, aspartylglucosaminuria, Niemann–Pick disease Type A, and multiple sulfatase deficiency. The facies in fucosidosis is different from what is known as the gargoyle facies and is characterized by bright eyes and a well-shaped nose without the depressed bridge and the upturned, flaring tip. Angiokeratoma (Table 13.4) is found in Fabry–Anderson disease, rarely in GM$_1$ gangliosidosis. In older children, dwarfism and bone deformities may resemble Sanfilippo (MPSD III) or Morquio syndromes (MPSD IV), and the finding of elevated keratan sulfate in urine may reinforce this impression. Skin or conjunctival biopsies are normal in MPSD IV. Special chromatographic techniques to demonstrate urinary oligosaccharides are simple and useful [57]. Urine in fucosidosis contains abundant material that does not migrate from the origin of the chromatogram.

Treatment

Prevention requires genetic counseling and prenatal diagnosis [10,45]. Curative therapy is not available. Bone marrow or organ transplantation does not seem to offer any chance of improvement in a disease with primary neuronal involvement. Techniques for enzyme replacement have not yet been successfully worked out.

References

1. Durand P, Philippart M, Borrone C, et al. Una nuova malattia da accumulo di glicolipidi. Minerva Pediatr 1967;19:2187–2196.
2. Freitag F, Kuchemann K, Blumcke S, et al. Hepatic

ultrastructure in fucosidosis. Virchows Arch (Cell Pathol) 1971;7:99–113.

3. Larbrisseau A, Brochu P, Ng Ying Kin NMK, et al. Première observation canadienne d'une fucosidose. Union Med Can 1978;107:968–980.

4. Loeb H, Tondeur M, Jonniaux G, et al. Biochemical and ultrastructural studies in a case of mucopolysaccharidosis "F" (fucosidosis). Helv Paediatr Acta 1969;24:519–537.

5. Matsuda I, Arashima S, Anakura M, et al. Fucosidosis. Tohoku J Exp Med 1973;109:41–48.

6. Troost J, Staal GEJ, Willemse J, et al. Fucosidosis. Neuropaediatrie 1977;8:155–162.

7. Staal GEJ, Troost J, van der Heijden MCM, et al. Two different families with α-L-fucosidase deficiency. Monogr Hum Genet 1978;10:56–61.

8. Libert J, Van Hoof F, Tondeur M. Fucosidosis: ultrastructural study of conjunctiva and skin and enzyme analysis of tears. Invest Ophthalmol 1976;15:626–639.

9. Libert J. La fucosidose: ultrastructure oculaire. J Fr Ophtalmol 1984;7:519–527.

10. Poenaru L, Dreyfus JC, Boue J, et al. Prenatal diagnosis of fucosidosis. Clin Genet 1976;10:260–264.

11. Garcia CA, McGarry PA, Duncan CM. Fucosidosis: neuropathology of one of two new cases resembling Alexander's disease. J Neuropathol Exp Neurol 1980;39:353.

12. Kolodny EH, Sotrol A, Cable W, et al. Fucosidosis presenting as a leukodystrophy. Ann Neurol 1980; 8:114.

13. Philippart M, Ashton N, Brown WJ. Fucosidosis with variable residual alpha-fucosidase activity. Presented at 10th Meeting of the Child Neurology Society, Minneapolis, 1981.

14. Sutton M, Blitzer MG, Miller JB, et al. A variant form of fucosidosis secondary to a low stability, α-fucosidase mutant. Am J Hum Genet 1983;35:55A.

15. Kousseff BG, Beratis MG, Strauss L, et al. Fucosidosis type 2. Pediatrics 1976;57:205–213.

16. Sovik O, Lie SO, Fluge G, et al. Fucosidosis: severe phenotype with survival to adult age. Eur J Pediatr 1980;135:211–216.

17. Prindiville DE, Stern D. Oral lesions in fucosidosis. J Oral Surg 1976;34:603–608.

18. Ikeda S, Kondo K, Oguchi K, et al. Adult fucosidosis: histochemical and ultrastructural studies of rectal mucosa biopsy. Neurology 1984;34:451–456.

19. Snodgrass MB. Ocular findings in a case of fucosidosis. Br J Ophthalmol 1976;60:508–511.

20. Landing BH, Donnell GN, Alfi OS, et al. Fucosidosis: clinical, pathologic, and biochemical studies of five patients. Adv Exp Med Biol 1976;68:147–165.

21. Patel V, Watanabe I, Zeman W. Deficiency of α-L-fucosidase. Science 1972;176:426–427.

22. Primrose DA. Mucopolysaccharidosis: a new variant? J Ment Defic Res 1972;16:167–172.

23. MacPhee GB, Logan RW, Primrose DAA. Fucosidosis: how many cases undetected? Lancet 1975;2:462–463.

24. MacPhee GB, Logan RW. Fucosidosis in a native-born Briton. J Clin Pathol 1977;30:278–283.

25. Borrone C, Gatti R, Trias X, et al. Fucosidosis: clinical, biochemical, immunologic, and genetic studies in two new cases. J Pediatr 1974;84:727–730.

26. Snyder RD, Carlow TJ, Ledman J, et al. Ocular findings in fucosidosis. Birth defects: original article series 1976;12(3):241–251.

27. Smith EB, Graham JL, Ledman JA, et al. Fucosidosis. Cutis 1977;19:195–198.

28. Romeo G, Borrone C, Gatti R, et al. Fucosidosis in Calabria: founder effect or high gene frequency? Lancet 1977;1:368–369.

29. Giovannini M, Riva E, Beluffi G, et al. Fucosidosi. Descrizione di un caso clinico. Minerva Pediatr 1978;30:1307–1313.

30. Porfiri B, Ricci R, Seminara D, et al. Ultrastructural studies of Type II fucosidosis. Arch Dermatol Res 1981;270:57–66.

31. Kessler RM, Altman DH, Martin-Jimenez R. Cranial CT in fucosidosis. AJNR 1981;2:591–592.

32. Boudet C, Maisongrosse G, Echenne B. A propos de deux nouveaux cas de fucosidose de type II. Bull Soc Ophtalmol Fr 1982;82:91–93.

33. Echenne B, Baldet P, Maire I, et al. Fucosidose de type II. Pediatrie 1982;37:501–510.

34. Christomanou H, Beyer D. Absence of α-fucosidase activity in two sisters showing a different phenotype. Eur J Pediatr 1983;140:27–29.

35. Schoonderwaldt HC, Lamers KJB, Kleijnen FM, et al. Two patients with an unusual form of type II fucosidosis. Clin Genet 1980;18:348–354.

36. Brill PW, Beratis NG, Kousseff BG, et al. Roentgenographic findings in fucosidosis type 2. AJR 1975;124:75–82.

37. Lee FA, Donnell GN, Gwinn JL. Radiographic features of fucosidosis. Pediatr Radiol 1977;5:204–208.

38. Kornfeld M, Snyder RD, Wenger DA. Fucosidosis with angiokeratoma. Electron microscopic changes in the skin. Arch Pathol Lab Med 1977;101:478–485.

39. Troost J, Straks W, Willemse J. Fucosidosis. II. Ultrastructure. Neuropaediatrie 1977;2:162–171.

40. Bugiani O, Borrone C. Fucosidosis: a neuropathological study. Riv Patol Nerv Ment 1976;97:133–141.

41. Playfer JR, Price-Evans DA. Enzyme activity in fucosidosis. Lancet 1976;2:1415–1416.

42. Bosmann HB. Glycoprotein degradation. Exp Cell Res 1969;43:217–221.

43. Beratis NG, Turner BM, Hirschhorn K. Fucosidosis: detection of the carrier state in peripheral blood leukocytes. J Pediatr 1975;87:1193–1198.

44. Durand P, Gatti R, Borrone C, et al. Detection of carriers and prenatal diagnosis for fucosidosis in Calabria. Hum Genet 1979;51:195–201.

45. Matsuda I, Arashima S, Oka Y, et al. Prenatal diagnosis of fucosidosis. Clin Chim Acta 1975;63:55–60.

46. Spooncer E, Fukuda M, Klock JC, et al. Isolation and characterization of polyfucosylated lactosaminoglycan from human granulocytes. J Biol Chem 1984; 259:4792–4799.

47. Strecker G, Fournet B, Montreuil J. Structure of the three major fucosyl-glycoasparagines accumulating in

the urine of a patient with fucosidosis. Biochimie 1978;60:725–734.

48. Nishigaki M, Yamashita K, Matsuda I, et al. Urinary oligosaccharides of fucosidosis. J Biochem (Tokyo) 1978;84:823–834.

49. McKibbin JM. Fucolipids. J Lipid Res 1978;19:131–147.

50. Philippart M. Fucosidosis: a novel neurovisceral sphingolipidosis. Neurology (NY) 1969;19:304.

51. Staal GEJ, van der Heijden MCM, Troost J, et al. Clin Chim Acta 1977;76:155–157.

52. Tao RVP, Shen U, Kovathana N, et al. A new family of fucose-containing gangliosides isolated from human senile cataracts. Biochim Biophys Acta 1983;753:89–96.

53. Vanier MT, Mansson JE, Svennerholm L. The occurrence of III³-α-fucosyllactoneotetraosylceramide in human brain. FEBS Lett 1980;112:70–72.

54. Greiling H, Stuhlsatz HW, Cantz M, et al. Increased urinary excretion of keratan sulfate in fucosidosis. J Clin Chem Clin Biochem 1978;16:329–334.

55. Durand P, Borrone C, Gatti R. On genetic variants in fucosidosis. J Pediatr 1976;89:688–690.

56. Wetzel W, Popov N, Lossner B, et al. Effect of L-fucose on brain protein metabolism and retention of a learned behavior in rats. Pharmacol Biochem Behav 1980;13:765–771.

57. Humbel R, Collart M. Oligosaccharides in urine of patients with glycoprotein storage diseases. Clin Chim Acta 1975;60:143–145.

Chapter 14

Phenylketonuria and Hyperphenylalaninemia

VIRGINIA V. MICHELS

Classic phenylketonuria (PKU) is an autosomal recessive inherited deficiency of the enzyme phenylalanine hydroxylase, which converts phenylalanine to tyrosine. The disease is characterized in the untreated state by elevated blood phenylalanine levels of over 20 mg/dl and by the abnormal urinary excretion of phenylalanine metabolites. Most untreated patients have pale blond hair, blue eyes, and fair skin and develop mental retardation with or without seizures. Many have eczema and a characteristic "mousy" odor. Fortunately, early treatment with a phenylalanine-restricted diet can prevent these complications. Treatment of pregnant women with PKU, whose fetuses are at risk for damage in utero, remains a therapeutic challenge.

Milder and transient hyperphenylalaninemic states must be distinguished from classic PKU, since the prognosis and need for treatment differ. Several types of hyperphenylalaninemia associated with abnormalities of biopterin metabolism have been recognized. These latter forms of hyperphenylalaninemia do not respond to dietary restriction, and in severe cases treatment with biopterin and neurotransmitter precursors may be required.

Historical Review

In 1934, the Norwegian physician Asbjörn Fölling evaluated a brother and sister with mental retardation in whom the mother had noted a peculiar odor. Fölling found that when ferric chloride was added to their urine a green color resulted, and he identified the compound responsible for this chemical reaction as phenylpyruvate. He then surveyed children in a mental institution, found eight additional cases, and proposed a new inherited defect of phenylalanine metabolism [1]. Penrose recognized the disorder to be inherited in an autosomal recessive fashion in 1935 [2]. In 1944, Bernheim demonstrated that the main catabolic pathway of phenylalanine was by parahydroxylation to tyrosine, and by 1953 the defect of phenylalanine hydroxylation was demonstrated in the liver of PKU patients. This laid the foundation of knowledge that led Bickel, in 1954, to treat PKU patients with a low phenylalanine diet. As expected, dietary treatment could not reverse brain damage, and it was realized that treatment would be more helpful when started early. Testing newborns' urine with ferric chloride often resulted in false-negative results, but in 1963 Guthrie developed the bacterial inhibition assay for blood phenylalanine that made newborn screening possible [1]. In the 1960s, several American states passed laws mandating such screening. Screening now is practiced in all 50 of the United States as well as in Japan and most European countries, although the criteria for diagnosis of classic PKU has changed over the years as milder forms of hyperphenylalaninemia were recognized [3].

In 1971 medical reports confirmed that early treatment could result in normal intellectual development, although it took time, trial, and error to determine the optimal range of blood phenylalanine that should be maintained. Horner, in 1962, reported a case in which therapy was discontinued early in childhood. Although it was generally thought to be safe to discontinue diet treatment at 4 to 5 years of age, as early as 1969 Murphy suggested that discontinuation could be harmful; this point continues to be debated [4]. Thus, tremendous advances in diagnosis and treatment of PKU have been made since the 1930s, and appropriate dietary management of PKU has prevented the severe mental retardation that previously occurred in this disease. Several challenges remain: (a) How can subtle deficiencies in school performance experienced by some intellectually normal PKU children be prevented? (b) When can diet safely be discontinued for PKU children, or how can one identify those at risk after diet discontinuation? (c) How can the threat of intrauterine damage to children of PKU women be eliminated? Work continues in these areas, and partial answers to these questions are beginning to emerge.

In 1974, Bartholome et al. [5] recognized that a few children had an unusual form of PKU that did not respond to dietary treatment. Kaufman et al. [6] described the first such case in which a different enzyme, dihydropteridine reductase, was deficient. Since then several other enzyme deficiencies of biopterin metabolism have been delineated. Significant advances have been made in identifying patients with these forms of hyperphenylalaninemia, but adequate treatment to prevent neurologic damage in the severe forms has not yet been found.

Classic Phenylketonuria

Clinical Symptoms and Signs

Infants with classic PKU are clinically normal at birth and during early infancy. Some infants vomit excessively and occasionally are diagnosed as having pyloric stenosis.

If PKU is left untreated, developmental delay usually becomes apparent some time after 6 months of age. Feeding problems and neurologic signs such as tremor, mild diplegia, hypertonia, and hyperactive deep tendon reflexes may develop. Myoclonic, akinetic, or other generalized seizures may either begin as early as the first year of life or later in childhood; the electroencephalogram is abnormal in 80% of affected patients and may show a hypsarrhythmia pattern or bursts of spike and wave activity [7].

Cerebral damage occurs most rapidly in the first 2 years of life, such that untreated or late-treated patients frequently have significant mental retardation. The intelligence quotient is less than 55 in over 90% of untreated cases, although occasionally it will fall within normal limits. Why some patients with classic PKU escape mental retardation is not known, but both retarded and intellectually normal individuals may exist within the same sibship.

The personality characteristics of retarded, institutionalized PKU patients include hyperactivity, restlessness, shyness, and fearfulness; they tend to be noisy and destructive and to have uncontrollable tempers. They may exhibit self-injurious behavior.

Some patients are lethargic. Both retarded and intellectually normal PKU patients may have schizoid personalities. The frequency of undetected PKU in psychiatric hospital populations is very low, and in several reported series no PKU patients were detected by a screening of more than 5,000 patients [2], although one study did find that 6 of 22,000 psychiatric patients were affected [8]. These researchers did not recommend general screening of psychiatric patients but suggested screening for those with mental retardation, pervasive developmental disorders, unexplained seizures, eczema, fair complexion for their family, or a family history of PKU.

Untreated patients have low levels of tyrosine, required in the biosynthetic pathway of melanin. Therefore, they usually have fair skin and hair and blue irides, which may result in mild photosensitivity. Skin, hair, and eye coloring is completely normal at birth and during early infancy; brown hair or eyes do not exclude the diagnosis of PKU. Many patients develop an eczematous skin rash within the first year of life and have excessive perspiration and a "mousy" odor that results from phenylacetic acid.

Untreated patients develop microcephaly and may be slightly smaller in height [9]. Bony changes, including slight decalcification of the long bones and a prominent maxilla, may be noted. Enamel hypoplasia with wide interdental spaces may be present.

Some patients develop cataracts at an early age, but it has been suggested that this is the result of medications or trauma rather than an intrinsic part of the disease [10].

Virtually all these tragic effects of PKU can be avoided by early treatment with a phenylalanine-restricted diet. Most infants born in civilized countries with a significant incidence of PKU are screened in the newborn period; however, it is important to realize that some infants are missed by screening programs. The clinician, therefore, must never assume that a patient does not have PKU because he or she was born in an area in which newborn screening is practiced. Any person with suspicious signs or symptoms should have a blood test to determine the phenylalanine level.

Biochemistry

Classic phenylketonuria is due to a deficiency of phenylalanine hydroxylase (E. C. 1.14.16.1), the enzyme required to convert phenylalanine to tyrosine (Figure 14.1). This reaction requires the presence of an active cofactor, tetrahydrobiopterin. Although the plasma phenylalanine level is normal at birth (<2

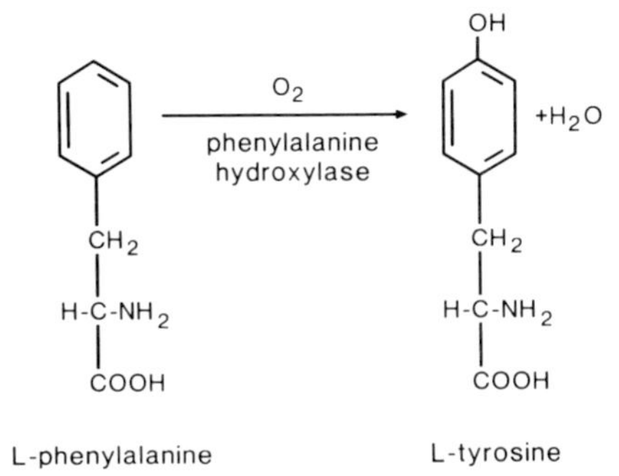

Figure 14.1. Conversion of phenylalanine to tyrosine by phenylalanine hydroxylase. This reaction requires the presence of the active cofactor tetrahydrobiopterin.

mg/dl) [11] deficiency of the enzyme causes the plasma phenylalanine to rapidly rise to over 20 mg/dl, usually within the first few days of life. Occasionally the rate of rise is more gradual, such that these levels may not be reached until 2 to 3 weeks of age. The plasma tyrosine is lower than normal; after an oral phenylalanine load, plasma tyrosine does not increase as it does in normal persons. The urinary excretion of phenylalanine is increased above normal.

When the blood concentration of phenylalanine is increased, metabolic pathways that are not important in normal persons become active and convert phenylalanine to phenylpyruvic acid, which in turn can be converted to phenylacetic acid, phenyllactic acid, phenylacetylglutamine, and phenylethylamine. Phenylpyruvic acid appears in the blood and is excreted in the urine where it can be detected by ferric chloride, dinitrophenylhydrazine, or Phenistix (a cellulose reagent strip impregnated with cyclohexylsulfamic acid and ferric and magnesium ions) [2]. However, the maturational delay in the enzyme system responsible for this conversion makes urine testing unsuitable for newborn screening. Because excretion of these compounds correlates directly with plasma phenylalanine levels, these compounds decrease dramatically when the patient is treated with a phenylalanine-restricted diet. Normal persons, even when given a phenylalanine load, do not excrete these compounds.

Since the phenylalanine hydroxylase enzyme normally is expressed only in the liver, the diagnosis of classic PKU usually is made on the basis of a persistently elevated plasma phenylalanine level of over 20 mg/dl. To be sure that the patient does not have transient hyperphenylalaninemia, approximately 3 months or later after diagnosis an oral phenylalanine challenge in a dosage of 180 mg/kg/day for 3 days is recommended. This loading test should result in a

sustained rise in phenylalanine to over 20 mg/dl and in increased urinary phenylalanine metabolites [12]. Some patients with milder hyperphenylalaninemia may have a peak level of plasma phenylalanine >20 mg/dl which then declines to less than 20 mg/dl as the challenge continues, possibly because of the induction of residual enzyme activity [13].

In classic PKU, liver phenylalanine hydroxylase activity may be less than 1% of normal; immunologic cross-reacting material may or may not be present [14,15]. Patients with milder hyperphenylalaninemia may have residual enzyme activity that is 3 to 6% of normal [16]. Some PKU patients have an enzyme with abnormal biochemical or kinetic characteristics, suggesting a structural gene mutation.

Except for elevated phenylalanine and low tyrosine, the plasma levels of other amino acids are normal or slightly low [17].

Cerebrospinal fluid phenylalanine is elevated in untreated PKU [17]. Slight decreases in CSF threonine, alanine, and arginine and slight increases in serine, isoleucine, and histidine have been observed. It has been speculated that these differences could have a significant effect on protein and lipoprotein synthesis [17,18]. However, in other reports, CSF threonine and other amino acids were said to be normal [18]. Despite low plasma tyrosine levels, there have been reports of both normal CSF tyrosine [17,18] and elevated CSF tyrosine [19]. Therefore, with the exception of elevated phenylalanine, there appears to be no consistent abnormality in the CSF amino acid concentrations, in spite of the fact that phenylalanine is believed to share a saturatable transport system across the blood–brain barrier with tyrosine and other large neutral amino acids [19].

Untreated PKU patients have decreased plasma, urine, and CSF levels of neurotransmitters such as epinephrine, norepinephrine, dopamine, serotonin, homovanillic acid, and 5-hydroxy-indoleacetic acid [20]. Levels of these compounds increase after dietary restriction of phenylalanine [6]. High phenylalanine levels may interfere with the hydroxylation of tyrosine and tryptophan, which could account for the decreased concentrations of neurotransmitters and their metabolites [21] (Figure 14.2).

Phenylalanine stimulates the biosynthesis of dihydroneopterin triphosphate, a precursor of tetrahydrobiopterin, the cofactor necessary for action of the phenylalanine, tyrosine, and tryptophan hydroxylases [1]. Consequently, the urine of untreated PKU patients contains higher than normal levels of biopterin, although the ratio of neopterin to biopterin usually is normal [22]. Occasionally, both normal infants and classic PKU patients have a transiently

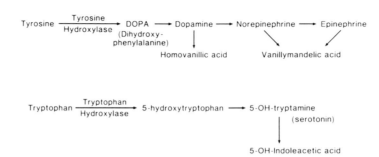

Figure 14.2. Hydroxylation of tyrosine and tryptophan as initial steps in synthesis of neurotransmitters and their metabolites. These hydroxylases require the presence of the active cofactor tetrahydrobiopterin.

elevated neopterin to biopterin ratio, which may relate to maturational changes [23]. This is important in distinguishing between classic PKU and variant forms of phenylketonuria, as discussed further under Abnormalities of Biopterin Metabolism.

In summary, most of the secondary biochemical changes observed in classic PKU can be reversed or ameliorated by treatment with a diet restricted in phenylalanine that contains adequate tyrosine, thus controlling the metabolic abnormalities that otherwise result in neurologic impairment.

Pathology

Most patients with untreated classic PKU have microcephaly, and the most consistent abnormality reported at autopsy is a brain weight that is 65 to 85% of normal [24]. There are no gross lesions or abnormalities in gyral configuration. However, histoanatomic studies suggest maturational delay, with a myelination pattern in adults comparable to that of 2- to 3-year-old children.

There are several reported cases of myelination abnormalities. In one report, pale staining of myelin suggestive of retarded myelination was most evident in fiber systems that had the most protracted postnatal cycles of myelination, while those systems with shorter cycles of myelination showed normal staining [24]. Some investigators have reported neuronal changes such as paucity of cortical neurons, faintly stained or immature appearance of neurons with decreased length and degree of arborization of dendritic processes and a decreased number of synaptic spines, dispersion of nuclear chromatin, and less distinct cerebral cortical lamination with increased cell packing density. Some of these changes also were interpreted to represent maturational delay, comparable to a 6- to 24-month age level. No significant gliosis, spongiform or atrophic changes, or myelenolysis were noted [24].

Rats made hyperphenylalaninemic have reduced brain weight with decreased myelin synthesis suggestive of maturational delay [25]. Several of the neuronal changes are similar to that observed in humans, but in rat models more marked cerebellar changes appear to exist [26].

Biochemical studies have demonstrated that untreated PKU patients have a less than normal amount of myelin; however, no gross change in the chemical composition of myelin in humans, or in rat models, has been demonstrated. Subtle differences may have gone undetected, however, and it has been suggested that high phenylalanine levels in the brain may restrict sulfatide formation in heavy myelin and that such small changes could significantly alter myelin stability and turnover. An increased rate of myelin and myelin protein turnover has been reported in a rat model [25].

It has been suggested that high plasma phenylalanine competes with other large neutral amino acids for transport into the brain and that subtle differences in amino acid concentrations may lead to decreased protein and lipoprotein synthesis [18]. The altered neurotransmitter concentrations of the CSF and brain also may be important in the pathogenesis of the neurologic abnormalities [20].

It is well known that elevated blood phenylalanine and its abnormal metabolites are associated with elevated CSF levels of these substances; however, the precise mechanism by which one or more of these agents leads to the observed pathologic changes is not known.

Treatment and Prognosis

The goal of dietary treatment is to limit oral phenylalanine intake while maintaining adequate amounts of other amino acids such as tyrosine, total protein, calories, and other nutrients to provide for normal growth and development. The plasma phenylalanine level should be maintained between 3 and 10 mg/dl, which is higher than the normal level of 0.4 to 1.5 mg/dl. The rationale for choosing this therapeutic range is twofold. First, attempts to keep the plasma phenylalanine level in the normal range sometimes inadvertently led to phenylalanine deficiency, which in turn led to anorexia, malnutrition, and even mental retardation or death [27]. Second, in the first phase of the collaborative study of PKU children, no difference in outcome was found in children assigned to two different treatment groups, one targeted to keep phenylalanine levels between 1.0 and 5.4 mg/dl, and the other at 5.5 to 9.9 mg/dl. Admittedly, many of the children's phenylalanine levels could not be maintained within these assigned ranges, and levels crossed over into the other groups' target range [28]. This demonstrates the impracticality of attempts at such strict control. However, persons with hyperphenylalaninemia whose levels are <10 or 12 mg/dl while ingesting a normal diet usually are mentally normal [11,29], adding support to the conclusion that phenylalanine levels between 3 and 10 mg/dl are satisfactory.

Children with PKU cannot ingest adequate protein without getting excess phenylalanine by only eating natural foods. To achieve dietary restriction, infants should be fed one of the commercial formulas such as Lophenalac, which contains a casein hydrolysate from which 95% of the phenylalanine has been removed. The formula is supplemented with corn syrup solids, corn oil, vitamins, and minerals to create a nutritionally complete infant formula [30]. The average PKU infant tolerates 58 ± 18 mg of phenylalanine/kg/day. As growth slows during infancy and childhood, the amount tolerated decreases by the age of 10 to 12 years to 30 ± 8 mg/kg/day. These are only guidelines, however, and the tolerance of each child must be monitored by serial plasma phenylalanine levels. Since Lophenalac contains only 0.08 gm of phenylalanine per 100 gm of powder, this formula does not contain sufficient phenylalanine for normal growth and development and must be supplemented by whole milk in infants or other protein-containing foods in older children. To allow a greater amount of protein in older children, an even lower phenylalanine protein product such as Phenyl-free may be utilized.

The diet of patients with PKU should be prescribed by a knowledgeable physician in collaboration with a nutritionist. Treatment should be initiated with Lophenalac, prepared in a way to meet the individual infant's nutritional and fluid needs. It should provide 85 to 90% of the protein requirement. The mother should never be told merely to purchase formula and prepare it according to the directions on the package. Plasma phenylalanine levels should be monitored daily, as levels can fall dramatically once the diet is started. As the levels approach 10 mg/dl, a supplemental source of phenylalanine (evaporated milk is convenient) should be added. Breast feeding is not contraindicated; human milk is lower in phenylalanine than is cow's milk or other commercial infant formulas. A Department of Health and Human Services publication [31] is available that describes techniques and problems for physicians and parents who are motivated to manage the diet of the PKU infant using a combination of breast milk and Lophenalac.

As discussed in the section Newborn Screening for Phenylketonuria, most infants who have a positive screen ultimately prove not to have classic PKU. It is extremely important that a significant elevation of phenylalanine is determined by a second blood test before dietary treatment is instituted. Some infants will have only a modest, transient elevation in phenylalanine of between 2 or 4 mg/dl (the cutoff point for a positive screen varies between states) and 12 mg/dl [32]. These individuals develop normally without dietary treatment, but repeated blood specimens must be obtained to ensure that levels do not increase further. No general agreement exists as to whether patients with persistent elevations greater than 12 or 15 mg/dl but less than 20 mg/dl need treatment [12]; however, there can be no argument that those with levels ≥20 mg/dl need therapy. Even within this latter group, a few children will later develop an increased dietary tolerance of phenylalanine, which is the reason why it has been recommended that children on treatment should be given a phenylalanine challenge at 3 to 6 months of age. If the results are equivocal, a repeat challenge may be performed at age 12 to 15 months [30].

When indicated, dietary treatment should be instituted as soon as possible. Infants whose treatment is instituted when they are less than 3 weeks of age usually have normal intelligence quotients [33–36]. In the PKU collaborative study, the treatment variable that was most strongly correlated with the child's IQ was the age at which treatment was initiated. Not unexpectedly, IQ also correlated with the mother's IQ [37]. The mean IQ of early treated children was comparable to that of unaffected siblings in some studies [33,35], but was slightly lower (IQ of 100 versus 107 in unaffected siblings) in the collaborative study [38]. In surveys conducted before widespread newborn screening, the later treatment began after the first month of life, the lower the IQ [28].

When the infant is ready for solid foods, cereals,

fruits, and vegetables can be added to the diet in a sequence similar to that for infants without PKU. However, these must be taken in prescribed amounts with an "exchange list" based on the phenylalanine content of the foods, analogous to the exchange lists of diabetics. Meat, eggs, and dairy products (other than the prescribed whole milk) are too high in phenylalanine to be included in the diet. The mother must keep a dietary record, and adjustments must be made to satisfy the child's appetite and to maintain the desired plasma phenylalanine level. Blood levels should be monitored weekly in the young infant and then tapered to monthly by the third year of life [30]. Low phenylalanine levels are due to insufficient dietary intake. High phenylalanine levels can result from acute febrile illnesses [39] or surgery when the baby is in a catabolic state [40], from insufficient protein or energy in the diet, or even from inadequate phenylalanine in the diet that results in breakdown of body proteins.

The results of the PKU collaborative study suggested that outcome is related to how well the patient adheres to the phenylalanine-restricted diet [41], determined in the study by the number of blood specimens with phenylalanine levels over 15 mg/dl.

The initial controversy about the value of dietary treatment of PKU, which stemmed from the finding that some PKU patients have normal intelligence, abated when population surveys revealed that this was a rare phenomenon [33]. No significant side effects have been caused by properly administered dietary treatment [36]. Physical growth, including head size, is normal in well-treated patients [9,27]. Treated children are neurologically normal. Although some have an abnormal electroencephalogram in infancy, this often becomes normal by 1 year of age. Those with an abnormal pattern had single repetitive or multiple spikes or sharp waves, focal or scattered, which rarely occurred in paroxysmal bursts. None had a hypsarrhythmia pattern. Those with an abnormal electroencephalogram tended to have a slightly higher phenylalanine level before treatment, but the abnormal electroencephalogram was not predictive of subsequent cognitive abilities or significant neurologic abnormality [42].

Extensive psychometric and school achievement testing has been performed in children considered adequately treated for PKU. An increased frequency of perceptual–motor dysfunction in PKU patients with normal IQ, as manifest by testing with the Bender–Gestalt Test, has been reported [43]. Other observers dispute these findings [44]. In the PKU collaborative study, children scored slightly lower in arithmetic for their grade level by the Wide Range

Achievement Test (WRAT) [4]. On the WRAT reading and spelling subtests, PKU patients did as well as their unaffected siblings and achieved results comparable to national norms [38]. Children with treated PKU did not have significant behavior problems [45]. There are conflicting reports as to whether PKU children with normal IQs have an increased frequency of learning disabilities [43,46–48]. However, some of the reports are difficult to interpret because they include older children who remained on dietary treatment as well as children who had discontinued treatment.

Originally it was thought that it was safe to discontinue the phenylalanine-restricted diet at approximately 5 years of age [33], although sporadic reports of deteriorated intellectual performance, behavioral changes, and abnormal electroencephalograms after diet discontinuation appeared as early as 1969 [4,33]. Waisbren [49] reviewed 19 published studies; approximately half of these reports, involving 288 subjects, suggested that intellectual performance decreased. The other reports, involving 123 subjects, suggested minimal if any change. In the second phase of the PKU collaborative study, 115 children were assigned randomly to continue or discontinue the phenylalanine-restricted diet at age 6 years. Those continuing on the diet were to have phenylalanine levels of 2 to 12 mg/dl. Unfortunately, the study design was compromised because some parents would not accept their child's randomized assignment and entered the converse group. Only 46% of those originally randomized remained in the assigned groups. Furthermore, it proved difficult to keep the phenylalanine levels in the assigned range, and the individual levels of those on and off the diet overlapped, although the mean levels were significantly different. The mean IQ of those remaining on the diet was 101 at age 6 (siblings 106) and 104 at age 8 years, compared to a mean sibling IQ score of 103. The mean IQ of those discontinuing the diet was 97 at age 6 (siblings 107) and 98 at age 8 years, compared to their siblings' mean IQ score of 111. Discontinuers performed less well in reading (WRAT scores 3.2 versus 3.9 in continuers) and spelling (WRAT scores 2.9 versus 3.3 in continuers), although these scores in both groups were above the childrens' grade level and were comparable to their baseline performance. Both groups scored slightly lower in arithmetic for grade level at age 8 compared to their performance at age 6 years [4,38]. In another study, all the PKU subjects had lower IQs at an older age, but there was a greater change for those who discontinued diet [46].

The performance of intellectually normal PKU subjects on psychometric tests negatively correlated with their plasma phenylalanine level on the day of testing [48]. The phenylalanine levels in the 6 months prior to testing also were negatively correlated with IQ and WRAT scores in the collaborative study [38]. These results were interpreted to support the evidence that children with PKU should continue the restricted diet, at least through their school years [38]. In another series of patients, IQs dropped by 10 points or more, and the degree of drop seemed related to how long the patient had been off the diet [50].

In an investigational setting, 10 treated PKU patients were given phenylalanine loads in a blinded, cross-over design; their performance was measured by the Computerized Choice Reaction Time Test for visual–perceptual integration. Plasma phenylalanine levels over 21 mg/dl resulted in reversible impairment of higher integrative function. It was suggested that these changes were mediated by inhibition of biogenic amine synthesis, as reflected by decreased dopamine excretion in the urine when phenylalanine levels were high [20]. There was no change in performance on the Grooved Pegboard Test to suggest that lower integrative function had been impaired.

In addition to reports of decreased intellectual functioning, some patients were reported to develop behavioral problems, hyperkinesis, eczema, and electroencephalographic changes after diet discontinuation [51].

These studies have led many to believe that the diet should be continued until additional data become available or until one can predict which patients will do poorly after diet discontinuation.

In a survey of diet policies in 90 United States clinics, it was found that in 1982, 15% of 4- to 5-year-old, 50% of 8- to 9-year-old, and 57% of 9- to 10-year-old PKU subjects were off the diet. The number of 6- to 8-year-olds maintained on the diet had increased markedly, and two-thirds of the clinics were recommending indefinite continuation of the low phenylalanine diet as compared to 1978 when only one-quarter had this policy [52]. Some patients have had their diet reinstituted because of poor school performance, behavioral or mood changes, or concern about the ill effects of diet discontinuation. In one survey, of those who resumed the diet, 42 of 72 subjects reported improvement, 19 of 72 reported no change, and 11 of 72 reported worsening of problems; 22 of 72 discontinued the diet again after 10 months because of poor diet control, poor tolerance of formula, or poor motivation on the part of patients or parents [53]. Although very palatable for children who have always been on a restricted diet, this diet and the special formula can be quite unpalatable for those who have become accustomed to a normal diet. Therefore, many patients may wish to remain on the diet until the question of how safe it is to discontinue it is resolved. Because of the special reproductive problems for women with PKU, females in particular may wish to continue the diet, a subject discussed in the section Maternal Phenylketonuria.

Alternative methods of PKU treatment are being investigated. Administration of branched-chain amino acids may competitively interfere with phenylalanine entry into the CNS, and thus has been suggested as a supplement to the phenylalanine-restricted diet for older PKU patients who are unwilling or unable to remain in control. This approach, however, has been tried only for short periods of time in a very small number of subjects [54]. Administration of membrane-protected phenylalanine–ammonia lyase capsules has been observed to reduce plasma phenylalanine in rats [55]. Neither of these treatment modalities should be considered alternatives to standard dietary treatment of PKU at this time.

Mild Hyperphenylalaninemia Variants

Transient Hyperphenylalaninemia

Transient hyperphenylalaninemia occurs in approximately 0.2% of live births and in 25 to 30% of premature infants who receive >4 mg protein/kg/day. This delay in enzyme maturation is related to gestational age and is not inherited. It results in no clinical abnormalities and resolves within the first few weeks of life. The importance of recognizing this entity lies in distinguishing it from other forms of hyperphenylalaninemia. The infants frequently have a normal or elevated plasma tyrosine. Plasma phenylalanine levels usually are not over 10 mg/dl but occasionally may rise to over 20 mg/dl.

Persistent Hyperphenylalaninemia

Persistent hyperphenylalaninemia of less than 20 mg/dl may be a heterogeneous group of disorders with an incidence of 1 in 22,000 [29]. In the PKU collaborative study, approximately 15% of subjects initially enrolled were subsequently eliminated from the study after their oral phenylalanine challenge for this reason. The mean IQ of these variant patients, who were not maintained on dietary treatment, was 102 [12]. Although some patients were reported to have mental impairment, there was ascertainment bias because such persons were more likely to be tested for a metabolic error. In patients identified by population screening [11] 13 persons with plasma phenylalanine of ≤12 mg/dl in infancy and ≤8 mg/dl later in life, and absence of phenylpyruvic acid in the urine, had normal IQs that were comparable to their unaffected siblings; all had done well in school. It was concluded that dietary treatment was not necessary for these individuals.

In another report of 20 subjects (ages 23 to 41 years) ascertained by population screening, 12 agreed to undergo psychometric testing by the Wechsler Adult Intelligence Scale, Bender–Gestalt Motor Integration Test, and California Personality Inventory. Six patients with phenylalanine levels of 3 to 9 mg/dl and no phenylketones in the urine had a mean IQ of 105. Six patients with phenylalanine levels of 10 to 16 mg/dl and phenylketones in the urine had a mean IQ of 97.3, but one of these women had a severe visual–motor deficit. As a combined group, the IQ scores ranged from 78 to 122. Their mean educational level was 12.6 years, and 25% were employed outside the home. The Hollingshed–Redlick Two-Factor Index of Social Position indicated 50% were in the lowest class, 33% in the middle, and 17% in the highest. Some showed signs of stress but none had serious emotional or psychiatric problems. It was concluded that no detrimental effect for persistent hyperphenylalaninemia of ≤16 mg/dl could be demonstrated [29]. In a third study, 21 patients with plasma phenylalanine levels of 4 to 15 mg/dl who had not been treated had a mean IQ of 104.2 [46].

Patients with hyperphenylalaninemia of this type usually have a partial defect in phenylalanine hydroxylase with 5 to 10%, and occasionally up to 30%, of residual activity. When given an oral phenylalanine challenge of 180 mg/kg/day, the plasma phenylalanine levels do not reach 20 mg/dl. Occasionally the levels peak at 20 to 30 mg/dl but then decrease below 20 mg/dl as the three-day challenge continues. Phenylketones are variably present in the urine. Levels in the newborn period may be 20 to 30 mg/dl or higher [12].

Newborn Screening for Phenylketonuria

Newborn screening for PKU was made possible by the Guthrie method for semiquantitative determination of phenylalanine concentration in a blood specimen dried on filter paper. Such screening was desirable because dietary therapy if started early prevented mental retardation, because of the relative frequency of the disease, and because the test could be performed efficiently and cost effectively in a large number of infants. Today, all of the United States and many other countries have screening programs. Some programs utilize a fluorometric or enzymatic assay rather than the Guthrie inhibition test [56]. Although variable, the majority of programs use ≥4 mg phenylalanine/dl as the cutoff for calling a screen positive; others use ≥2 mg/dl [56,57].

In PKU infants blood phenylalanine levels are normal to minimally increased [58] at birth, thus cord blood is not acceptable for screening. The levels rise postnatally from oral ingestion of phenylalanine and from breakdown of endogenous protein [59].

All healthy infants, regardless of age or feeding status, should be screened as close as possible to the time of hospital discharge. If the infant is screened before 24 hours of age, rescreening before 3 weeks of age is recommended [60].

Although it often had been stated that infants should ingest milk for 24 hours prior to screening [61], many affected infants have shown phenylalanine levels of ≥4 mg/dl before feeding is instituted [59]. It is not clear if feeding practices influence the accuracy of screening in the first 3 days of life, but the Genetics Committee of the American Academy of Pediatrics believes that this factor is "only of minor importance" and that recommendations for only rescreening infants tested within the first 24 hours of life need be followed regardless of the feeding protocol [60]. Breast-fed PKU infants may have a slower rise in phenylalanine levels after birth, such that a level of 20 mg/dl may not be reached until other higher protein foods are introduced [30,61]. Therefore, it has been recommended that infants with persistent hyperphenylalaninemia who are taking breast milk be serially monitored or given a phenylalanine challenge to ensure that a diagnosis of classic PKU is not missed [61]. There is no proof, however, that these infants will be missed by newborn screening because they are taking breast milk [61,62].

Premature or ill hospitalized newborns should be screened on the seventh day of life [60], regardless of the type of nutrition or antibiotic treatment they are receiving [63]. Newborn siblings of PKU patients should be given special attention in screening [60]. Older siblings of newly detected cases should be tested, even if they appear normal.

False-negative screening results can occur because of biological variation [58], inadequate specimen collection, or clerical or analytical laboratory error. Inadequate follow-up by the laboratory, physician, or family can also result in missed cases. Therefore, the physician must remember that a screening program is not the same as diagnostic testing, and infants who have signs or symptoms suggestive of PKU should have their blood phenylalanine level determined.

All babies with persistent hyperphenylalaninemia, regardless of the exact level, should be investigated for tetrahydrobiopterin-deficient diseases, discussed in the section Abnormalities of Biopterin Metabolism.

Maternal Phenylketonuria

As females treated for PKU only during childhood entered their reproductive years, it became evident that they were at significant risk for damaging their infants in utero, as manifest by intrauterine growth retardation, microcephaly, and mental retardation [64]. Some of these babies had additional birth defects that included vertebral malformations, congenital heart defects, and esophageal atresia. Most of these infants did not have phenylketonuria.

Although there is no question that women with classic PKU are at high risk for having children with birth defects, what lower level of maternal hyperphenylalaninemia is safe is not known. In an international survey of reproductive outcome in women with classic PKU, 95% had at least one mentally retarded child and 81% had all mentally retarded children. Ninety percent of offspring had microcephaly, and 19% had congenital heart defects [65].

Initial reports of women with mild to moderate hyperphenylalaninemia and abnormal children were misleading because of the biased ascertainment of these mothers [66]. In 1983, a study was performed on children born to mothers with hyperphenylalaninemia who were identified by population screening; none of the women was under treatment for hyperphenylalaninemia. Any of their children with PKU or persistent hyperphenylalaninemia were excluded from analysis. Eleven women had phenylalanine levels of 10 to 20 mg/dl and a mean IQ of 99; 23% of their children were microcephalic at birth but only one was microcephalic at subsequent examination. The mean IQ of these children was 95, and the lowest was 69; 11% had visual–motor coordination delay. Nine women had phenylalanine levels of 2.7 to 10 mg/dl and a mean IQ of 105; the mean IQ of their children was 116. Children's IQ scores correlated with maternal IQ and maternal phenylalanine levels. Since mentally retarded offspring were observed only when the maternal phenylalanine level was ≥18 mg/dl, it was concluded that women with

classic PKU or severe hyperphenylalaninemia should be offered dietary treatment during pregnancy [67]. For less severe degrees of hyperphenylalaninemia, the decision on whether to treat should be based on consideration of the possible, subtle, ill effects of dietary treatment versus its potential benefit [67,68].

A national collaborative study has been initiated to determine what effects dietary therapy has on reproductive outcome in women with PKU [69]. In an international survey of outcome in women with PKU who were treated with diet during pregnancy, only 3 initiated the diet before conception. Two women were in good control and had normal children. One woman with poor dietary compliance had a microcephalic child with an IQ of 80. Eleven women started treatment in the first trimester. Of these, 4 children died from congenital heart defects and 2 of these were microcephalic; 1 child had esophageal atresia, microcephaly, and a developmental quotient of 85; 5 children were normal. One child had an IQ less than 75 but he also had PKU. When treatment was started in the second trimester, only 4 of 16 children were normal [70]. Recently, 12 pregnancies in 7 PKU women were reported; in 3 pregnancies diet was initiated before conception, and the children were normal [71,72]. Thus, the number of pregnancies in which the diet was initiated before conception and was well followed is small, but the results appear promising. For women who present after conception and who understand that birth defects already may have occurred but wish to continue their pregnancy, diet should be offered since it may still prevent or ameliorate brain damage [70,72,73].

Many PKU women are not aware of these reproductive hazards. Therefore, it has been recommended that registries for PKU patients be created so that these persons can be advised of their risks. Some families and PKU clinic personnel plan to continue the diet in female children until after they have completed childbearing. Although routine screening of pregnant women for PKU in obstetrical clinics is not generally advocated, one should consider screening women with unexplained mental retardation or who have a family history of mental retardation, microcephaly or PKU [68,74].

Dietary treatment of the PKU woman who is planning a pregnancy or who is already pregnant should maintain plasma phenylalanine levels of 3 to 12 mg/dl. The diet must provide adequate calories, protein, vitamins, and minerals for proper maternal and fetal nutrition. To accomplish this, a product such as Phenyl-free must be used. Dietary guidelines have been published [75]. Plasma phenylalanine and tyrosine must be measured weekly while other parameters of nutritional status can be measured less frequently [75].

Epidemiology and Genetics

The incidence of classic PKU in Caucasians ranges from 1 in 3,000 to 1 in 5,000 in Ireland to 1 in 28,000 in Belgium [1]. The overall incidence is 1 in 8,000 in Western Europe [1] and 1 in 11,000 [76] to 1 in 16,000 in the United States [20]. The disorder is less frequent in Finland, Japan [77], and in American blacks [78].

The carrier frequency in Caucasians is approximately 1 in 50 to 1 in 55 [57,79]. Heterozygotes are clinically normal. Many methods to identify PKU heterozygotes have been proposed, including determination of their plasma:tyrosine ratio, analysis of phenylalanine and tyrosine by linear or quadratic discriminant function, and phenylalanine clearance after intravenous or oral loading tests [76]. However, none of these tests definitely assigns heterozygosity for the PKU gene. A superior method for heterozygosity testing based on analysis at the DNA level has been made possible by the work of Woo et al. [79]. In most families with a PKU patient, this technique can be utilized to assign carrier status of close relatives. It is not, however, useful in population screening for PKU heterozygosity. A cDNA probe for the phenylalanine hydroxylase structural gene was identified and used to analyze DNA from PKU families by restriction fragment length polymorphisms (RFLPs) created by bacterial enzyme cleavage. These RFLPs are normal variants in the DNA sequence of the phenylalanine hydroxylase gene of normal and PKU subjects; they do not identify the mutation site within the gene that causes PKU. Therefore, a PKU patient must be available for analysis, and the parents must be informative by being heterozygous for one of the RFLPs; if not informative the mutation cannot be traced in the family. This technique also can be used for prenatal diagnosis, not previously possible because the enzyme normally is expressed only in the liver and not in the amniocytes. It has been estimated that more than 85% of families have informative RFLPs and could have such testing if they desired. Since PKU is a treatable disease, many families may not wish to have testing of this type.

This DNA work confirms that the mutation that causes PKU is in the structural gene for phenylalanine hydroxylase and that the disease is not caused by deletion of the entire gene [79]. The phenylalanine hydroxylase gene has been mapped to chromosome 12q22-24.1.

Analysis for phenylalanine hydroxylase mRNA in the liver of two PKU patients showed different results; in one, abundant mRNA was detected, suggesting that the disease was due to a defective or unstable enzyme. In the second case, there were negligible amounts of mRNA, suggesting decreased gene transcription or decreased mRNA stability. This finding was compatible with previous reports by enzyme immunoassay of both cross-reacting positive and cross-reacting negative forms of PKU, and confirms the genetic heterogeneity of PKU at the intragenic level [80].

The incidence of persistent hyperphenylalaninemia not due to classic PKU is approximately 1 in 17,000 [12] to 1 in 25,000 [11]. The exact gene defect leading to the reduced phenylalanine hydroxylase activity in these patients has not been identified.

Abnormalities of Biopterin Metabolism

The group of diseases due to abnormalities in biopterin metabolism has been referred to by a variety of names including "variant," "atypical," or "malignant" PKU. These terms are not used consistently in the literature and should be replaced by reference to the specific enzymatic or metabolic abnormality. There are two clinically similar groups of biopterin defects: (a) dihydropteridine reductase deficiency and (b) synthesis defects ("dihydrobiopterin synthetase" and guanosine triphosphate cyclohydrolase deficiencies).

Dihydropteridine Reductase Deficiency

In 1975, Kaufman et al. [6] reported a patient who developed severe neurologic impairment in spite of early detection and treatment of hyperphenylalaninemia. The child seemed normal until 7 months of age, when he developed seizures and began to show developmental delay and neurologic deterioration. A hypsarrhythmia pattern was seen on electroencephalogram. By 14 months of age, he had almost constant myoclonus, central hypotonia, increased peripheral tone, and episodes of hyperpnea. He was found to have a deficiency of dihydropteridine reductase (Figure 14.3). Since this report, at least 26 additional patients [23] have been identified. The enzyme deficiency can be demonstrated in liver, brain, cultured skin fibroblasts [6], and white and red blood cells [81]. The median age of onset of neurologic problems has been 4 months, with progressive deterioration and death by 6 to 7 years of age if un-

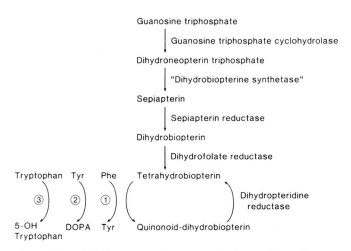

Figure 14.3. Synthesis pathway of tetrahydrobiopterin. The enzyme dihydropteridine reductase is required to keep this cofactor in its active form. Active cofactor is required for the activity of (1) phenylalanine hydroxylase, (2) tyrosine hydroxylase, and (3) tryptophan hydroxylase.

treated. In addition to the abnormalities described in the first case, some patients experience irritability, drowsiness, hypersalivation, hyperthermic crises, swallowing problems, and microcephaly. Some patients have elevated phenylalanine levels in the same range as classic PKU, while others have only mild elevations of 4 to 10 mg/dl [23]. The plasma phenylalanine levels can be controlled by diet, but this does not alter the clinical course. Neurotransmitter synthesis is decreased because of deficient tyrosine and tryptophan hydroxylation caused by deficiency of the active tetrahydrobiopterin cofactor (Figure 14.3). Several patients have been shown to have abnormally low plasma, urine, and CSF levels of neurotransmitters and their metabolites; for example, dopamine, serotonin, 5-hydroxy-indoleacetic acid (5HIAA), homovanillic acid [82], and 3-methoxy-4-hydroxy-phenolglycol [83,84].

Several forms of treatment have been tried. In one patient administration of large amounts of a reducing substance (ascorbate 5 gm/day) in an effort to accelerate nonenzymatic reduction of quinonoid dihydrobiopterin was unsuccessful [6].

Treatment with tetrahydrobiopterin (BH$_4$) and neurotransmitter precursors (L-dopa and 5-OH tryptophan) may be helpful in some patients if started early, but few patients have been treated before neurologic damage occurred. In one child, treated since 2 months of age by a phenylalanine-restricted diet, folinic acid, 5-OH tryptophan, L-dopa, and carbidopa (a peripheral dopa decarboxylase inhibitor that allows one to give smaller doses of L-dopa), normalization of CSF neurotransmitter metabolites and

only mild gross motor delay at 14 months of age was reported [83]. Subsequently another patient had improved outcome attributed to addition of folinic acid to the treatment regimen, leading Kaufman [85] to conclude that "there is no longer any reason why therapy with folinic acid or 5-CH$_3$ tetrahydrofolsate should not be included in the treatment for all dihydropteridine reductase-deficient patients." Another patient with 10% residual activity of dihydropteridine reductase was said to be neurologically and mentally normal. Thus, response to treatment may be related to severity of the enzyme defect [85].

There is strong evidence that dihydropteridine reductase deficiency is inherited in an autosomal recessive pattern. The synthesis defects may be inherited in the same way, but less information is available.

Dihydrobiopterin Synthesis Defects

The second class of abnormalities of biopterin metabolism are defects in dihydrobiopterin synthesis. These include deficiencies of guanosine triphosphate cyclohydrolase and of "dihydrobiopterin synthetase." This latter "enzyme" may represent two or more sequential enzymatic steps (Figure 14.3). The clinical presentation of all these synthesis defects is similar to that of dihydropteridine reductase [22]. Twenty-two patients with "dihydrobiopterin synthetase" deficiency and two with guanosine triphosphate cyclohydrolase deficiency have been reported [23,86].

"Dihydrobiopterin Synthetase" Defect(s)

The majority of patients with "dihydrobiopterin synthetase" deficiency have severe disease, but milder forms with approximately 10% residual enzyme activity exist [23]. A few patients had peripheral forms of the disease with normal CSF biopterin levels while receiving no treatment other than a phenylalanine-restricted diet; these children remained clinically normal [23]. In severe forms of the disease, with enzyme levels of 0.6 to 2.3% of normal, most patients had plasma phenylalanine levels of over 20 mg/dl, but at least two infants had moderate elevations of 14 mg/dl, and two had levels of <5 mg/dl. Patients with the partial form of the disease had levels of 7 to 20 mg/dl in the newborn period. In both groups, phenylalanine tolerance may increase with age, and this process occurs more quickly in those with partial enzyme deficiency [23]. Cerebrospinal fluid and plasma levels of neurotransmitters and metabolites are low in the severe forms of the disease [87]. One patient was successfully treated with a low dose of BH$_4$ (2.5 mg/kg/day). Treatment with higher doses of BH$_4$ (8 to 20 mg/kg/day) results in markedly increased plasma, urine, and cerebrospinal BH$_4$ levels. Slight clinical neurologic improvement [89], and some increase in CSF neurotransmitters and metabolites may be seen [87] in some patients, but others do not respond at all [85].

Since the cerebrospinal levels of neurotransmitters may not reach normal, treatment with neurotransmitter precursors also may be needed and seem to result in some neurologic improvement in some patients [89]. For example, in one patient, treatment with BH$_4$ alone (20 to 40 mg/kg) resulted in clinical deterioration, while treatment with L-dopa, 5-OH tryptophan, carbidopa, and BH$_4$ resulted in improvement. In a few other patients, neurotransmitter therapy seemed to result in no further improvement over BH$_4$ alone [84]. It is possible that this difference in response depends on the severity of the enzyme deficiency. Despite the early treatment provided in a few cases, all patients with severe forms of the disease are neurologically and mentally impaired [84]. Patients with the peripheral form of the disease, who have normal CSF pterin levels, may need no treatment except for phenylalanine restriction [88]. It is possible that some patients who have been reported to have done well on BH$_4$ or neurotransmitter precursor therapy have had either the peripheral or "transient" form of the disease. There is controversy over whether a transient form exists; this is discussed below.

Guanosine Triphosphate Cyclohydrolase Defect

Two patients with guanosine triphosphate cyclohydrolase deficiency have been reported; they have low cerebrospinal fluid, plasma, and urine levels of neopterin and biopterin, but the relative proportions are normal [82]. Administration of BH$_4$ has resulted in lowering of plasma phenylalanine and some neurologic improvement, but both patients have severe neurologic impairment.

Differentiation of Biopterin Disorders from Classic PKU

It has been estimated that approximately 0.5 to 3.0% of infants with persistent hyperphenylalaninemia have a disorder of biopterin metabolism [60]. Because the prognosis is different from that of classic PKU, and since the chance for successful treatment is increased when therapy is started early, it has been recommended that all patients with persistent hyperphenylalaninemia be evaluated for biopterin defects [60]. In the United States, central laboratories have been testing the urine of hyperphenylalaninemic children for biopterin defects since 1980 [60]. The urine can be spotted on filter paper [90] and mailed to one of the screening centers [Naylor EW: personal communication, 1985]. Patients with these cofactor defects have abnormal amounts of neopterin or biopterin in the urine that allows them to be distinguished from classic PKU patients (Table 14.1). In classic PKU, administration of a phenylalanine load results in a rise in biopterin through stimulation of synthesis [91]. Therefore, the urine specimen to be analyzed for biopterin defects should be obtained after the plasma phenylalanine has been lowered by dietary treatment [23].

Patients with dihydropteridine reductase defects have no tetrahydrobiopterin in the liver, although total liver and plasma biopterin levels may be normal and may increase after a phenylalanine load. In the urine there sometimes are normal or low levels of BH$_4$ and neopterin (N) and a high level of biopterin (B) so that the N:B ratio is lower than the normal ratio of 2 to 8 in newborns [85] and 0.2 to 2.0 in adults [22]. Since standard measurement of the N:B ratio alone may miss the dihydropteridine reductase deficiency [91], a filter paper blood specimen for the reductase enzyme assay should also be submitted for all infants with persistent hyperphenylalaninemia [Naylor EW: personal communication, 1985; 92]. In some patients, but not all, oral

Table 14.1. Comparison of Biochemical Parameters in Classic Phenylketonuria and Abnormalities in Biopterin Metabolism

| | Classic PKU (Phenylalanine Hydroxylase) | Biopterin Defects | | |
| | | Synthesis Defects | | Tetrahydrobiopterin Reductase |
		"Biopterin Synthetase"	Guanosine Triphosphate Hydrolase	
Plasma Phe	↑↑	↑ or ↑↑	↑↑	↑ or ↑↑
CSF BH$_4$	N	N (peripheral forms) to ↓	↓	↓
CSF neurotransmitters	N[a]	N (peripheral forms) to ↓	↓	↓
BH$_4$ load— plasma Phe response	−	↓↓	↓↓	↓↓ or ↓
Phe load— biopterin response	↑	− to ↑	−	− to ↑
Urine neopterin	N[a]	↑	↓	↓
Urine biopterin	N[a]	↓	↓	↑
Urine neopterin: biopterin ratio	0.2:8.0[a]	↑	N	N to ↓

Phe = phenylalanine
N = normal
↑ = increased
↓ = decreased
− = no change
[a]When plasma phenylalanine levels are lowered to normal

administration of 7.5 mg of BH$_4$/kg lowers the plasma phenylalanine level to normal within 4 to 6 hours [23]. (In classic PKU, the phenylalanine remains elevated.) Patients with partial phenylalanine hydroxylase deficiency may be difficult to distinguish from reductase deficient patients by this technique. This is another reason why all suspected cases of dihydropteridine reductase deficiency should be confirmed by enzyme assay.

Patients with "dihydrobiopterin synthetase" defects have decreased plasma and urinary biopterin and increased neopterin [88]. Their N:B ratio is elevated from 6 to infinity (one patient had no detectable biopterin) [88,93]. However, the ratio may overlap with that seen in normal newborns who may have a maturational delay in this enzyme system [85]. These patients more consistently achieve lowering of elevated plasma phenylalanine when given BH$_4$ [84], which also results in a lower urine N:B ratio. In severely affected patients a phenylalanine challenge causes no increase in plasma biopterin, but in patients with an incomplete enzyme block a moderate rise may result [88].

Transient forms of dihydrobiopterin synthesis defects have been reported. These infants had elevated urine N:B ratios of 8 to 16 that decreased to normal by 3 to 24 weeks of age; they were later shown to have classic PKU [93]. Other investigators have suggested that these changes reflect developmental maturation of the enzyme system rather than a transient dihydrobiopterin synthesis defect, especially since some of these patients had little change in their plasma phenylalanine levels when given BH$_4$ [23]. This enzyme system can be measured only in the liver.

In conclusion, newborn screening and dietary treatment of classic PKU have resulted in prevention of mental retardation in most patients, but new problems in management of maternal PKU have arisen. The understanding and treatment of the biopterin abnormalities that result in hyperphenylalaninemia are progressing, but outcome in all but the mildest and peripheral forms remains unsatisfactory.

References

1. Guttler F. Phenylketonuria: 50 years since Folling's discovery and still expanding our clinical and biochemical knowledge. Acta Paediatr Scand 1984; 73:705–716.
2. Reveley AM, Reveley MA. Screening for adult phenylketonuria in psychiatric inpatients. Biol Psychiatry 1982;17:1343–1345.

3. Holtzman NA, Mellits ED, Kallman CH. Neonatal screening for phenylketonuria: II. Age dependence of initial phenylalanine in infants with PKU. Pediatrics 1974;53:353–357.

4. Koch R, Azen CG, Friedman EG, et al. Preliminary report on the effects of diet discontinuation in PKU. J Pediatr 1982;100:870–885.

5. Bartholome K, Byrd DJ, Kaufman S, et al. Atypical phenylketonuria with normal phenylalanine hydroxylase and dihydropteridine reductase activity in vitro. Pediatrics 1977;59:757–761.

6. Kaufman S, Holtzman NA, Milstien S, et al. Phenylketonuria due to a deficiency of dihydropteridine reductase. N Engl J Med 1975;293:785–790.

7. Batshaw ML, Valle D, Bessman SP. Unsuccessful treatment of phenylketonuria with tyrosine. J Pediatr 1981;99:159–160.

8. Szymanski HV, Friedman S, Guthrie R. Screening for phenylketonuria in chronic psychiatric inpatients. Hosp Commun Psychiatr 1984;35:936–938.

9. Chang P-N, Weisberg S, Fisch RO. Growth development and its relationship to intellectual functioning of children with phenylketonuria. Dev Behav Pediatr 1984;5:127–131.

10. Zwaan J. Eye findings in patients with phenylketonuria. Arch Ophthalmol 1983;101:1236–1237.

11. Levy HL, Shih VE, Karolkewicz V, et al. Persistent mild hyperphenylalaninemia in the untreated state: a prospective study. N Engl J Med 1971;285:424–429.

12. O'Flynn ME, Holtzman NA, Blaskovics M, et al. The diagnosis of phenylketonuria: a report from the collaborative study of children treated for phenylketonuria. Am J Dis Child 1980;134:769–774.

13. Hsieh MC, Berry HK, Bofinger MK, et al. Comparative diagnostic value of phenylalanine challenge and phenylalanine hydroxylase activity in phenylketonuria. Clin Genet 1983;23:415–421.

14. Woo SLC. Prenatal diagnosis and carrier detection of classic phenylketonuria by gene analysis. Pediatrics 1984;74:412–423.

15. Tourian A, Sidbury JB. Phenylketonuria and hyperphenylalaninemia. In: Stanbury JB, Wyngaarden JB, Fredrickson DS, et al., eds. The metabolic basis of inherited disease. 5th ed. New York: McGraw–Hill, 1983:271–272.

16. Friedman PA, Fisher DB, Kang ES, et al. Detection of hepatic phenylalanine 4-hydroxylase in classical phenylketonuria. Proc Natl Acad Sci USA 1973;70:552–556.

17. Synderman SE, Sansaricq C, Norton PM, et al. Plasma and cerebrospinal fluid amino acid concentrations in phenylketonuria during the newborn period. J Pediatr 1981;99:63–67.

18. Berry HK, Bofinger MK, Hunt MM, et al. Reduction of cerebrospinal fluid phenylketonuria after oral administration of valine, isoleucine, and leucine. Pediatr Res 1982;16:751–755.

19. Ratzmann GW, Grimm U, Jahrig K, et al. On the brain barrier system function and changes of cerebrospinal fluid concentrations of phenylalanine and tyrosine in human phenylketonuria. Biomed Biochim Acta 1984;43:197–204.

20. Krause W, Halminski M, McDonald L, et al. Biochemical and neuropsychological effects of elevated plasma phenylalanine in patients with treated phenylketonuria: a model for the study of phenylalanine and brain function in man. J Clin Invest 1985;75:40–48.

21. Perry TL, Hansen S, Tischler B, et al. Glutamine depletion in phenylketonuria. N Engl J Med 1970;282:761–766.

22. Matalon R, Michals K, Lee C-L, et al. Screening for biopterin defects in newborns with phenylketonuria and other hyperphenylalaninemias. Ann Clin Lab Sci 1982;12:411–414.

23. Dhondt J-L. Tetrahydrobiopterin deficiencies: preliminary analysis from an international survey. J Pediatr 1984;104:501–508.

24. Bauman ML, Kemper TL. Morphologic and histoanatomic observations of the brain in untreated human phenylketonuria. Acta Neuropathol (Berl) 1982;58:55–63.

25. Hommes FA, Eller AG, Taylor EH. Turnover of the fast components of myelin and myelin proteins in experimental hyperphenylalaninemia: relevance to termination of dietary treatment in human phenylketonuria. J Inher Metab Dis 1982;5:21–27.

26. Huether G, Neuhoff V, Kaus R. Brain development in experimental hyperphenylalaninemia: disturbed proliferation and reduced cell numbers in the cerebellum. Neuropediatrics 1983;14:12–19.

27. Acosta PB, Trahms C, Wellman NS, et al. Phenylalanine intakes of 1- to 6-year-old children with phenylketonuria undergoing therapy. Am J Clin Nutr 1983;38:694–700.

28. Dobson J, Koch R, Williamson M, et al. Cognitive development and dietary therapy in phenylketonuric children. N Engl J Med 1968;278:1142–1144.

29. Waisbren SE, Schnell R, Levy HL. Intelligence and personality characteristics in adults with untreated atypical phenylketonuria and mild hyperphenylalaninemia. J Pediatr 1984;105:955–958.

30. United States Department of Health, Education and Welfare. Management of newborn infants with phenylketonuria. (DHEW Publication No (HSA) 79-5211) 1978:1–75.

31. Ernest AE, McCabe ERB, Neifert MR, et al. United States Department of Health and Human Services. Guide to breast feeding the infant with PKU. (DHHS publication No (HSA) 79-5110) 1980:1–50.

32. Berry HK, Porter LJ. Newborn screening for phenylketonuria (letter). Pediatrics 1982;70:505–506.

33. Kang ES, Sollee ND, Gerald PS. Results of treatment and termination of the diet in phenylketonuria (PKU). Pediatrics 1970;40:881–890.

34. Lonsdale D, Foust M. Normal mental development in treated phenylketonuria: report of ten cases. Am J Dis Child 1970;119:440–446.

35. O'Grady DJ, Berry HK, Sutherland BS. Cognitive de-

velopment in early treated phenylketonuria. Am J Dis Child 1971;121:20–23.

36. Dobson JC, Kushida E, Williamson M, et al. Intellectual performance of 36 phenylketonuria patients and their nonaffected siblings. Pediatrics 1976;58:53–56.

37. Williamson ML, Koch R, Azen C, et al. Correlates of intelligence test results in treated phenylketonuric children. Pediatrics 1981;68:161–167.

38. Koch R, Azen C, Friedman EG, et al. Paired comparisons between early treated PKU children and their matched sibling controls on intelligence and school achievement test results at eight years of age. J Inher Metabol Dis 1984;7:86–90.

39. Hunt MM, Sutherland BS, Berry HK. Nutritional management in phenylketonuria. Am J Dis Child 1971;122:1–6.

40. Fiedler AE, Miller MJ, Bickel H, et al. Phenylalanine levels in PKU following minor surgery. Am J Med Genet 1982;11:411–414.

41. Williamson M, Dobson JC, Koch R. Collaborative study of children treated for phenylketonuria: study design. Pediatrics 1977;60:815–827.

42. Blaskovics M, Engel R, Podosin RL, et al. EEG pattern in phenylketonuria under early initiated dietary treatment. Am J Dis Child 1981;135:802–808.

43. Koff E, Boyle P, Pueschel SM. Perceptual-motor functioning in children with phenylketonuria. Am J Dis Child 1977;131:1084–1087.

44. Zartler AS. Linguistic development in PKU. J Pediatr 1981;99:501.

45. Schor DP. PKU and temperament: rating children three through seven years old in PKU families. Clin Pediatr 1983;22:807–811.

46. Netley C, Hanley WB, Rudner HL. Phenylketonuria and its variants: observations on intellectual functioning. Can Med Assoc J 1984;131:751–754.

47. Melnick CR, Michals KK, Matalon R. Linguistic development of children with phenylketonuria and normal intelligence. J Pediatr 1981;98:269–272.

48. Brunner RL, Jordan MK, Berry HK. Early-treated phenylketonuria: neuropsychologic consequences. J Pediatr 1983;102:831–835.

49. Waisbren SE, Schnell RR, Levy HL. Diet termination in children with phenylketonuria: a review of psychological assessments used to determine outcome. J Inher Metab Dis 1980;3:149–150.

50. Seashore MR, Friedman E, Novelly RA, et al. Loss of intellectual function in children with phenylketonuria after relaxation of dietary phenylalanine restriction. Pediatrics 1985;75:226–232.

51. Parker CE, Shaw KNF, Mitchell JB, et al. Clinical experience in dietary management of phenylketonuria with a new phenylalanine-free product. J Pediatr 1977; 91:941–943.

52. Schuett VE, Brown ES. Diet policies of PKU clinics in the United States. Am J Pub Health 1984;74:501–503.

53. Schuett VE, Brown ES, Michels K. Reinstitution of diet therapy in PKU patients from twenty-two US clinics. Am J Pub Health 1985;75:39–42.

54. Jordan MK, Brunner RL, Hunt MM, et al. Preliminary support for the oral administration of valine, isoleucine and leucine for phenylketonuria. Dev Med Child Neurol 1985;27:33–39.

55. Bourget L, Chang TMS. Phenylalanine ammonia-lyase immobilized in semipermeable microcapsules for enzyme replacement in phenylketonuria. Fed Eur Biochem Soc 1985;180:5–8.

56. Committee on Genetics. Screening for congenital metabolic disorders in the newborn infant: congenital deficiency of thyroid hormone and hyperphenylalaninemia. Pediatrics 1977; (suppl)60:389–404.

57. Griffin RF, Humienny ME, Hall EC, et al. Classic phenylketonuria: heterozygote detection during pregnancy. Am J Hum Genet 1973;25:646–654.

58. McCabe ERB, McCabe L, Mosher GA, et al. Newborn screening for phenylketonuria: predictive validity as a function of age. Pediatrics 1983;72:390–398.

59. Frechette AL, Russo PK. Prospective study of early neonatal screening for phenylketonuria. N Engl J Med 1981;304:294–296.

60. Committee on Genetics. New issues in newborn screening for phenylketonuria and congenital hypothyroidism. Pediatrics 1982;69:104–106.

61. Binder J, Johnson CF, Saboe B, et al. Delayed elevation of serum phenylalanine level in a breast-fed child. Pediatrics 1979;63:334–336.

62. Holtzman NA, Meek AG, Mellits ED. Neonatal screening for phenylketonuria. JAMA 1974;229:667–669.

63. Fisch RO, Anthony BF, Bauer H, et al. The effect of antibiotics on the results of the Guthrie test given to phenylketonuric patients. J Pediatr 1968;73:685–689.

64. Fisch RO, Doeden D, Lansky LL, et al. Maternal phenylketonuria: detrimental effects on embryogenesis and fetal development. Am J Dis Child 1969;118:847–858.

65. Lenke RR, Levy HL. Maternal phenylketonuria and hyperphenylalaninemia. N Engl J Med 1980;20:1202–1208.

66. Brown ES, Waisman HA. Mental retardation in four offspring of a hyperphenylalaninemic mother. Pediatrics 1971;48:401–410.

67. Levy HL, Waisbren SE. Effects of untreated maternal phenylketonuria and hyperphenylalaninemia on the fetus. N Engl J Med 1983;309:1269–1274.

68. Holtzman NA, Howell RR, Lawson WG, et al. Maternal phenylketonuria. Pediatrics 1985;76:313–314.

69. University of Colorado Health Sciences Center. National maternal PKU collaborative study. IMD Newsletter 1985;3:2.

70. Lenke AR, Levy HL. Maternal phenylketonuria—results of dietary therapy. Am J Obstet Gynecol 1982;142:548–553.

71. Murphy D, Saul I, Kirby M. Maternal phenylketonuria and phenylalanine restricted diet: studies of 7 pregnancies and of offsprings produced. Irish J Med Sci 1985;154:66–70.

72. Bush RT, Dukes PC. Women with phenylketonuria: successful management of pregnancy and implications.

N Z Med J 1985;98:181–183.

73. Michels VA, Justice CL. Treatment of phenylketonuria during pregnancy. Clin Genet 1982;21:141–144.

74. Practice perspectives: need for follow-up counseling. AGOG Newsletter (Sept 1984):5.

75. Acosta PB, Blaskovics M, Boberg OT, et al. Nutrition in pregnancy of hyperphenylalaninemic women. J Am Diet Assoc 1982;80:443–450.

76. Freehauf CL, Lezotte D, Goodman SI, et al. Carrier screening for phenylketonuria: comparison of two discriminant analysis procedures. Am J Hum Genet 1984;36;1180–1189.

77. Kutter D, Thoma J. Frequency of phenylketonuria carriers. Biochem Med 1982;28:285–289.

78. Kirkman HN, Carroll CL, Moore EG, et al. Fifteen-year experience with screening for phenylketonuria with an automated fluorometric method. Am J Hum Genet 1982;34:743–752.

79. Woo SLC, Lidsky AS, Guttler F, et al. Cloned human phenylalanine hydroxylase gene allows prenatal diagnosis and carrier detection of classical phenylketonuria. Nature 1983;306:151–155.

80. DiLella AG, Ledley FD, Rey F, et al. Detection of phenylalanine hydroxylase messenger RNA in liver biopsy samples from patients with phenylketonuria. Lancet 1985;1:160–161.

81. Narisawa K, Arai N, Hayakawa H, et al. Diagnosis of dihydropteridine reductase deficiency by erythrocyte enzyme assay. Pediatrics 1981;68:591–592.

82. Niederwieser A, Blau N, Wang M, et al. GTP cyclohydrolase I deficiency: a new enzyme defect causing hyperphenylalaninemia with neopterin, biopterin, dopamine, and serotonin deficiencies and muscular hypotonia. Eur J Pediatr 1984;141:208–214.

83. Irons M, O'Flynn M, Stock C. Results of early treatment of dihydropteridine reductase deficiency with neurotransmitter replacement and folinic acid (abstr). Am J Hum Genet 1984;(suppl)36:135.

84. Endres W, Niederwieser A, Curtius HC, et al. Atypical phenylketonuria due to biopterin deficiency. Helv Paediatr Acta 1983;37:489–498.

85. Kaufman S. Unsolved problems in diagnosis and therapy of hyperphenylalaninemia caused by defects in tetrahydrobiopterin metabolism. J Pediatr 1986;109:572–578.

86. Matalon R, Rouse B. Neopterin deficiency: a cause for hyperphenylalaninemia (abstr). Pediatr Res 1984;(suppl)18:223A.

87. Kaufman S, Kapatos G, Rizzo WB, et al. Tetrahydropterin therapy for hyperphenylalaninemia caused by defective synthesis of tetrahydrobiopterin. Ann Neurol 1983;14:308–315.

88. Hoganson G, Berlow S, Kaufman S, et al. Biopterin synthesis defects: problems in diagnosis. Pediatrics 1984;74:1004–1011.

89. Kaufman S, Kapatos G, McInnes RR, et al. Use of tetrahydropterins in the treatment of hyperphenylalaninemia due to defective synthesis of tetrahydrobiopterin: evidence that peripherally administered tetrahydropterins enter the brain. Pediatrics 1982; 70:376–380.

90. Narisawa K, Arai N, Hayakawa H, et al. Diagnosis of dihydropteridine reductase deficiency by erythrocyte enzyme assay. Pediatrics 1981;68:591–592.

91. O'Brien D. Screening for biopterin disorders in PKU. Pediatrics 1980;66:813.

92. Nobuhiro A, Narisawa K, Hayakawa H, et al. Hyperphenylalaninemia due to dihydropteridine reductase deficiency: diagnosis by enzyme assays on dried blood spots. Pediatrics 1982;70:426–430.

93. Matalon R. Current status of biopterin screening (editorial). J Pediatr 1984;104:579–581.

Chapter 15

Homocystinuria due to Cystathionine Synthase Deficiency

PAUL R. DYKEN

Homocystinuria, due to cystathionine synthase deficiency, is a genetically determined inborn error of methionine transsulfuration characterized clinically by typical features and biochemically by an excess of homocystine–homocysteine in plasma and urine and of methionine in plasma.

The term homocystinuria indicates a biochemical abnormality and not a specific symptom, syndrome, or enzymatic defect. It is now clear that a variety of disorders, the majority of which are listed in Table 15.1, can be associated with this abnormality. The clinical characteristics of these disorders vary between those that are symptom-free and those that severely impair different systems. Homocystinuria, besides being a manifestation of cystathionine synthase deficiency, is associated with at least three other genetically determined conditions as well as several nongenetic ones [1]. These clinical and biochemical complexities were identified after the introduction in 1962 of the term homocystinuria. Two groups of investigators separately identified the clinical, pathologic, genetic, and biochemical syndromes now called homocystinuria for its consistent and characteristic biochemical abnormality: the first group, from northern Ireland, reported two sisters with characteristic neurocutaneous features [2,3], thus placing this disorder among the neurocutaneous diseases; the second group, from Wisconsin, reported an infant with severe systemic abnormalities [4,5]. The enzymatic defect, that is, cystathionine synthase deficiency, was not discovered in a patient with clinical symptoms and homocystinuria until 1964 [6]. Several nosologic entities associated with homocystinuria have been recognized since that time. Only the homozygotic forms of homocystinuria due to cystathionine synthase deficiency with characteristic neurologic and dermatologic manifestations are discussed here as examples of neurocutaneous diseases.

Clinical and Pathological Features

Homocystinuria due to cystathionine synthase deficiency may be classified into three main types, listed in Table 15.1 in decreasing order of severity and clinical specificity [7–9]. The major clinical features of the homozygotic homocystinurias due to cystathionine synthase deficiency are in order of importance: neurocutaneous, ocular, musculoskeletal, and cardiovascular (Table 15.2). Although these clinical features are intertwined, they are discussed separately. Figures 15.1, 15.2, and 15.3 illustrate some of the clinical features.

Neurologic Features

Mental retardation is the most common neurologic manifestation of cystathionine synthase deficiency. In each of the original cases, and in subsequent early reported series, mental retardation was prominent. In later reported series, this feature has been less consistent. Such variation is expected with the identification of asymptomatic newborns, asymptomatic individuals with partial enzyme deficiency, and after treatment became available. Mild clinical forms of cystathionine synthase deficiency are found in individuals with genetic heterogeneity. The vitamin B_6 nonresponsive form is clinically more severe, especially in mental symptoms, than the vitamin B_6 responsive form, regardless of treatment [7,8]. Recognizing symptoms of the heterozygous state of

Table 15.1. Disorders Associated with Clinical Homocystinuria

Cystathionine synthase deficiencies
    Homozygotic vitamin B_6 nonresponsive form
    Homozygotic vitamin B_6 responsive form
    Heterozygotic forms
    Peripheral arterial and venous occlusive disease
    Cerebrovascular arterial and venous occlusive disease
    Schizophrenia and other psychoneuroses
    Cataract, refractive errors, and other ocular
        disturbances
    Hypopigmentation and premature graying
    Isolated neurologic symptomatology
Other homocystinurias
    Failure to accumulate methylcobalamin
    Decreased 5,10-methylene tetrahydrofolate reductase
    Imersulund's syndrome (defective vitamin B_{12}
        absorption) with cystathioninuria
    Related to 6-azauridine triacetate administration
    Bacterial conversion of urinary cystathionine to
        homocysteine

homocystinuria has added another clinical entity, thus widening clinical variability [9].

Developmental delay, one of the first signs of cystathionine synthase deficiency, is detectable in the first months of life [5] (Figure 15.1). This delay is evenly distributed, although at first motor retarda-

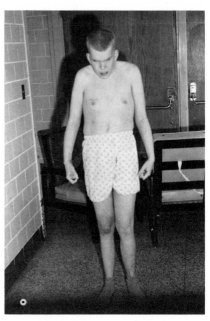

Figure 15.2. A 22-year-old young adult with severe mental retardation and homocystinuria. Patient has subluxation of lens, genu valgum, and marfanoid habitus.

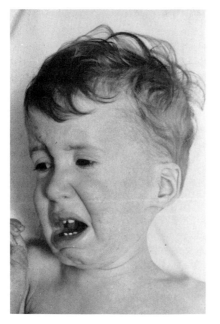

Figure 15.1. Child of 10 months of age with mild developmental delay and presumed homocystinuria. Observe the marfanoid facies, dysplastic ears, hand deformity, and the faint but typical mildly developed malar flush. Patient has no ectopia lentis.

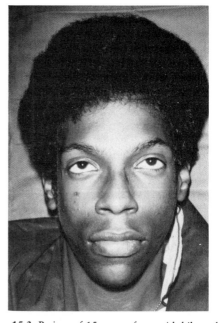

Figure 15.3. Patient of 15 years of age with bilateral ectopia lentis and homocystinuria. The patient has a mild learning disability without mental retardation and is responsive to vitamin B_6. No major cutaneous disturbance exists.

Table 15.2. Clinical Features of Homocystinuria due to Cystathionine Synthase Deficiency

System Involvement	Examples of Symptoms and Signs	Estimated Involvement*
Neurocutaneous	Mental retardation	Usually
	Developmental delay	
	Seizures	
	Behavioral–psyche disturbances	
	Neurologic defects	
	Hair and cutaneous abnormalities	
	Stroke	
Ophthalmologic	Subluxation of lens	Very frequent
	Cataracts	
	Glaucoma	
	Myopia	
	Buphthalmos, staphyloma	
	Retinal degeneration	
	Optic atrophy	
	Central artery thrombosis	
Musculoskeletal	Osteoporosis	Very frequent
	Joint or bony deformity	
	Marfanoid characteristics	
	Kyphoscoliosis	
	Pathologic fractures	
	Microcephaly	
	Myopathy	
	Abnormal collagen	
Cardiovascular	Arteriosclerosis	Common
	Thrombophlebitis	
	Pulmonary arterial occlusion	
	Venous thrombosis	
	Platelet adhesiveness	
	Coronary arterial occlusion	
	Renal arterial occlusion	
	Hypertension	
	Atherosclerosis	
	Aortic aneurysm	
Other	Fatty liver	Sometimes
	Inguinal hernia	
	Hyperinsulinemia	
	Increased growth hormone	
	Hepatomegaly	
	Gastrointestinal bleeding	

*According to recent questionnaire on 472 patients reported by Mudd et al [8], ectopia lentis was found in 86%; mental disturbances, developmental retardation and seizures in 84% marfanoid characteristics and bony abnormality in 60%; all others in 27%. There is overlap in the figures reported here.

tion precedes mental delay. In late childhood the patient has frank mental retardation. The intelligence quotient (IQ) of patients with homocystinuria, when studied in large groups, usually ranged between 30 and 70. A slight correlation exists between normal intelligence in certain patients and no elevation of plasma methionine concentration. This correlation also exists for the B_6 responsive group. Higher intelligence correlates with more favorable responses to vitamin B_6 administration. The majority (55.7%) of reported patients with homocystinuria, not ascertained through a neonatal screening program, had mental retardation [8]. An additional large segment of this population (22.5%) had developmental retardation. The authors of this study concluded that about 20% of the reported cases were of normal or near normal intelligence. On the other hand, of those patients not diagnosed by their neurologic features (that is, ectopia lentis) as many as 50% were found to be of normal intelligence [7].

The extent of intellectual handicaps is not fully explained by the data that exist on the incidence of mental retardation and developmental delay in homocystinuric patients. Mudd et al. [8] found that 5.7% of patients with late-detected cystathionine synthase deficiency, although of average or above average global intelligence, suffered from learning disabilities. Although available data are conflicting, it appears that intellectual deficit represents one of the most common clinical expressions of the homozygotic forms of cythathionine synthase deficiency. This is particularly true for the vitamin B_6 nonresponsive form, the most severe, of these diseases.

Seizures frequently occur in patients with cystathionine synthase deficiency. Their incidence varies according to methods of ascertainment. In a recent review [8] only 0.2% of patients had seizures as a presenting symptom. Yet in 3% of patients, the presence of seizures contributed to the investigation. In this review, newborns and siblings excluded, 114 of 536 patients were said to have had seizures. The patients with the vitamin B_6 nonresponsive form had a higher incidence of seizures (23.4%) than those with the vitamin B_6 responsive form (16.8%).

Seizures may be an early symptom and are often partial or unilateral, suggesting focal brain disease. In fact, these seizures are associated with frequent focal neurologic findings such as a hemiparesis, which is indicative of thromboembolic cerebrovascular occlusion. Otherwise patients may have generalized seizures not associated with focal neurologic findings. Generalized tonic–clonic seizures account for 69% of the seizures experienced by symptomatic patients with cystathionine synthase deficiency [8]. Patients with the vitamin B_6 nonresponsive form are more susceptible to generalized seizures than the vitamin B_6 responsive patients, despite their higher incidence of thromboembolic phenomena. In addition, seizures in patients with cystathionine synthase deficiency are also not limited to major seizure types. So-called diencephalic seizures characterized by flushing and other autonomic features, have been reported [10], as have myoclonic seizures [11] and other types of generalized seizures [12,13].

Electroencephalographic abnormalities have been found in patients with or without clinical seizures. These abnormalities take the form of excessive slow activity or paroxsymal spike and sharp-wave discharges. Electroencephalographic abnormalities have also been seen in those patients with or without cerebral thromboembolic episodes [8].

Other neurologic abnormalities are usually associated with cerebrovascular thromboembolic disease or with focal seizures. As one might expect, both focal and diffuse neurologic abnormalities may occur including hypo- or hypertonia, hypo- or hyperreflexia, truncal or appendicular ataxia, cranial nerve or sensory deficits, and paresis or paralysis. Our experience and that of others suggest that paresis, incoordination, ataxia, microcephaly, and sensory disturbances are not uncommon. Patients with the vitamin B_6 nonresponsive forms have a greater chance of suffering severe neurologic symptoms. This is apparently related to an increased incidence of thromboembolic phenomena. An interesting clinical observation, made early in young children, is a peculiar Chaplinesque gait. Psychiatric disturbances, seen especially in the more severely involved patients, include excessive withdrawal, hyperexcitability, apathy, depression, autistic behavior, attention deficits, and other mental derangements not related to mental retardation.

Brain infarctions are found in different stages. Of the histologic patients, cystic changes are particularly evident. Some patients have shown extensive cystic changes that are unrelated to strokes but form a widespread spongy degeneration. There is extensive demyelination of the white matter of the cerebrum, cerebellum, brain stem, and cervical spinal cord, which is difficult to explain on the basis of separate strokes [14]. In most cases there is greater alteration of the gray than the white matter of the brain. Focal necrosis and gliosis are frequently encountered. Selective neuronal loss in the cerebral cortex and hippocampus has also been reported [15]. Although the majority of postmortem studies have shown infarctions due to arterial occlusion in the cerebrum, cerebellum, midbrain, and thalamus, thrombosis of the dural sinuses and other venous channels are not uncommon [16].

Cutaneous Features

In early reports concerning Caucasian patients, skin and hair findings were prominently described features of homocystinuria. Carson et al. [17] reported 10 patients, 90% of whom had a characteristic malar flush (Figure 15.1). The malar flush is often intense and has a somewhat cyanotic or dusky hue, particularly at its periphery where it blends into normal skin. The skin lesion may become more dusky after excessive crying or exposure to cold. The flush is distributed over the middle face but in locations somewhat dissimilar to the distribution of malar rashes seen in other neurocutaneous and systemic diseases. It often extends to the zygoma and beyond into the temporal fossae and even to the ears themselves, a feature not seen in other neurocutaneous diseases. The lower eyelids are usually spared, giving the impression in photographs that the rash begins as a narrow band that widens laterally as it extends toward the ears [17,18]. The malar flush may curve over the cheeks to the oral line and often to the chin. The tip of the nose and the forehead are usually spared. This sometimes highly characteristic skin lesion appears to be of a vascular type—it blanches with pressure. Although the skin lesions may be unique and characteristic of the majority of Caucasian patients with homocystinuria reported early on, more recent reports tend to ignore it since many patients do not have it (Figure 15.2). Mudd et al. [8] reported that at least 50% of affected individuals had both malar flush and livedo reticularis, but in the original report by Carson et al. [3], in which a malar flush was reported in 90% of the patients, livedo reticularis was found in only 60%. In this group of patients, malar flush was more often associated with fine, fair hair. McKusick noted a distinct difference in the incidence of malar flushing between patients reported from the United Kingdom and the United States [7]. He believed this feature was more common in cases from the United Kingdom because of the lack of central heating there. The cause of both malar flush and livedo reticularis is probably an abnormality of the peripheral circulation.

Abnormal nail fold capillaries and abnormal telangiectasia around scars have been reported [19]. The hair in cystathionine synthase deficiency has been described as sparse, fine, and brittle. The hair may be very light and may darken after vitamin B_6 therapy and diet [20]. The facial skin in the older patient is usually thin and has large pores [21,22]. One of the original cases and a few observed later had premature graying of hair [17].

The malar flush and livedo reticularis are possible manifestations of vascular lesions. There is some evidence to support a cellular disturbance in melanogenesis. Melanotrichia has been observed in response to pyridoxine administration in some patients [20]. Although the skin lesions may be particularly prominent in fair-complected Caucasian patients, similar cutaneous symptoms, except for a less intense malar flush, may also appear in well-pigmented individuals (see Figure 15.3). The enzyme cystathionine synthase is as deficient in the skin as it is elsewhere.

Ocular Features

Clinical eye findings are ectopia lentis, myopia, glaucoma (with and without pupil-block), buphthalmos, staphyloma, cataract, retinal detachment, and optic atrophy. By far the most common eye finding in cystathionine synthase deficiency is ectopia lentis, which consists of inferior and anterior lenticular subluxation. Subluxation is due to disrupted zonular fibers that normally hold the lens in place. The subluxation of the lens in cystathionine synthase deficiency, different from Marfan's syndrome, is not usually present at birth but is usually acquired later in life and is progressive. In a series of 83 patients [7], all with subluxation of the lens, the earliest detection was at age 3 years, but in a patient who had a mild form, it was not recognized until 24 years. In another series [8], ectopia lentis represented the most common clinical feature of 472 patients. In this study, 20.6% of patients had ectopia lentis as the only symptom leading to the search for homocystinuria, and in 85.6% ectopia lentis was either the sole or an additional feature leading to the investigation. In both of these series, subluxation of the lens was the most common clinical feature of cystathionine synthase deficiency. Neither one of these series included newborns or patients' siblings identified by screening. Both presented data biased toward ophthalmologic means of screening. In comparison, screening of stroke or mental deficient patients would be expected to show a different distribution of symptoms [9]. Ectopia lentis may develop late in many patients and some never develop it. When ectopia lentis occurs, it is usually detected by 10 years of age [7]. Before the subluxation becomes evident, mild to severe myopia may be noted. This may be caused by either an inherited excessively long eye globe or an improper accommodation due to faulty zonular ligament contraction and control.

When glaucoma is associated with ectopia lentis it is usually a complication of lens displacement. After the lens is severely displaced anteriorly, pupil-block may occur, causing glaucoma by entrapment. However, glaucoma has also been reported without pupillary entrapment. Buphthalmos and staphyloma may occur even at low intraocular pressure and without strict glaucoma. This alteration of the global shape is thought to be caused by a defect in scleral collagen. Retinal detachment may occur either spontaneously or as a complication of surgery performed to remove displaced lenses. Optic atrophy may occur secondary to glaucoma or to thromboembolism of the central retinal artery and subsequent venous thrombosis.

Frayed and disrupted zonular fibers are present in patients with ectopia lentis. This pathologic event leads to subluxation of the lens. Postmortem study shows that fractured zonular fibers recoil on the surface of the ciliary body. Other histopathologic changes in the eye include peripheral pigmentary retinal degeneration and atrophy of the nonpigmented ciliary epithelium. Occlusion of the retinal vessels is regularly found. The posterior sclera may be thin and the choroid atrophic [23,24].

Musculoskeletal Features

Musculoskeletal features consist of osteoporosis, pathologic fractures, kyphoscoliosis, pectus excavatum and carinatum, genu valgum, rocker bottom feet, arachnodactyly, dolichostenomelia, humerus varus, large knobby knees, high arched narrow palate, enlargement of distal femoral epiphysis, thickened calvaria, microcephaly, large paranasal sinuses, limitation of joint mobility, platyspondylisis, spondylolisthesis, degenerative nucleus pulposus, widening of femoral and tibial condyles, pes cavus and planus, calcifications in radial and ulnar epiphyses, retarded lunate development, and enlargement of other carpal bones (capitate, hamate, triquetral). Many of these skeletal abnormalities produce the marfanoid habitus, characterized by some similarities to Marfan's syndrome but also by differences (Figure 14.3). One characteristic contrast is the limitation of joint extensibility seen in cystathionine synthase deficiency instead of the hyperelastic joints seen in Marfan's syndrome.

Myopathy has been noted as a feature of cystathionine synthase deficiency but it was only detected by electromyographic study [25].

Osteoporosis is said to be present in almost all patients with cystathionine synthase deficiency and explains the pathologic fractures. In a large well-done study [7], radiographic studies revealed that 25 of 26 patients had porotic vertebral bodies, and in 19 of these the vertebral end plates were concave. Scoliosis was seen in 17, kyphosis in 2, and spondylolisthesis in 2 patients. Needless to say, chronic back pain is a major problem in patients with these musculoskeletal defects. Even if the musculoskeletal symptoms may not be a prominent complaint, a large number of these patients exhibit abnormalities. A recently reported series [8] found that marfanoid features and bony abnormalities were the only initial symptoms of homocystinuria in only 0.9% and 0.2% of patients, respectively. Yet, these features were contributors to the diagnosis in 60.4% of the cases.

Microcephaly is present in a large number of patients, many of whom are mentally retarded.

Radiographic and histologic studies of the vertebral bodies reveal rarefaction of spongy bone. These studies suggest that an ossification defect exists. Many of the manifestations of cystathionine synthase deficiency are due to abnormal connective tissue. Structural abnormalities of collagen and elastin are probably secondary to defective cross-linking of collagen [26,27].

Cardiovascular Features

Thromboembolism and its manifestations represent the major clinicopathologic complications of cystathionine synthase deficiency [28–31]. Either large or small arteries or veins may be affected. The greatest risks to life and disability result from cerebral, carotid, coronary, pulmonary, and renal arterial occlusions. Vascular occlusions may occur at any time in life, but it has been observed that the large thromboses of the cerebral arteries and venous sinuses may be particularly prone to occur in infancy, whereas insults from occluded cerebral, coronary, pulmonary, and renal arteries occur later in life.

Several clinical syndromes, characteristic of vascular pathology, may occur. Thrombophlebitis is a source of sudden pulmonary embolism. Renal arterial stenosis leads to arterial hypertension but may also reflect diffuse vascular changes that occur without renal involvement [31]. Fatal coronary occlusion, as well as incapacitating angina pectoris, have occurred in teenagers.

A recent study [9] showed that over 25% of two groups of patients, with either occlusive peripheral or cerebrovascular arterial disease, were determined by methionine loading responses and cystathionine synthase measurements from skin fibroblast cultures to be heterozygotes for cystathionine synthase deficiency. Thus, it appears that the clinical features of both the homozygous and heterozygous forms of cystathionine synthase deficiency are very important in understanding these disorders and possibly in gauging the sites of primary deficit.

Heart failure has most often been due to cor pulmonale or to thromboembolism of the pulmonary arterial tree, related to or aided by ischemic heart disease [9,21]. Pulseless disease, acute gangrene or ulceration of limbs, gastrointestinal bleeding, and mesenteric artery occlusion have been recorded. Complications of cerebral angiography, probably due to thrombosis, were reported prior to the availability of more modern angiographic techniques. There have been no reports of contrast-induced thrombosis with computer-assisted tomography.

Several processes are important in the production of vascular lesions seen in cystathionine synthase deficiency. Medial degeneration of the aorta and other elastic arteries resemble the vascular lesions seen in Marfan's syndrome. More widely occurring are internal hyperplasia and fibrosis, which occur in arteries of all sizes and which lead to the formation of pads and ridges [21]. This process also leads to recurrent venous thrombosis and consequent infarcts in various parts of the body. An increased incidence of hypercoagulability of the blood also exists. Excessive adhesiveness of platelets has been suspected but has not been proved [32].

Thrombi and emboli have been reported in almost every major artery or vein and in many smaller vessels. The central nervous system is a preferential site for infarctions. Coronary artery occlusion, pulmonary artery occlusion, and embolisms from thrombophlebitis and renal artery occlusion occur frequently. Studies of arterial walls show marked fibrous thickening of the intima. Coarctation of the aorta from intimal fibrosis has been reported [28,29]. The thickening may be either symmetrical or patchy. In the media of the artery, muscle fibers are found to be frayed and split and contain increased amounts of interstitial collagen. The elastic fibers of large arteries also may be frayed and fragmented. There are often changes in the internal elastic lamina. Advanced atherosclerotic degenerative changes have been found in a large abdominal aortic aneurysm [29]. Endocardial fibroelastosis of the left atrium has been reported [30,31].

The pathogenesis of the thrombotic tendency in cystathionine synthase deficiency of both homozygotic and heterozygotic types is not clearly understood. It is believed that the elevated plasma homocystine, rather than hypermethioninemia, is a factor in the thrombotic tendency that exists in these patients [31–33].

Biochemistry

Methionine is the major donor of methyl groups in the body (Figure 15.4). In the steps of transsulfuration, methionine is converted to S-adenosylmethionine and then to S-adenosylhomocysteine. The major product of the adenosyl pathway is homocysteine, which is oxidized rapidly to the disulfide, homocystine. Under normal conditions the homocysteine–homocystine complex is not present in the plasma and is present only in very low quantities in the ur-

ine, whereas methionine is present in relatively low amounts in the plasma and is barely detectable in the urine. The body attempts to replenish methionine by the methylation of homocysteine. Remethylation is accomplished by a tetrahydrofolate circuit in which vitamin B_{12} and folate are important contributors. Vitamin B_{12} acts as a coenzyme, and betaine and choline are important methyl donors to this reaction. Defects in this methylation process account for several other defects of metabolism whose primary biochemical feature is homocystinuria. These disorders block methionine synthesis. Thus, homocystinuria, in the face of abnormally low levels of serum methionine, is the characteristic biochemical feature of these disorders. In the normal process, the homocysteine–homocystine complex contributes to cystathinione formation by combining with serine in the presence of cystathionine synthase. Vitamin B_6, or pyridoxine, acts as a cofactor for cystathionine synthase activity. Cystathionine is found in highest quantities in the brain, for as yet unexplained reasons. It is later converted to cysteine, then to its disulfide cystine, and then to free sulfate. This pathway represents the major source of sulfate's excretion in the body. Thus, the breakdown of methionine, through its adenosyl products to homocysteine, then to cystathionine, and finally to cysteine and sulfate are the major sources of transsulfuration.

In cystathionine synthase deficiency several biochemical events occur. Due to the impediment or stoppage of cystathionine's formation not only is cystathionine deficient but cysteine is not formed. Therefore, in these circumstances, cystine becomes an essential amino acid. In addition, homocysteine accumulates in large quantities, and thus more is converted to homocystine. The homocysteine–homocystine complex increases in the plasma and in large part is excreted since no renal absorptive process exists to help conserve it. Therefore, most of the homocystine offered to the kidneys is excreted, unlike amino acids such as phenylalanine or methionine even. These amino acids with their renal reabsorptive mechanisms must reach plasma levels above the renal threshold before they are excreted in the urine ("overflow mechanism"). Because the tetrahydrofolate pathway is stimulated as much as it can be, methionine accumulates in greater amounts in the plasma. At levels above the renal threshold, the amino acid overflows into the urine. With even more available methionine, the homocysteine—homocystine complex also increases in the plasma but is excreted in particularly large amounts in the urine since there is no renal mechanism to help conserve it. Homocystinuria due to cystathionine synthase de-

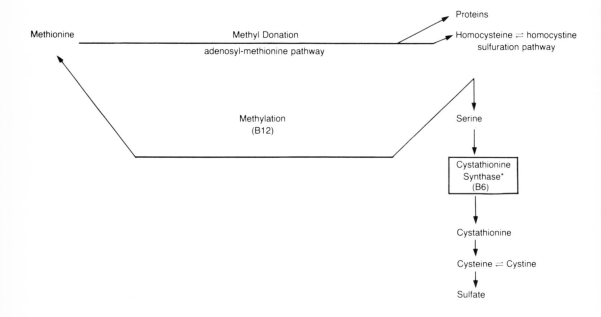

*Absent in severest forms of homocystinuria due to cystathionine synthase deficiency and mildly deficient in many heterozygotic conditions.

Figure 15.4. Simplified methionine metabolism pathway.

ficiency is an example of a "combination" type of aminoaciduria—caused by both the "no-threshold" mechanism for homocystine and an "overflow" mechanism for methionine. The major end result is hypermethioninemia and homocystinuria. The extent to which homocystinemia is elevated may be responsible for the thromboembolic phenomena. In most patients hypocystinemia is also present.

It is believed that some of the mild forms of cystathionine synthase deficiency exist because a heterogeneous, limited amount of cystathionine synthase present in the body allows some of the metabolic events to occur. This small amount of enzyme is stimulated by large amounts of vitamin B_6, allowing the maximum function possible. To be beneficial, vitamin B_6 is required in amounts much larger than a normal person would require. Thus vitamin B_6 responsiveness in homocystinuria due to cystathionine synthase deficiency is a vitamin-dependent condition.

In the many clinical conditions believed to be related to the heterozygotic state of cystathionine synthase deficiency enough enzyme is available to reasonably carry out normal multisystem functions except under stressful conditions.

Epidemiology

The epidemiology of cystathionine synthase is complicated by many potential biases. There are now at least 672 reported cases of probable homozygotic homocystinuria due to cystathionine synthase deficiency [8]. Earlier reported data on the number of patients with the disorder are subject to error by the previous lack of specificity in diagnosis. Several of the earlier reported patients may have been reported only because of the biochemical phenomenon of homocystinuria or because of the more unique clinical manifestations, such as ectopia lentis, profound mental retardation, marfanoid habitus, and childhood stroke, among others. The natural history of cystathionine synthase deficiency is still somewhat unclear. The age of onset and the severity of clinical manifestation are known to vary widely among affected individuals, and thus the prevalence and natural history of each of the variable features remain uncertain. The effects of genetic heterogeneity, such as expressed by vitamin B_6 responsiveness or nonresponsiveness, are still not universally accepted even though they are now specifically defined, nor are the wide clinical manifestations of the purely heterozygotic forms accepted. The variable clinical presentations of the heterozygotic forms that are possible, such as isolated coronary or cerebral vascular occlusive accidents, unexplained cataracts, schizophrenia or other psychotic and neurotic behaviors, and isolated neural or cutaneous clinical presentations may go unreported. The effect of excessive methionine and its relationship to schizophrenia was suggested long before the discovery of homocystinuria due to cystathionine synthase deficiency [34–36]. Disturbances in methionine breakdown, its effect on neurotransmitter systems, and the effect of various toxins on these pathways are of great importance [36] and could alter our current view on the epidemiology of these disorders.

Cystathionine synthase deficiency has been found in practically every part of the world, including the Americas, Europe, and Asia, and in all races, including Negroes, Caucasians, and Orientals, and in many different small ethnic populations. In the first 10 years of the disease, only 100 patients were reported [22], compared to the well over 500 additional patients that have accumulated within the last 13 years. This vastly expanded experience must cast doubt on some of the early epidemiologic generalizations. The reported incidence of this disorder varies a great deal, chronologically and geographically, depending on the method of ascertainment. In Northern Ireland the estimated prevalence was 1 in 24,000, whereas in New South Wales it was 1 in 58,000. Prevalence rates, based on newborn screening methods, suggest incidences from 1 in 57,000 in Northern Ireland to 1 in 824,000 in Scotland and to the extreme case of Belgium, where no cases were found among 945,566 newborns. Even still, McKusick [37], using logical correction factors, estimated the general prevalence to be roughly 1 in 45,000. Mudd [31] suggested that a minimum prevalence rate in screened newborn infants is 1 in 200,000 worldwide. Some estimates indicate that the carrier frequency or gene frequency for cystathionine synthase deficiency is more like 1 in 70 at the most [7]. If heterozygotes are more subject to the possible risk factors for the multisystem disease previously discussed, a more accurate study of the heterozygote condition is needed.

Genetics

Cystathionine synthase deficiency is inherited as an autosomal recessive trait. Several studies of obligatory carriers of the trait have found that these individuals have less than 50% of the cystathionine synthase that normal controls possess. Among affected individuals, residual cystathionine synthase activities range from 0 to 10% of mean control activity [33,38]. Additionally, a variable amount of enzyme activity in different homozygotic individuals (which is influenced appreciably by pyridoxine) strongly indicates that there is much genetic heterogeneity in this disorder. In the series reported by McKusick et al. [7], 45 kindreds were studied. In all instances, both parents of affected patients were clinically normal. Parental consanguinity was known in 4 cases and suspected in at least 7 others. Although it is a rule that autosomal enzymopathies usually cause clinical manifestations only in homozygotes, this may not hold true given the possible symptomatology associated with presumed heterozygotes. However, no evidence for two generation transmission has ever been conclusively reported. It is now accepted that evidence of pathologic homocystinemia after methionine loading along with cystathionine beta-synthase deficiency determined by skin fibroblast cultures, is adequate for the diagnosis of the heterozygotic or carrier state, even without clinical symptomatology.

Diagnosis

Diagnostic studies helpful in the laboratory confirmation of homocystinuria due to cystathionine synthase deficiency range from simple urinary procedures all the way to the analysis of enzyme levels. One ubiquitous test that is still used as a screen is the urinary cyanide–nitroprusside test. Here, 2 ml of urine is mixed with 1 ml of 5% sodium cyanide solution and is left to react at room temperature for about 10 minutes. After the addition of a few drops of 5% sodium nitroprusside solution, a positive reaction is indicated by the appearance of a bright red beet color. This reaction is a test for disulfides. Thus, a positive cyanide–nitroprusside test does not absolutely confirm the diagnosis of homocystinuria, let alone the diagnosis of cystathionine synthase deficiency. Further evaluation is therefore necessary. One of these, the so-called silver nitroprusside test, separates the standard reactivity of homocystine and cystine. Since homocystine will be elevated in both the urine and serum in cystathionine synthase deficiency, a variety of procedures can be used to isolate homocystine from both urine and serum. This can be achieved by paper or thin-layer chromatography, high-voltage paper electrophoresis, and two-way sequential paper chromatography. Quantitation of the amino acid profile is accomplished by column chromatography.

The latter procedure accurately measures plasma methionine and homocystine, which, when elevated, rule out the other clinical conditions associated with homocystinuria not due to cystathionine synthase deficiency.

When the activity of the enzyme cystathionine synthase is demonstrated to be absent or markedly reduced the diagnosis of homocystinuria due to cystathionine synthase deficiency is confirmed. Enzymatic analysis of the liver, cultured phytohem-agglutinin-stimulated lymphocytes, and cultured fibroblasts are the most commonly used tissues for study.

Management

Management of patients with cystathionine synthase deficiency varies according to the form of the disease, the various tissues involved, and the complications of the disease. Since the identification of the presymptomatic or minimally symptomatic but potentially severe heterozygotic form, management principles have become even more complex. Two general treatment approaches must be considered in all forms of cystathionine synthase deficiency. First, an effort should be made to control or eliminate the biochemical abnormalities in order to prevent development of clinical disease, to prevent progression of existing clinical defects, and to ameliorate potentially reversible clinical manifestations. Second, efforts should be made to treat medical complications. In a classical sense these approaches include institution of both curative and palliative forms of treatment.

Diet

The standard diet used in the treatment of cystathionine synthase deficiency is low in methionine and contains supplemental cystine. Its goal is to maintain normal plasma levels of methionine and of the homocysteine–homocystine complex. Cystine supplements are given to supply the body with a now essential amino acid. Several commercial types of diets can be used. The amount of methionine in the diet can be adjusted to eliminate homocystine and to maintain blood methionine levels within the normal range of less than 0.04 μmol/ml. Cystine supplementation is usually set at 150 to 200 mg/kg/day. It is now accepted that dietary restrictions begun in infancy may prevent severe mental retardation as well as many of the other progressive aspects of the disease [31].

Vitamins

Large amounts of vitamin B_6 or pyridoxine have been effective in reducing or eliminating the biochemical abnormalities in many of the patients with cystathionine synthase deficiency. The dose used is much greater than the normal daily requirement of 1 to 2 mg and has been set as high as 1,200 mg per day in certain cases. Between 250 and 500 mg/day originally was used but others have cautioned that a patient should not be considered a vitamin B_6 nonresponder until a dose of at least 500 to 1,000 mg per day has been given for a matter of weeks [1,39,40]. Vitamin B_{12} should be maintained if it is found to be deficient.

The palliative treatments of the clinical manifestations of cystathionine synthase deficiency are quite extensive and include ophthalmologic and orthopedic procedures. Psychiatric and behavioral modification therapies and chemotherapies are important. Antithrombotic therapy with dipyridamole and acetylsalicylic acid have been advocated [31]. Closely regulated anticonvulsant management is essential.

Late treatment with diet or large amounts of vitamin B_6 can produce behavioral improvement, which suggests that mental disturbance may be reversible in some cases, although improvement of the IQ is minimal. Betaine, which lowers homocysteine–homocystine by accelerating its methylation, has been shown, in recent studies, to be useful in patients not responsive to pyridoxine.

The avoidance of surgery and angiography whenever possible is important in the management of patients with cystathionine synthase deficiency. Oral contraceptives should not be used, and pregnancy should probably be avoided in most homozygous forms of cystathionine synthase deficiency.

References

1. Mudd SH. Disorders of transsulfuration. In: Stanbury JB, Wyngaarden JB, Fredrickson DS, et al., eds. The metabolic basis of inherited disease. New York: McGraw–Hill, 1983;5:522–559.
2. Field CMB, Carson NAJ, Cusworth DC, et al. Homocystinuria. A new disorder of metabolism. Xth Internat Congr Paed 1962;(abstr):274.
3. Carson NAJ, Neill DW. Metabolic abnormalities detected in a survey of mentally backward individuals in Northern Ireland. Arch Dis Child 1962;37:505–513.
4. Gerritsen T, Vaughn JG, Waisman HA. The identification of homocystine in the urine. Biochem Biophys Res Commun 1962;9:493–496.
5. Gerritsen T, Waisman HA. Homocystinuria: an error

in the metabolism of methionine. Pediatrics 1962;33: 413–420.

6. Mudd SH, Finkelstein JD, Irreverre F, et al. Homocystinuria: an enzymatic defect. Science 1964;143:1443–1445.

7. McKusick VA, Hall JG, Char F. The clinical and genetic characteristics of homocystinuria. In: Carson NAJ, Raine DN, eds. Inherited disorders of sulfur metabolism. Edinburgh, London: Churchill Livingstone, 1971:179–204.

8. Mudd SH, Skovby F, Levy HL, et al. The natural history of homocystinuria due to cystathionine beta synthase deficiency. Am J Hum Genet 1985;37:1–31.

9. Boers GHJ, Smals AGH, Trijbels FJM, et al. Heterozygosity for homocystinuria in premature peripheral and cerebral occlusive arterial disease. N Engl J Med 1985;313:709–715.

10. Kennedy C, Shih VE, Rowldan LP. Homocystinuria: a report in two siblings. Pediatrics 1965;35:736–741.

11. Kang ES, Byers RK, Gerald PS. Homocystinuria response to pyridoxine. Neurology 1970;20:503–507.

12. Gaull GE, Sturman JA, Schaffner F. Homocystinuria due to cystathionine synthase deficiency: enzymatic and ultrastructural studies. J Pediatr 1974;84:381–390.

13. Gaull GE, Schaffner F. Electron microscopic changes in hepatocytes of patients with homocystinuria. Pediatr Res 1971;5:23–32.

14. Chou SM, Waisman HA. Spongy degeneration of the central nervous system. Case of homocystinuria. Arch Pathol 1965;79:357–363.

15. Gaull GE, Carson NAJ, Dent CE, et al. Homocystinuria: clinical and pathological description of 10 cases. In: Oester J, ed. Proceedings of the international congress on the scientific study of mental retardation. Copenhagen, 1964;1:91.

16. Gibson JB, Carson NAJ, Neill DW. Pathological findings in homocystinuria. J Clin Pathol 1964;17:427–437.

17. Carson NAJ, Dent CE, Field CMB, et al. Homocystinuria: clinical and pathological review of ten cases. J Pediatr 1965;66:565–583.

18. Dyken PR, Miller M. Facial features of neurologic syndromes. St. Louis: CV Mosby, 1980:449.

19. Price J, Vickers CFH, Brooker BK. A case of homocystinuria with noteworthy dermatological features. J Ment Defic Res 1968;12:111–117.

20. Shelley WB, Dawnsley HM, Morrow G. Pyridoxine-dependent hair pigmentation in association with homocystinuria. Arch Dermatol 1972;106:228–230.

21. Dunn HG, Perry TL, Dolman CL. Homocystinuria: a recently discovered cause of mental defect and cerebrovascular thrombosis. Neurology 1966;16:407–420.

22. Gerritsen T, Waisman HA. Homocystinuria: cysta-

thionine synthase deficiency. In: Stanbury JB, Wyngaarden JB, Fredrickson DS, eds. The metabolic basis of inherited disease. 3rd ed. New York: McGraw–Hill, 1972;3:404–412.

23. Ramsey MS, Yanoff M, Fine BS. The ocular histopathology of homocystinuria. A light and electron microscopic study. Am J Ophthalmol 1972;74:377–385.

24. Henkind P, Ashton N. Ocular pathology in homocystinuria. Trans Ophthalmol Soc UK 1965;85:21–38.

25. Hurwitz LJ, Chopra JS, Carson NAJ. Electromyographic evidence of a muscle lesion in homocystinuria. Acta Paediatr Scand 1968;57:401–404.

26. Meynadier J, Guilhou JJ, Thorel M, et al. Homocystinurie: étude histologique et ultrastructurale. Dermatologica (Basel) 1981;163:34–41.

27. Schedewie H, Willich E, Gröbe H, et al. Skeletal findings in homocystinuria: a collaborative study. Pediatr Radiol 1973;1:12–23.

28. Gaull GE. Homocystinuria. Adv Teratology 1967; 2:101–126.

29. Almgren B, Eriksson I, Hemmingsson A, et al. Abdominal aortic aneurysm in homocystinuria. Acta Chir Scand 1978;144:545–548.

30. Schimke RN, McKusick VA, Huang T, et al. Homocystinuria. JAMA 1965;193:711–719.

31. Mudd SH. Homocystinuria. In: Wyngaarden JB, Smith LH, eds. Cecil textbook of medicine. 16th ed. Philadelphia: Saunders, 1985:1131–1132.

32. McDonald L, Bray C, Field C, et al. Homocystinuria, thrombosis and the blood-platelets. Lancet 1964;1:745–746.

33. Uhlendorf BW, Conerly EB, Mudd SH. Homocystinuria: studies in tissue culture. Pediatr Res 1973;7:645–658.

34. Osmond H, Smythies JR. Schizophrenia: a new approach. J Ment Sci 1952;98:309–315.

35. Pollin W, Cardon PV, Katy SS. Effect of amino acid feedings in schizophrenic patients treated with iproniazid. Science 1961;133:104–105.

36. Bracken P, Coll P. Homocystinuria and schizophrenia: literature review and case report. J Nerv Ment Dis 1985;173:51–55.

37. McKusick VA. Heritable disorders of connective tissue. St. Louis: CV Mosby, 1972:333.

38. Fowler B, Sardharwalla IB. Homocystinuria: cystathionine synthase activity in cultured skin fibroblasts. In: Cockburn F, Gitzelmann R, eds. Inborn errors of metabolism in humans. New York: Alan R. Liss, 1982.

39. Barber GW, Spaeth GL. Pyridoxine therapy in homocystinuria. Lancet 1967;1:337.

40. Perry TL. Homocystinuria. In: Myhan WL, ed. Heritable disorders of amino acid metabolism. New York: John Wiley & Sons, 1974:395.

Chapter 16
Citrullinemia and Arginosuccinicaciduria

STUART B. BROWN

Citrullinemia and arginosuccinicaciduria represent two metabolic disorders that result from enzymatic impairment in steps 3 and 4 of the urea cycle. The urea cycle represents a series of enzyme-mediated reactions that result in ammonia detoxification and waste nitrogen excretion through the production of urea. There are five steps in the cycle, each mediated by an individual enzyme. In step 1, ammonia and bicarbonate are converted to carbamoyl phosphate by the enzyme carbamoyl phosphate synthetase. The carbamoyl group is then transferred from carbamoyl phosphate to ornithine in step 2, by the enzyme ornithine carbamoyl transferase, to form citrulline. Citrulline in turn reacts with aspartate and is catalyzed in step 3 by the enzyme arginosuccinic acid synthetase to form arginosuccinic acid. In step 4, arginosuccinic acid is cleaved by the enzyme arginosuccinase (arginosuccinic lyase) to form arginine and fumaric acid. A molecule of urea is split off by the enzyme arginase, in step 5, and ornithine is regenerated for the next turn of the cycle.

Inhibition or deficiency of each particular enzyme in the urea cycle has resulted in the production and subsequent identification of a disease state. Deficiency in arginosuccinic acid synthetase has produced the disorder citrullinemia. Deficiency in arginosuccinase has resulted in arginosuccinicaciduria [1].

Citrullinemia

Deficiency in arginosuccinic acid synthetase causes a metabolic disorder characterized by a markedly elevated plasma citrulline level and an elevated plasma ammonia concentration without acidosis.

The neonatal form of this disorder is character-ized by an infant, normal at birth, who develops lethargy, poor suck, altered muscle tone, grunting or rapid respirations, hypothermia, and convulsions [1–3]. These signs begin within a few days of birth and often are noted at early feedings. A rapid progression of the lethargic state to coma and death occurs. The laboratory findings indicate a markedly elevated plasma citrulline level, greater than 1,000 μmol/L (normal 6 to 20 μmol/L), absence of plasma arginosuccinic acid, elevated blood ammonia concentration (600 to 1,000 μmol/L; normal is 15 to 35 μmol/L), low serum urea nitrogen and arginine levels, and increased urinary citrulline and orotic acid levels [2,3]. Fibroblast enzyme assay reveals that less than 10% of normal arginosuccinic acid synthetase activity occurs [3].

Genetic heterogeneity in citrullinemia has caused both a subacute and adult form of the disorder. The subacute form is due to a partial arginosuccinic acid synthetase deficiency. Children afflicted with this disorder exhibit intermittent symptomatic hyperammonemia, characterized in infancy by a gradual onset of feeding difficulties and recurrent vomiting. These are associated with lethargy, altered consciousness, tremor, ataxia, seizures, and psychomotor retardation [1].

An adult-onset form of citrullinemia has been described in Japan. It is characterized by intermittent bizarre behavior, manic episodes, psychosis, dysarthria, papilledema, motor weakness, hepatomegaly, and subsequent dementia [4–7].

Arginosuccinicaciduria

Deficiency in arginosuccinase results in a metabolic disorder characterized by moderately elevated plasma citrulline levels, hyperammonemia without acidosis, and increased levels of plasma and urine arginosuccinic acid.

The neonatal form of this disorder presents with poor feeding and lethargy, tachypnea, respiratory distress, seizures, and ultimately coma and death [1]. The infant with arginosuccinicaciduria, as with citrullinemia, is normal at birth and then exhibits symptoms 24 to 48 hours after birth.

The degree of hyperammonemia in this disorder is similar in quantity to that seen in citrullinemia. However, the elevation of plasma citrulline (100 to 300 μmol/L) is only a fraction of that seen in citrullinemia. Elevation of plasma and urinary arginosuccinic acid, not seen in citrullinemia, is present in this disorder [3].

Not all patients manifest arginosuccinicaciduria as neonates. An indolent or subacute form is seen in infants and is characterized by feeding problems, failure to thrive, seizures, and hepatomegaly. With time these patients develop intermittent ataxia, developmental delay, and mental retardation. The intellectual slowing may not be apparent until 2 years of age. Seizures associated with abnormal electroencephalograms, and episodes of intermittent ataxia occur throughout childhood, often provoked by infection or increased protein intake. The majority of patients reported with arginosuccinic acid fall into this form of the condition, with diagnosis often made through amino acid screening of retarded children with seizures. Their histories, however, indicate that many of these children have had periods of irritability, failure to thrive, feeding difficulties, or intermittent ataxia earlier in their life, beginning in infancy [1].

Clinical Features

In approximately one-half of patients with the subacute or late-onset form of arginosuccinicaciduria a type of abnormal hair, trichorrhexis nodosa, is seen. The scalp hair is sparse, dry, brittle, and friable. Minute nodes are formed in the hair shafts. This morphological abnormality causes the hair to fracture leaving a paintbrush-like end at the fracture site [1,8,9]. Another structural hair defect, pili torti, has been reported in both arginosuccinicaciduria and citrullinemia. Characterized by a flattened hair shaft with a 180° rotation or twist in several places along the length of the shaft, it causes the hair to be quite friable and to break easily when plucked. Pili torti has been seen in both scalp hair and hair from the eyebrows. When seen in patients with citrullinemia

this hair abnormality is said to occur most frequently in blond females. It is most prominent by 2 to 3 years of age and although it may be replaced by normal hair by late childhood it may be a lifelong affliction [10,11].

Trichorrhexis nodosa and pili torti have rarely been described in the neonatal form of either of these metabolic disorders. Both of these structural hair defects have been described in other clinical syndromes and therefore are not a pathognomonic characteristic of urea cycle abnormalities. There does not appear to be any relationship between the hair abnormality and the severity of either of these disorders.

The etiology of the hair abnormalities is controversial. Batshaw has suggested that it is caused by an arginine deficiency, and he indicates that the hair abnormality will disappear within 1 to 2 months following arginine dietary supplementation [3]. Potter et al., who have reported normal arginine content in the hair of their patient, therefore question the relationship of arginine and the hair shaft abnormalities [12]. They have indicated that the quality of their patient's hair improved over a several year period and that this improvement appeared to be related to an increase in hair cystine content with a concomitant increase in the tensile strength of the hair [13].

A generalized erythematous maculopapular skin rash has been noted in patients with childhood arginosuccinicaciduria and citrullinemia. This rash is thought to be related to arginine deficiency and has been found to disappear within a matter of days after dietary arginine supplementation [3].

Diagnosis

The diagnosis of neonatal-onset forms of citrullinemia or arginosuccinicaciduria requires clinical acumen to assess the patient's symptomatology and laboratory expertise to define the exact biochemical abnormality producing these symptoms. In the newborn period the major symptoms are nonspecific. Vomiting, lethargy, poor feeding, hypotonia, respiratory difficulties, and seizures may be seen in neonatal sepsis, intracranial hemorrhage, or perinatal asphyxia. Gastrointestinal obstruction, congenital heart disease, or pulmonary abnormalities also require diagnostic consideration. However, the presence of a normal clinical state in the first 24 to 72 hours following birth with subsequent deterioration that often coincides with feedings should suggest a metabolic etiology as the basis for the patient's symptoms. Urea cycle abnormalities, organic acidemias, and congenital lactic acidosis are the major metabolic considerations. The laboratory finding of hyperammonemia supports the diagnosis of a metabolic problem. Congenital lactic acidosis and organic acidemias are the most likely diagnoses if the hyperammonemia is associated with ketosis or acidosis. If associated with a respiratory alkalosis, then a urea cycle disorder is the primary diagnostic consideration.

In pursuing the diagnosis of a urea cycle disorder, the measurement of plasma citrulline is essential and permits the differentiation of these disorders. An absence of citrulline is anticipated in step 1 (carbamoyl phosphate synthetase) or step 2 (ornithine carbamoyl transferase) enzyme deficiencies of the urea cycle since citrulline is the product of these reactions. Elevated citrulline indicates an enzyme deficiency in step 3 (arginosuccinic acid synthetase) or step 4 (arginosuccinase lyase) of the cycle as citrulline production precedes these two metabolic steps in the cycle. A marked elevation of citrulline indicates citrullinemia and a moderate elevation, one-third the magnitude seen in citrullinemia, indicates arginosuccinicaciduria. The diagnosis of arginosuccinicaciduria is then made when the presence of arginosuccinic acid is found in blood and urine [14].

In the childhood-onset forms of these two disorders the symptoms are those of intermittent vomiting, lethargy, irritability, ataxia, or behavioral changes. The diagnostic approach to the metabolic problem in these children is the same as in the neonate, except that Reye's syndrome, systemic carnitine deficiency, and liver disease are also diagnostic considerations in hyperammonemia associated with acidosis or ketosis. In the hyperammonemic state without acidosis, citrulline again is quite elevated in step 3 and step 4 urea cycle enzyme deficiencies. When these disorders are seen in childhood citrulline is found in low concentrations, rather than absent, as it is in the neonatal form of the step 1 and step 2 urea cycle abnormalities [3].

Radiologic findings in patients with urea cycle abnormalities have been nonspecific and have consisted of ventricular enlargement and widening of the subarachnoid space with sulcal widening over the cortex. These findings indicate cerebral atrophy. Diffuse parenchymal hypodensity has been seen in subcortical areas through the use of computerized tomography [15].

Electroencephalographic findings in patients with urea cycle abnormalities have consisted of nonspecific slowing in theta frequency with multifocal spike, spike and wave, and sharp and slow wave discharges over both hemispheres. Triphasic waves, which have been reported in patients with hepatic encephalopathy, were not in evidence in these patients. Electroencephalographic abnormalities were associated with all degrees of ammonia elevation. Electroencephalograms were normal when ammonia levels were normal or only slightly elevated. Thus, although electroencephalogram abnormalities may be seen in patients with urea cycle problems they do not manifest any particular specific pattern [6,16].

Neuropathologic findings in step 3 and step 4 urea cycle disorders consist of generalized impairment of myelin formation along with brain swelling in the neonatal form of these disorders. In the more indolent forms, the ventricular system has been enlarged, and Type II Alzheimer astrocytes have been noted in the basal ganglia, pontine nuclei, and Purkinje cell layer of the cerebellum. These findings in both the early- and late-onset forms of these two disorders are not pathognomonic for either condition.

Treatment

Treatment of citrullinemia and arginosuccinicaciduria, as with other urea cycle disorders, consists of prevention of hyperammonemic events and treatment of episodic hyperammonemia and acute hyperammonemic coma. Because these patients have a limited ability to excrete waste nitrogen as urea, long-term therapy is directed toward limitation of nitrogen ingestion through reduction of protein intake. Protein synthesis and growth is maintained and promoted by supplying essential amino acids or their nitrogen-free ketoacid analogues [17,18]. Alternative metabolic pathways have been exploited to further assist in nitrogen waste excretion. Both arginosuccinic acid and citrulline are nitrogenous substances whose synthesis and excretion are promoted by dietary arginine supplementation [19]. Such supplementation enhances nitrogen excretion without the need to achieve excretion of urea. In citrullinemia, the oral administration of sodium benzoate further increases nitrogen excretion through the formation of urinary hippuric acid, a substitute for urea as a waste nitrogen product. Sodium phenylacetate is also given orally to increase urinary nitrogen excretion in the form of phenylacetylglutamine. These metabolic maneuvers have enhanced control of these disorders [14,20].

Intermittent hyperammonemic episodes or hyperammonemic coma occurs when control is lost. Treatment of such an event is similar in the neonate, infant, or child. Initially protein intake is stopped. Intravenous arginine, sodium benzoate, and phenylacetate are administered to achieve acute nitrogen excretion. All three substances are administered in citrullinemia, whereas arginine alone suffices in arginosuccinicaciduria. Intravenous hypertonic glucose is given to provide calories in a non-nitrogenous form and at the same time to suppress endogenous protein breakdown. These methods are generally effective in the acute treatment of the hyperammonemia associated with these two disorders. If hyperammonemia is refractory peritoneal dialysis or hemodialysis is used. Both of these dialysis methods appear more effective than exchange transfusion in removing accumulated nitrogen from the body [3,20].

In the neonate with hyperammonemic coma, phenylacetate administration is not used. Peritoneal or hemodialysis is used acutely in addition to intravenous arginine and benzoate administration to effect rapid reduction in the ammonia level while a definitive etiology for the increased ammonia is sought. This is necessary because of the catastrophic results that can occur in the potentially lethal neonatal forms of the urea cycle disorders [3,21].

Prognosis

Prognosis, especially in the neonatal form of the urea cycle disorders, has been extremely poor. Ten years ago the chance of surviving 1 year was 14%. However, early diagnosis and aggressive treatment, using alternative pathway therapy for ammonia reduction and nitrogen excretion, has brought the 1-year survival rate for neonatal hyperammonemic states due to urea cycle abnormalities to 92% [15]. Morbidity remains quite significant; mental retardation, cerebral palsy, and seizures were reported in 79% of a group of 26 patients with urea cycle enzyme deficiencies who survived 1 year following the onset and diagnosis of their problems [15]. IQ scores in these patients were found to correlate directly with the duration of the neonatal hyperammonemic coma. Patients who were in coma less than 3 days subsequently had average intelligence, but those whose coma lasted more than 5 days had a poor outcome. The height of the peak ammonia level did not seem to correlate with the IQ the patients attained [3,15].

Inheritance

Citrullinemia and arginosuccinicaciduria are inherited as autosomal recessive entities with genetic heterogeneity accounting for the variable degree of enzyme deficiency and variable clinical presentation

[2]. The carrier or heterozygote state is identifiable by enzyme determination in cultured fibroblasts. Such carriers have 50% normal enzyme activity, and their intracellular and extracellular levels of amino acids proximal to the enzymatic block may be increased [22]. Prenatal diagnosis has been carried out by enzyme assay of arginosuccinic acid synthetase and arginosuccinase in cultured amniotic fluid cells. Arginosuccinic acid and citrulline levels may be measured in the amniotic fluid [2]. Chorionic villi biopsy has also been used for prenatal diagnosis of arginosuccinicaciduria [23]. A neonatal screening test has been devised and tested to detect patients with citrullinemia, arginosuccinicaciduria, and argininemia [24]. Since the results of the test are not available early enough to permit diagnosis and treatment of acute neonatal hyperammonemia [3], the test's major applicability appears to be in those children with the more indolent-onset subacute form of these metabolic disorders.

References

1. Shih VE. Urea cycle disorders and other congenital hyperammonemic syndromes. In: Standury JB, Wyngaarden JB, Fredrickson DS, eds. Metabolic basis of inherited disease. 4th ed. New York: McGraw–Hill, 1978:362–387.
2. Nyhan WL. Abnormalities in amino-acid metabolism in clinical medicine. Norwalk, Conn.: Appleton–Century–Crofts, 1984:267–293.
3. Batshaw ML. Hyperammonemia. Curr Probl Pediatr 1984;14:1–69.
4. Miyazaki M, Fukuda S, et al. Hepatic encephalomyelopathy associated with citrullinemia. Brain Nerve (Tokyo) 1971;23:19–25.
5. Kooka T, Higashi Y, et al. A special form of hepatocerebral degeneration with citrullinemia. Neurol Med 1977;6:47. Cited by Nyhan WL. See reference 2 above.
6. Origuchi Y, Ushijima T, et al. Citrullinemia presenting as uncontrollable epilepsy. Brain Dev 1984;6:328–331.
7. Hayasaka S, Kiyosawa M, et al. Papilledema in late-onset citrullinemia. Am J Ophthalmol 1984;97:242–243.
8. Lee EB. Metabolic diseases and the skin. Pediatr Clin North Am 1983;30:597–608.
9. Coulter D, Beals TF, Allen RJ. Neurotrichosis: hairshaft abnormalities associated with neurological diseases. Dev Med Child Neurol 1982;24:634–644.
10. Phillips ME, Barrie H, Cream JJ. Arginosuccinicaciduria with pili torti. J R Soc Med 1981;74:221–222.
11. Patel HP, Unis ME. Pili torti in association with citrullinemia. J Am Acad Dermatol 1985;12:203–226.
12. Potter JL, Timmons GD, et al. Arginosuccinicaciduria: the hair abnormality. Am J Dis Child 1974; 127:724–727.

13. Potter JL, Timmons GD, Silvida AA. Arginosuccinic-aciduria: the hair abnormality revisited. Am J Dis Child 1980;134:1095–1096.

14. Batshaw ML, Thomas GH, Brusilow SW. New approaches to the diagnosis and treatment of inborn errors of urea synthesis. Pediatrics 1981;68:290–297.

15. Msall M, Batshaw ML, et al. Neurologic outcome in children with inborn errors of urea synthesis: outcome of urea cycle enzymopathies. N Engl J Med 1984; 310:1500–1505.

16. Verma SP, Hart ZH, Kooi KA. Electroencephalographic findings in urea-cycle disorders. Electroencephalogr Clin Neurophysiol 1984;57:105–112.

17. Thoene J, Batshaw ML, et al. Neonatal citrullinemia: treatment with ketoanalogues of essential amino acids. J Pediatr 1977;90:218–224.

18. Batshaw ML, Brusilow S, et al. Treatment of inborn errors of urea synthesis: activation of alternative pathways of waste nitrogen synthesis and excretion. N Engl J Med 1982;306:1387–1392.

19. Brusilow SW, Batshaw ML. Arginine therapy of arginosuccinase deficiency. Lancet 1979;1:124–127.

20. Brusilow S, Batshaw ML, Waber L. Neonatal hyperammonemic coma. Adv Pediatr 1982;29:69–103.

21. Brusilow S, Danney M, et al. Treatment of episodic hyperammonemia in children with inborn errors of urea synthesis. N Engl J Med 1984;310:1630–1634.

22. Ng WG, Oizumi J, et al. Carrier detection of urea cycle disorders. Pediatrics 1981;68:448–452.

23. Vimal CM, Fensom AH, et al. Prenatal diagnosis of arginosuccinicaciduria by analysis of cultured chorionic villi. Lancet 1984;2:521–522.

24. Talbot HW, Sumlin AB, et al. A neonatal screening test for arginosuccinic acid lyase deficiency and other urea cycle disorders. Pediatrics 1982;70:526–531.

Chapter 17

Biotin-responsive Multiple Carboxylase Deficiency

HERBERT M. SWICK

Skin lesions can be an integral part of a neurocutaneous disease, as in tuberous sclerosis and neurofibromatosis, or may reflect an underlying pathophysiologic process in which both the skin and the nervous system are involved. The biotin-responsive multiple carboxylase deficiencies, which fall into the latter category, are a group of metabolic disorders whose clinical features include a skin rash and striking neurologic signs.

In man, neurologic problems can result from a deficiency of any of several vitamins, including vitamin A, niacin, thiamine, pyridoxine, or biotin. Symptoms occur secondary either to a dietary deficiency or to a specific inborn error of metabolism. Criteria for a vitamin-responsive inherited metabolic disorder include genetic etiology, a specific clinical or biochemical abnormality, and response to pharmacologic doses of a single vitamin [1]. Biotin-responsive multiple carboxylase deficiency meets each of these criteria.

A brief review of the biochemical role of biotin is necessary to understand the clinical manifestations of the biotin-responsive diseases.

The Biochemistry of Biotin

Biotin is widely distributed in most foods, with relatively high concentrations found in liver, egg yolk, cooked grains, cow's milk, and human milk; it is also synthesized by intestinal flora [2–4]. The recommended dietary allowance of 35 μg/day for neonates and 100 to 200 μg/day for adults [5], therefore, is usually easily met by exogenous and endogenous

sources. Little is known about the mechanisms of biotin absorption, transport, or intracellular distribution.

Biotin's major role is to serve as a coenzyme in a number of carboxylation reactions. The biotin-dependent carboxylases include β-propionyl-CoA carboxylase (E.C. 6.4.1.4, PCC), β-methylcrotonyl-CoA carboxylase (E.C. 6.4.1.3, MCC), pyruvate carboxylase (E.C. 6.4.1.1, PC), and acetyl-CoA carboxylase (E.C. 6.4.1.2, ACC) [6]. These carboxylases catalyze steps in gluconeogenesis (PC), amino acid catabolism (PCC and MCC), organic acid metabolism (PCC), and long chain fatty acid biosynthesis (ACC) [7]. Three of these enzymes are found in the mitochondria, while the fourth (ACC) is cytosolic [7].

The important metabolic pathways utilizing the biotin-dependent carboxylases are shown schematically in Figure 17.1. A block in one or more of these pathways leads to the production of organic acids. Thus, deficient MCC activity leads to increased production of β-methylcrotonylglycine and β-hydroxyisovaleric acid. A deficiency of PCC activity prevents the conversion of propionyl-CoA to D-methylmalonyl-CoA, with production of methylcitric and 3-hydroxypropionic acids and propionylglycine. A block in PC or ACC activity may cause excessive lactic acid production.

The biologically active holocarboxylases are synthesized from biotin and an apoenzyme in a reaction that requires holocarboxylase synthetase (Figure 17.2). Whether there is a single holocarboxylase that catalyzes the reaction in both the cytosol and the mitochondrion is not certain, but at least some com-

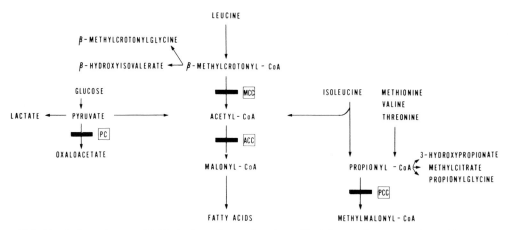

Figure 17.1. Metabolic pathways with biotin-dependent carboxylases. Black bars indicate sites of possible enzyme block. PC = pyruvate carboxylase; MCC = β-methylcrotonyl-CoA carboxylase; ACC = acetyl-CoA carboxylase; PCC = propionyl-CoA carboxylase. Note that deficient carboxylase activity leads to production of several abnormal organic acids. (Adapted from Wolf et al. [8].)

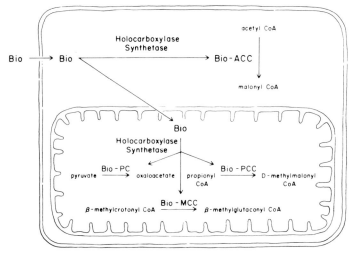

Figure 17.2. Schematic diagram of holocarboxylase synthetase's role in linking biotin to carboxylase apoenzymes. (See Figure 17.1 for abbreviations.) (Reproduced with permission from Stanbury JB et al. eds. The metabolic basis of inherited disease. 5th ed. New York: McGraw–Hill, 1983:479.)

ponents may be shared by cytosolic and mitochondrial elements [9]. More than one carboxylase can be linked covalently to biotin by the same holocarboxylase synthetase [6,10].

Degradation of the active holocarboxylase occurs by removal of biotin from biocytin (epsilon-N-biotinyl-L-lysine), a lysine moiety of the carboxylase [11]. This reaction requires biotinidase (E.C. 3.5.1.2) [12], which "permits the recycling of biotin for reutilization in the activation of apocarboxylases to active holocarboxylases" [13, p.236].

Clinical Problems

Biotin-responsive diseases present with one of several clinical patterns, depending upon the specific pathophysiologic mechanisms involved, but the signs usually reflect defective carboxylase activity. Clinical problems might be expected to occur under one of several conditions: dietary biotin deficiency, a defect in the absorption or transport of biotin, absent holocarboxylase synthetase activity, an isolated inherited deficiency of one of the carboxylases, or biotinidase deficiency. Three major clinical patterns have been defined, two of which represent primary defects in biotin metabolism while the third results from a nutritional deficiency of biotin.

Neonatal Multiple Carboxylase Deficiency: An Absence of Holocarboxylase Synthetase

Neonatal multiple carboxylase deficiency (MCD) typically presents in the first several days of life, heralded by vomiting and lethargy [6,8,14–18]. Neurologic signs indicate a severe diffuse metabolic disturbance, with hypotonia, seizures, and coma. The occurrence of a rash is variable; many children in this group have no rash, possibly because they die in profound acidosis before there has been time for a rash to develop [19]. A fine, scaly erythematous rash has been described in other children with neonatal MCD.

A persistent metabolic acidosis is present. Lactic acidosis [20] and hyperammonemia [8,21] have been noted in some patients. Cowan et al. [22] reported one family with MCD associated with immunologic defects related to T-cell and B-cell function. However, immunologic abnormalities do not comprise a common feature of neonatal MCD.

Patients with neonatal MCD excrete excessive amounts of abnormal organic acids in their urine. The pattern of organic acid excretion confirms defective activity of multiple carboxylases [6,16]. Beta-methylcrotonylglycine, β-hydroxyisovalerate, 3-hydroxypropionate, and methylcitrate are all excreted in excessive amounts, indicating a block in both MCC and PCC [16].

The neonatal form of MCD is caused by absent holocarboxylase synthetase activity [23,24]. Serum biotin is normal. However, biotin cannot be linked to the several apoenzymes to synthesize the active holocarboxylases. For that reason, carboxylase activity is low when measured in cultured leukocytes or fibroblasts, but enzyme activity returns to normal or nearly normal levels when biotin is added to the culture medium [6,25].

Some degree of clinical heterogeneity is characteristic of all varieties of the biotin-responsive diseases. Although most patients with absent holocarboxylase synthetase activity present early in the newborn period, children may remain asymptomatic until weeks or occasionally even months of age [26].

Infants with an isolated defect in a single carbox-

ylase may have signs that mimic those of holocarboxylase synthetase deficiency. Each of the isolated deficiencies is rare. Propionyl-CoA carboxylase deficiency, or propionic acidemia, is characterized by vomiting, lethargy, and hypotonia beginning in the neonatal or early infancy period [6]. Ketoacidosis and organic aciduria are often exacerbated by intercurrent illness or high protein loads [27,28]. Isolated PCC deficiency has been described in one asymptomatic sibling of an affected infant [29].

Most patients initially thought to have an isolated MCC deficiency have subsequently been shown to have multiple carboxylase deficiency. One infant with probable MCC deficiency presented with a clinical illness that resembled spinal muscular atrophy; her urine had a peculiar smell that resembled cat's urine [30].

Only a single case of suspected ACC deficiency has been reported in a newborn with hypotonia and evidence of defective fatty acid synthesis [31].

Common clinical features of PC deficiency are hypotonia, developmental delay, and seizures, noted from early infancy [6,32]. Metabolic acidosis reflects elevation of serum lactate and pyruvate levels.

Because of the similarity of symptoms—hypotonia, vomiting, lethargy, seizures, and metabolic acidosis—a defect in a single carboxylase must be considered in the differential diagnosis. Most infants, however, will have MCD related to absent holocarboxylase synthetase activity.

Infantile (Late-Onset) Multiple Carboxylase Deficiency: An Absence of Biotinidase

In contrast to neonatal MCD, the symptoms of infantile, or late-onset, MCD develop less acutely [12,13,33–37]. The onset may be as early as 1 week or as late as 2 years, but most patients develop symptoms at a few months of age (mean: 5.7 months) [33]. Cutaneous changes are a more prominent part of the clinical picture in late-onset MCD than in neonatal MCD. The first sign is often a skin rash, characterized initially by a fine scaly dermatitis and progressing to a nonspecific erythematous rash that is most prominent over the face and extremities. Hair loss is the initial symptom in about 20% (Figure 17.3), and alopecia develops in most children at some time during the course of their illness [33]. Conjunctivitis and mucocutaneous lesions commonly occur.

The neurologic signs in late-onset MCD are somewhat variable. The most common neurologic find-

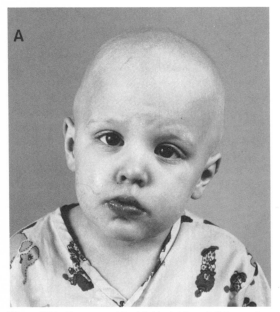 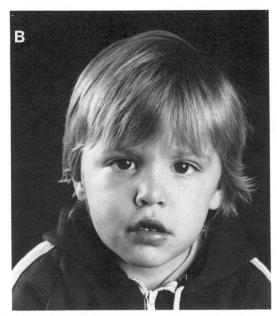

Figure 17.3. Two-year-old with biotinidase deficiency shown before treatment with biotin *(A)* and six months after treatment with biotin *(B)*. (Reproduced with permission of the New York Academy of Sciences. From Swick and Kien [40].)

ings are seizures, which are the initial symptom in about 60%, ataxia, and hypotonia [33]. Many children are quite irritable. Late-onset MCD is associated with a high-frequency neurosensory hearing loss in about 40% of the patients [33,38,39], and some children have had visual problems or optic atrophy [33].

Serum biotin is low in patients with infantile MCD [6,18]. Carboxylase activity is low in leukocytes but normal in cultured fibroblasts; carboxylase activity becomes normal when biotin is added to the culture medium [6].

Most children with infantile MCD have a metabolic acidosis and organic aciduria, reflecting a block in the various carboxylase pathways. However, metabolic acidosis is not always present and at least four children have been reported without organic aciduria [13,36,40].

Late-onset MCD is caused by biotinidase deficiency [12,19,34,35]. Because patients are unable to cleave biotin from biocytin, biotin cannot be reutilized to synthesize active holocarboxylases. Patients with biotinidase deficiency lose an excessive amount of biotin and biocytin in the urine [41,42] and seem to have impaired intestinal absorption of biotin [43,44]. This apparent defect in absorption probably results from inhibition by biocytin, which is a potent competitive inhibitor of biotin absorption [13].

Table 17.1 summarizes the differences between the neonatal and infantile forms of MCD.

Nutritional Biotin Deficiency

Although not genetically determined, dietary biotin deficiency deserves brief mention because its clinical signs and biochemical abnormalities are similar to those seen in the inherited varieties of MCD.

Clinical illness related to an insufficient dietary supply of biotin is quite rare, because biotin is present in many foods and is also synthesized by intestinal flora. In 1942 Sydenstricker et al. produced biotin deficiency in human volunteers [45]. After 4 to 6 weeks of a biotin-deficient diet, a fine, scaly dermatitis developed. Neurologic symptoms included depression, lassitude, and irritability. All signs were promptly reversed by the administration of biotin.

Biotin deficiency can develop in patients who receive large amounts of raw egg white [46,47], which contains avidin, a protein that prevents the absorption of biotin by binding it in the intestine. Williams [48] reported biotin deficiency in a 66-year-old man whose diet consisted almost entirely of red wine, to each glass of which he added a raw egg. So prodigious was this man's appetite for this concoction that

Table 17.1. Neonatal versus Late-Onset Multiple Carboxylase Deficiency

Feature	Neonatal	Late-Onset
Major clinical features	Vomiting, lethargy, hypotonia, seizures	Rash, alopecia, seizures, ataxia, developmental delay
Major biochemical features	Metabolic acidosis, organic aciduria, hyperammonemia	Metabolic acidosis, organic aciduria
Serum and urinary biotin levels	Normal	Low
Leukocyte carboxylase activity[a]	Deficient	Deficient
Fibroblast carboxylase activity[a]	Deficient	Normal
Defect	Holocarboxylase synthetase	Biotinidase

Source: adapted from Wolf et al. [8].
[a]Carboxylase activities become normal when biotin is added to culture media.

he moved to a chicken farm, simply to ensure his daily requirement of two to six dozen eggs!

Dietary biotin deficiency most often occurs in patients who have had major segments of their small intestine removed and who are on total parenteral alimentation without supplemental biotin [49–52]. In these patients, dietary deficiency and lack of endogenous synthesis combine to create clinical illness. Cutaneous manifestations include a scaly, erythematous or eczematous rash that develops after several weeks of parenteral alimentation [53,54]. Mucocutaneous candidiasis may develop and be quite severe [49]. Neurologic symptoms include depression, lability in mood, memory loss, and hyperesthesias [54,55]. These patients usually have organic aciduria secondary to inactivity of the carboxylase pathways.

Pathologic Findings

Little information is available about the pathologic changes associated with biotin-responsive MCD. Changes in the skin, while clinically often severe, are rather nonspecific on pathologic examination [48,49,56]. Williams reported "a sharp distinction between the corium and epidermis . . . there is hyperkeratinization; masses of keratinized material are separated from the underlying epidermis . . . The sebaceous glands are absent, the hair follicles atrophic . . . [A] vasculitis involves chiefly the superficial vessels . . . The vessels in the upper cutis are increased in number and show endothelial proliferation" [48, p.249]. In a patient with nutritional biotin deficiency, skin changes included "superficial dermal edema, hyperkeratosis . . . minimal perivascular chronic inflammatory response in the dermis [and] mild ectasis of the superficial papillary dermal vessels" [49, p.548]. The changes in the skin are thought to reflect deficient acetyl-CoA carboxylase activity, which is necessary for fatty acid metabolism and hence maintenance of skin integrity [31].

Even less information is available about the pathologic changes in the nervous system. Biotinidase activity in human cerebrospinal fluid is 0.53% that of serum, and activity in cerebral tissue is also low [57]. The brain is probably dependent on a continuing supply of biotin from the serum [57]. Although PC activity is better preserved in the brain than in the liver of biotin-deficient rats [58], decreased brain PC activity resulting from biotin deficiency could lead to accumulation of lactate in the brain [57,59] with subsequent toxicity. Alternatively, biotin may have some role in metabolism distinct from its role as a cofactor for the carboxylases. Vesely [60] demonstrated in the rat that biotin enhances guanylate cyclase activity in several organs, including the cerebellum. Therefore, the ataxia seen in patients with biotinidase deficiency might relate to some defect in cerebellar guanosine metabolism. One patient with MCD had chronic cerebellar degeneration and a subacute necrotizing myelopathy on postmortem examination [61]. Finally, accumulation of organic acids or biotinyl peptides could be toxic to the nervous system. This mechanism has been postulated as the reason for the sensorineural deafness that has been noted in children with biotinidase deficiency [38].

Diagnosis

The diagnosis of biotin-responsive MCD or of dietary biotin deficiency may be suspected from the characteristic pattern of signs and symptoms. Holocarboxylase synthetase deficiency should be considered in neonates or young infants with lethargy, vomiting, and hypotonia, especially if a rapidly progressive illness with seizures and coma ensues. The presence of a rash is not a prerequisite for the diagnosis of neonatal MCD.

Biotinidase deficiency, in contrast, is frequently characterized by a rash and alopecia. The rash may resemble that seen in acrodermatitis enteropathica

[19], zinc deficiency, or essential fatty acid deficiency [52]—conditions sometimes considered in the differential diagnosis. Neurologic signs often develop after the rash, although seizures can antedate the development of the dermatitis [33]. Irritability, hypotonia, ataxia, and hearing loss are other common neurologic findings.

Dietary biotin deficiency is almost solely restricted to patients with severe gastrointestinal disease on total parenteral nutrition.

Most infants affected with MCD will have a metabolic acidosis or lactic acidosis, so serum pH, pCO_2, bicarbonate, and lactate should be determined. In some patients serum ammonia is elevated. If MCD is suspected, the urine should be assayed for the presence of abnormal amounts of organic acids, specifically β-methylcrotonylglycine, β-hydroxyisovaleric acid, 3-hydroxypropionic acid, and methylcitric acid. Although most patients with either neonatal or late-onset MCD have organic aciduria, measurement of urinary organic acids is not sufficient for the diagnosis since a few patients with biotinidase deficiency have not had excessive excretion of urinary organic acids.

Definitive diagnosis requires the determination of serum and urine biotin levels. Serum biotin levels are normal (200 to 500 pg/ml) in infants with absent holocarboxylase synthetase activity, while patients with biotinidase deficiency or with dietary biotin deficiency will have low serum levels (often 10 to 20 pg/ml). Urinary biotin levels are normal in neonatal MCD but low in the infantile form. Biotinidase can be measured in the serum [12]. In controls, normal serum biotinidase activity is 5.80 ± 0.89 nmol/min/ml; homozygous individuals often have undetectable amounts of biotinidase, while their heterozygous parents have about half normal values (3.25 ± 0.51 nmol/min/ml) [12]. Carboxylase activities can be measured in cultured leukocytes or fibroblasts [62], and this is helpful in confirming the diagnosis of holocarboxylase synthetase or an isolated carboxylase deficiency.

Treatment

The principles of treatment are similar for each of the clinical patterns. Patients with MCD respond to pharmacologic doses of biotin, whether the underlying etiology is holocarboxylase synthetase or biotinidase deficiency. An abnormally low urinary biotin excretion and the characteristic pattern of organic aciduria are good criteria for predicting response to treatment with biotin [52]. The dose of biotin is not clearly established, but most patients have received oral biotin 10 mg daily. The dose of 10 mg is empiric, and many patients probably require less [12,52]. There are no proven toxic effects from pharmacologic doses of biotin, although massive doses may affect reproductive growth and development in rats [62]. Because MCD can be life threatening, however, large doses have been recommended.

Response to treatment has been dramatic. Metabolic acidosis often disappears within 24 to 48 hours; skin lesions resolve in 1 to 2 weeks, with resumption of hair growth that leads to a full growth of hair in about 2 months; and neurologic signs improve rapidly, often to complete recovery within several weeks. However, the neurologic signs, especially hearing loss, may not resolve completely [12,33,52]. Response to treatment should be monitored not only by clinical improvement, but also by resolution of the metabolic acidosis and disappearance of organic aciduria. In patients with biotinidase deficiency, audiometric evaluation for possible neurosensory hearing loss is important, and this should be monitored periodically.

Treatment of biotin-responsive MCD needs to be continued indefinitely, although a lower dose of biotin might be considered after the initial response is established.

Multiple carboxylase deficiency can be diagnosed and treated prenatally [63,64]. Determination of maternal urinary organic acid excretion is not helpful [64], but amniocentesis permits measurement of organic acids in the amniotic fluid. More reliably, carboxylase activities can be measured in cultured amniotic fluid cells [63]. If the diagnosis of MCD is made in utero, the mother should be given biotin, 10 mg/day. Potential teratogenic effects of pharmacologic doses of biotin are not known, so treatment should not begin until the second trimester. In one pregnancy, maternal treatment began in the twenty-third week of gestation, without adverse effects [63]. Infants in whom the diagnosis was made prenatally and whose mothers received biotin have been born with no evidence of clinical disease. Continuing treatment with biotin after birth has prevented the development of clinical illness, although one infant who was not supplemented postnatally did develop ketoacidosis at 3 months of age [65].

Biotinidase deficiency can also be detected in mass neonatal screening programs. In a pilot program conducted by Wolf et al. [66], newborn infants were screened by using the same blood-impregnated filter paper employed for detecting other metabolic diseases. Two cases of biotinidase deficiency were identified among 81,243 infants screened; in addition, 2 mildly affected older siblings of one of the probands were subsequently found to have biotinidase deficiency.

Techniques of prenatal diagnosis and neonatal screening hold promise for the early detection and effective treatment of biotin-responsive MCD.

References

1. Rosenberg LE. Vitamin-responsive inherited metabolic disorders. Adv Hum Genet 1976;6:1–74.
2. Roth KS. Biotin in clinical medicine—a review. Am J Clin Nutr 1981;34:1967–1974.
3. Bonjour JP. Biotin in man's nutrition and therapy—a review. Int J Vit Nutr Res 1977;47:107–117.
4. Bonjour JP. Biotin in human nutrition. Ann NY Acad Sci 1985;447:97–104.
5. National Research Council. Recommended dietary allowances. 9th ed. Washington, D.C.: National Academy of Sciences, 1980.
6. Wolf B, Feldman GL. The biotin-dependent carboxylase deficiencies. Am J Hum Genet 1982;34:699–716.
7. Rosenberg LE. Disorders of propionate and methylmalonate metabolism. In Stanbury JB, Wyngaarden JB, Fredrickson DS, et al., eds. The metabolic basis of inherited disease. 5th ed. New York: McGraw–Hill, 1983:474–497.
8. Wolf B, Hsia E, Sweetman L, et al. Multiple carboxylase deficiency: clinical and biochemical improvement following neonatal biotin treatment. Pediatrics 1981;68:113–118.
9. Packman S, Caswell N, González-Ríos MC, et al. Acetyl CoA carboxylase in cultured fibroblasts: differential biotin dependence in the two types of biotin-responsive multiple carboxylase deficiency. Am J Hum Genet 1984;36:80–92.
10. Achuta Murthy PN, Mistry SP. Synthesis of biotin-dependent carboxylases from their apoproteins and biotin. Biochem Rev 1972;43:1–10.
11. Wolf B, Grier RE, Allen RJ, et al. Biotinidase deficiency: the enzymatic defect in late-onset multiple carboxylase deficiency. Clin Chim Acta 1983;131:273–281.
12. Wolf B, Heard GS, McVoy JRS, et al. Biotinidase deficiency. Ann NY Acad Sci 1985;447:252–262.
13. Wolf B, Grier RE, Allen RJ, et al. Phenotypic variation in biotinidase deficiency. J Pediatr 1983;103:233–237.
14. Roth KS, Yang W, Foreman JW, et al. Holocarboxylase synthetase deficiency: a biotin-responsive organic acidemia. J Pediatr 1980;96:845–849.
15. Gompertz D, Draffan GH, Watts JL, et al. Biotin-responsive β-methylcrotonylglycinuria. Lancet 1971;2:22–24.
16. Packman S, Sweetman L, Baker H, et al. The neonatal form of biotin-responsive multiple carboxylase deficiency. J Pediatr 1981;90:418–420.
17. Bartlett K, Ng H, Leonard JV. A combined defect of three mitochondrial carboxylases presenting as biotin-responsive 3-methylcrotonylglycinuria and 3-hydroxyisovaleric aciduria. Clin Chim Acta 1980;100:183–186.
18. Thoene J, Baker H, Yoshino M, et al. Biotin-responsive carboxylase deficiency associated with subnormal plasma and urinary biotin. N Engl J Med 1981;308:817–820.
19. Nyhan WL. Clinical problems relating to biotin. Ann NY Acad Sci 1985;447:222–224.
20. Munnich A, Saudubray JM, Cotisson A, et al. Biotin-dependent multiple carboxylase deficiency presenting as a congenital lactic acidosis. Eur J Pediatr 1981;137:203–206.
21. Packman S, Sweetman L, Wall S. Biotin-responsive multiple carboxylase deficiency in a child with congenital lactic acidosis. Am J Hum Genet 1979;31:58A.
22. Cowan MJ, Packman S, Wara DW, et al. Multiple biotin-dependent carboxylase deficiencies associated with defects in T-cell and B-cell immunity. Lancet 1979;2:115–118.
23. Saunders ME, Sherwood WG, Dutine M, et al. Evidence for a defect of holocarboxylase synthetase activity in cultured lymphoblasts from a patient with biotin-responsive multiple carboxylase deficiency. Am J Hum Genet 1982;34:590–601.
24. Burri BJ, Sweetman L, Nyhan WL. Heterogeneity of holocarboxylase synthetase in patients with biotin-responsive multiple carboxylase deficiency. Am J Hum Genet 1985;37:326–337.
25. Bartlett K, Ghneim HK, Stirk J-H, et al. Enzyme studies in combined carboxylase deficiency. Ann NY Acad Sci 1985;447:235–251.
26. Sherwood WG, Saunders M, Robinson BH, et al. Lactic acidosis in biotin-responsive multiple carboxylase deficiency caused by holocarboxylase synthetase deficiency of early and late onset. J Pediatr 1982;101:546–550.
27. Shafai T, Sweetman L, Weyler W, et al. Propionic acidemia with severe hyperammonemia and defective glycine metabolism. J Pediatr 1978;92:84–86.
28. Wolf B, Hsia YE, Sweetman L, et al. Propionic acidemia: a clinical update. J Pediatr 1981;99:835–846.
29. Wolf B, Paulsen EP, Hsia YE. Asymptomatic propionyl CoA carboxylase deficiency in a 13-year-old girl. J Pediatr 1979;95:563–565.
30. Stokke O, Eldjarn L, Jellum E, et al. Beta-methylcrotonyl-CoA carboxylase deficiency: a new metabolic error in leucine degradation. Pediatrics 1972;49:726–735.
31. Blom W, DeMuinck Keizer SMPF, Stolte HR. Acetyl-CoA carboxylase deficiency: an inborn error of de novo fatty acid synthesis. New Engl J Med 1981;305:465–466.
32. Saudubray JM, Marsac C, Charpentier C, et al. Neonatal congenital lactic acidosis with pyruvate carboxylase deficiency in two siblings. Acta Paediatr Scand 1976;65:717–724.

33. Wolf B, Heard GS, Weissbecker KA, et al. Biotinidase deficiency: initial clinical features and rapid diagnosis. Ann Neurol 1985;18:614–617.

34. Thoene J, Wolf B. Biotinidase deficiency in juvenile multiple carboxylase deficiency. Lancet 1983;2:398.

35. Wolf B, Grier RE, Parker WD, et al. Deficient biotinidase activity in late-onset multiple carboxylase deficiency. N Engl J Med 1983;308:161.

36. Swick HM, Kien CL. Biotin deficiency with neurologic and cutaneous manifestations but without organic aciduria. J Pediatr 1983;103:265–267.

37. Charles BM, Hosking G, Green A, et al. Biotin-responsive alopecia and developmental regression. Lancet 1979;2:118–120.

38. Taitz LS, Green A, Strachan I, et al. Biotinidase deficiency and the eye and ear. Lancet 1983;2:918.

39. Wolf B, Grier RE, Heard GS. Hearing loss in biotinidase deficiency. Lancet 1983;2:1365–1366.

40. Swick HM, Kien CL. Biotin deficiency without organic aciduria. Ann NY Acad Sci 1985;447:430–433.

41. Baumgartner R, Suormala T, Wick H, et al. Infantile multiple carboxylase deficiency: evidence for normal intestinal absorption but renal loss of biotin. Helv Paediatr Acta 1982;37:499–502.

42. Baumgartner ER, Suormala T, Wick H, et al. Biotinidase deficiency associated with renal loss of biocytin and biotin. Ann NY Acad Sci 1985;447:272–287.

43. Munnich A, Saudubray JM, Carré G, et al. Defective biotin absorption in multiple carboxylase deficiency. Lancet 1981;2:263.

44. Thoene JG, Lemons R, Baker H. Impaired intestinal absorption of biotin in juvenile multiple carboxylase deficiency. N Engl J Med 1983;308:639–642.

45. Sydenstricker VP, Singal SA, Briggs AP, et al. Observations on the "egg white injury" in man and its cure with a biotin concentrate. JAMA 1942;118:1199–1200.

46. Scott D. Clinical biotin deficiency ("egg white injury"). Report of a case with some remarks on serum cholesterol. Acta Med Scand 1958;162:69–70.

47. Sweetman L, Surh L, Baker H, et al. Clinical and metabolic abnormalities in a boy with dietary deficiency of biotin. Pediatrics 1981;68:553–558.

48. Williams RH. Clinical biotin deficiency. N Engl J Med 1943;228:247–252.

49. Kien CL, Kohler E, Goodman SI, et al. Biotin-responsive in vivo carboxylase deficiency in two siblings with secretory diarrhea receiving total parenteral nutrition. J Pediatr 1981;99:546–550.

50. McClain CJ, Baker H, Onstad GR. Biotin deficiency in an adult during home parenteral nutrition. JAMA 1982;247:3116–3117.

51. Gillis J, Murphy FR, Boxall LBH, et al. Biotin deficiency in a child on long-term TPN. J Parent Ent Nutr 1982;6:308–310.

52. Mock DM, Baswell DL, Baker H, et al. Biotin deficiency complicating parenteral alimentation: diagnosis, metabolic repercussions, and treatment. J Pediatr 1985;106:762–769.

53. Mock DM, DeLorimer AA, Liebman WM, et al. Biotin deficiency: an unusual complication of parenteral alimentation. N Engl J Med 1981;304:820–822.

54. Khalidi N, Wesley JR, Thoene JG, et al. Biotin deficiency in a patient with short bowel syndrome during home parenteral nutrition. J Parent Ent Nutr 1984;8:311–314.

55. Levenson JL. Biotin-responsive depression during hyperalimentation. J Parent Ent Nutr 1983;7:181–183.

56. Fitzpatrick TB, Eisen AZ, Wolff K, et al. Dermatology in general medicine. 2nd ed. New York: McGraw–Hill, 1979:1029.

57. Suchy SF, Secor McVoy J, Wolf B. Neurologic symptoms of biotinidase deficiency: possible explanation. Neurology 1985;35:1510–1511.

58. Sander JE, Packman S, Townsend JJ. Brain pyruvate carboxylase and the pathophysiology of biotin-dependent diseases. Neurology 1982;32:878–880.

59. DiRocco MA, Superti-Furga A, Durand P, et al. Different organic acid patterns in urine and in cerebrospinal fluid in a patient with biotinidase deficiency. J Inher Metab Dis 1984;7;119–120.

60. Vesely DL. Biotin enhances guanylate cyclase activity. Science 1982;216:1329–1330.

61. Sander JE, Malamud N, Cowan MJ, et al. Intermittent ataxia and immunodeficiency with multiple carboxylase deficiency: a biotin-responsive disorder. Ann Neurol 1980;8:544–547.

62. Paul PK. Effect of nutrient toxicities in animals and man: biotin. In Rechcigl M, ed. Handbook of nutrition and food. Boca Raton, Fla.: CRC Press, 1978:47–58.

63. Packman S, Golbus MS, Cowan MJ, et al. Prenatal treatment of biotin-responsive multiple carboxylase deficiency. Lancet 1982;1:1435–1438.

64. Roth KS. Prenatal treatment of multiple carboxylase deficiency. Ann NY Acad Sci 1985;447:263–270.

65. Roth KS, Allan L, Yang W, et al. Serum and urinary biotin levels during treatment of holocarboxylase synthetase deficiency. Clin Chim Acta 1981;109:337–340.

66. Wolf B, Heard GS, Jefferson LG, et al. Clinical findings in four children with biotinidase deficiency detected through a statewide neonatal screening program. N Engl J Med 1985;313:16–19.

Chapter 18
Cerebrotendinous Xanthomatosis

JAMES R. SCHIMSCHOCK

Cerebrotendinous xanthomatosis, while not strictly a neurocutaneous disease, is a unique disorder in which remote biochemical mischief produces progressively devastating effects upon the nervous system. Simultaneously with the development of these nervous system lesions, prominent tendon xanthomas develop, affording early students of this disease a convenient but unique name for the disorder. Recently, biochemical insight into this disorder has uncovered a surprising series of consequences of this enzyme deficiency in bile metabolism that reminds one of the progressive calamities which followed a missing horseshoe nail in the famous allegory about lost kingdoms.

History

In the dark turbulent years prior to World War II, van Bogaert, Scherer, and Epstein published an extensive monograph meticulously describing a progressive, eventually fatal, neurologic disorder beginning with ataxia, dementia, and subsequent spasticity in a male who also exhibited large tendon xanthomas and cataracts [1]. This original exhaustive monograph, published in 1937, described similar but less severe clinical findings in an affected but otherwise healthy female paternal cousin. Extensive descriptions of the postmortem findings in the first case were presented. Multiple xanthomas were found in the brain, particularly in the cerebellum, and in the lung, tendons, and bone. Subsequently, a few additional case reports appeared in the world literature, but these consisted of new case descriptions, and no significantly new pathologic information about this disease appeared until the biochemical

characterization of this disorder was reported by Menkes et al. in 1968 [2].

In the two cases reported by Menkes et al., normal serum cholesterol levels and the selective tissue accumulation of cholestanol, a cholesterol metabolite, gave this disease a biologic profile [2]. In the following year Philippart and van Bogaert affirmed the presence of cholestanol in tissues from the first patient described in van Bogaert's original monograph as well as in serum from the second patient who was still living at the time of their report. They proposed that an elevated serum cholestanol level provided the basis for an accurate diagnosis during the patient's lifetime [3]. The disease appeared to be an autosomally inherited disorder of cholestanol metabolism presumably due to a cellular defect in cholesterol metabolism as proposed by Menkes. However, as will be discussed later, the cause of this rare disease probably stems from events distant from the nervous system.

Clinical Symptoms and Prognosis

This unique disease with its unusual association of progressive neurologic disorder, pulmonary insufficiency, tendon xanthomas, cataracts, and xanthelasma seems at first to be an improbable collage of unrelated lesions. The early neurologic symptoms of insidious development can be those of dementia. Alternatively, mental retardation is often present early in the course of the disease; however, affected adults with normal intelligence have been reported [4]. Ataxia and long tract signs have been reported frequently in adolescents and young adults. Progressive spasticity and ataxia leading to incapacitation characterize the third and fourth decades of the patient's life. The symptoms of the final stages of this relentlessly progressive disease include tremor, long tract motor and sensory deficits, and pseudobulbar palsy ending with death.

The tendon xanthomas usually appear in the second decade. The Achilles-tendon xanthomas are typical of the disease (Figure 18.1), but have been absent in four cases [5]. Tendon xanthomas have been found on tibial tuberosities, finger extensor tendons, and in the triceps, and may be indistinguishable from those seen in familial hypercholesterolemia. Palpebral xanthelasma may also be present.

The cataracts encountered in this disorder are described as zonular cortical lens cataracts [6]. They ordinarily appear in the second decade and frequently require removal in early adulthood.

This disease is unquestionably an autosomal recessive disorder. Berginer and Abeliovich have described a series of six patients from families who are Sephardic Jews of Moroccan origin [7]. They concluded that these families represented an ethnic subgroup with a high cerebrotendinous xanthomatosis gene frequency, estimated to be 1 in 108. Although the remaining cases in the world's literature are of multiracial origin, the majority are Caucasian.

Laboratory Studies

The diagnosis of cerebrotendinous xanthomatosis should be considered in any young person developing cataracts and xanthoma, since these findings may precede the neurologic manifestations of this disease. Elevated serum cholestanol levels are the major diagnostic laboratory finding. Reported values from affected individuals range from 1.3 to 15 mg/dl, 3 to 20 times the reported normal mean levels for serum cholestanol. Serum cholesterol levels are typically normal as are serum triglyceride levels. Low or normal range plasma cholesterol levels in individuals with cataracts and tendon xanthomas with or without neurologic signs mandates the determination of cholestanol levels according to the method of Salen et al. [8]. In individuals with normal lipid levels or hyperlipidemia, cholestanol does not exceed 1 mg/dl. Higher values should suggest the diagnosis of cerebrotendinous xanthomatosis. Biliary cholestanol is also elevated in this condition, and biliary chenodeoxycholic acid is very low. Other laboratory studies are nonspecific. Motor nerve conduction velocities may reveal nonspecific slowing, and nerve biopsy shows marked loss of myelinated axons and large amounts of cholestanol [9]. The diagnosis truly rests upon a high index of suspicion in those observing persons with early-onset tendon xanthomas and cataracts, or childhood ataxia and dementia with either xanthomas or cataracts.

Cerebrotendinous xanthomatosis is not the only disease in which prominent tendon xanthomas occur. Individuals with hypercholesterolemia, sitosterolemia, and eosinophilic granuloma may exhibit large tendon xanthomas and cutaneous xanthomata [10]. However, cerebrotendinous xanthomatosis is distinguished by its neurologic symptomatology.

Figure 18.1. Large, firm distal Achilles-tendon xanthomas.

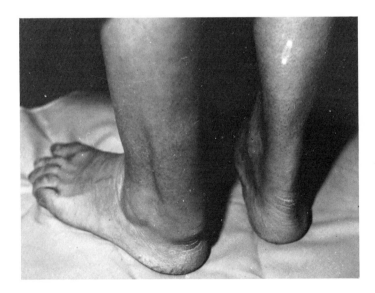

Radiology and Other Imaging

Computed tomography studies reveal diffuse areas of white matter hypodensity above and below the tentorium [11]. A recently reported magnetic resonance imaging scan in an affected individual showed an abnormally high intensity signal from periventricular white matter, suggesting demyelination [12]. Magnetic resonance imaging appears to detect the demyelinating changes in the brain before they are evident with CT. Radiographs of the extremities may show the xanthomas within the tendons.

Biochemistry

In 1973, Salen and Grundy reported decreased bile acid production in patients with this disease and further documented increased serum cholestanol levels in an increasing cohort of individuals with cerebrotendinous xanthomatosis [13]. It became apparent that markedly decreased amounts of chenodeoxycholic acid, a bile acid, was a unique and consistent finding in these individuals. The primary defect appears to be in the bile acid synthesis, which results in increased neutral sterol production in the liver and subsequent deposition of those sterols in certain tissues, including brain, tendons, lung, and bone. Defective bile acid synthesis due to an enzymatic block in the distal steps of the process of converting cholesterol to bile acids results in incomplete oxidation of the cholesterol side chain. Oftebro et al. presented evidence that a mitochondrial cholesterol side-chain oxidation 26-hydroxylase defect causes accumulating substrate to be converted to bile alcohols and cholic acid by a microsomal 25-hydrolylase cholesterol side-chain oxidation pathway [14]. This pathway is far less efficient than the usual preferred mitochondrial oxidation system, accounting for the low levels of cholic acid found in affected individuals. An alternative explanation by Salen et al. proposes that the defect is that of cholesterol side-chain 24-S-hydroxylase in the mitochondrial system. He and his coworkers have also demonstrated elevated bile alcohols and other bile acid precursors in the serum of individuals with cerebrotendinous xanthomatosis [8].

The absence of chenodeoxycholic acid apparently deprives hepatic systems producing neutral sterols of a negative feedback system to modulate neutral sterol production. Elaborate isotope kinetic techniques have demonstrated elevated cholesterol and cholestanol synthesis in individuals with cerebrotendinous xanthomatoses [15]. This increased amount of cholesterol and cholestanol then accumulates in certain tissues having been transported to them by low-density lipoproteins that carry both cholesterol and cholestanol nonpreferentially. The removal of these hepatic-produced sterols from body tissues is effected by high-density lipoproteins. Recent work by Shore et al. suggests that these high-density lipoproteins are defective in individuals with cerebrotendinous xanthomatosis, and in fact, transport cholesterol less efficiently than normal [16]. These abnormalities of high-density lipoproteins are not yet understood but may be linked to the genetic defect in bile acid synthesis. Cholesterol and cholestanol generally seem to be transported with equal efficiency by this system but with higher concentrations of cholestanol retained in the brain, tendons, and bile where it is found in concentrations of 10 to 40% of the total sterol content as opposed to a 1 to 3% concentration in red cells and plasma lipoproteins. According to Shore's explanation, decreased selective tissue sterol efflux could be related to defective high-density lipoproteins. The functions of these lipoproteins include the transport of cholesterol and cholestanol from peripheral tissues to the liver as well as the control of low-density lipoprotein sterol tissue uptake by modulating the binding of low-density lipoproteins to membrane receptor sites and transendothelial sterol transport. Defective high-density lipoproteins may explain the sequestration of these sterols in certain tissues.

While these insights into the kinetics of sterol transport have greatly advanced our understanding of this rare disorder, recent attention to cellular sterol production has indicated that we may not be able to attribute this disease solely to the mischief created by defective chenodeoxycholic metabolism. Recent work by Barron et al. has shown increased cholestanol production in fourth passage fibroblasts cultured from the skin of an individual with cerebrotendinous xanthomatosis, suggesting de novo tissue production of cholestanol in affected individuals. The work of Barron et al. raises the possibility that a biochemical defect in tissue might exist in cholestanol metabolism [17], as postulated by Menkes et al. when the biochemical profile of this disease was first elaborated [2].

Pathology

The pathologic findings in this disease are, as one might expect, most elaborately demonstrated in the nervous system and tendons and, in varying degrees, in other organ systems. In the nervous system, the cerebellum typically shows extensive white matter lesions that have a granulomatous cystic appearance

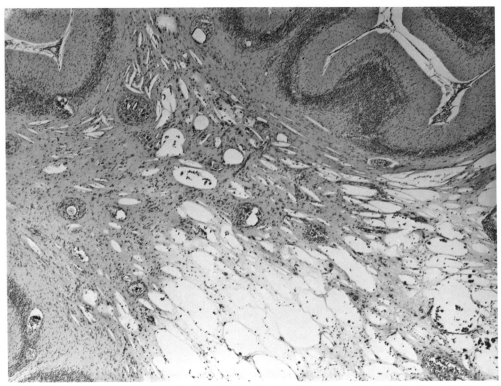

Figure 18.2. A low-power photomicrograph of cerebellum showing white matter disruption by the needle-shaped cleft and areas of necrosis. (Courtesy of P. D. Swanson.)

with microscopically apparent needle-like clefts (Figure 18.2). Microscopic examination reveals large mononuclear cells surrounding cystic spaces and needle-shaped clefts that are birefringent to polarized light. Oil Red O staining of frozen sections shows abundant quantities of fat around blood vessels and in the cystic spaces.

The cerebral hemispheres exhibit similar, though less extensive, areas of demyelination as well as perivascular collections of mononuclear cells. Similar findings have been reported in the spinal cord. In peripheral nerves, axonal degeneration and regeneration are typically present. Achilles tendons are grossly enlarged with distal tendon thickening (Figure 18.1). Microscopic examination shows birefringent crystalline clefts surrounded by multinucleated giant cells with foamy cytoplasm. These xanthomata contain large amounts of cholestanol, but cholesterol accounts for 90% of their total sterol content. Granulomatous lesions have been found in lung and bone. Like those found in the brain, these lesions contain the multinucleated giant cells and foamy appearing cells that surround crystalline clefts. Hepatocytes containing light golden brown pigmentation have

been seen in the liver on low magnification light microscopy. Electron microscopy showed diffuse amorphous electron dense material enveloped by free-floating endoplasmic reticulum or free-floating bodies in the cytosol.

Treatment

Treatment of this condition with chenodeoxycholic acid has been recently shown to arrest and in some cases reverse the progress of the disease. On the basis of the biochemical understanding of the disease treatment has been proposed by Berginer et al. [18]. These investigators have given subjects replacement chenodeoxycholic acid by oral administration of 750 mg per day. Salen recently reported promising results in 17 affected individuals who had received long-term treatment (several years) with this regimen. While tendon xanthomas and cataracts did not disappear, all these patients exhibited some degree of improvement ranging from arrested progress of the disease to measurable improvement in neurologic symptomatology. All individuals showed reduced plasma cholestanol levels. However, not all patients have responded to treatment, as recently reported cases seem refractory to therapy [12,19].

This disease has been extensively studied in the course of one generation and while rare, it is not an entity to be considered a neurologic museum piece. As a consequence of Salen's singularly determined efforts to illuminate the mechanisms of this extremely unusual syndrome, in which mischief in the hepatic biliary system is reflected in distant, apparently passively involved tissues, including those of the brain and tendons, the biochemical profile of this disorder has been identified and treatment proposed. While the disease is not truly neurocutaneous in the sense that it is truly of ectodermal origin, the neurologist is in a unique position to appreciate and diagnose this disorder that is now treatable—unlike most of the other neurocutaneous syndromes. The thoughtful clinician should include this rare disorder in the assessment of individuals with tendon xanthomas, cataracts, and neurologic symptoms.

References

1. Van Bogaert L, Scherer HJ, Epstein E. Une forme cérébrale de la cérébrotendineuse xanthomatosis généralisée. Paris: Masson et Cie, 1937.
2. Menkes JH, Schimschock JR, Swanson PD. Cerebrotendinous xanthomatosis: the storage of cholestanol within the nervous system. Arch Neurol 1968;19:47–53.
3. Philippart M, van Bogaert L. Cholestanolosis (cerebrotendinous xanthomatosis): a followup study on the original family. Arch Neurol 1969;21:603–610.
4. Salen, G. Cholestanol reposition in cerebrotendinous xanthomatosis: a possible mechanism. Ann Intern Med 1971;75:843–851.
5. Salen G, Shefer V, Berginer V. Familial diseases with storage of sterols other than cholesterol: cerebrotendinous xanthomatosis, sitosterolemia with xanthomatosis. In: Stanbury JB, Wyngaarden JB, Fredrickson DS, et al., eds. The metabolic basis of inherited disease. 5th ed. New York: McGraw–Hill, 1983:713–730.
6. Seland J, Slagovold JE. The ultrastructure of lens and iris in cerebrotendinous xanthomatosis. Acta Ophthalmol 1977;55:201–207.
7. Berginer V, Abeliovich D. Genetics of cerebrotendinous xanthomatosis (CTX): an autosomal recessive trait with high gene frequency in Sephardim of Moroccan origin. Am J Med Genet 1981;10:151–157.
8. Salen G, Shefer S, Cheng FW, et al. Cholic acid biosynthesis: the enzymatic defect in cerebrotendinous xanthomatosis. J Clin Invest 1979;63:38–44.
9. Katz D, Scheinberg L, Horoupian D. Peripheral neuropathy in cerebrotendinous xanthomatosis. Arch Neurol 1984;42:1008–1010.
10. de Yong JGY, van Gent CM, Delleman JW. Cerebrotendinous xanthomatosis in relation to other cerebral xanthomatoses. Clin Neurol Neurosurg 1977;79:253–272.
11. Berginer V, Berginer J, Salen G, et al. Computed tomography in cerebrotendinous xanthomatosis. Neurology 1981;31:1463–1465.
12. Swanson PD, Cromwell LD. Magnetic resonance imaging in cerebrotendinous xanthomatosis. Neurology 1986;36:124–126.
13. Salen G, Grundy S. The metabolism of cholestanol, cholesterol and bile acids in cerebrotendinous xanthomatosis. J Clin Invest 1973;52:2822–2835.
14. Oftebro H, Bjorkhem I, Stirmer FC, et al. Cerebrotendinous xanthomatosis: defective liver mitochondrial hydroxylation of chenodeoxycholic acid precursors. J Lipid Res 1981;22:632–640.
15. Setoguchi T, Salen G, Tint GS, et al. A biochemical abnormality in cerebrotendinous xanthomatosis: impairment of bile acid synthesis associated with incomplete degradation of the cholesterol side chain. J Clin Invest 1974;53:1393–1401.
16. Shore V, Salen G, Cheng FW, et al. Abnormal high density lipoproteins in cerebrotendinous xanthomatosis. J Clin Invest 1981;68:1295–1304.
17. Barron JL, Maxwell JU, Rutherford GS. Cerebrotendinous xanthomatosis: a defect in cellular sterol biosynthetic control. J Inher Metab Dis 1982;5:91–93.
18. Berginer V, Salen G, Shefer S. Long term treatment of cerebrotendinous xanthomatosis with chenodeoxycholic acid. N Engl J Med 1984;311:1649–1652.
19. Hinman RC. Cerebrotendinous xanthomatosis in Hawaii: a therapeutic failure. Hawaii Med J 1984;43:472–473, 477–478.

Chapter 19
Familial Dysautonomia

FELICIA B. AXELROD and JOHN PEARSON

Familial dysautonomia is the most extensively described of the disorders known as congenital sensory neuropathies [1]. In the original report of familial dysautonomia by Riley and Day in 1949 [2], the disorder was called central autonomic dysfunction with defective lacrimation. Over the past 35 years, knowledge of the disorder has expanded so that genetic transmission has been studied [3,4], diagnostic tests have been devised [5–7], and consistent pathologic findings have been described [8]. In addition, treatment programs, resulting in improved survival, have developed [9].

Two statistical studies of cases in North America [3] and in Israel [4] estimate the incidence of disease frequency in Ashkenazi Jews to be 1 in 10,000 to 1 in 20,000. This extrapolates to a carrier rate of 1 in 50, closely approximating that of Tay-Sachs disease in the same population. Rare reports of non-Jewish cases [1,10,11] have appeared but probably represent other types of congenital sensory neuropathies. Although these cases are phenotypically very similar, our own experience indicates subtle differences, and we assume they involve different genetic abnormalities.

Clinical Symptoms

Although the major known anatomic abnormality in familial dysautonomia is due to anatomic depletion of sensory and autonomic neurons [8], it is the clinical manifestations that are the concern of the treating physician. The widespread influence of the autonomic nervous system results in protean functional abnormalities best described for clinical management purposes in a systems-oriented approach (Table 19.1). Even when using this approach, one cannot completely isolate the cause of all symptoms since one system dysfunction has repercussions on another.

Signs of the disorder are present from birth, and neurologic function exhibits a slow and variable deterioration with age such that symptoms and problems alter with time [12,13].

Gastrointestinal

Gastrointestinal problems are among the earliest symptoms [12]. Oropharyngeal incoordination results in a poor to absent suck reflex that impedes feeding and proper nutrition and results in slow weight gain and growth. Aspiration due to misdirected swallows leads to recurrent pneumonias. If not treated early, bronchiectasis, atelectasis, and even lung abscesses will develop as will eventual decreased pulmonary function and chronic hypoxemia. Gastroesophageal reflux [14] occurs in approximately 67% of patients and can further increase the risk of aspiration or can result in hematemesis. Vomiting crises associated with irritability, negativistic behavior, hypertension, tachycardia, blotchy erythema of skin, and diaphoresis occur in 40% of patients [13]. If a patient has this problem, the crises usually start by 3 years of age. They can occur as often as weekly and can last for days.

Respiratory

Pneumonias can be difficult to diagnose due to the paucity of clinical signs [15]. Fever is not always present, and tachypnea is rarely seen as the patients do not respond normally to hypoxia and hypercapnic states [16,17]. Lethargy, anorexia, and respiratory congestion may be the only initial signs. Breath-holding to the point of cyanosis, syncope, and decerebrate posturing are fairly common from 15 months to 6 years of age [13]. We have seen these

200

Table 19.1. Clinical Symptoms in Familial Dysautonomia

System	Symptom	Complications
Gastrointestinal	Oropharyngeal incoordination	Aspiration pneumonias
	Gastroesophageal reflux	Difficulty feeding
	Episodic vomiting	Poor nutrition, slow weight gain and growth
		Hematemesis
Respiratory	Aspiration pneumonias	Bronchiectasis, atelectasis
	Insensitivity to hypoxia and hypercapnea	Syncope at high altitudes
		Hypoxemia
Orthopedic	Unrecognized fractures	Bony deformities
	Kyphoscoliosis	Decreased pulmonary function
	Aseptic necrosis	Short stature
	Charcot joints	
Ophthalmologic	Decreased tearing	Keratitis
	Corneal hypoesthesia	Decreased blink frequency
		Corneal ulceration
	Optic atrophy	Myopia
	Muscular imbalance	Strabismus
Dermatologic	Excessive sweating	Excessive fluid loss
	Blotching	
	Hypersecretion of oil glands	Seborrhea
		Cradle cap, excessive cerumen
Vascular	Postural hypotension	Weakness, micturition syncope
	Peripheral vasoconstriction	Cold hand and feet, cutis marmorata
	Episodic hypertension	
Renal	Azotemia	Renal insufficiency and failure
	Ischemic-type glomerulosclerosis	
Neurologic	Insensitivity to pain	Self-injury
	Insensitivity to heat	Unrecognized burns
	Motor incoordination	Ataxic gait
	Hypotonia	Delayed developmental milestones

episodes increase during times of fatigue or increased respiratory congestion.

Orthopedic

There is a high incidence of juvenile scoliosis in familial dysautonomia [12,18,19]. Spinal curvature will develop in 95% of patients by 16 years of age. Left thoracic curves occur more frequently than in idiopathic scoliosis. In addition to contributing to short stature, kyphoscoliosis causes restrictive chest deformities that further compromise pulmonary function.

Decreased pain sensitivity results in unrecognized injuries including fractures. Aseptic necrosis and Charcot joints have been observed [19,20].

Ophthalmologic

Lack of overflow or emotional tearing is one of the cardinal signs of the disorder [1,2,12]. When evalu-

ating this sign, it should be recalled that alacrima may be normal up to 10 months of age. Baseline or reflex tearing varies among patients, which may explain why some patients require less use of topical eye lubricants. Affected individuals will vary also in degree of corneal hypoesthesia, which influences blink frequency. Corneal deepithelialization, ulceration, and scarring with opacification often occur.

Dermatologic

The skin manifestations of this disorder are a direct reflection of the neurologic deficit. Decreased temperature and pain appreciation result in unrecognized burns and injuries. In 15% of infants with this disorder incessant rubbing of the tongue against the saw-edged surface of newly erupting teeth causes tongue ulcers with granulomatous edges [12]. Autonomic dysfunction results in erythematous blotching of the skin during eating or emotional excitement, predominantly on the face, neck, chest, and upper arms. Emotional excitement can cause profuse sweating over the head and trunk but spares the hands and feet. We have noted excessive sweating in many patients during the initial phases of sleep. Only a few patients will have gustatory sweating and then it tends to be limited to the bridge of the nose and forehead. Among our patients, hypersecretion of oil glands on the scalp and eyebrows has resulted in seborrhea and persistence of "cradle cap" well into the teen and adult years.

Vascular

Poor peripheral perfusion as well as supersensitivity to intermittent surges of catecholamines results in mottling of extremities. Cutis marmorata and cold, red hands and feet are particularly prominent in infants. In older patients, dependent extremities will show signs of venous stasis.

Vascular problems become more debilitating with age as problems of postural hypotension become more apparent [12]. Lightheadedness, weakness, blurred vision, and even micturition syncope can limit function. Yet with excitement or brief exertion, blood pressures can quickly rise to hypertensive ranges.

Renal

Progressive diminution of renal function with age is a frequent observation [21]. Prerenal azotemia is an early sign and more likely to be noted in the patient whose fluid intake is inadequate. Creatinine clearance decreases and many individuals have subnormal renin excretion. Renal failure has occurred and resulted in the demise of some patients. Renal biopsies and autopsies have revealed ischemic-type glomerulosclerosis and tubular atrophy. The cause of these pathologic lesions is unknown but may be due to autonomic denervation, resulting in poor vascular control.

Nocturnal enuresis persisting into the teen years is not unusual, and overflow incontinence has been observed [12]. Obstructive uropathy from neurogenic incompetence has not been reported.

Neurologic

Overall, these patients have normal intelligence with a general tendency for better verbal than motor performance [22]. Motor and coordination problems are the primary cause of the commonly delayed developmental milestones. Walking begins beyond 18

months of age in 68%, and only 25% have intelligible speech by the age of 3½ years [12].

Epileptiform discharges in the electroencephalograms have been reported [12]. Seizures simulating decerebrate posturing can follow breath-holding spells even in children whose encephalograms are normal.

Endocrine

Somatic growth is usually poor. Sexual maturity is commonly delayed in both males and females, but primary and secondary sexual characteristics eventually develop in both sexes. Fertility has been demonstrated in both males (Axelrod FB: personal observations 1982) and females [23].

Physical Findings

The penetrance of the genetic disorder varies such that the clinical picture and severity of symptoms differ widely among individuals and in any one individual with age. The most consistent physical findings are found on neurologic assessment and aid in diagnosis.

Neurologic

Physical findings on neurologic examination demonstrate both sensory and autonomic dysfunction as well as incoordination. Varying degrees of hypotonia that contribute to a delay in motor milestones will be noted in the infant and young child. In the ambulatory individual, the gait is often broad based and mildly ataxic, causing special difficulties when performing rapid movements or turning. Many of our patients walk listing forward with a compensatory increased stiffness in shoulders and neck that leads to protracted shoulders. In the adult, the ataxic gait is often more pronounced. Oral incoordination causes feeding problems and dysarthria [12]. Characteristically, the speech is hypernasal and dysarthric.

Decreased sensation to pain is demonstrated by dampened response to pin prick. The hypoalgesia is *not* universal and spares the hands, soles of feet, the neck, and genital areas. Lower extremities are more affected than the upper ones, and older individuals have greater losses than do the younger patients. Temperature appreciation is also less on the trunk and lower extremities. The patellar and corneal reflexes are depressed. Progressive sensory deficits develop in the older individual; vibration sense and joint position are reduced and Romberg sign may be noted [13].

Absent fungiform papillae [5] containing gustatory receptors indicate a defect in the sensory neurons with cell bodies in the geniculate ganglion. Fungiform papillae normally are concentrated toward the tip of the tongue. To the naked eye, they appear as pinhead-sized red projections interspersed among the gray-white filiform papillae. The red color results from their being highly vascularized. In the dysautonomic patient, the fungiform papillae are sparse and rudimentary (Figure 19.1) so that the tongue often appears smooth and pale.

Autonomic dysfunction becomes apparent during the examination, especially if the child is agitated; excessive sweating and blotching may be noted. Distal vasoconstriction in the peripheral skin causes cutis marmorata accompanied by hypertension and tachycardia. Blood pressures are often in the hyper-

tensive range when the patient is in the supine position, especially in adult patients, but postural hypotension occurs without compensatory tachycardia when the standing position is assumed.

Ophthalmologic

Examination of the eye also reveals neurologic dysfunction. Alacrima or lack of overflow tears is very unusual in the normal infant after the first few months of life and is almost always present in the dysautonomic. It is one of the useful diagnostic criteria [7,12]. History is usually sufficient to document this finding but semiquantitation of the deficiency can be obtained by the Schirmer filter paper test or by trying to provoke tearing, emotionally or with an irritant. Corneal hypoesthesia not only results in absent corneal reflexes but decreased blinking frequency and

Figure 19.1. (A) The tip of the tongue of a normal child. The dark spots are blood vessels seen through the clear epithelium of the fungiform papillae. (B) In familial dysautonomia the tongue appears relatively smooth, and there are no fungiform papillae.

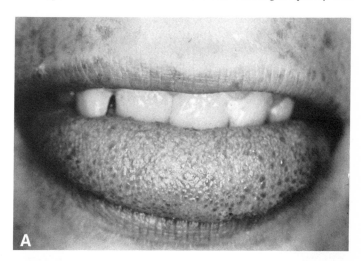

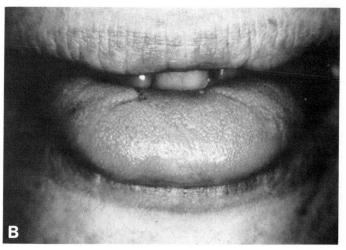

contributes to the common staring, wide-eyed expression. The neurotrophic abnormalities are compounded by undetected trauma and exposure that contribute to frequent keratitis and corneal ulceration. Early signs of keratitis can be detected by fluorescein stain. Other common findings are myopia, exotropia, and optic nerve pallor. Pupillary reaction to accommodation and light adaptation is intact [24].

Dermatologic

In addition to the skin's autonomic instability, another manifestation of poor peripheral perfusion is dystrophic nails. Insensitive skin can result in decubiti and unrecognized bruises and burns. Healing is normal. Hypersecretion of oil glands, causing excessive cerumen in ear canals and seborrhea, is frequently noted.

Orthopedic

Spinal curvature is a frequent finding and contributes to the short stature of patients with this disorder. Average heights and weights are more than two standard deviations below normal third percentiles [12]. The degree of scoliosis [18] varies considerably, from mild curves to severe deformities. The forward list and protracted shoulders are early signs of kyphosis.

Diagnosis

As a specific biochemical abnormality has not yet been described for familial dysautonomia, diagnosis relies on clinical criteria (Table 19.2). The diagnosis should be suspected by history and physical examination, which can provide much of the essential information. Confirmation is then obtained by performing the tests described below.

Histamine Test

In the normal individual, the intradermal injection of histamine phosphate 1:10,000 produces pain and local erythema. This is followed, within minutes, by the development of a central wheal surrounded by the axon flare [25], a diffuse poorly demarcated zone of erythema that is best appreciated 15 minutes postinjection (Figure 19.2). The flare is usually sustained for over 30 minutes and slowly resolves as peripheral

Table 19.2. Diagnostic Criteria for Familial Dysautonomia

Signs of sensory dysfunction
    Absence of fungiform papillae on the tongue
    Absence of flare after intradermal histamine
    Decreased or absent deep tendon reflexes
    Decreased or absent corneal reflexes
    Decreased response to pain and temperature
Signs of autonomic dysfunction
    Absence of overflow tears
    Miosis following intraocular administration of dilute
        2.5% methacholine or 0.0625% pilocarpine
    Postural hypotension
    Blotching
    Increased sweating

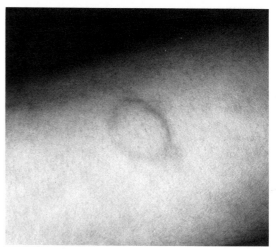

Figure 19.2. Shown is response to intradermal histamine in a dysautonomic subject. The normally diffuse axon flare that should surround the wheal is replaced by a thin areola with sharply demarcated margins.

pallor invades the central erythema. Although the initial local area of erythema is noted in the dysautonomic patient [6], the pain is not appreciated, and the flare does not appear. The central wheal is surrounded only by a narrow violaceous areola that is sharply demarcated.

Methacholine Test

The instillation of 2.5% methacholine or 0.0625% pilocarpine, which has no observable effect on the normal pupil, causes miosis in almost all patients with familial dysautonomia [7]. First, both pupils are carefully examined for symmetry, and then the dilute parasympathomimetic agent is instilled in one eye with the other serving as a control. The pupils are compared at 5-minute intervals over a 30-minute period. At least 20 minutes will pass before miosis appears.

The combination of the five cardinal criteria, that is, alacrima, absent fungiform papillae, depressed patellar reflexes, abnormal histamine test, and an abnormal methacholine test in an individual of Ashkenazi Jewish extraction is usually sufficient to make the diagnosis [12]. Other criteria, listed in Table 19.2, can be used for confirmation. Further supportive evidence of autonomic dysfunction may be seen on cinesophagrams [26,27], which may reveal delay in cricopharyngeal closure, tertiary contractions of the esophagus, gastroesophageal reflux, and delayed gastric emptying. Sural nerve biopsy is rarely required unless one of the five cardinal criteria is not present, or the patient is not of Jewish extraction.

Pathology and Pathogenesis

Pathologically familial dysautonomia is a congenital developmental disorder onto which a prolonged degenerative process is superimposed. A common causative deficiency, which affects both production and maintenance of neurons in this autosomal recessive condition, is likely to be found [28]. Trophic factors, their receptors, or the associated intracellular responder systems are hypothetical explanations. The known lesions of autonomic, skeletal muscle motor and sensory neurons provide a structural basis for many of the biochemical and clinical features of the disease and help distinguish it from syndromes that are closely related phenotypically; however, they leave unexplained the dysfunctions of the higher central nervous system that are prominent in some patients.

Severe depletion of sensory neurons [29], including some that contain the putative neurotransmitter peptide substance P [30], which is thought to be involved in pain pathways [31,32], accounts for the marked, but incomplete, blunting of pain sensitivity and the more profound loss of temperature sensitivity observed in familial dysautonomia. The loss of axons that conduct pain information leads in turn to the development of Charcot joints and skin ulceration. Loss of sensory neurons, which continues into adulthood, along with accumulation of degenerative nodules in dorsal root and trigeminal ganglia and associated progressive loss of myelinated axons from spinal cord dorsal columns, provides a basis for the diminution of proprioception observed with aging in

familial dysautonomia. Since taste buds wither in the absence of their corresponding sensory nerves, atrophy of fungiform lingual papillae in familial dysautonomia [33] can be explained by the severe sensory neuron depletion in the geniculate ganglion.

Marked diminutions of sympathetic ganglia neurons [34] and their vascular terminals [35] provide an explanation for the postural hypotension that is a prominent feature of familial dysautonomia. Sympathetic dysfunction with vasodilation also accounts for the characteristic blotchy erythema. Renal sympathetic denervation may produce hemodynamic changes that precipitate the commonly seen progressive glomerulosclerosis [21]. Extreme depletion of parasympathetic sphenopalatine ganglion neurons [36] causes the lack of overflow tears. Some autonomic reflexes may have anatomically abnormal sensory components, evidenced by the degenerative changes observed in the vagal sensory nodose ganglion.

Ganglionic neuronal losses are indicated by changes in the axon distribution of the sensory sural nerve [37,38]. While this is not the place to discuss the pathology of the spectrum of developmental disorders of the sensory nervous system, it is worth noting that the disease which most closely mimics familial dysautonomia clinically is associated with a distinctive sural nerve pathology [1]. The disease, which we have termed "congenital autonomic dysfunction with universal pain loss" has all the clinical features of familial dysautonomia, but loss of pain is total and the facial bones are abnormally prominent; the sural nerve shows severe loss of myelinated axons and large numbers of unmyelinated fibers persist, whereas in familial dysautonomia, by contrast, myelinated axons are relatively well preserved, and unmyelinated axons are markedly depleted [1].

The pharmacologic anomalies are, to a large extent, attributable to anatomic defects in the peripheral nervous system. Thus the abnormally low proportion of urinary catecholamine metabolites attributable to norepinephrine catabolism [39], and the severe blunting of the norepinephrine surge in the blood that should normally occur on standing [40], can be accounted for by severe depletion of the norepinephrinergic peripheral sympathetic neurons. Denervation supersensitivity is the cause of the anomalous and exaggerated hypertension and tachycardia that result when low doses of sympathomimetic agents are infused [41]. This sympathetic denervation also accounts for the lack of appropriate reflex tachycardia in response to hypotension [42] and the blunting of renin secretion on standing [43]. The parasympathetic denervation supersensitivity associated with sphenopalatine neuron loss [36] causes the return of tearing seen with dilute, normally subthreshold, levels of infused cholinomimetics [42], but, since the ciliary ganglion is little affected [36], such denervation cannot account for the anomalous sensitivity of the pupil to topical mecholyl [7]. Normal responses to light and accommodation [24] confirm that the cholinergic innervation of the pupil is intact. It has been suggested that the abraded cornea may be unduly permeable to conjunctively instilled mecholyl. The ability of cholinomimetics to restore tendon reflexes may rest in the supersensitivity of denervated muscle spindles that result from gamma motoneuron loss [44].

The morphologically and functionally intact adrenal gland provides a pathway that allows the abnormally intense responses to stress to release catecholamines into the blood stream where they act on supersensitive blood vessels. Unless adrenal metabolism is abnormal, however, the adrenal gland cannot be thought of as the source of the very high levels of dopamine detected in some dysautonomic crises. That the vomiting and hypertension associated with the crises respond to diazepam and chlorpromazine therapy suggests that dopaminergic neurotransmission, probably central in location, may be abnormal in familial dysautonomia.

The absence or severe depletion of the sensory neurons that contain the vasodilator peptide substance P [30] is an anatomic basis for the lack of axon-reflex flare that accompanies the intradermal infusion of histamine.

The observation in one patient of diminished numbers of the spinal-cord gamma motoneurons that drive muscle spindles [44] provides a possible basis for the hypotonia, the shuffling, forward-leaning gait, and the difficulty in making rapid movements that are observed in patients with familial dysautonomia. A motor dysfunction of intrafusal skeletal muscle fibers may well be the cause of the depressed tendon reflexes, since the large myelinated axons of the type that subserve tendon and spindle proprioceptive afferent conduction are not markedly diminished in young patients. Furthermore, tendon reflexes return when cholinomimetic agents are infused, which, given current knowledge, do not seem likely to affect sensory neurons.

Nevertheless, a spindle dysfunction cannot account for the imbalance of ocular muscles and the frequent strabismus that occurs in many patients with this disorder and which would seem to indicate higher central nervous system disease. Similarly, although the esophagogastric uncoordination and delayed cricopharyngeal closure, the tertiary esophageal contractions, and the delayed gastric emptying might be caused in some part by sensory dysfunction, it is possible that neurons forming the efferent component of the vagus in the medulla are involved. Certainly the vomiting crises, which respond to diazepam and chloral hydrate therapy, must involve a central nervous system dysfunction. The sweating that can be observed on the nasal bridge and forehead of some patients while eating also suggests anomalous central reflex control, which may involve the nucleus of the tractus solitarius and related structures. Abnormal control of the medullary salivary nuclei is evidenced by sialorrhea which, in some patients, increases with advancing age. Anomalies of peripheral chemoreceptors could be involved in the decreased responses of patients to hypoxia and hypercapnia, but the deficit, which may be so profound that it can cause death at high altitudes or permit a child to willfully suspend breathing until unconscious, suggests that medullary autonomic centers are involved. The diaphoresis that occurs with emotion and early sleep suggests that not only are the cholinergic sudomotor sympathetic neurons which control most of the skin spared, but also that the central systems which govern the appropriate sweating responses are malfunctioning. This abnormality of centrally controlled responses is also evidenced by the excessive hypertension, tachycardia, and peripheral cutis marmorata that may occur in response to excitement and which may require that chlorpromazine also be given to control vomiting crises. The absence of fever during infection suggests hypothalmic dysfunction.

Thus far no structural central nervous system anomalies have been determined, but with the advent of methods for immunocytochemical detection of neurotransmitter-specific neurons in human tissue and of computer-assisted methods for their enumeration, it is possible that anatomic defects will be detected. Increasing evidence for the role in the central nervous system of trophic factors and their receptors, notably for nerve growth factor, which is known to be required for the development and to some extent the maintenance of many of the neural crest neurons affected in familial dysautonomia, suggests that a single, peripherally and centrally acting deficit may be involved in producing the entire range of clinical effects in this disorder [28,45].

Treatment

The disease process cannot be arrested. Treatment is preventive, symptomatic, and supportive [12,46] and must be directed toward specific problems, which vary considerably among patients and at different ages.

Oropharyngeal incoordination is compensated for

with various maneuvers to improve feeding and nutrition and to avoid aspiration. If the use of thickened formula and different nipples is ineffective, then gastrostomy may be necessary. In those patients with gastroesophageal reflux, medical management is tried first but if pneumonia, hematemesis, or apnea persist, then the surgical procedure of fundoplication is required [14,47]. Vomiting crises [28] have been managed most effectively with a combination of intravenous or rectally administered diazepam (0.2 mg/kg q3hr) and chloral hydrate suppositories (30 mg/kg q6hr) and the prevention of dehydration and aspiration. Chlorpromazine is used only when hypertension is refractory to the above treatment.

Respiratory problems are avoided when gastrointestinal dysfunction is well managed. For those individuals who already have had pneumonia and who have developed chronic lung disease, daily chest physiotherapy, which consists of nebulization, bronchodilators, and postural drainage, is recommended [15]. Suctioning is often required in the individual who has an ineffective cough. Breath-holding episodes are usually self-limited and decrease in frequency as the child matures.

An annual spinal examination allows early diagnosis of scoliosis and permits appropriate institution of brace and exercise therapy [18], the latter of which is helpful in correcting or preventing secondary contractures in shoulders and hips. Extreme care is required in fitting braces as decubiti may develop on the insensitive skin at pressure points. Braces may also inhibit respiratory excursion and may induce gastroesophageal reflux if there is a high epigastric projection. If rapid progression of the spinal curve or severe curvature is present at the time of first examination, spinal fusion is recommended.

The regular use of artificial tear solutions containing methylcellulose and the maintenance of normal body hydration have contributed to the decreasing number of corneal complications. Artificial tears [12] are instilled three to six times daily, depending on the child's own baseline eye moisture, environmental conditions, and whether the child is febrile or dehydrated. Moisture chamber spectacle attachments help to maintain eye moisture and to protect the eye from wind and foreign bodies. Tarsorrhaphy has been reserved for unresponsive and chronic situations. Soft contact lenses also help to promote corneal healing. Corneal transplants have had limited success.

Postural hypotension is treated with attention to adequate hydration monitored by serum blood urea nitrogen levels. Exercise to increase lower extremity muscle tone and to promote venous return is encouraged. Elastic stocking and Florinef (fludrocortisone, a mineralocorticoid) have also been of some benefit in our experience.

Prognosis

Dysautonomia can no longer be considered only a disease of childhood. Greater understanding of the disorder and the development of treatment programs have markedly improved survival statistics [18] such that an increasing number of patients are reaching adulthood. Despite physical and emotional developmental lags, intelligence is normal, and many of the adults are able to function independently. Some patients have even married and produced phenotypically normal offspring, despite their obligatory heterozygous state.

Causes of death are still predominantly pulmonary, indicating that more aggressive treatment is still needed in this area. Another large group has succumbed to unexplained deaths, which may have been the result of unopposed vagal stimulation. A few adult patients have died of renal failure.

References

1. Axelrod FB, Pearson J. Congenital sensory neuropathies: diagnostic distinction from familial dysautonomia. Am J Dis Child 1984;138:947–954.
2. Riley CM, Day RL, Greeley D McL, et al. Central autonomic dysfunction with defective lacrimation: report of five cases. Pediatrics 1949;3:468–477.
3. Brunt PW, McKusick VA. Familial dysautonomia: a report of genetic and clinical studies with a review of the literature. Medicine 1970;49:343–374.
4. Moses SW, Rotem Y, Jogoda N, et al. A clinical, genetic and biochemical study of familial dysautonomia in Israel. Isr J Med Sci 1967;3:358–371.
5. Smith AA, Farbman A, Dancis J. Absence of taste buds in familial dysautonomia. Science 1965;147:1040–1041.
6. Smith AA, Dancis J. Response to intradermal histamine in familial dysautonomia: a diagnostic sign. J Pediatr 1963;64:889–894.
7. Smith AA, Dancis J, Brienen G. Ocular responses to autonomic drugs in familial dysautonomia. Invest Ophthalmol 1965;4:358–361.
8. Pearson J, Axelrod FB, Dancis J. Current concepts of dysautonomia: neuropathological defects. Ann NY Acad Sci 1974;228:288–300.
9. Axelrod FB, Abularrage JJ. Familial dysautonomia: a prospective study of survival. J Pediatr 1982;101:234–236.
10. Levine SL, Maniello RL, Farel PM. Familial dysautonomia: unusual presentation in an infant of non-Jewish ancestry. J Pediatr 1977;90:78–81.

11. Orbeck H, Oftedal G. Familial dysautonomia in a non-Jewish child. Acta Paediatr Scand 1977;66:777–781.

12. Axelrod FB, Nachtigall R, Dancis J. Familial dysautonomia: diagnosis, pathogenesis and management. In: Schulman I, ed. Advances in pediatrics. Chicago: Year Book Medical Publishers, 1974;21:75–96.

13. Axelrod FB, Iyer K, Fish I, et al. Progressive sensory loss in familial dysautonomia. Pediatrics 1981;67:517–522.

14. Axelrod FB, Schneider KM, Ament ME, et al. Gastroesophageal fundoplication and gastrostomy in familial dysautonomia. Ann Surg 1982;195:253–258.

15. Axelrod FB. Familial dysautonomia. In: Kendig E, Chernick V, eds. Disorders of the respiratory tract in children. Philadelphia: Saunders, 1983;4:872–876.

16. Filler J, Smith AA, Stone S, et al. Respiratory control in familial dysautonomia. J Pediatr 1965;66:509–516.

17. Edelman NH, Cherniack NS, Lahiri S, et al. The effects of abnormal sympathetic nervous function upon the ventilatory response to hypoxia. J Clin Invest 1970;41:1153–1165.

18. Levine DB. Orthopedic aspects of familial dysautonomia. In: Zorab PA, ed. Scoliosis and muscle. London: Spastics International Medical Publishers, 1974;143–150.

19. Yoslow W, Becker M, Bartels J, et al. Orthopedic defects in familial dysautonomia: a review of 65 cases. J Bone Joint Surg 1971;53A:1541–1550.

20. Mitnick JS, Axelrod FB, Genieser NB, et al. Aseptic necrosis in familial dysautonomia. Radiology 1982;142:89–91.

21. Pearson J, Gallo G, Gluck M, et al. Renal disease in familial dysautonomia. Kidney Int 1980;17:102–112.

22. Welton W, Clayson D, Axelrod FB, et al. Intellectual development and familial dysautonomia. Pediatrics 1979;63:708–712.

23. Porges RF, Axelrod FB, Richards M. Pregnancy in familial dysautonomia. Am J Obstet Gynecol 1978;132:485–488.

24. Korczyn AD, Rubenstein AE, Yahr MD, et al. The pupil in familial dysautonomia. Neurology 1981;31:628–629.

25. Thomas LT. The blood vessels of the human skin and their responses. London: Shaw & Sons, 1927.

26. Margulies SI, Brunt PW, Donner MW, et al. Familial dysautonomia: a cineradiographic study of the swallowing mechanism. Radiology 1968;90:107–112.

27. Gyepes M, Linde L. Familial dysautonomia: the mechanism of aspiration. Radiology 1968;91:471–475.

28. Pearson J. Developmental neurobiology of human disease: familial dysautonomia and related diseases. In: Blach IB, ed. Cellular and molecular biology of neuronal development. New York: Plenum, 1984:341–354.

29. Pearson J, Pytel B, Grover-Johnson N, et al. Quantitative studies of dorsal root ganglia and neuropathological observations on spinal cords in familial dysautonomia. J Neurol Sci 1978;35:77–92.

30. Pearson J, Brandeis L, Cuello AC. Depletion of substance P-containing axons in substantia gelatinosa of patients with diminished pain sensitivity. Nature 1982;295:61–63.

31. Henry J. Relation of substance P to pain transmission: neurophysiological evidence. In: Porter R, O'Connor M, eds. Substance P in the nervous system (Ciba Foundation Symposium). London: Pitman, 1982:206–224.

32. Lembeck F, Gamse R. Substance P in peripheral sensory processes. In: Porter R, O'Connor M, eds. Substance P in the nervous system (Ciba Foundation Symposium). London: Pitman, 1982:35–48.

33. Pearson J, Finegold M, Budzilovich G. The tongue and taste in familial dysautonomia. Pediatrics 1970;45:739–745.

34. Pearson J, Pytel B. Quantitative studies of sympathetic ganglia and spinal cord. Intermedio-lateral gray columns in familial dysautonomia. J Neurol Sci 1978;39:47–59.

35. Grover-Johnson N, Pearson J. Deficient vascular innervation in familial dysautonomia: an explanation for vasomotor instability. Neuropathol Appl Neurobiol 1976;2:217–224.

36. Pearson J, Pytel B. Quantitative studies of ciliary and sphenopalatine ganglia in familial dysautonomia. J Neurol Sci 1978;39:123–130.

37. Aguayo AJ, Nair CPV, Bray GM. Peripheral nerve abnormalities in the Riley–Day syndrome: findings in a sural nerve biopsy. Arch Neurol 1971;24:106–116.

38. Pearson J, Dancis J, Axelrod F, et al. The sural nerve in familial dysautonomia. J Neuropathol Exp Neurol 1974;34:413–424.

39. Goodall G, Gitlow S, Alton H. Decreased noradrenaline synthesis in familial dysautonomia. J Clin Invest 1971;50:2734–2740.

40. Ziegler M, Lake R, Kopin I. Deficient sympathetic nervous response in familial dysautonomia. N Engl J Med 1976;294:630–633.

41. Smith AA, Dancis J. Exaggerated response to infused norepinephrine in familial dysautonomia. N Engl J Med 1964;270:704–707.

42. Smith A, Hirsch J, Dancis J. Responses to infused metacholine in familial dysautonomia. Pediatrics 1969;36:225–230.

43. Rabinowitz D, Landau H, Rosler A, et al. Plasma renin activity and aldosterone in familial dysautonomia. Metabolism 1974;23:1–5.

44. Kawamura Y, Dyck PJ, Low PA, et al. The number and sizes of reconstructed peripheral autonomic, sensory and motoneurons in a case of dysautonomia. J Neuropathol Exp Neurol 1978;37:741–755.

45. Pearson J. Familial dysautonomia: a brief review. J Autonom Nerv Syst 1979;1:119–126.

46. Axelrod FB. Familial dysautonomia. In: Gellis SC, Kagan BM, eds. Current pediatric therapy. Philadelphia: Saunders, 1984;11:81–83.

47. Axelrod FB, Maayan C, Hazzi C, et al. Case report: bradycardia associated with hiatal hernia and gastroesophageal reflux relieved by surgery. Am J of Gastroenterology 1987;82:159–161.

Chapter 20
Chediak–Higashi Syndrome

PHILIP VAN HALE

The Chediak–Higashi syndrome is a rare lethal autosomal recessive syndrome characterized by partial oculocutaneous albinism, photophobia, nystagmus, neurologic deficit, recurrent pyogenic infections, and gigantism of cytoplasmic organelles associated with immunologic and coagulation deficits. The disorder ultimately evolves into a phase characterized by widespread tissue infiltration by lymphohistiocytic cells. Death usually occurs at an early age from infection, bleeding, or possibly by malignant transformation.

Historical Background

Beguez-Cesar first reported 3 cases of the syndrome in 1943 [1]. Steinbrick reported 1 case in 1948 [2]. In 1952 Chediak [3] reported 4 cases in 13 Cuban siblings, and in 1954 Higashi [4] described 4 cases in 7 Japanese siblings. In these cases the parents were related; however, subsequent cases have not necessarily involved related parents. No sex linkage has been demonstrated. The eponym Chediak–Higashi syndrome was first used by Sato in 1955 [5]. The 59 cases reported in the world literature as of 1972 were reviewed by Blume and Wolff [6]. Numerous animal models for the disorder have been studied and reported [7], and various culture systems have been employed to study affected cells [8,9]. The genetic and biochemical basis for the disorder remains elusive in spite of the multiple functional and cytologic defects described. A defect in membrane fluidity is present in association with lysosomal abnormalities that ultimately affects leukocyte, pigment cell, neural, platelet, and other cellular functions [10–13].

Clinical Presentation

Clinically, the Chediak–Higashi syndrome may become manifest by fever, failure to thrive, recurrent infection, neurologic or ophthalmologic symptoms, or bleeding. Febrile episodes are generally caused by infection, which may include orbital cellulitis, pharyngitis, sinusitis, otitis media, bronchitis, bronchopneumonia, subcutaneous abscess, or cellulitis [5,6,14–16]. The skin may be susceptible to hyperhidrosis and severe sunburns [14]. Postinfection atrophic scars or areas of cutaneous ulceration may be present [17]. Photophobia, squint, nystagmus, sensory deficit [15,18], or gait ataxia may be present [14,15]. Headaches or emotional lability may occur, occasionally in a setting of mental retardation. Bruising, gastrointestinal bleeding, or epistaxis may be present, although this usually heralds the more accelerated phase of the syndrome.

Patients with Chediak–Higashi syndrome have a partial oculocutaneous albinism. This pigment dilution, which involves the skin, hair, and eyes, is secondary to the aggregation of melanin into giant melanosomes [6,19]. The skin is a slate gray color [17], and the hair has a silvery tint with a silken sheen [20]. Mild exposure to sunlight may result in burning. Recurrent pyogenic infections in the lower extremities may resemble pyoderma gangrenosum. Ophthalmoscopic examination may reveal pale irides and fundi due to decreased iridian and retinal pigmentation, although ocular bulb transillumination will show that some pigment is present in the iris [21]. Papilledema is rarely observed. Decreased lacrimation when crying has been reported [14].

Peripheral neuropathy is manifested by paresthesia, transitory pareses, and sensory deficit of the glove-stocking type [15,18,20]. It may begin early in childhood and progress to complete loss of muscle stretch reflexes, weakness, atrophy, and sensory deficits. Ataxia with a broad-based gait and dysdiadochokinesia, seizures, and behavioral abnormalities also occur. The patient may become bedridden and totally incapacitated. Hepatosplenomegaly and lymphoadenopathies are characteristic of the disease. Visceral involvement caused by lymphohistiocytic cellular infiltration may include, in the accelerated phase of the disease, in addition to the liver and spleen, the kidneys, the aorta, and the adrenal glands [6]. Other features of this disease are hemolytic anemia, neutropenia, and life-threatening thrombocytopenia.

Diagnosis

Diagnosis is based on demonstration of abnormal giant granulations in affected cells combined with partial albinism, a history of infection, and in the more advanced cases, hepatosplenomegaly and pancytopenia. Giant granulation is usually demonstrated in granulocytes or monocytes on a peripheral blood smear (Figure 20.1) or in the bone marrow [6]. A ring-shaped lysosome may be seen in circulating monocytes [22]. Lysosomal abnormalities have been described in a wide variety of hematopoietic and extrahematopoietic cell lines, including granulocytes, monocytes, megakaryocytes, platelets, fibroblasts, melanocytes, neurons, type II pneumonocytes, hepatocytes, renal tubular cells, and the chief and parietal cells of the gastric glands [12,23,24]. Granulocytes show multiple inclusion bodies in myelo-

cytes and in the more differentiated cells, which are Sudan black-positive, peroxidase-positive (Figure 20.2), and PAS-negative. The abnormal granules in Chediak–Higashi neutrophils have been shown to contain both azurophilic markers (myeloperoxidase, elastase, and cathepsin G) and specific granule markers (lactoferrin, lysozyme) within the abnormal granules, suggesting a membrane abnormality or a defect of microtubular function leading to inappropriate granule fusion [25]. Granule fusion is related to cell maturation, and many giant granules are believed to undergo transformation to secondary lysosomes, incapable of degranulation and variable in the intensity of their cytochemical reactivity [26]. In addition to their other defects, the large granules are believed to interfere with cellular locomotion on a mechanical basis. Pelger-Huët changes have occasionally been seen [17,27]. Giant granules resembling the Chediak–Higashi abnormality and termed the pseudo-Chediak–Higashi anomaly, have been described in granulocytic precursors in acute granulocytic leukemia, acute myelomonocytic leukemia, and in a case of evolving myelodysplastic syndrome [28–33]. Eosinophils also demonstrate enlarged granules, especially in the accelerated phase. In the nonaccelerated phase serum immunoglobulin levels, complement levels, and cutaneous sensitization are usually normal [20]. Prolonged bleeding times, abnormal platelet aggregation, and a defect of platelet storage granules may be seen [34,35]. Studies of such patients support the existence of a marked deficiency in the storage pool of platelet adenine nucleotides. Abnormal leukocyte migration has been demonstrated both in vivo and in vitro [20]. Peripheral blood subpopulations of lymphocytes are affected heterogeneously by the Chediak–Higashi abnormality. Al-

Figure 20.1. Chediak–Higashi leukocytes and large granules demonstrated by Wright's stain on peripheral smear. (From: Maguire R, Selle J, Beju D. Chediak–Higashi Disease. American Society of Clinical Pathologists, Check Sample (H 81-9) 1981:9. With permission.)

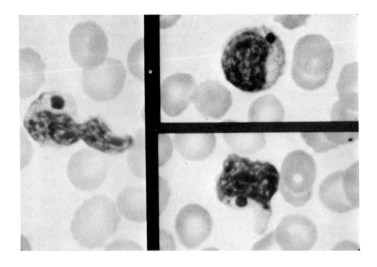

Figure 20.2. Large peroxidase-positive granules in bone marrow of patient with pseudo-Chediak—Higashi syndrome.

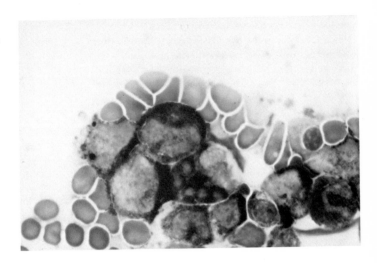

though antibody-dependent cell-mediated cytotoxicity and natural killer function seem impaired [36–41], some T-cell functions such as mitogen responses and lectin-induced cytotoxicity may be within normal limits [42]. The lysosomal defect is expressed as lysosomal fusion in B-lymphocytes after activation and differentiation. Similar abnormalities are seen in granular lymphocytes with surface markers characteristic of natural killer cell lineage. The Chediak—Higashi abnormality has not been noted in non-natural killer target-binding lymphocytes with T-cell markers, and no T-cell functional abnormality has been demonstrated in Chediak—Higashi patients [43].

Scattered neurologic function abnormalities are characteristic of the Chediak—Higashi syndrome, the most common of these being peripheral neuropathy [6]. Giant lysosomes are present in the cytoplasm of the Schwann cells of myelinated peripheral nerve axons. Histologic studies support the association between peripheral neuropathy and the cellular infiltrates of the accelerated phase of the syndrome [44,45]. In the Blume and Wolff review, mental retardation appeared to be independent of other neurologic involvement and was thought to be related to the high incidence of consanguineous marriages in the affected patient population [6]. Cerebrospinal fluid studies show a slight pleocytosis with minimally elevated protein levels. Electroencephalographic study may reveal generalized background dysrhythmia without focal abnormalities. Reduced rates of nerve conduction with a myopathic pattern may be seen on electromyography. Denervation atrophy may be seen on muscle biopsy [6]. Neurologic abnormalities, in Blume's review, were thought to best correlate with infiltrative lesions associated with the accelerated phase.

Natural History and Treatment

Recurrent infections in the Chediak—Higashi patient reportedly respond to appropriate antimicrobial therapy. However, prophylactic antibiotics such as cloxacillin have not been proven to be of benefit in preventing infection in such patients [20,46]. Ascorbic acid in high doses (200 mg/day in infants and 6 g/day in adults) has been suggested as being of some value in preventing infection [47], and studies in the beige mouse animal model of the disease have shown significant protection from a *Candida albicans* challenge [48]; however, in vivo and in vitro studies have not shown such therapy to improve immune defenses of adult humans [48]. Cholinergic agonists have been reported to be effective in correcting characteristic abnormalities of granule morphology and microtubule function [49]. Cholinergic agonists apparently were associated with decreased quantities of abnormal granules in affected monocytes. Likewise, certain aspects of Chediak—Higashi leukocyte dysfunction have been reported to be improved by cyclic guanosine monophosphate [50]. The practical utility of such therapy in a clinical setting remains unclear. The onset of the accelerated phase may occur at any age and may be correlated with rising liver function tests, new problems with hemostasis, pancytopenia, abnormalities in cellular immunity, and infections unresponsive to antibiotics. Vincristine and glucocorticoid therapy have been used in such circumstances and although, paradoxically, improvement in a peripheral neuropathy was noted in one case (transiently), the efficacy of such therapy remains to be established [6]. Although some references have referred to the accelerated phase of the disease as a neoplastic process, the bulk of the cases described have revealed a reactive process [6,51–53]. The exact etiology of the accelerated phase of the syndrome is unknown; however, several reports have suggested a possible association with a recent viral infection. Virus-like particles have been described in the leukocytes of two patients in the accelerated phase, based on electron microscopic studies [54]. High titers to Epstein–Barr viral (EBV) capsid antigen and EBV-associated nuclear antigens have also been described in isolated cases [55]. Recently Rubin et al. and Risdall et al. have proposed that the accelerated phase of the Chediak–Higashi syndrome may actually represent one form of the virus associated hemophagocytic syndrome [56,57]. Nonetheless, definitive proof of a causative agent responsible for the accelerated phase remains to be established. Bone marrow transplantation may offer the best hope for correcting the immunologic defects in the Chediak–Higashi syndrome [58,59].

References

1. Beguez-Cesar A. Neutropenia crónica maligna familar con granulaciones atípicas de los leucocitos. Bol Soc Cuban Pediatr 1943;15:900–922.
2. Steinbrinck W. Über eine neue Granulations-anomalie der Leukocyten. Dtsch Arch Klin Med 1948;193:577–581.
3. Chediak M. Nouvelle anomalie leucocytaire de caractère constitutionnel et familial. Rev Hematol 1952; 7:362–367.
4. Higashi O. Congenital gigantism of peroxidase granules: first case ever reported of qualitative abnormality of peroxidase. Tohoku J Exp Med 1954;59:315–332.
5. Sato A. Chediak and Higashi's disease. Probable identity of "new leucocytal anomaly (Chediak)" and "congenital gigantism of peroxidase granules (Higashi)." Tohoku J Exp Med 1955;61:201–210.
6. Blume RS, Wolff SW. The Chediak–Higashi syndrome: studies in four patients and a review of the literature. Medicine 1972;51:247–280.
7. Prieur DJ, Collier LL. Animal model: the Chediak–Higashi syndrome of animals. Am J Pathol 1978; 90:533–536.
8. Newburger PE, Speier C, Stock JL, et al. Chediak–Higashi syndrome: studies in long term bone marrow culture. Exp Hematol 1985;13:117–122.
9. Ostlund RE, Tucker RW, Leung JT, et al. The cytoskeleton in Chediak–Higashi syndrome fibroblasts. Blood 1980;56:806–811.
10. Haak RA, Ingraham LM, Balfhner RL, et al. Membrane fluidity in human and mouse Chediak–Higashi leukocytes. J Clin Invest 1979;64:138–144.
11. Oliver JM. Cell biology of leukocyte abnormalities membrane and cytoskeletal function in normal and defective cells: a review. Am J Pathol 1978;93:221–270.

12. Spicer SS, Sato A, Vincent R, et al. Lysosomal enlargement in the Chediak–Higashi syndrome. Fed Proc 1981;40:1451–1455.
13. Rendu F, Breton-Gorius J, Lebret M, et al. Evidence that abnormal platelet functions in human Chediak–Higashi syndrome are the lack of dense bodies. Am J Pathol 1983;111:307–314.
14. Donohue WL, Bain HW. Chediak–Higashi syndrome: a lethal familial disease with anomalous inclusions in the leukocytes and constitutional stigmata: report of a case with necropsy. Pediatrics 1957;20:416–430.
15. Kritzler RA, Terner JY, Lindenbaum J, et al. Chediak–Higashi syndrome: cytologic and serum lipid observations in a case and family. Am J Med 1964;36:583–594.
16. Pagett GA, Reiquam CW, Henson JB, et al. Comparative studies of susceptibility to infection in Chediak–Higashi syndrome. J Pathol Bacteriol 1968;95:509–522.
17. Weary PE, Bender AS. Chediak–Higashi syndrome with severe cutaneous involvement. Arch Intern Med 1967;119:381–386.
18. Lockman LA, Kennedy WR, White JG. The Chediak–Higashi syndrome: electrophysiologic and electron microscopic observations on the peripheral neuropathy. J Pediatr 1967;70:942–951.
19. Windhorst DB, Zelickson AS, Good RA. A human pigmentary dilution based on a heritable subcellular structural defect—the Chediak–Higashi syndrome. J Invest Dermatol 1968;50:9–18.
20. Wolf SM, Dale DC, Clark RA, et al. The Chediak–Higashi syndrome: studies of host defenses (NIH Conference). Ann Intern Med 1972;76:293–306.
21. Witkop CJ, Quevedo WC, Jr, Fitzpatrick TB. Disorders of amino acid metabolism: Chediak–Higashi syndrome. In: Stanbury JB, Wyngaarden JB, Fredrickson DS, et al., eds. The metabolic basis of inherited disease. 5th ed. New York: McGraw–Hill, 1983:324–328.
22. White JG, Clawson CC. Chediak–Higashi syndrome: ring shaped lysosomes in circulating monocytes. Am J Pathol 1979;96:781–798.
23. White JG, Clawson CC. The Chediak–Higashi syndrome: nature of giant neutrophil granules and their interactions with cytoplasm and foreign particulates. Am J Pathol 1980;98:151–196.
24. Parmley RT, Poon M, Crist W, et al. Giant platelet granules in a child with the Chediak–Higashi syndrome. Am J Hematol 1979;6:51–60.
25. Rausch PG, Pryzwansky KB, Spitznagel JK. Immunocytochemical identification of azurophilic and specific granule markers in the giant granules of Chediak–Higashi neutrophils. N Engl J Med 1978;298:693–698.
26. White JG, Clawson CC. Chediak–Higashi syndrome: variable cytochemical reactivity of giant inclusions in polymorphonuclear leukocytes. Ultrastruct Pathol 1980;1:223–236.
27. Saraiva LG, Azevedo M, Correa JM, et al. Anomalous panleukocytic granulation. Blood 1959;14:1112–1127.
28. Van Slyck EJ, Rebuck JW. Pseudo-Chediak–Higashi

anomaly in acute leukemia: a significant morphologic coronary. Am J Clin Pathol 1974;62:673–678.

29. Gorman AM, O'Connel LG. Pseudo-Chediak–Higashi anomaly in acute leukemia. Am J Clin Pathol 1976;65:1030–1031.

30. Tulliez M, Vermat JP, Breton-Gorius J, et al. Pseudo-Chediak–Higashi anomaly in a case of acute myeloid leukemia: electron microscopic studies. Blood 1979; 54:863–871.

31. Efrati P, Nir E, Kaplan H, et al. Pseudo-Chediak–Higashi anomaly in acute leukemia. Acta Hematol 1979;62:264–271.

32. Payne CM, Harrow EJ. A cytochemical and ultrastructural study of acute myelomonocytic leukemia exhibiting the pseudo-Chediak–Higashi anomaly of leukemia and "splinter type" Auer rods. Am J Clin Pathol 1983;80:216–223.

33. Gallardo R, Kronwinkel RN. Pseudo-Chediak–Higashi anomaly. Am J Clin Pathol 1984;83:127–129.

34. Buchanan GR, Handin RI. Platelet function in the Chediak–Higashi syndrome. Blood 1976;47:941–948.

35. Boxer GJ, Holmsen H, Robbin L, et al. Abnormal platelet function in Chediak–Higashi syndrome. Br J Hematol 1977;35:521–533.

36. Haliotis T, Roder J, Klein M, et al. Chediak–Higashi gene in humans. I. Impairment of natural-killer function. J Exp Med 1980;151:1039–1048.

37. Roder JC, Haliotis T, Kleim M, et al. A new immunodeficiency disorder in humans involving NK cells. Nature 1980;284:553–555.

38. Roder JC, Duwe AD. The beige mutation in the mouse selectively impairs natural killer cell function. Nature 1979;278:451–453.

39. Abo T, Roder JC, Abo W, et al. Natural killer (HNK-1+) cells in Chediak–Higashi patients are present in normal numbers but are abnormal in function and morphology. J Clin Invest 1982;70:193–197.

40. Targan SR, Oseas R. The "lazy" NK cells of Chediak–Higashi syndrome. J Immunol 1983;130:2671–2674.

41. Merino F, Klein GO, Henle W, et al. Elevated antibody titers to Epstein–Barr virus and low natural killer cell activity in patients with Chediak–Higashi syndrome. Clin Immunol Immunopathol 1983;27:326–339.

42. Klein M, Roder J, Haliotis T, et al. Chediak–Higashi gene in humans. II. The selectivity of the defect in natural-killer and antibody-dependent cell-mediated cytotoxicity function. J Exp Med 1980;151:1049–1058.

43. Grossi CE, Crist WM, Abo T, et al. Expression of the Chediak–Higashi lysosomal abnormality in human peripheral blood subpopulations. Blood 1985;65:837–844.

44. Sung JH, Okada K. Neuronal inclusions in Aleutian mink: a light and electron microscopic study. J Neuropathol Exp Neurol 1969;28:160–161.

45. Sung JH, Meyers JP, Stadlan EM, et al. Neuropathological changes in Chediak–Higashi disease. J Neuropathol Exp Neurol 1969;28:86–118.

46. Dale DC, Alling DW, Wolff SM. Cloxacillin prophylaxis in the Chediak–Higashi syndrome. J Infect Dis 1972;125:393–397.

47. Boxer LA, Watanabe AM, Rister M, et al. Correction of leukocyte function in Chediak–Higashi syndrome by ascorbate. N Engl J Med 1976;295:1041–1045.

48. Gallin JI, Elin RJ, Hubert RT, et al. Efficacy of ascorbic acid in Chediak–Higashi syndrome (CHS): studies in humans and mice. Blood 1979;53:226–234.

49. Oliver JM, Zurier RB. Correction of characteristic abnormalities of microtubule function and granule morphology in Chediak–Higashi syndrome with cholinergic agonists. J Clin Invest 1976;57:1239–1247.

50. Boxer LA, Rister M, Allen JM, et al. Improvement of Chediak–Higashi leukocyte function by cyclic guanosine monophosphate. Blood 1977;49:9–17.

51. Dent PB, Fish LA, White JG, et al. Chediak–Higashi syndrome: observations on the nature of the associated malignancy. Lab Invest 1966;15:1634–1642.

52. Kruger GRF, Bedoya V, Grimely PM. Lymphoreticular tissue lesions in Steinbrinck–Chediak–Higashi syndrome. Virchows Arch A [Path Anat] 1971;353:273–288.

53. Pagett GA, Reiquam CW, Gorham JR, et al. Comparative studies of the Chediak–Higashi syndrome. Am J Pathol 1967;51:553–571.

54. White JG. Virus-like particle in the peripheral blood cells of two patients with Chediak–Higashi syndrome. Cancer 1966;19:877–884.

55. Merino F. Immunodeficiency to Epstein–Barr virus in Chediak–Higashi syndrome. In: Purtillo DT, ed. Immune deficiency and cancer: Epstein–Barr virus and lymphoproliferative malignancies. New York: Plenum, 1984:143–164.

56. Rubin CM, Burke BA, McKenna RW, et al. The accelerated phase of Chediak–Higashi syndrome: an expression of the virus associated hemophagocytic syndrome. Cancer 1985;56:524–530.

57. Risdall RJ, McKenna RW, Nesbit ME, et al. Virus associated hemophagocytic syndrome: a benign histiocytic proliferation distinct from malignant histiocytosis. Cancer 1979;44:993–1002.

58. Virelizier J, Lagrue A, Durancy A, et al. Reversal of natural killer defect in a patient with Chediak–Higashi syndrome after bone marrow transplantation (letter). N Engl J Med 1982;306:1055–1056.

59. Griscelli C, Virelizier J. Bone marrow transplantation in a patient with Chediak–Higashi syndrome. Birth Defects 1983;19:333–334.

Chapter 21
Neuroichthyosis

RAMON RUIZ-MALDONADO

The term ichthyosis should be reserved for a group of genetically determined alterations of keratinization clinically characterized by persistent, clinically evident scales on the skin surface.

There are various forms of ichthyosis, depending on the mode of inheritance, clinical and pathologic features, and the basic defect involved: (a) autosomal dominant ichthyosis vulgaris (ichthyosis simplex)—incidence 1 in 5,300; (b) X-linked recessive ichthyosis (ichthyosis nigricans)—incidence 1 in 13,500 or 1 in 6,190 males; and (c) autosomal recessive ichthyosis (lamellar ichthyosis, nonbullous ichthyosiform erythroderma)—incidence 1 in 300,000 [1]. Inherited ichthyosis is also part of various complex syndromes.

Ichthyosiform dermatosis is the name applied to a heterogeneous group of skin disorders characterized by different degrees of hyperkeratosis, scaling, and erythema. Lesions with capricious designs are often found in ichthyosiform dermatoses. Most conditions included in this group are separate nosologic entities unrelated to true ichthyosis. They are known as ichthyosiform dermatoses because of their superficial clinical resemblance to true ichthyosis. There is still insufficient knowledge about their nature and nosology. Some ichthyosiform dermatoses are genetically determined and others are acquired.

Neuroichthyosis refers to those conditions associating ichthyosis or ichthyosiform dermatoses to central or peripheral nervous system involvement.

Ichthyosis and Nervous System Involvement

Several well-recognized diseases and a few infrequently reported syndromes strongly support the concept that the association between ichthyosis, ichthyosiform dermatoses, and nervous system pathology is not coincidental. At the National Institute of Pediatrics in Mexico City we retrospectively reviewed 101 genetically determined cases of ichthyosis seen between January 1970 and September 1983. Eighty of the 101 patients were available for neurologic examination. Thirty-five of them (44%) had autosomal recessive lamellar ichthyosis, 25 patients (31%) had X-linked dominant ichthyosis, and 20 patients (25%) had autosomal dominant ichthyosis vulgaris. This large number of patients with lamellar ichthyosis is apparently the result of our institution being a third-level national referral center.

After clinical studies we performed the following examinations on our patients with ichthyosis: psychometrics or developmental assessment, head radiographs, electroencephalogram, audiometry or brain stem auditory evoked responses. Out of 80 patients with ichthyosis, 10 had the Sjögren–Larsson syndrome. In the remaining 70 patients the neurologic symptoms we found included seizures in 5 patients (7.1%) while in the general pediatric population in the same area the percentage was only 4%. Psychometric testing revealed that 45% were subnormal (IQ or DQ under 69). Whether this is genetically determined as part of an ichthyosis-associated disorder or is the consequence of familial or other environmental factors was not determined.

The head radiograph was abnormal in 11% of patients. In two of these patients there was a correlation between the radiologic and the neurologic findings (microcephaly and seizures; agenesis of cochlea and deafness).

Six percent of patients had sensorineural deafness.

A majority of children with ichthyosis (81%) had an abnormal EEG. However, for most of them (63%) there was no correlation between the EEG and the clinical features.

Our findings suggest that patients with ichthyosis are at high risk of having central nervous system involvement.

Ichthyosiform Dermatoses

Table 21.1 summarizes the differential diagnostic features of these disorders. The Sjögren-Larsson syndrome is discussed in Chapter 22, and Refsum's syndrome in Chapter 23.

Rud's Syndrome

Ruds syndrome is inherited as an autosomal recessive trait. As of 1985, only 18 cases of this syndrome, whose main features are ichthyosis and hypogonadism, has been reported [2]. Less constant alterations are hypoplastic teeth and nails, polyneuropathy, sensorineural deafness, and nystagmus. Various degrees of developmental retardation have been observed in almost all patients (Figure 21.1). The histopathologic changes in the skin have not been found consistently. Its pathogenesis remains unknown.

Treatment is directed toward control of the seizures; application of mild keratolytic agents to the skin, such as 20% urea cream, 5% salicylic acid, or 5% lactic acid; and rehabilitation measures in order to improve physical activity.

Brittle Hair, Ichthyosis, and Dwarfism (BID Syndrome)

Only recently described, this syndrome is apparently of autosomal recessive inheritance. Its main clinical features are lamellar-type ichthyosis, dwarfism, microcephaly, abnormal teeth and nails, pili torti and trichoschisis, punctate lenticular cataracts, poor sexual maturation, peculiar facies, and mental retardation [3]. Treatment of the ichthyotic skin requires oral retinoids or keratolytic agents (see Rud's syndrome).

Ichthyosis and Neutral Lipid Storage Disease

This condition is inherited as an autosomal recessive trait. Its substrate is a disorder of lipid metabolism,

Table 21.1. Differential Diagnoses of Main Syndromes of Neuroichthyosis

Syndrome	Inheritance	Underlying Alteration	Usual Type of Ichthyosis	Neurologic Alterations	Mental Retardation	Other Associated Defects
Sjögren–Larsson	Autosomal recessive	Fatty acid metabolism defect	Lamellar	Spasticity, seizures	+	Ocular, dermatoglyphic, osseus, dental
Refsum's	Autosomal recessive	Phytanic acid oxidase deficiency	Vulgaris-like	Peripheral neuropathy, ataxia, sensory alterations	−	Hyposomia, ocular, cardiac, skeletal, cerebrospinal fluid protein increase
Rud's	Autosomal recessive	Unknown	Vulgaris-like	Polyneuropathy, sensorineural deafness, seizures	+	Hypogonadism, short stature
Brittle hair, ichthyosis, dwarfism (BID syndrome)	Autosomal recessive	Unknown	Lamellar	Microcephaly	+	Dwarfism, abnormal hair, teeth, and nails
Keratitis, ichthyosis, deafness (KID syndrome)	Autosomal recessive	Inborn error of glycogen metabolism?	Keratoderma	Sensorineural deafness	−	Hypotrichosis, keratitis, peculiar facies, etc.
Ichthyosis, neutral lipid storage (Williams [4])	Autosomal recessive	Alteration of lipid metabolism	Lamellar	Sensorineural deafness, ataxia	+ −	Cataracts, myopathy, intracellular lipid vacuoles
Tay	Autosomal recessive	Sulfur-containing amino acids defect	Lamellar	Microcephaly, ataxia, spasticity calcification of basal ganglia	+	Progeroid aspect, hypogonadism, cataracts, etc.
Migratory ichthyosis neuro-ocular defects (Zunich [7])	Autosomal recessive?	Unknown	Figurate, migratory	Seizures, cerebral atrophy, conductive hearing loss	+	Retinal colobomas, abnormal dermatoglyphics, etc.

Abbreviations: + = present; − = absent

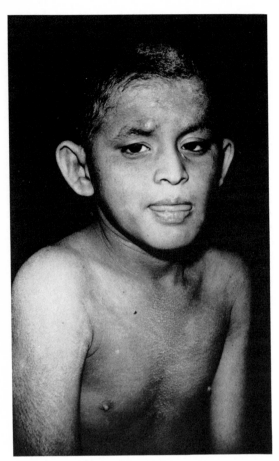

Figure 21.1. Mental retardation and ichthyosis in a patient with Rud's syndrome.

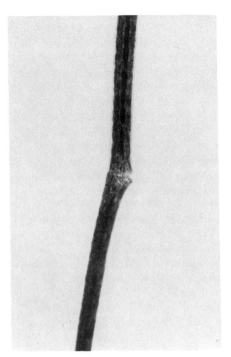

Figure 21.2. Trichorrhexis nodosa-like fracture (trichoschisis) in ichthyosis with trichothiodystrophy or Tay syndrome.

possibly of intracellular fatty acid catabolism. The main clinical features exhibited by patients with this disorder are congenital ichthyosiform erythroderma, sensorineural deafness, cataracts, myopathy, inconstant developmental delay, and prominent cytoplasmic vacuoles in granulocytes and monocytes. Heterozygotes may be detected through the presence of lipid vacuoles within eosinophilic leukocytes [4]. Management of the skin is similar as for Rud's syndrome. Cataracts may be surgically treated.

Tay Syndrome

This unusual ichthyotic syndrome of autosomal recessive inheritance is characterized by pili torti and a tricorrhexis nodosa-like alteration whose substrate is trichothiodystrophy (Figure 21.2). Skin alterations compatible with nonbullous congenital ichthyosiform erythroderma are seen. Hair is extremely brittle. The hair shafts under polarizing light show alternating light and dark banding. Associated clinical features include short stature, abnormal nails, hypoplasia of subcutaneous tissue, prematurely aged facial appearance, hypogonadism, cataracts, osteosclerosis, dysphonia, and increased susceptibility to infection. The neurologic findings are mental retardation, microcephaly, ataxia, limb spasticity, delayed neuromuscular development, and radiographic basal ganglia calcification [5]. No treatment is available for the hair abnormalities. The ichthyosis is controlled as in Rud's syndrome.

Keratitis, Ichthyosis, and Deafness (KID Syndrome)

KID syndrome is apparently inherited as an autosomal recessive trait. That glycogen is stored in various tissues of patients with KID syndrome suggests that this syndrome is caused by a lysosomal enzyme deficiency [6].

Its clinical features are generalized ichthyosiform dermatosis with thickened and hyperkeratotic skin but without the scales characteristic of the ichthyotic disorders; palmar–plantar keratoderma; sparse or absent scalp hair, eyebrows, and eyelashes; dystrophic nails; vascularized keratitis; and sensorineural deafness. Patients with KID syndrome also have a peculiar facies (Figure 21.3). Inconstant findings include short heel cords, hypohidrosis, propensity to skin infections, particularly to *Candida* species, and carcinoma of the tongue. The skin changes respond well to 1 to 2 mg/kg/day of oral etretinate.

Other Syndromes

A syndrome of migratory ichthyosiform dermatosis with neurologic and ocular abnormalities, present since birth, has recently been described. Its main clinical features are sharply demarcated erythematous and scaly plaques that erupt unpredictably, migrate over uninvolved skin, and spontaneously resolve in a period of days to weeks. These lesions are histologically and ultrastructurally different from erythrokeratodermia figurata variabilis. Other features are thickened palms and soles, sparse hair, conduction deafness, retinal colobomas, seizures, severe

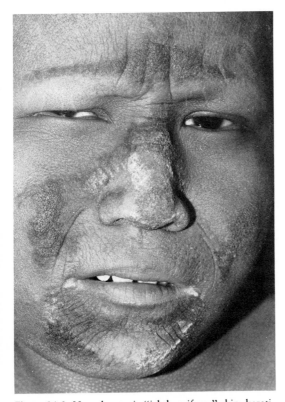

Figure 21.3. Hyperkeratotic "ichthyosiform" skin, keratitis, and alopecia exhibited in a 12-year-old patient with KID syndrome.

mental retardation, cerebral atrophy, and peculiar facies [7].

A syndrome probably inherited as an autosomal recessive trait associates the following features: congenital ichthyosiform skin, neurosensory deafness, mental retardation, dental aplasia, brachydactyly, clinodactyly, accessory cervical ribs, and carcinoma of the thyroid [8].

Atypical erythrokeratodermia variabilis, deafness, peripheral neuropathy, and physical retardation have been described by Beare et al. [9].

Erythrokeratoderma present since infancy in association with slowly progressive severe gait ataxia after the age of 40 in a French Canadian family has been described by Giroux and Barbeau [10].

The association of congenital ichthyosis, hypoplastic teeth, mental retardation, spasticity of all limbs, and renal hypertension in three siblings has been described by Rayner et al. [11].

Reported in two brothers by Dykes et al. [12] was an atypical ichthyosis with desmosomal complexes in the granular cell layer and adjoining corneal cells, progressive ataxia, paresis of upward gaze, dementia, corticospinal tract involvement, cerebellar atrophy, and hepatosplenomegaly. A third affected brother was reported later [13]. The disease is either of X-linked recessive or of autosomal recessive inheritance.

Congenital ichthyosis, dystrophic nails and teeth, dwarfism, mental retardation, and renal impairment have been described by Paswell et al. [13] in three members of an Iranian family.

Cullen et al. [14] described a syndrome the main components of which are congenital ichthyosis, ectromelia, enlargement of the cerebral ventricular system, and mental retardation.

Congenital ichthyosiform erythroderma, deafness, psychomotor retardation, prematurity, and hepatic failure in three patients have been reported by Desmons et al. [15].

A patient with congenital ichthyosis, mental retardation, short stature, and deficient growth hormone has been described by Sibertin–Blanc et al. [16].

Anosmia, ichthyosis, hypogonadism, and various neurologic manifestations with deficiency of steroid sulfatase and arylsulfatase c was the name given by Sunohara et al. [17] to a recently described disease characterized by congenital ichthyosis, hypogonadism, anosmia, nystagmus, decreased vision, strabismus, hypopigmented irides, and mirror movements of hands and feet. The condition seems to be of X-linked recessive inheritance. Steroid sulfatase and arylsulfatase c activity in leukocytes and fibroblasts were markedly diminished in the affected patients.

The association of ichthyosis, thrombocytopenia, myasthenia, miosis, asplenia, migraine, and dyslexia has been recently reported [18].

A new syndrome of anosmia, ichthyosis, and hypogonadism with deficiency of steroid sulfatase and arylsulfatase c has been recently reported by Sunohara, Sakuragawa, Satoyoshi, Tanae, and Shapiro and is described in Chapter 33.

References

1. Wells RS. Clinical features of autosomal dominant and sex linked ichthyosis in an English population. Br Med J 1966;1:947–950.
2. Marxmiller J, Trenkle I, Ashwal S. Rud syndrome revisited: ichthyosis, mental retardation, epilepsy and hypogonadism. Dev Med Child Neurol 1985;27:335–343.
3. Jorizzo JL, Crounse RG, Wheeler CE. Lamellar ichthyosis: dwarfism, mental retardation and hair shaft abnormalities. J Am Acad Dermatol 1980;2:309–317.
4. Williams ML, Koch TK, O'Donnel JJ, et al. Ichthyosis and neutral lipid storage disease. Am J Med Genet 1985;20:711–726.
5. Happle R, Traupe H, Grobe H, et al. The Tay syndrome (congenital ichthyosis with tricothiodystrophy). Eur J Pediatr 1984;142:233–234.
6. Jurecka W, Abreer E, Mainitz M, et al. Keratitis, ichthyosis, and deafness syndrome with glycogen storage. Arch Dermatol 1985;121:799–801.
7. Zunich J, Esterly NB, Holbrook KA, et al. Congenital migratory ichthyosiform dermatosis with neurologic and ophthalmologic abnormalities. Arch Dermatol 1985;121:1149–1156.
8. Ruzicka T, Goerz G, Anton-Lamprecht I. Syndrome of ichthyosis congenita, neurosensory deafness, oligophrenia, dental aplasia, brachydactyly, clinodactyly, accessory cervical ribs and carcinoma of the thyroid. Dermatologica 1981;162:124–136.
9. Beare JM, Froggatt NP, Kernohan DC, et al. Atypical erythrokeratoderma with deafness, physical retardation, and peripheral neuropathy. Br J Dermatol 1982;87:308–311.
10. Giroux JM, Barbeau A. Erythrokeratoderma with ataxia. Arch Dermatol 1972;106:183–188.
11. Rayner A, Lampert RP, Rennert OM. Familial ichthyosis, dwarfism, mental retardation and renal disease. J Pediatr 1978;92:766–768.
12. Dykes PJ, Marks R, Harper PS. Syndrome of ichthyosis, hepatosplenomegaly, and cerebellar degeneration-steroid sulphatase activity. Br J Dermatol 1980; 102:353–354.
13. Paswell JH, Goodman RM, Ziporowski M, et al. Congenital ichthyosis, mental retardation, dwarfism and renal impairment. New syndrome. Clin Genet 1975; 8:59–65.
14. Cullen SI, Harris DF, Carter CH, et al. Congenital unilateral ichthyosiform erythroderma. Arch Dermatol 1969;99:724–729.
15. Desmons F, Bar J, Chevillard Y. Erythrodermie ichthyosiforme congénitale sèche, surdi-mutité, hépatomégalie, de transmission récessive autosomique. Étude d'une famille. Bull Soc Fr Dermatol Syph 1971;78:585–591.
16. Sibertin-Blanc D, Ferrari P, Duche DJ. À propos d'un cas de débilité mentale associé à un retard staturale et à une ichthyose. Rev Neuropsychiatr Infant 1975;23:207–215.
17. Sunohara N, Sakuragawa N, Satoyoshi E, et al. A new syndrome of anosmia, ichthyosis, hypogonadism, and various neurological manifestations with deficiency of steroid sulfatase and arylsulfatase C. Ann Neurol 1986;19:174–181.
18. Stormorken HO, Sjaastad A, Langstet I, et al. A new syndrome: thrombocytopenia, muscle fatigue, asplenia, miosis, migraine, dyslexia and ichthyosis. Clin Genet 1985;314:367–374.

Chapter 22

Sjögren–Larsson Syndrome

ENRIQUE CHAVES-CARBALLO

Mental retardation in combination with congenital ichthyosis and spastic disorders was defined as a distinctive syndrome by Sjögren [1] in 1956 and by Sjögren and Larsson [2] in 1957 (Figure 22.1). Although earlier descriptions [3–7] of the syndrome have been found, the Swedish cohort, consisting of 58 patients among 41 families, remains the largest and most completely studied group [8]. The inheritance pattern, based on nearly complete ascertainment of the Swedish cases, is consistent with autosomal-recessive transmission and almost complete penetrance. More than 200 cases [9] of Sjögren–Larsson syndrome have been reported from 24 countries [8], and several comprehensive reviews [8,10,11] have appeared.

The clinical features (Table 22.1), laboratory and radiologic data, pathologic findings, clinical course, and genetic aspects of Sjögren–Larsson syndrome are reviewed in this chapter.

Clinical Features

Skin involvement is the earliest sign to appear in affected individuals [9]. At birth the skin may be erythematous and later becomes thickened and scaly (congenital nonbullous ichthyosiform erythroderma). The ichthyosis develops to its full extent during infancy. The distribution of the lesions is generalized, with predilection for the neck (Figure 22.2), elbows, and knees, and, to a lesser extent, for the face, hands, and feet. Hair and nails are uninvolved, and the ability to sweat is unaffected [12].

A second cardinal feature of Sjögren–Larsson syndrome is mental retardation. With few exceptions, all patients show evidence of severe intellectual impairment. Intelligence test scores are below 50 in the majority, and the patients are classified as severely mentally retarded [13]. About one-third of

IQ scores are between 50 and 60 [13], and only rarely are scores above 70 [14].

Spasticity is usually manifested as diplegia or tetraplegia between the age of 4 and 30 months [13]. Among 111 cases reviewed by Theile [11], 64 had spastic diplegia or Little's disease, 25 had spastic quadriplegia, 12 had a "stiff gait," and 4 had insufficient information. Contractures eventually develop at the knees, hips, and ankles (Figure 22.3), giving these patients the typical appearance of walking on the tips of their toes [11]. Despite orthopedic treatment with braces and surgery, nearly 75% cease to ambulate without assistance. As expected, deep tendon reflexes are exaggerated, clonus is easily elicited, and plantar responses (Babinski) are extensor.

In addition to the cardinal triad of ichthyosis, mental retardation, and spasticity, patients with Sjögren–Larsson syndrome may develop retinal lesions, speech defects, and seizures.

Sjögren and Larsson [2] found macular degeneration in only 3 of 12 patients examined ophthalmologically. However, subsequent reports suggest that eye involvement may be more common. Among 76 cases reviewed by Theile [11], 38 had normal fundi, 24 had macular degeneration, 15 had "glistening spots," and 9 had retinitis pigmentosa. Jagell et al. [15] examined personally all 35 living Swedish patients with Sjögren–Larsson syndrome and found "glistening dots" in all fundi examined. They concluded that retinal lesions probably originate from early childhood and are stationary. Thus, the presence of retinal glistening spots may become a useful diagnostic finding in Sjögren–Larsson syndrome.

Visual acuity is difficult to measure due to mental retardation and poor cooperation. Nevertheless, this was estimated in 12 patients to be between 0.2 and 0.5, with most at about 0.4 [15]. Other eye findings include myopia, blepharitis and conjunctivitis, cor-

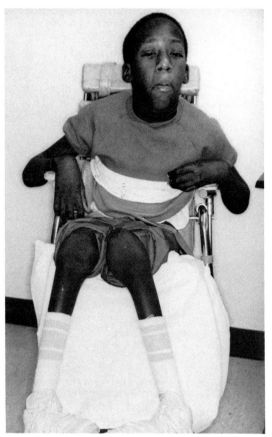

Figure 22.1. A 13-year-old male with ichthyosis, spastic diplegia, and mental retardation consistent with Sjögren–Larsson syndrome.

Table 22.1. Clinical Features in Sjögren–Larsson Syndrome

Main features
  Mental retardation
  Congenital ichthyosis
  Spastic disorders
  Retinal lesions (glistening dots)
Secondary features
  Speech defects
  Seizures
  Kyphosis
  Small stature
  Dental enamel hypoplasia

neal lesions ranging from punctate epithelial erosions to gray stromal opacities with vascularization, and photophobia [15].

According to Sjögren and Larsson [2], speech defects are not uncommon and consist of stammered, single, often incomprehensible syllables. Most patients are able to answer simple questions but only seldom speak of their own accord [11]. It is difficult to determine whether these speech abnormalities are due to intellectual impairment or to a separate neurologic component.

Epileptic seizures occurred in 11 of 35 Swedish patients [13] and in 24 of 40 patients reviewed by Theile [11]. The electroencephalogram is abnormal in the majority of patients with seizures but the findings are nonspecific, usually showing generalized epileptiform activity.

Other secondary features described in some patients include kyphosis, small stature, and dental enamel hypoplasia [16].

Figure 22.2. Congenital ichthyosis (nonbullous ichthyosiform erythroderma) in Sjögren–Larsson syndrome affecting the neck region.

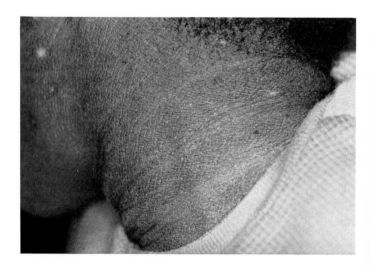

Figure 22.3. Talipes equinovarus due to severe spastic diplegia in Sjögren–Larsson syndrome.

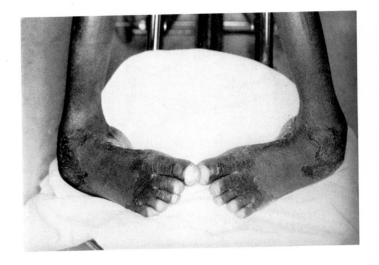

Laboratory and Radiologic Findings

The results of routine blood and urine studies, such as complete blood count, glucose, electrolytes, urea nitrogen, and urinalysis, are usually normal [11]. Serum copper and zinc levels [17], as well as urinary 17-ketosteroids [11], amino acids, and organic acids [18], are unremarkable. Blood amino acid profiles, on the other hand, were abnormal in 26 of 38 patients but without any recognizable pattern [11,19].

Routine radiographic studies of the skull, thorax, spine, pelvis, and extremities are normal except for an occasional finding of kyphosis [11]. Bone age was measured in 19 patients, and only a few had significant delay in skeletal maturation [11].

Neuroradiographic studies have included pneumoencephalography in 12 patients; of these, 7 showed generalized brain atrophy [11]. On the other hand, CT scans have not been helpful [20]. Radionuclide brain scans in 2 patients were normal [11].

Few neurophysiologic studies, with the exception of electroencephalograms, have been reported in Sjögren–Larsson patients. Electromyography in 12 patients detected no abnormality in 7 and was abnormal in 5 [11]. Electroretinograms were normal in 5 patients studied [11]. Brain stem auditory evoked responses showed bilateral prolongation of interwave II–III latency in one patient [21].

Chromosomal analysis showed normal karyotypes in 25 patients [11]. Dermatoglyphic studies in 13 patients showed abnormalities in 2 but without consistency [22].

A defect in fatty acid metabolism has been suspected by several authors. Nevertheless, Hernell et al. [23] found no significant abnormality in the fatty acid composition of plasma phospholipids, cholesterol esters, triglycerides, and free fatty acids. The normal concentration of linolenic acid ($18:2\omega6$) in plasma phospholipids suggests that the disorder does not involve a dietary essential fatty acid deficiency or a defect in the absorption of linolenic acid. However, the metabolites derived from $\Delta6$ desaturation were reduced to 3% of control values. Avigan et al. [24] found the relative concentration of linolenic, eicosatrienoic, and arachidonic acids, as well as the ability of cells to desaturate linoleic acid, to be normal in skin fibroblasts from patients with Sjögren–Larsson syndrome.

Pathology

Pathologic examination of the central nervous system has been reported in few cases and with disparate results. Barr and Galindo [25] found asymmetrical atrophy of the caudate and status marmoratus of the right corpus striatum. Of lesser importance were findings of neuronal loss in the caudate, lentiform nuclei, and hypothalamus, as well as of small patches of demyelination in the frontal lobes along with marked gliosis of central gray and in the cortical–subcortical boundaries. In contrast, Sylvester [26] observed no apparent loss of neurons in the caudate, lentiform nuclei, or hypothalamus. Instead, the number of Betz cells was reduced in the precentral gyrus, and most of those present had shrinkage and condensation of Nissl substance. Considerable loss of myelin and axis cylinders was noted in the centrum semiovale. Astrocytes were increased in number. There was degeneration of the corticospinal and vestibulospinal tracts, and both medullary pyramids showed poor myelin content. Posterior columns, anterior horn cells, and Clarke's column cells were intact. There was a slight loss of Purkinje cells. McLennan et al. [27] found an almost total absence of myelin that resulted in severe, symmetrical atrophy of the cerebrum, brain stem, cerebellum, and spinal cord. Silva et al. [28] found neither neuronal degeneration nor demyelination in the cerebral cortex, internal capsule, basal ganglia, and pons. In the medulla there was diffuse and marked demyelination of the corticospinal tracts. The spinal cord also evidenced demyelination of ascending and descending tracts, including anterior and lateral corticospinal tracts, dorsal funiculi, and spinocerebellar and vestibulospinal tracts. The variability in the neuropathologic findings reported by Sylvester [26], McLennan et al. [27], and Silva et al. [28] may differ more in severity than in type and distribution of lesions, a reflection perhaps of the different ages of patients at the time of study.

The peripheral nervous system was uninvolved in the patients of McLennan et al. [27]. Maia [29] found, in two patients, destruction of axons and vacuolation and fragmentation of myelin sheaths with partial tumefaction of axons (sausage appearance) in sural nerves.

Pathologic examination of the eye has been reported by McLennan et al. [27] in one case. There was a reduction in the number of ganglion cells in the posterior segment, particularly in the section passing through the perimacular area. The number of axons in the retina and optic nerve was reduced, especially at the margin of the optic disc. There was no visible myelin in the optic nerve, and the area of the optic nerve was markedly reduced. No evidence of pigmentary lesion was seen in the macula. The lateral geniculate bodies showed diffuse and marked loss of neurons as well as disruption of the laminar pattern. The parvocellular portions were almost completely depopulated, with some preservation of neurons in the magnicellular portion.

Hofer and Jagell [30] examined histologically the skin of 36 patients with Sjögren–Larsson syndrome. All had moderate to pronounced hyperkeratosis (Figure 22.4). Additional findings not previously emphasized were follicular hyperkeratosis, thickened stratum granulosum, and acanthosis. Papillomatosis was frequently noted. There was also vasodilation and perivascular round cell infiltration. Electron microscopy by Matsuoka et al. [31] showed concentric lamellar membranous figures within cornified cells. These were thought to be remnants of cementosomes (keratinosomes). Large number of mitochondria and prominent Golgi bodies were also apparent in keratinosomes. Increased DNA synthesis of the epidermis and an increased production of horny layer were reported by Jagell and Lidén [12]. Brown et al. [32] found cholesterol sulfate accumulated in the stratum corneum.

Clinical Course and Treatment

The clinical course in patients with Sjögren–Larsson syndrome is one of slow progression leading eventually to impaired ambulation due to spasticity and contractures of the lower extremities. Early physical therapy and orthopedic intervention may prolong functional mobility. Despite vigorous therapy, most patients require braces or wheelchair assistance. Infant stimulation and remedial tutoring may be indicated when the diagnosis is recognized early.

Figure 22.4. Skin biopsy in Sjögren–Larsson syndrome shows thickened stratum corneum (hyperkeratosis), papillomatosis, thickened stratum granulosum, and acanthosis (original magnification × 400).

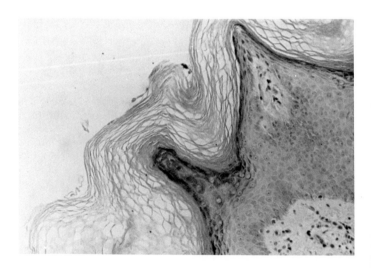

Ichthyosis has been treated with emollients, steroids, vitamins, and various time-honored creams and ointments without significant improvement. Some parents and patients consider ichthyosis to be the most important part of the syndrome because of its constant demand for attention and treatment. More recently, treatment with etretinate, an aromatic retinoid (initial dose 1 mg/kg daily), has yielded encouraging results [33].

Medium-chain triglycerides have been used empirically in four patients [21,34,35]. All experienced reduction in skin dryness and scaliness but neurologic improvement occurred in only two patients [35].

In 13 of 23 Swedish patients the cause of death was respiratory (pneumonia, tuberculosis, whooping cough, and influenza) [8]. The mean age at death was 22 years (15 years for males and 26 years for females). All patients born after 1939 were still alive in 1981; only three patients have died in Sweden during the last 20 years [8].

Epidemiology and Genetics

Genealogical data from relatives, hospitals, parish registers, and county archives allowed for almost complete ascertainment of the Sjögren–Larsson syndrome patients in Sweden, most of whom originated from the northern county of Västerbotten [8]. Sjögren and Larsson [2] calculated the incidence for the period of 1891 to 1959 as 1 in 10,000 births in Västerbotten. For the whole of Sweden, the incidence for the period 1901 to 1977 was 0.6 per 100,000 births (10.2 for Västerbotten) [8]. The prevalence of the syndrome on December 31, 1978, was 0.4 per 100,000 for the Swedish population and 8.3 for the county of Västerbotten. Approximately 1 person in 200 of the Swedish population is a carrier of the Sjögren–Larsson syndrome gene, while in Västerbotten the frequency of gene carriers is 1 in 50. Owing to the marked decline in the death rate of Sjögren–Larsson syndrome patients in Sweden since 1940, prevalence figures would be expected to increase [8].

Witkop and Henry [36] reported the only other population study among the Haliwas of Halifax and Warren counties in North Carolina, an inbred group of Caucasian, black, and American Indian stock. However, most of the infants had normal skin at birth and when ichthyosis appeared between 4 and 8 months of age, it was acral in distribution and mainly involved the hands, shoulders, and trunk. According to Jagell et al. [8], this condition probably represents a different clinicopathologic entity.

Prenatal diagnosis of Sjögren–Larsson syndrome has been accomplished by fetal skin biopsy using fetoscopy at 23 weeks' gestation [37].

References

1. Sjögren T. Oligophrenia combined with congenital ichthyosiform erythrodermia, spastic syndrome and macular-retinal degeneration. A clinical and genetic study. Acta Genet Stat Med 1956;6:80–91.
2. Sjögren T, Larsson T. Oligophrenia in combination with congenital ichthyosis and spastic disorders. A clinical and genetic study. Acta Psychiatr Neurol Scand 1956–1957; (suppl) 113:1–108.
3. Pardo-Castelló V, Faz H. Ichthyosis—Little's disease. Arch Dermatol Syph (Chicago) 1932;26:915.
4. Pisani D, Cacchione A. Frenastenia e dermatosi. Riv Sper Freniat 1935;58:722–736.
5. Laubenthal F. Über einige Sonderformen des "angeborenen Schwachsinns." Z Ges Neurol Psychiatr 1938;163:233–238.
6. Bredmose GV. Et tilfaelde af mongoloid idioti og ichthyosis med neurohistologiske forandringer. Nord Med 1940;5:440–442.
7. Söderhjelm AL, Enel H. Iktyos, spastik diplegi i nedre extremiteterna och oligofreni—ett särskilt syndrom. Nord Med 1957;17:624–625.
8. Jagell S, Gustavson K-H, Holmgren G. Sjögren–Larsson syndrome in Sweden. A clinical, genetic and epidemiological study. Clin Genet 1981;19:233–256.
9. Liden S, Jagell S. The Sjögren–Larsson syndrome. Int J Dermatol 1984;23:247–253.
10. Richards BW. Sjögren–Larsson syndrome. In: Handbook of Neurology. Vinken PJ, Bruyn GW, eds. Amsterdam: North–Holland, 1972;13:468–482.
11. Theile U. Sjögren–Larsson syndrome. Oligophrenia–Ichthyosis–Di/Tetraplegia. Humangenetik 1974;22:91–118.
12. Jagell S, Lidèn S. Ichthyosis in the Sjögren–Larsson syndrome. Clin Genet 1982;21:243–252.
13. Jagell S, Heijbel J. Sjögren–Larsson syndrome: physical and neurological features. A survey of 35 patients. Helv Paediatr Acta 1982;37:519–530.
14. Selmanowitz VJ, Porter MJ. The Sjögren–Larsson syndrome. Am J Med 1967;42:412–422.
15. Jagell S, Polland W, Sandgren O. Specific changes in the fundus typical for the Sjögren–Larsson syndrome. An ophthalmological study of 35 patients. Acta Ophthalmol (Copenh) 1980;58:321–330.
16. Forsberg H, Jagell S, Reuterving CO. Oral conditions in Sjögren–Larsson syndrome. Swed Dent J 1983;7:141–151.
17. Jagell S, Hallmans G, Gustavson K-H. Zinc and copper concentration in serum of patients with congenital ichthyosis, spastic di- or tetraplegia and mental retardation (Sjögren–Larsson syndrome). Upps J Med Sci 1981;86:291–295.

18. Holmgren G, Jagell S, Seeman H, et al. Urinary amino acids and organic acids in the Sjögren–Larsson syndrome. Clin Genet 1981;20:64–66.

19. Ionasescu V, Stegink L, Mueller S, et al. Amino acid abnormality in Sjögren–Larsson syndrome. Arch Neurol 1973;28:197–199.

20. Probst FP, Jagell S, Heijbel J. Cranial CT in the Sjögren–Larsson syndrome. Neuroradiology 1981;21:101–105.

21. Chaves-Carballo E, Frank LM, Bason WM. Treatment of Sjögren–Larsson syndrome with medium-chain triglycerides. Ann Neurol 1981;(abstr.)10:294.

22. Gustavson K-H, Jagell S. Dermatoglyphic patterns in the Sjögren–Larsson syndrome. Clin Genet 1980;17:120–124.

23. Hernell O, Holmgren G, Jagell SF, et al. Suspected faulty essential fatty acid metabolism in Sjögren–Larsson syndrome. Pediatr Res 1982;16:45–49.

24. Avigan J, Campbell BD, Yost DA, et al. Sjögren–Larsson syndrome: Δ5- and Δ6- fatty acid desaturases in skin fibroblasts. Neurology 1985;35:401–403.

25. Barr HS, Galindo J. Pathology of the Sjögren–Larsson syndrome. J Maine Med Assoc 1965;56:223–226.

26. Sylvester PE. Pathological findings in Sjögren–Larsson syndrome. J Ment Defic Res 1969;13:267–275.

27. McLennan JE, Gilles FH, Robb RM. Neuropathological correlation in Sjögren–Larsson syndrome. Oligophrenia, ichthyosis and spasticity. Brain 1974;97:693–708.

28. Silva CA, Saraiva A, Gonçalves V, et al. Pathological findings in one of two siblings with Sjögren–Larsson syndrome. Eur Neurol 1980;19:166–170.

29. Maia M. Sjögren–Larsson syndrome in two sibs with peripheral nerve involvement and bisalbuminaemia. J Neurol Neurosurg Psychiatry 1974;37:1306–1315.

30. Hofer PA, Jagell S. Sjögren–Larsson syndrome: a dermato-histopathological study. J Cutan Pathol 1982; 9:360–376.

31. Matsuoka LY, Kousseff BG, Hashimoto K. Studies of the skin in Sjögren–Larsson syndrome by electron microscopy. Am J Dermatopathol 1982;4:295–301.

32. Brown BE, Williams WL, Elias PM. Stratum corneum lipid abnormalities in ichthyosis. Arch Dermatol 1984;120:204–209.

33. Jagell S, Lidèn S. Treatment of the ichthyosis of the Sjögren–Larsson syndrome with etretinate (Tigason). Acta Dermatol Venereol (Stockh) 1983;63:89–91.

34. Hooft C, Kriekemans J, van Acker K, et al. Sjögren–Larsson syndrome with exudative enteropathy. Influence of medium-chain triglycerides on the symptomatology. Helv Paediatr Acta 1967;22:447–458.

35. Guilleminault C, Harpey JP, Lafourcade J. Sjögren–Larsson syndrome. Report of two cases in twins. Neurology 1973;23:367–373.

36. Witkop CJ, Henry FV. Sjögren–Larsson syndrome and histidinemia: hereditary biochemical diseases with defects of speech and oral functions. J Speech Hear Dis 1963;28:109–123.

37. Kouseff BG, Matsuoka LY, Stenn KS, et al. Prenatal diagnosis of Sjögren–Larsson syndrome. J Pediatr 1982;101:998–1001.

Chapter 23
Refsum's Disease

SIGVALD REFSUM and ODDVAR STOKKE

Refsum's disease (heredopathia atactica polyneuritiformis) is a biochemically well-defined disease for which there is a specific dietary treatment. It was first described by Refsum in 1945 [1], who also emphasized that it was most probably a distinct nosological entity, a *morbus sui generis* [2]. This conclusion was later substantiated by biochemical studies. The disease is an autosomal recessive inborn error of metabolism. Diagnosis is based on a constellation of clinical symptoms and signs combined with a disturbance of phytanic acid metabolism.

One hundred twenty cases of Refsum's disease have been reported, and more than 20 autopsied cases have been recorded. The disease has been observed in many countries, but mainly in Norway, northern France, the British Isles, and Ireland.

Clinical Manifestations

The disease is characterized by pigmentary retinal degeneration (retinitis pigmentosa), chronic polyneuropathy, ataxia, and an increase in cerebrospinal fluid protein with normal cell content. Refsum [1,2] originally considered this tetrad as the essential manifestations of the disease. In most cases sensorineural (cochlear) impairment of hearing, anosmia, and cardiopathy also have been present. Additional signs are pupillary abnormalities, lens opacities, skin changes (sometimes ichthyosis), and skeletal malformations.

Since Refsum's original description, several cases have been observed without definite cerebellar signs, while a peripheral neuropathy has been the dominating neurologic feature. In a recent review of 17 cases of Refsum's disease, with clearly increased serum phytanic acid levels and reduced α-oxidation capacity of phytanic acid in fibroblast cultures, two-thirds of the patients were reported as having no

cerebellar signs [3]. Such observations have led to speculations about a possible genetic heterogeneity.

Clinical Course

In some cases with predominant peripheral neuropathy, the signs have occurred in distinct attacks with a remarkable recovery in between, thus mimicking relapsing polyneuropathy or Guillain–Barré syndrome. A patient described by Veltema and Verjaal [4] had nine attacks of polyneuropathy over a 25-year-period with almost complete remission after each episode. Behan [5] observed a family in which three of ten children were affected with Refsum's disease. These patients had multiple attacks of an illness, following viral infections, that was indistinguishable from Guillain–Barré syndrome. In between the early attacks, there was complete clinical remission; however, one girl died during the fifth episode. Serum phytanic acid levels were the same in or out of the attacks. Immunologic studies of two patients revealed cell-mediated hypersensitivity and low-titer humoral antibodies to whole peripheral nerve antigen. Behan postulated that the individuals are "primed" and, under certain circumstances, such as viral infection, develop organ-specific damage. This hypothesis is supported by evidence from animal experiments.

The age of onset has varied from early childhood to the second and third decade and even later. The onset of the disease seems in most cases to be insidious; therefore, it is difficult to ascertain its actual start. An early onset of the disease does not necessarily indicate a particularly poor prognosis as to life span. Incomplete early syndromes, particularly retinitis pigmentosa, have been described in patients already showing storage of phytanic acid. In some cases the onset has been acute and precipitated by infections [5]. Other precipitating or aggravating factors described are surgery, pregnancy, and childbirth.

The course has in many cases been characterized by very marked exacerbations and remissions, sometimes without obvious antecedent cause. This observation made Refsum conclude, in his earliest report, that in addition to the hereditary factor, environmental factors interacted. In other cases, the course seems to have remained stationary for long periods of time. A few patients have led an active and enjoyable life for 20 years after the onset of symptoms; other cases have shown steady progression. Sudden unexpected death has occurred in several cases (see below).

Ocular and Neurologic Abnormalities

The funduscopic changes are illustrated in Figure 23.1. In some cases the retinal disturbance is characterized as "retinitis pigmentosa sine pigmento."

Ataxia and other cerebellar signs have been prominent in many cases, and sometimes unsteadiness of gait has been the only presenting symptom. This was the case in the first patient with this disease, observed in 1937 [1,2]. On admission one diagnosis of this patient was "tabes dorsalis." Initially many cases have been diagnosed as Friedreich's disease or other forms of cerebellar ataxia. Many reports by competent observers confirm that the unsteadiness of gait has been out of proportion to motor and sensory losses. Nystagmus and intention tremor have been observed in several cases and have sometimes been marked.

Hyposmia or anosmia is common and may be an early finding and even one of the earliest symptoms. However, patients rarely complain about it. The hearing loss is of cochlear type and may become almost complete. Vestibular function is, as a rule, unimpaired.

The peripheral neuropathy is sometimes preceded for several years by visual and auditory dysfunction. The neuropathy is generally symmetrical, and, at the onset, chiefly affects the distal parts of the limbs with muscular weakness and atrophy (Figure 23.2). Over the course of years, muscular weakness can become widespread and disabling, involving not only the limbs but also the trunk musculature.

Sensory disturbances are frequent. Deep sensation is impaired in most cases, particularly with regard to vibration and position–motion in distal parts of the lower limbs. Less striking is the loss of superficial sensation, but cutaneous hypoesthesia of the glove and stocking type is common. Paresthesias, dysesthesias, and spontaneous pains occur in some cases. The peripheral nerves (ulnar, peroneal, and great auricular) may be palpably enlarged and firm, but not in all cases, even when hypertrophic changes can be histologically detected in the nerve sections.

There is progressive diminution and finally loss of deep (myotatic) reflexes, starting with those of the ankle. The superficial abdominal reflexes are usually preserved, but may be decreased or even absent. Generally the plantar responses are flexor or absent.

Neurophysiologic studies have revealed reduced motor and sensory nerve conduction velocity. The reduction sometimes becomes very marked. Before one of our patients received dietary treatment, a mo-

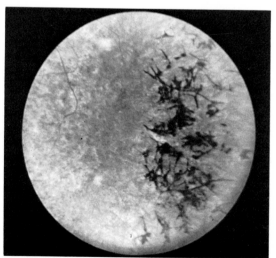

Figure 23.1. Funduscopic pictures. *(Left)* Secondary optic atrophy with a yellowish pale disc color and pathologically narrow arteries. *(Right)* Typical bone corpuscle retinal pigmentation.

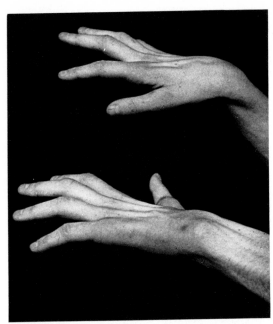

Figure 23.2. Marked bilateral atrophy of the small muscles of the hand.

tor conduction velocity in the ulnar nerve of 7 meters per second was recorded. Following treatment it increased to 30 meters per second [6]. Electromyography has shown evidence of denervation.

There are usually no signs of pyramidal or extrapyramidal system involvement. Intelligence levels appear to be the same as in the general population. Epileptic seizures are not part of the typical clinical picture. The electroencephalogram is normal in most cases, but in some a mild to moderate dysrhythmia with a slight slowing of activity has been recorded. In a few cases psychoses, particularly paranoid psychosis, have occurred. These have been considered chiefly reactive and may be related to sensory deprivation and chronic disability.

Cardiac and Skeletal Changes

Cardiac manifestations are encountered in the majority of cases in the form of tachycardia, enlargement of the heart, conduction disturbances, and electrical changes compatible with myocardial lesions. Cardiomyopathy has probably been the most frequently reported cause of sudden death in both young and middle-aged patients.

Skeletal malformations—symmetrical epiphyseal dysplasia of the knee joints, elbows, and shoulders—were found in the patients in the first families ob-

served [1,2]. Skeletal malformations have been recorded in about half of the cases of Refsum's disease. Pes cavus and hammer toes are frequently reported. The most common finding appears to be bilateral shortening or elongation of the metatarsal bones, particularly the third and fourth metatarsal.

Skin Changes

Many patients with Refsum's disease experience skin changes. Cutaneous changes have sometimes led physicians to the correct diagnosis of Refsum's disease. These changes are variously described as dry, scaly, xerodermic, or hyperkeratotic; a "scaly pigmented rash," ichthyosis-like changes, or ichthyosis. The descriptions of the appearance and course of skin changes are often inadequate.

Skin changes may be one of the presenting symptoms. The first patient, observed in 1937 [1,2], had no skin changes. His sister, the second patient observed, reported that for 3 years before admission she had been troubled by a skin disease—she "changed the skin" on her entire body. On examination coarse desquamation was present everywhere except on the face and scalp. The dermatologic diagnosis was ichthyosis [2]. All four children first reported, who belonged to three unrelated families, exhibited marked skin changes [7].

The history of these four children was very similar, the symptoms presenting at ages 4 to 7. The onset was insidious with anorexia, unsteady gait, and dry scaling skin; hearing loss developed later. In one child, the skin over the patella and elbow was thickened and of a dirty brown color. The scales were large and some were brown. A steady progression occurred; she became bedridden and the condition of her skin grew worse (Figure 23.3). After 6 months, however, a remarkable remission occurred. She gained weight, her arms and legs became stronger, and the muscle stretch reflexes, which had been completely abolished, returned. Concomitantly, her skin showed marked improvement and the ichthyotic changes finally disappeared entirely. These patients were observed before the dietary treatment was known. A similar striking parallelism between general condition, neurologic manifestations, including CSF findings, and skin changes, has been observed in several cases reported later. The skin changes have sometimes been accompanied by pruritus.

In a review of the reported cases of Refsum's disease with skin changes, Refsum [8] has emphasized that even if the pathogenesis of the skin changes was unknown, their parallel course with other clinical

Figure 23.3. Skin changes in a child with Refsum's disease [7].

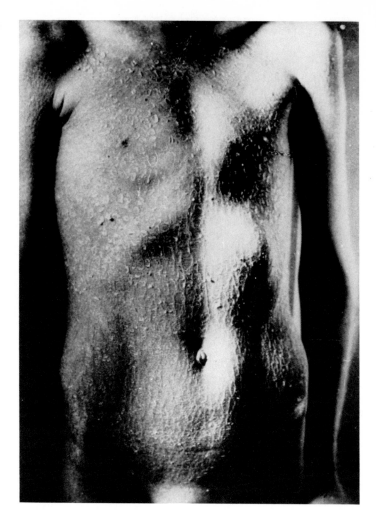

manifestations suggests that the skin changes, although not always present, are an important clinical feature of the disease and are probably caused by the same biochemical defect responsible for the other clinical manifestations.

All seven British patients with Refsum's disease recently reported by Gibberd et al. [9] had ichthyosis at some stage. The ichthyosis changed rapidly with the clinical state and correlated well with the plasma phytanic acid level. As the plasma phytanic acid level improved so did the skin.

The phytanic acid content of subcutaneous fat prior to dietary treatment was found by Refsum and Eldjam [10] to be 1.6% of the total fatty acids in one of our patients and 0.7% in another. After dietary treatment the phytanic acid content was reduced to 0.25 and 0.2%, respectively. None of these patients had ichthyosis at the time of examination.

In a female patient with Refsum's disease, but without ichthyosis, the proportion of phytanic acid in skin and serum was 15% of the total fatty acid, while in the peripheral subcutaneous fat it was 4.5%. The phytanic acid content of three xanthomas on her neck and thorax was 60% of their total fatty acid. Phytanic acid has not been demonstrable in skin from controls [11].

Skin Pathology

Only a few histologic examinations of the skin in Refsum's disease have been reported. Hyperkeratosis with atrophy of the granular layer and of the stratum Malpighi was reported by Flament–Durand et al. [12] and hyperkeratotic epidermis by Fryer et al. [13]. The skin of one of our patients was examined histologically postmortem by Cammermeyer [14]. Hyperkeratosis with sloughing of the horn layer and moderate atrophy of the epidermis was found although no previous skin changes had been noted.

The keratinization disturbance in Refsum's disease has been investigated by Anton–Lamprecht and Kahlke [15] by means of electron microscopy and compared to the keratinization pattern of the common inherited ichthyoses. The main observations from epidermal differentiation and ultrastructure clearly distinguish Refsum's disease from autosomal dominant ichthyosis vulgaris and X-linked recessive ichthyosis. In the lower epidermal strata, lipid droplets (liposomes) are associated with endoplasmic reticulum and abnormal or giant mitochondria. Their degree of extraction by routine preparation technique favors a high content of neutral lipids or of lipids rich in saturated fatty acids. The epidermal liposomes are thus supposed to be the morphological substrate of the cellular accumulation of phytanic acid, possibly as cholesteryl esters and triglycerides. Quantitative deviations in the granular and horn layers result in a moderate orthohyperkeratosis. The granular layer is reduced in depth to one single cellular stratum with decreased amounts of keratohyalin, which is structurally normal. Keratinosomes are found in normal numbers. Hyperkeratosis is formed by about 30 to 40 flat horny cells that show in part a typical keratin pattern. The dissolution of desmosomal disks is obviously retarded and begins around the twenty-fifth horn cell layer. No structural abnormalities are found in the desmosomes, tonofibrils, or keratinosomes.

A patient, aged 37, with Refsum's disease reported by Davies et al. [16] had a marked generalized ichthyosis. She became bedridden, greatly underweight and wasted, and died suddenly. Studies by light microscopy and transmission electron microscopy showed lipid deposits in the basal layer of the epidermis, similar to the findings of Anton–Lamprecht and Kahlke [15]. Furthermore, the patient showed hypergranulosis and a strikingly increased nonspecific esterase activity in the upper epidermis. The results of kinetic and other metabolic studies showed markedly increased epidermopoiesis and metabolic activity. Scanning electron microscopy performed on skin surface biopsies showed a profound disruption in overall scale pattern and at higher magnification, the suggestion of a microvillous pattern on individual keratinocytes. This latter finding is, according to Davies et al. [16], often seen in scaling conditions characterized by high output epidermopoiesis, which their patient had.

Large amounts of phytanic acid were found in all epidermal lipid subfractions. Analysis of the phospholipid subfractions showed a striking reduction in linoleic acid content (approximately one-sixth of normal). A similar, though less marked, reduction was observed in the arachidonic acid levels in the epidermal phospholipid subfraction. Both linoleic and arachidonic acid are essential fatty acids in man and animals, their deficiency producing an ichthyosis-like scaling dermatosis. It would appear that in Refsum's disease the epidermis substitutes phytanic acid for essential fatty acid in all lipid subfractions and especially in phospholipids. The above findings suggest that the abnormal epidermal findings in Refsum's disease result from the failure of these cells to degrade the phytanic acid which has been incorporated. Plasma postheparin lipase is incapable of splitting glyceryl triphytanate whereas glyceryl tripalmitate is easily hydrolysed.

In both essential fatty acid deficiency and in Refsum's disease an altered phospholipid profile exists, and in contrast with other "nonerythematous" ichthyotic states, there is a marked elevation of epidermopoiesis. All membranes contain much phospholipid. The above observation and the localization of 5-nucleotidase activity in the plasma membrane suggest a particular relationship between this structure and mitotic activity [16].

A patient with Refsum's disease and skin changes, recently reported by Lorand et al. [17], had a palmar–plantar hyperkeratosis and an ichthyosiform condition characterized by fine scales and an accumulation of brown scales in the elbow region. The scales were thicker and larger on the abdomen and thighs. After 3 weeks of strict dietary treatment, the skin changes disappeared and after 6 months improvement of the peripheral neuropathy and cardiomyopathy and a normalization of serum phytanic acid level was noted. Her younger brother also suffered from visual and auditory impairment, and his skin condition was described as a diffuse xerosis.

Biochemistry

The main events which led to the biochemical elucidation of Refsum's disease took place in less than 10 years, from 1963 to about 1970. The first biochemical approach was made by Klenk and Kahlke [18] who reported finding large amounts of phytanic acid (3,7,11,15-tetramethylhexadecanoic acid) in postmortem tissues of a 7-year-old girl suffering from Refsum's disease. Shortly afterward Kahlke [19] showed that phytanic acid had accumulated in the serum of all nine patients with this disease that he had been able to trace. These reports raised a series of questions. Where does phytanic acid originate?

What is the nature of the metabolic defect? Is there any causal relationship between accumulated phytanic acid and clinical symptoms? If so, would this give a clue to an efficacious treatment? Several research groups took up these problems, and within a few years much new and important knowledge had been gathered. Extensive review articles have been written by Eldjarn et al. [6], Steinberg [20], and Stokke and Eldjarn [21].

Origin of Phytanic Acid

The polyisoprenoid structure of phytanic acid led Kahlke [19] to propose that an excessive endogenous synthesis—a divergent path from the mevalonic acid–squalene–cholesterol biosynthetic pathway—occurred in these patients. Shortly afterward it was, however, conclusively shown that no endogenous synthesis of phytanic acid took place, and that the phytanic acid that had accumulated in the patients stemmed from exogenous sources [22].

Small amounts of preformed phytanic acid are found in food derived from fish oils and ruminant animals. Furthermore, it has been shown that free phytol (Figure 23.4) is easily transformed to phytanic acid in mammals. Phytol is a constituent of the chlorophyll molecule and is present in all types of green vegetables and fruits. This chlorophyll-bound phytol is, however, liberated in the intestines only to a small extent. More important as a source of phytanic acid in the patients is probably free phytol in plant fats. Other isoprenoid structures, like dihydrophytol and phylloquinone, also may be precursors of phytanic acid in mammals. As will be discussed later, the preformed phytanic acid of animal fat and fish fat seems, however, to be the most significant source.

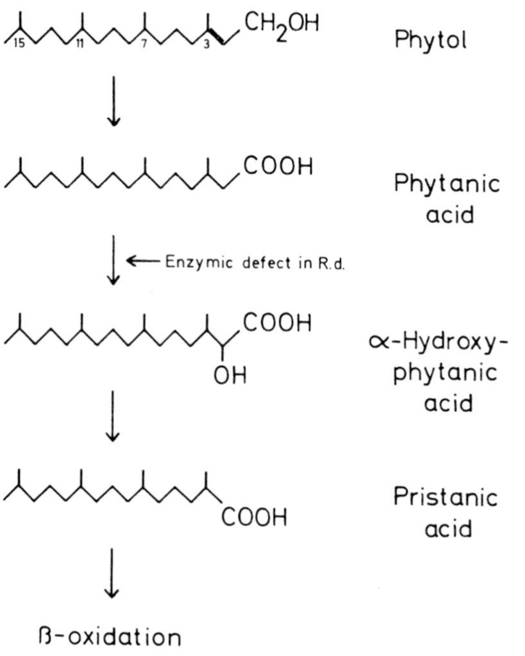

Nature of the Metabolic Defect

The mammalian organism is able to degrade phytanic acid at a considerable rate. The fact that phytanic acid stems from exogenous sources implies that the accumulation of phytanic acid in patients must be caused by a defect in the degradation mechanism. The normal degradation route for phytanic acid was, however, unknown.

In 1966 it was shown independently in three different laboratories that the main degradation pathway for β-methyl substituted fatty acids was an α-oxidation. Shorland et al. [23] and Avigan et al. [24] were able to demonstrate an accumulation of small amounts of pristanic acid (2,6,10,14-tetramethyl-

Figure 23.4. Chemical structures and main metabolic route of phytol, phytanic acid, and pristanic acid.

pentadecanoic acid) in rats fed phytanic acid. Eldjarn et al. [25,26] isolated 2,5-dimethylheptanoic acid from the urine after 3,6-dimethyloctanoic acid was administered to healthy men, thus proving that an α-oxidation had taken place. Furthermore, patients with Refsum's disease failed to excrete any 2,5-dimethylheptanoic acid, revealing a defect in their α-oxidation mechanism.

In an elegant piece of work, Steinberg et al. [22] and Mize et al. [27] showed the conversion, in mouse liver, of phytanic acid to pristanic acid, to 4,8,12-trimethyltridecanoic acid, to 2,6,10-trimethylundecanoic acid, and to 4,8-dimethylnonanoic acid, thus demonstrating that an initial α-oxidation of the compound was followed by consecutive β-oxidations [24,27]. In addition, α-hydroxyphytanic acid was found to be a probable intermediate in the α-decarboxylation mechanism [28].

Cultures of skin fibroblasts demonstrated that the rate of oxidation of phytanic acid in patients was less than 1% of that found in fibroblasts from normal skin. Pristanic acid and α-hydroxyphytanic acid were, however, oxidized at a normal rate in the patients' cultures [29,30]. It may be concluded that the enzyme deletion in patients with Refsum's disease involves a system for α-hydroxylation of β-methyl fatty acids (Figure 23.4). On the basis of in vitro experiments, it is reasonable to believe that this enzyme system is located in the mitochondria [31,32].

Pathogenetic Role of Phytanic Acid

On an ordinary diet patients with Refsum's disease run the risk that their intake of phytanic acid is greater than their degradation capacity. In such a situation stores of phytanic acid build up in the body lipids. In addition to their presence in plasma lipids, large amounts of phytanic acid have been found in the liver and kidney [18], in both the central and peripheral nervous systems [33], and in the skin [16]. It would not be unlikely that some, if not all, of the clinical symptoms of Refsum's disease could be traced back to a toxic effect of phytanic acid.

Both clinical data and data from experimental animals show that large amounts of phytanic acid, bringing serum phytanic acid values to above 100 mg/100 ml, may cause toxic symptoms. These symptoms are nonspecific. The subject loses weight and fails to thrive. Increasing fatigue follows, and death appears to occur when the serum levels of phytanic acid are in the range of 200 to 250 mg/100 ml. In rats skin symptoms have also been provoked [34–36]. It has, however, been impossible to mimic the chronic symptoms of Refsum's disease in animals. In spite of high concentrations of phytanic acid both in serum and in the liver and kidney, only trace amounts were found in the lipids of the central and peripheral nervous systems of the animals [37].

It is the observations made on patients following successful dietary treatment that make us believe that most, if not all, of the symptoms of Refsum's disease are caused by phytanic acid accumulation. This is true for nerve conduction velocity, the protein content of cerebrospinal fluid, electrocardiographic disturbances, and probably for the ichthyosiform skin changes as well. Of particular significance is the fact that, in our two Norwegian patients who have been kept free of phytanic acid for many years (a total of 20 patient-years of observation), no relapses of symptoms and signs of the disease have been observed, although observation has been careful and continuous [21]. However, the biochemical basis of this relationship between phytanic acid and the symptoms remains to be clarified.

Diagnostic Significance of Phytanic Acid

The clinical diagnosis of Refsum's disease may be difficult. No symptom is pathognomonic for the disease, and the various symptoms and signs may develop in succession at different times. However, until now, the detection of phytanic acid in serum has been considered diagnostic for the disease [6,9,38].

Several reports limit, however, the significance of phytanic acid accumulation as the decisive criterion for the diagnosis. Two mothers of patients with Refsum's disease have been reported in whom serum phytanic acid was considerably increased but who had no clinical symptoms [39,40]. A few patients, successfully treated by a diet low in phytanic acid, have normalized their pattern of fatty acids in serum [21]. Patients who happen to live on a diet with a very low fat content may thus suffer from Refsum's disease without showing any accumulation of phytanic acid. Furthermore, several patients with phytanic acid accumulation in serum, but with clinical pictures clearly different from Refsum's disease, have been reported. Clinical designations such as infantile Refsum's syndrome, Zellweger's syndrome, and neonatal adrenoleukodystrophy have been used on this group of patients [41–45].

Measurement of α-Oxidation Capacity

The ability to degrade phytanic acid by α-oxidation is retained also in fibroblasts cultured from skin biopsies from healthy individuals, while those from patients with Refsum's disease have almost no such activity [30]. The expression of the enzymatic defect of the patients in cultured fibroblasts has made it possible to establish in vitro tests in order to measure the defect directly. It is done by adding [1-^{14}C]-phytanic acid to the medium of fibroblasts growing in monolayer. After an incubation for several days the amount of ^{14}CO$_2$ produced is trapped and measured [46,47]. By this method control fibroblasts have a phytanic acid oxidase activity of about 80 pmol phytanic acid degraded per hour per mg of cell protein, while cells from patients with Refsum's disease show a residual activity of about 4 pmol per hour per mg of protein [47]. Those patients who have been successfully treated, and who have emptied their phytanic acid stores, show the same low residual activity as the others. This technique thus makes it possible to diagnose Refsum's disease independent of any storage of phytanic acid in the patients.

Patients with Zellweger's syndrome, neonatal adrenoleukodystrophy, and so-called infantile Refsum's syndrome, who may show accumulation of phytanic acid, are characterized by a lack of peroxisomes in the cells [48], and these are therefore often called peroxisomal disorders. Fibroblasts from these patients show the same defective metabolism of phytanic acid as do the cells from patients with Refsum's disease [3,47]. Patients with peroxisomal disorders also have, however, a number of other biochemical abnormalities. They accumulate pathologic bile acids and very long straight-chain fatty acids; they have a defective synthesis of plasmalogens; some of them excrete increased amounts of pipecolic acids in the urine; and recently the excretion of a large number of epoxy acids has been described [49].

It is now our conclusion that neither the clinical symptoms and signs, nor an elevated level of phytanic acid in serum, nor a defective α-oxidation capacity of the skin fibroblasts can alone be considered diagnostic for Refsum's disease. The diagnosis of Refsum's disease can only be made when all three types of criteria are taken together.

Diagnosis

The diagnosis is based on the clinical picture, the demonstration of an increased level of phytanic acid in serum, and a decreased capacity for α-oxidation of phytanic acid.

Many patients with Refsum's disease have carried the diagnosis of retinitis pigmentosa or Usher's syndrome. One patient in whom cerebellar signs became very marked was diagnosed as having a cerebellar tumor and had a craniotomy before the correct diagnosis finally was established. Other common misdiagnoses are Friedreich's disease or cerebellar ataxias, chronic progressive or relapsing polyneuropathy, or Guillain–Barré syndrome.

Abetalipoproteinemia (Bassen–Kornzweig syndrome) shares some of the features of Refsum's disease, but also presents marked differences. The clinical picture is characterized by the association of atypical pigmentary degeneration of the retina with a neurologic disorder resembling Friedreich's ataxia. In addition, the erythrocytes are malformed (acanthocytosis). Fat malabsorption is present from birth. Chronic diarrhea, profound hypocholesterolemia, and the absence of low-density lipoproteins in the serum are typical signs. Chylomicrons and triglycerides are also lacking; other plasma lipids are markedly reduced [50]. Peripheral sensory neuropathy has also been reported [51]. Abetalipoproteinemia is an autosomal recessive disorder; approximately 25% of the cases have been reported in Ashkenazi Jews.

A syndrome of anosmia, ichthyosis, hypogonadism, and neurologic manifestations was reported by Satoyoshi et al. [52] (see Chapter 33, this volume). In one family three affected members were observed. They presented with congenital ichthyosis, congenital anosmia, congenital nystagmus with decreased visual acuity, strabismus, hypopigmentation of the iris, mirror movements of hands and feet, and hypogonadism. The syndrome appeared to be X-linked recessive. Karyotype was normal. Steroid sulfatase and arylsulfatase c activities in leukocytes and fibroblasts were markedly reduced. The syndrome appears so distinct that a confusion with Refsum's disease should easily be avoided, even if the two disorders have some features in common.

Therapy and Prognosis

The fact that phytanic acid stems exclusively from exogenous sources makes it possible to arrest further accumulation in patients and also, since the degradation capacity is not totally lacking, to reduce the body stores. A dietary treatment was first started in 1965 at Rikshospitalet in Oslo [53]. Since then several other patients have been subjected to dietary treatment at various clinics. By the use of a diet low in phytanic acid and its precursors it has been possible to remove the body stores of phytanic acid to such an extent that the serum level of phytanic acid has become completely normal [3,6,21].

The amount of phytol and phytanic acid has been determined in commonly used food items; phytanic acid has been found in a great variety of fats of animal origin, and appreciable amounts of free phytol are present in plant lipids. A detailed study of the phytanic acid content in foods has recently been published by Masters-Thomas et al. [54]. Furthermore, it has been shown that free phytol is easily transformed into phytanic acid in the mammalian organism, but that the phytol that is bound to chlorophyll is liberated only to a small extent in the intestines, and is therefore probably of minor importance as a source of phytanic acid in the patient. These facts have formed the basis for the dietary approach. Further details on dietary treatment have been given elsewhere [6,9,21].

It is well known that very high serum levels of phytanic acid (above 100 mg/dl) may precipitate toxic and life-threatening symptoms. Several patients have shown such a reaction [55]. Toxic symptoms may also easily be reproduced by feeding experiments in animals [34–36,56]. Thus, it is of great importance to develop procedures that can lower these high levels of phytanic acid as rapidly as possible. As an emergency measure, patients with very high levels of phytanic acid may be treated by plasmapheresis, as suggested by Lundberg et al. [57]. Once a week, over a period of several months, 400 ml of plasma was removed and the blood corpuscles were reinjected into the patient. This technique was found to be an excellent supplement to the dietary treatment. The decrease of the serum phytanic acid concentration took place considerably more rapidly than would have been expected by dietary means alone.

The evidence of a direct relationship between the accumulation of phytanic acid and the clinical picture of the disease is now strong enough to merit intensive dietary treatment of the patient. How rapidly phytanic acid stores are reduced is mainly a question of how completely phytanic acid and its precursors can be excluded from the diet.

The prognosis of untreated cases of Refsum's disease is bad. Ten of the eleven patients registered in Norway before the dietary treatment had been introduced were practically blind. Half of the untreated patients have died before the age of 30 years. Cardiomyopathy has probably been the most frequent cause of sudden death, both in young and middle-aged patients. The dietary treatment has to a large extent changed the natural course of the disease. To our knowledge, no serious clinical relapses have occurred in any of the patients on dietary treatment with a significant lowering of the serum phytanic acid level. The well being and the general condition of the patients have become remarkably good.

References

1. Refsum S. Heredopathia atactica polyneuritiformis—et tidligere ikke beskrevet familiært syndrom? Nord Med 1945;28:2682–2685.
2. Refsum S. Heredopathia atactica polyneuritiformis: a familial syndrome not hitherto described. A contribution to the clinical study of the hereditary diseases of the nervous system. Acta Psychiatr Scand 1946; (suppl) 38:1–303.
3. Skjeldal OH, Stokke O, Refsum S, et al. Clinical and biochemical heterogeneity in conditions with phytanic acid accumulation. J Neurol Sci 1987;77:87–96.
4. Veltema AN, Verjaal A. Sur un cas d'hérédopathie ataxique polynévritique. Maladie de Refsum. Rev Neurol (Paris) 1961;104:15–23.
5. Behan PO. Immunological mechanisms in Refsum's disease. Acta Neurol Scand 1983;67:191.
6. Eldjarn L, Stokke O, Try K. Biochemical aspects of Refsum's disease and principles for the dietary treatment. In: Vinken PJ, Bruyn GW, eds. Handbook of Clinical Neurology. Amsterdam: North–Holland, 1976;27:519–541.
7. Refsum S, Salomonsen L, Skatvedt M. Heredopathia actactica polyneuritiformis in children. J Pediatr 1949;35:335–343.
8. Refsum S. Heredopathia atactica polyneuritiformis. Phytanic acid storage disease (Refsum disease). In: Vinken PJ, Bruyn GW, eds. Handbook of Clinical Neurology. Amsterdam: North–Holland, 1975;21: 181–229.
9. Gibberd FB, Billimoria JD, Goldman JM, et al. Heredopathia atactica polyneuritiformis: Refsum's disease. Acta Neurol Scand 1985;72:1–17.
10. Refsum S, Eldjarn L. Heredopathia atactica polyneuritiformis—an inborn defect in the metabolism of branched-chain fatty acids. In: Bammer HG, ed. Zukunft der Neurologie. Stuttgart: Georg Thieme, 1967;36–45.
11. Kark RAP, Engel WK, Blass JP, et al. Heredopathia atactica polyneuritiformis (Refsum's disease). A second trial of dietary therapy in two patients. In: Bergsma D, McKusick V, eds. The Nervous System. New York: National Found Birth Defects Original Art Series, 1971;7:53–55.
12. Flament–Durand J, Noël P, Rutsaert J, et al. A case of Refsum's disease: clinical, pathological, ultrastructural and biochemical study. Pathol Eur 1971;6:172–191.
13. Fryer DG, Winckleman AC, Ways PO, et al. Refsum disease. A clinical and pathological report. Neurology 1971;21:162–167.
14. Cammermeyer J. Refsum's disease. Neuropathological aspects. In: Vinken PJ, Bruyn GW, eds. Handbook of Clinical Neurology. Amsterdam: North–Holland, 1975;21:231–261.
15. Anton-Lamprecht A, Kahlke W. Zur Ultrastruktur hereditärer Verhörnungsstörungen. V. Ichthyosis beim Refsum-Syndrom (Heredopathia atactica polyneuritiformis). Arch Dermatol Forsch 1974;250:185–206.
16. Davies MG, Reynolds DJ, Marks R, et al. The epidermis in Refsum's disease (heredopathia atactica polyneuritiformis). In: Marks R, Dykes PJ, eds. The Ichthyoses. Lancaster, England: MTP, 1978;51–64.
17. Lorand T, Piérard–Franchimont C, Delcour CH, et al. Maladie de Refsum. Ann Dermatol Venereol 1983;110:733–734.
18. Klenk E, Kahlke W. Über das Vorkommen der 3,7,11,15-Tetramethyl-Hexadecansäure (Phytansäure) in den Cholesterinestern und anderen Lipoidfraktionen der Organe bei einem Krankheitsfall unnbekannter Genese. (Verdacht auf Heredopathia atactica polyneuritiformis [Refsum-Syndrom]). Hoppe Seylers Z Physiol Chem 1963;333:133–139.
19. Kahlke W. Refsum-Syndrom. Lipoidchemische Untersuchungen bei 9 Fällen. Klin Wochenschr 1964;42: 1011–1016.
20. Steinberg D. Phytanic acid storage disease (Refsum's disease). In: Stanbury JB, Wyngaarden JB, Fredrickson DS, et al., eds. The Metabolic Basis of Inherited Disease. New York: McGraw–Hill, 1983;731–747.
21. Stokke O, Eldjarn L. Biochemical and dietary aspects of Refsum disease. In: Dyck PJ, Thomas PK, Lambert EH, et al., eds. Peripheral neuropathy. Philadelphia: Saunders, 1984;2:1684–1703.
22. Steinberg D, Mize CE, Avigan J, et al. Studies on the metabolic error in Refsum's disease. J Clin Invest 1967;46:313–322.
23. Shorland FB, Hansen RP, Prior IAM. The effect of phytanic acid on the fatty acid composition of the lipids of the rat with further observations on its metab-

olism. Proceedings of the Seventh International Congress on Nutrition. Braunschweig: Vieweg & Sohn. 1966;5:399–407.

24. Avigan J, Steinberg D, Gutman A, et al. Alpha-decarboxylation, an important pathway for degradation of phytanic acid in animals. Biochem Biophys Res Commun 1966;24:838–844.

25. Eldjarn L, Stokke O, Try K. Alpha-oxidation of branched chain fatty acids in man and its failure in patients with Refsum disease showing phytanic acid accumulation. Scand J Clin Lab Invest 1966;18:694–695.

26. Stokke O, Try K, Eldjarn L. α-Oxidation as an alternative pathway for the degradation of branched-chain fatty acids in man, and its failure in patients with Refsum disease. Biochim Biophys Acta 1967;144:271–284.

27. Mize CE, Steinberg D, Avigan J, et al. A pathway for oxidative degradation of phytanic acid in mammals. Biochem Biophys Res Commun 1966;25:359–365.

28. Tsai SC, Herndon JH, Jr, Uhlendorf BW, et al. The formation of alpha-hydroxy phytanic acid from phytanic acid in mammalian tissues. Biochem Biophys Res Commun 1967;28:571–577.

29. Steinberg D, Herndon JH, Jr, Uhlendorf BW, et al. Refsum disease: nature of the enzyme defect. Science 1967;156:1740–1742.

30. Herndon JH, Jr, Steinberg D, Uhlendorf BW, et al. Refsum's disease: characterization of the enzyme defect in cell culture. J Clin Invest 1969;48:1017–1032.

31. Stokke O. α-Oxidation of a β-methyl-substituted fatty acid in guinea-pig liver mitochondria. Biochim Biophys Acta 1968;152:213–216.

32. Tsai SC, Avigan J, Steinberg D. The pathway for mitochondrial oxidation of phytanic acid (3,7,11,15-tetramethyl-hexadecanoic acid). Fed Proc 1968;27:648.

33. MacBrinn MC, O'Brien JS. Lipid composition of the nervous system in Refsum's disease. J Lipid Res 1968;9:552–561.

34. Klenk E, Kremer GJ. Untersuchungen zum Stoffwechsel des Phytols, Dihydrophytols und der Phytansäure. Hoppe Seylers Z Physiol Chem 1965;343:39–51.

35. Steinberg D, Avigan J, Mize CE, et al. Effects of dietary phytol and phytanic acid in animals. J Lipid Res 1966; 7:684–691.

36. Stokke O. Alpha-oxidation of fatty acids in various mammals, and a phytanic acid feeding experiment in an animal with a low alpha-oxidation capacity. Scand J Clin Lab Invest 1967;20:305–312.

37. Stokke O. The effect of phytanic acid feeding on the fatty acid composition of organ lipids in the polecat (Mustela putorius). In: Try K, Stokke O, eds. Biochemical and dietary studies in Refsum's disease (heredopathia atactica polyneuritiformis). Oslo: Universitetsforlaget, 1969.

38. Try K. Heredopathia atactica polyneuritiformis (Refsum's disease). The diagnostic value of phytanic acid determination in serum lipids. Eur Neurol 1969;2:296–314.

39. Kahlke W, Richterich R. Refsum's disease (heredopathia atactica polyneuritiformis). An inborn error of lipid metabolism with storage of 3,7,11,15-tetramethylhexadecanoic acid. Am J Med 1965; 39:237–241.

40. Nevin NC, Cumings JN, McKeown F. Refsum's syndrome. Heredopathia atactica polyneuritiformis. Brain 1967;90:419–428.

41. Kahlke W, Goerlich R, Feist D. Erhöhte Phytansäurespiegel in Plasma und Leber bei einem Kleinkind mit unklarem Hirnschaden. Klin Wochenschr 1974; 52:651–653.

42. Scotto JM, Hadchouel M, Odievre M, et al. Infantile phytanic acid storage disease, a possible variant of Refsum's disease: three cases, including ultrastructural studies of the liver. J Inher Metab Dis 1982;5:83–90.

43. Poulos A, Pollard AC, Mitchell JD, et al. Patterns of Refsum's disease. Phytanic acid oxidase deficiency. Arch Dis Child 1984;59:222–229.

44. Stokke O, Skrede S, Ek J, et al. Refsum's disease, adrenoleucodystrophy, and the Zellweger syndrome. Scand J Clin Lab Invest 1984;44:463–464.

45. Poulos A, Sharp P, Whiting M. Infantile Refsum's disease (phytanic acid storage disease): a variant of Zellweger's syndrome? Clin Genet 1984;26:579–586.

46. Poulos A. Diagnosis of Refsum's disease using 1-^{14}C phytanic acid as substrate. Clin Genet 1981;20:247–253.

47. Skjeldal OH, Stokke O, Norseth J, et al. Phytanic acid oxidase activity in cultured skin fibroblasts. Diagnostic usefulness and limitations. Scand J Clin Lab Invest 1986;46:283–287.

48. Goldfischer S, Moore CL, Johnson AB, et al. Peroxisomal and mitochondrial defects in the cerebrohepatorenal syndrome. Science 1973;182:62–64.

49. Stokke O, Jellum E, Kvittingen EA, et al. Epoxy acids in peroxisomal disorders. Scand J Clin Lab Invest 1986;46:95–96.

50. Rowland LP. Abetalipoproteinemia. In: Vinken PJ, Bruyn GW, eds. Handbook of Clinical Neurology. Amsterdam: North–Holland, 1981;42:511–512.

51. Wichman A, Buchthal F, Pezeshkpour GH, et al. Peripheral neuropathy in abetalipoproteinemia. Neurology 1985;35:1279–1289.

52. Satoyoshi E, Sunohara N, Sakuragawa N, et al. Abstracts of the XIII world congress of neurology, Hamburg, September 1985. J Neurol 1985; (suppl) 232:288.

53. Eldjarn L, Try K, Stokke O, et al. Dietary effects on serum-phytanic acid levels and on clinical manifestations in heredopathia atactica polyneuritiformis. Lancet 1966;1:691–693.

54. Masters-Thomas A, Bailes J, Billimoria JD, et al. 2. Estimation of phytanic acid in foods. J Hum Nutr 1980;34:251–254.

55. Stokke O, Eldjarn L. Toxicity of phytanic acid in Refsum's disease. In: Vinken PJ, Bruyn GW, eds. Handbook of Clinical Neurology. Amsterdan: North–Holland, 1979;36:347–349.

56. Hansen RP, Shorland FB, Prior IAM. The fate of phytanic acid when administered to rats. Biochim Biophys Acta 1966;116:178–180.

57. Lundberg A, Lilja I-G, Lundberg PO, et al. Heredopathia atactica polyneuritiformis (Refsum's disease). Experiences of dietary treatment and plasmapheresis. Eur Neurol 1972;8:309–324.

Chapter 24

Giant Axonal Neuropathy

BRUCE O. BERG

A 6-year-old girl with a chronic progressive poly-neuropathy and remarkably frizzly hair was reported in 1972 (Figure 24.1). Sural nerve biopsy showed a reduced nerve fiber population and of those remaining fibers, about one-half were greatly enlarged. On biopsy, longitudinal sections demonstrated that the axonal enlargements were segmental, and electron microscopic preparations showed that these swollen segments were filled with closely packed swirls of neurofilaments which, on occasion, appeared to tie into granular electron opaque condensations. This progressive polyneuropathy, called giant axonal neu-ropathy, was thought to be of genetic origin [1,2].

A similarly affected 3-year-old boy was reported shortly thereafter, and it was suggested that the two cases represented a definite disease entity with char-acteristic changes of hair, as well as peripheral nerve, that were probably a manifestation of an inborn er-ror of metabolism [3,4]. Then a third case with closely related clinical characteristics revealed structural ab-normalities of the sural nerve on biopsy. It appeared that the neuronal degeneration was part of a gener-alized disorder with the accumulation of large dis-crete masses of cytoplasmic filaments in endoneurial fibroblasts, endothelial cells, Schwann cells, perineu-rial cells, and cultured skin fibroblasts [5,6]. That both the peripheral and central nervous systems were involved was evidenced by an abnormal electroen-cephalogram in the first patient and reportedly ab-normal plantar responses in the second [1,3,4,7].

Since that time, 20 patients with similar symp-toms, signs, clinical courses, and structural changes revealed by sural nerve biopsies have been reported. All except 2 patients had notably frizzly hair without evidence of pili torti [8,9] and 1 other patient with straight hair was described as having a congenital form of giant axonal neuropathy [10].

Parental consanguinity was present in 3 cases, persuasive evidence that giant axonal neuropathy is inherited as an autosomal recessive trait [5,7,11]. In addition, there is one report of 2 affected siblings [12]. The inheritance of a similar disease process in dogs, canine giant axonal neuropathy, is firmly es-tablished as an autosomal recessive trait [13–15].

Clinical Course and Features

The early motor development of affected patients is usually normal, and not until they reach the age of 2 to 4 years are they noted to be inordinately clumsy. One patient was hypotonic at birth, had progressive weakness, and died at 15 months of age from car-diorespiratory arrest [10].

Although some patients appear mentally normal when initially evaluated, most patients have im-paired mental function. Speech is commonly affected and has been described as abnormally slow, nasal, scanning, or dysarthric. Pallor of the optic discs has been observed in some patients, and nystagmus or coarse ocular movements are common. Neuro-ophthalmic function of 4 patients was assessed by electroretinography, demonstrating abnormal retinal function; visual evoked potentials showed abnor-malities of both optic nerves and retrochiasmal path-ways. Ocular motility, evaluated by electro-oculography, was characterized by defective pursuit, inability to maintain eccentric gaze with gaze paretic and rebound nystagmus, abnormal optokinetic nys-tagmus, and failure of fixation to suppress the ves-tibulo-ocular reflex [16]. One patient had an external ophthalmoplegia [17].

As the disease progresses, most patients experi-ence facial weakness. Other cranial nerves are gen-

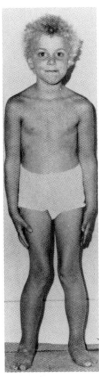

Figure 24.1. Original patient with giant axonal neuropathy showing remarkably frizzly hair. (Reproduced with permission from Berg et al. [1].)

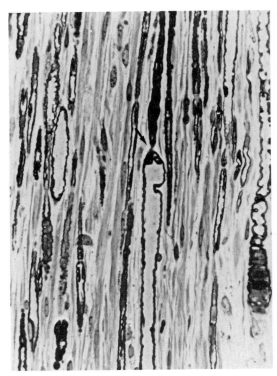

Figure 24.2. Sural nerve in longitudinal section. The segmental nature of the axonal enlargement *(arrow)* is noted. The swollen axon contains glossy appearing material, a characteristic light microscopic feature of neurofilamentous masses. (Courtesy of Dr. Arthur K. Asbury.)

erally not as affected, although one patient had poor elevation of the palate and ultimately became aphonic [17]. The gait is unsteady and broad-based and patients commonly walk on the medial aspects of their feet.

Early in the course of the disease muscle tone is normal to decreased, but as time passes progressive hypotonia, muscle weakness, and variable degrees of muscle atrophy are experienced. One patient, noted to have moderate hypertonia of the lower limbs when 3 years of age, within several years became markedly hypotonic and weak with absent stretch reflexes [17, Michaud J: personal communication 1986]. The stretch reflexes range from active (normal) to absent, depending upon the stage of the disease, and are generally more active in the arms than legs. The plantar response has been variably reported as flexor, nonreactive, or extensor.

Progressive impairment of sensation, greater in the arms than in the legs, is usually of the stocking-glove type in distribution, affecting touch, pain, and proprioception. Precocious puberty has been reported in 2 patients [7,12,18].

Laboratory Findings

In patients with giant axonal neuropathy complete blood counts, urinalyses, and a wide variety of biochemical tests have all been unremarkable, including serum electrolytes, calcium, phosphorus, magnesium, manganese, blood urea nitrogen, creatinine, liver function tests, serum protein and lipoprotein electrophoreses, cholesterol, triglycerides, vitamin A, carotene, and D-xylose absorption tests. Both serum and urine copper studies are normal, as are urine quantitative amino acids, including cystine screen and assays for heavy metals (arsenic, lead, mercury).

Cerebrospinal fluid examination, including cells, protein, protein electrophoresis, and glucose, are normal. Electrophysiologic studies have been variably interpreted as showing normal to decreased motor and sensory fibers with normal to decreased conduction velocities [2,4,5,9,11,17,19–21].

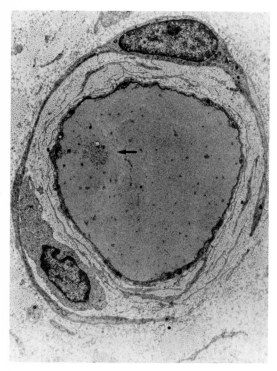

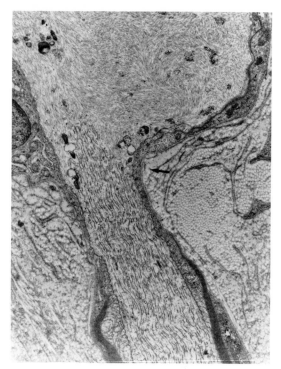

Figure 24.3. Electron micrograph of an enlarged axon in transverse section. The axon is filled with masses of neurofilaments and some small clusters of neurotubules and mitochondria *(arrow)*. A thin coat of Schwann cell cytoplasm invests the axon; other Schwann cell processes centrifugally placed, make up an onion bulb formation (original magnification × 4800). (Reproduced with permission from Asbury et al. [2].)

Figure 24.4. Electron micrograph of A node of Ranvier showing the beginning of an axonal enlargement *(arrow)*. At right, terminal loops of myelin appear in normal array. At left, the axon abruptly enlarges and is filled with masses of neurofilaments in whorled patterns. The narrow portion of the axon *(right)* contains primarily neurotubules and only rare neurofilaments (original magnification × 4800). (Reproduced with permission from Asbury et al. [2].)

Pathology

Sural nerve biopsies demonstrate decreased numbers of myelinated and unmyelinated fibers with abundant swollen axonal segments that electron microscopy reveals to be packed with aggregates of neurofilaments (Figures 24.2, 24.3, 24.4). Both myelinated and unmyelinated fibers are affected, and onion bulb formations are seen [2,4,6,17,19]. Similar axonal changes have been reported following chronic exposure to some neurotoxins [23–28].

Electron microscopy has shown that neurotubules, mitochondria, and cisternae of smooth endoplasmic reticulum may be either reduced or absent and may be displaced to peripheral areas near the axolemma [2,19].

Axonal swellings are found in both the central and peripheral nervous systems and assume a spheroid, fusiform, or transitional configuration [19,

29,30]. They are observed in the brain stem and cerebral cortex and have also been demonstrated in limited areas of the cerebellum. Abundant Rosenthal fibers are present, sometimes in association with axonal swellings, but usually where axonal pathology is less apparent. This proliferation of Rosenthal fibers is similar to that seen in Alexander's disease. Subependymal swollen astrocytes form bulging protrusions or pseudotumors and areas of demyelination are present [29,30; Michaud J: personal communication 1986].

The autonomic nervous system also shows axonal swelling, and perikaryal inclusions are found in myenteric neurons. Ultrastructural studies reveal abnormal cytoplasmic accumulations of structurally normal intermediate filaments in axons, Schwann cells, astrocytes, ependymal cells, arachnoidal cells, perikaryon of myenteric neurons, endothelial cells, fibroblasts, and melanocytes [6,19,29–32, Michaud

J: personal communication 1986]. No abnormal accumulations of intermediate fibers have been found in visceral epithelial cells [17,29, Michaud J: personal communication 1986].

Management

The disease process is relentlessly progressive, and ambulation, usually made worse by thoracolumbar scoliosis, ultimately becomes impossible. No specific treatment for giant axonal neuropathy exists. Patients must receive vigorous medical support, including orthopedic care, physical therapy, and meticulous attention to pulmonary function. The life span of affected patients is generally less than two decades.

References

1. Berg BO, Rosenberg SH, Asbury AK. Giant axonal neuropathy. Pediatrics 1972;49:894–899.
2. Asbury AK, Gale MK, Cox SC, et al. Giant axonal neuropathy—a unique case with segmental neurofilamentous masses. Acta Neuropathol (Berl) 1972; 20:237–247.
3. Carpenter S, Karpati G, Andermann F, et al. Giant axonal neuropathy—a second case. Neurology 1973; (abstr)23:429.
4. Carpenter S, Karpati G, Andermann F, et al. Giant axonal neuropathy: a clinically and morphologically distinct neurologic disease. Arch Neurol 1974;31:312–316.
5. Ouvrier RA, Prineas J, Walsh JC, et al. Giant axonal neuropathy—a third case. Proc Austral Assoc Neurol 1974;11:137–144.
6. Prineas JW, Ouvrier RA, Wright RG, et al. Giant axonal neuropathy—a generalized disorder of cytoplasmic microfilament formation. J Neuropathol Exp Neurol 1976;35:458–470.
7. Igisu H, Ohta M, Tabira T, et al. Giant axonal neuropathy: a clinical entity affecting the central as well as peripheral nervous system. Neurology 1975;25:717–721.
8. Boltshauser E, Bischoff A, Isler W. Giant axonal neuropathy: report of a case with normal hair. J Neurol Sci 1977;31:269–278.
9. Jedrzejowska H, Drac H. Infantile chronic peripheral neuropathy with giant axons: report of a case. Acta Neuropathol (Berl) 1977;37:213–217.
10. Kinney RB, Gottfried MR, Hodson AK, et al. Congenital giant axonal neuropathy. Arch Pathol Lab Med 1985;109:639–641.
11. Gambarelli D, Hassoun J, Pellissier JF, et al. Giant axonal neuropathy: involvement of peripheral nerve, myenteric plexus and extra-neural area. Acta Neuropathol (Berl) 1977;39:261–269.
12. Takeba Y, Koide N, Takahashi G. Giant axonal neuropathy: report of two siblings with endocrinological and histological studies. Neuropediatrics 1981;12:392–404.
13. Duncan ID, Griffiths IR. Peripheral nervous system in a case of canine giant axonal neuropathy. Neuropathol Appl Neurobiol 1979;5:25–39.
14. Griffiths IR, Duncan ID. The central nervous system in canine giant axonal neuropathy. Acta Neuropathol (Berl) 1979;46:169–172.
15. Duncan ID, Griffiths IR, Carmichael S, et al. Inherited canine giant axonal neuropathy. Muscle Nerve 1981;4:223–227.
16. Kirkham TH, Guitton D, Coupland SG. Giant axonal neuropathy: visual and oculomotor deficits. Can J Neurol Sci 1980;7:177–184.
17. Larbrisseau A, Jasmin G, Hausser C, et al. Generalized giant axonal neuropathy—a case with features of Fazio–Londe disease. Neuropaediatrie 1979;10:76–86.
18. Mizuno Y, Otsuka S, Takano Y, et al. Giant axonal neuropathy: combined central and peripheral nervous system disease. Arch Neurol 1979;36:107–108.
19. Peiffer J, Schlote W, Bischoff A, et al. Generalized giant axonal neuropathy: a filament-forming disease of neuronal, endothelial, glial, and Schwann cells in a patient without kinky hair. Acta Neuropathol (Berl) 1977;40:213–218.
20. Koch TK, Schultz P, Williams R, et al. Giant axonal neuropathy: a childhood disorder of microfilaments. Ann Neurol 1977;1:438–451.
21. Fois A, Balestri P, Farnetani MA, et al. Giant axonal neuropathy: endocrinologic and histological studies. Eur J Pediatr 1985;144:274–280.
22. Dooley JM, Oshima Y, Becker LE, et al. Clinical progression of giant axonal neuropathy over a twelve year period. Can J Neurol Sci 1981;8:321–323.
23. Sayre LM, Autillio-Gambetti L, Gabetti P. Pathogenesis of experimental giant neurofilamentous axonopathies: a unified hypothesis based on chemical modifications of neurofilaments. Brain Res Rev 1985;10:69–83.
24. Duckett S, Williams N, Francis S. Peripheral neuropathy associated with inhalation of methyl m-butyl ketone. Experientia 1974;30:1283.
25. Korobkin R, Asbury AK, Sumner AJ, et al. Glue sniffing neuropathy. Arch Neurol 1975;32:158–162.
26. Saida K, Mendell JR, Weiss HS. Peripheral nerve changes induced by methyl n-butyl ketone and potentiation by methyl ethyl ketone. J Neuropathol Exp Neurol 1976;35:207–225.
27. Spencer PS, Schaumburg HH. A review of acrylamide neurotoxicity. Part 2. Experimental animal neurotoxicity and pathologic mechanisms. Can J Neurol Sci 1974;1:152–169.
28. Suzuki K, Pfaff LD. Acrylamide neuropathy in rats. Acta Neuropathol (Berl) 1973;24:197–213.
29. Dubeau F, Michaud J, Lamarre L, et al. Giant axonal neuropathy: a complete autopsy study. J Neuropathol Exp Neurol 1985(abstr)44:355.

30. Kretzchmar HA, Berg BO, Davis RL. Giant axonal neuropathy—a neuropathologic study. Acta Neuropathol (Berl) 1987;73:138–144.

31. Pena SD. Giant axonal neuropathy: an inborn error of organization of intermediate filaments. Muscle Nerve 1982;5:166–172.

32. Ionesescu V, Searby C, Rubenstein P, et al. Giant axonal neuropathy: normal protein composition of neurofilaments. J Neurol Neurosurg Psychiatry 1983; 46:551–554.

Chapter 25
Werner's Syndrome

MAKOTO GOTO

Werner's syndrome (adult progeria) is a rare, recessively inherited illness characterized by growth retardation, premature graying of hair, alopecia, cataracts, diabetes mellitus, leg ulcers, muscle atrophy, osteoporosis, soft tissue calcification, and a high incidence of malignancy. Its clinical features are comparable to the natural aging process, thus it has been called "progeria of the adult" or "a caricature of aging."

Recent laboratory studies, including fibroblast cultures and immunologic examinations [1–3], have served to make Werner's syndrome an ideal model for human aging and for certain geriatric diseases such as diabetes mellitus, malignancy, arteriosclerosis, and osteoporosis.

Historical Background

In 1904 Werner [4] described this disorder in his doctoral thesis in which he reported four siblings who had cataract associated with scleroderma.

Oppenheimer and Kugel [5,6] published reviews in 1934 and 1941 of this peculiar illness in which they included a report of the first postmortem examination of a patient with the disorder and renamed it "Werner's syndrome." Thannhauser [7] reviewed the reported cases and provided a list of 12 major characteristics including premature senility and tendency for it to occur in brothers and sisters. The diminished life span of cultured fibroblasts in Werner's syndrome was first reported by Martin et al. [8]. The fibroblast cultures from a 48-year-old woman with this disease could not be successfully transferred more than 2 or 3 times, while cultures from healthy middle-aged women actively proliferated well in more than 10 transfers and infant fibroblasts in more than 20 transfers. Cultures from an 83-year-old healthy woman could be successfully transferred only twice.

Epstein et al. [9] in an extensive review article included 125 cases of Werner's syndrome, defined the natural history of the disease, and thoroughly described its pathologic and histologic changes. In 1968 Zucker–Franklin et al. [10] analyzed 10 cases of Werner's syndrome and added several endocrinological and metabolic abnormalities including hyperthyroidism, hypercholesterolemia, and hyperuricemia. Tokunaga et al. [11] identified as a new characteristic of Werner's syndrome excessive excretion of hyaluronic acid in the urine, for which they coined the term hyaluronuria. Goto and Murata confirmed this phenomenon in 1978 [12]. No hyaluronic acid was detected in urine from healthy individuals of any age.

Werner [4] recognized the hereditary nature of Werner's syndrome. Pedigree analysis by Epstein et al. [9] and Goto et al. [13] confirmed the autosomal recessive inheritance of the disease. Salk [14] reviewed the published research to 1982.

Its etiology is unknown, although the finding of excessive urinary excretion of hyaluronic acid in Werner's syndrome patients suggests that an enzymatic defect in mucopolysaccharide metabolism is the cause [12].

Epidemiology and Genetics

About 400 cases of Werner's syndrome have been reported throughout the world, half of whom are of Japanese origin [13]. Seven unrelated cases were apparently of Jewish origin in the report by Epstein et al. [9]. Italian investigators identified 10 affected members in 3 unrelated families [15,16]. The high incidence of consanguineous marriage among these three ethnic groups (Japanese, Jewish, and Italian) may be responsible for this patient aggregation.

Representative pedigree charts are presented in

Figure 25.1. The sex ratio of Werner's syndrome was equal. An autosomal recessive type of inheritance is well established [13]. The prevalence of Werner's syndrome is estimated at three in one million in Japan and 0.3 in one million in the United States [9,13].

Chromosomal analysis has revealed no abnormality. There is no significant association between any of the HLA specificities and Werner's syndrome [13].

Clinical Features

There are several major characteristic signs and symptoms of Werner's syndrome: characteristic habitus and stature, scleroderma-like skin changes, precocious aging, endocrinologic abnormalities, malignancy, mental or neurologic abnormalities, and consanguinity.

Werner's syndrome is recognized by a characteristic habitus and constitutional-type or short stature (Figure 25.2). The short stature and small body weight, resulting from lack of adolescent growth, are common findings. All patients appear to be normal before adolescence, but growth stops shortly thereafter. Body parts are proportional in size although the extremities are slender, and the trunk is stocky

in most patients. Atrophy of subcutaneous tissue and muscle are constant features.

Scleroderma-like skin changes are the following: atrophic skin, subcutaneous tissue, and muscle; circumscribed hyperkeratosis, especially of the soles; atrophic or deformed nails; tight skin over metatarsal bones; skin ulcers and leg-gangrene; and localized soft-tissue calcification over the Achilles tendons, knees, and elbows (Figures 25.3, 25.4).

Because skin changes and a high incidence of antinuclear antibodies are similar in both Werner's syndrome and progressive systemic scleroderma, misdiagnosis sometimes occurs [1]. However, unlike progressive systemic scleroderma, Werner's syndrome is not characterized by Raynaud's phenomenon, esophageal dilatation, lung fibrosis, pulmonary hypertension, renal dysfunction, or sicca syndrome.

Chronic ulceration over pressure points on the feet has frequently led to gangrene and amputation. Flat feet, occasionally complicated by hallus valgus, and painful calluses may result from sclerotic skin and foot weakness.

All patients have an accelerated form of at least one of the clinical manifestations of premature aging, which include canities, alopecia, skin hyperpigmentation, hoarse voice, arteriosclerosis, cataracts, and osteoporosis (Figure 25.4). The patients exhibit

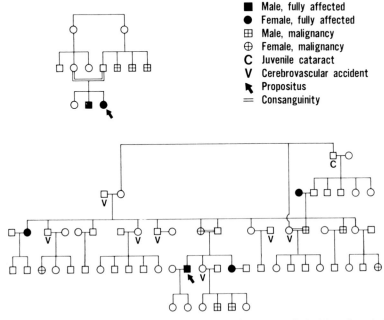

Figure 25.1. Representative pedigree charts of Werner's syndrome and key to symbols. The relatively high incidence of cancer deaths, juvenile cataracts, and diabetes mellitus among families may indicate the presence of an incomplete form, so-called forme fruste.

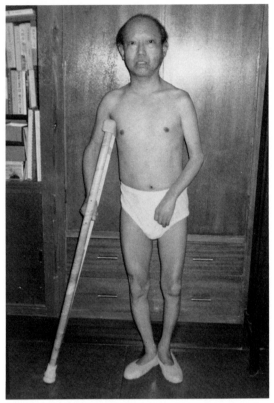

Figure 25.2. A 48-year-old patient with characteristic habitus and stature. Distal muscular atrophy is noted.

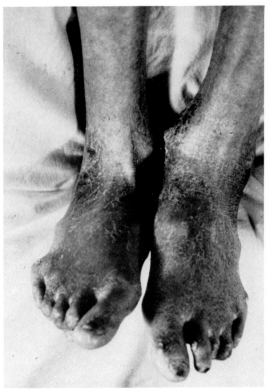

Figure 25.3. Typical scleroderma-like skin changes are shown here: atrophic skin, circumscribed hyperkeratosis, atrophic or deformed nails, tight skin over the bone of the foot, and skin ulcers.

Figure 25.4. Osteoporosis and subcutaneous calcifications over the Achilles tendons in a 43-year-old patient.

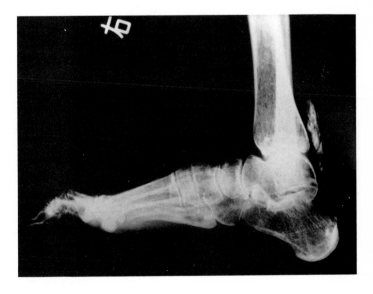

a bird-like appearance, gray hair, alopecia, cataracts (usually posterior polar type), caries, and atrophic auricles. Several common features found in natural aging such as diminished hearing, presbyopia, prostatic hypertrophy, parkinsonism, and senile dementia have been rarely reported in patients with Werner's syndrome.

Diabetes mellitus and hypogonadism are frequently associated with Werner's syndrome. Most diabetic patients are controlled with small doses of sulfonylurea or biguanide. There is a poor response to exogenous insulin.

Male hypogonadism was found in half of the reported patients [13,17]: 60% showed a hypogonadotropic type with high urinary levels of gonadotropin, aspermatogenesis, and an increase in Sertoli's cells. Gynecomastia has been noted in 22% of the hypergonadotropic hypogonadism patients. Amenorrhea, early onset of menopause, and sterility have been recognized on occasion.

Six percent of the patients had malignant tumors; there was preponderance of those with a mesenchymal origin. A relatively high incidence of malignant tumors among family members of propositi with Werner's syndrome has also been described [13].

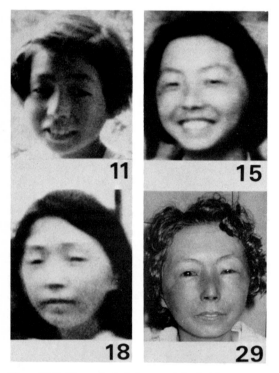

Figure 25.5. Chronological change of the facial expression of a patient with Werner's syndrome (numbers indicate the patient's age).

The neurologic and psychologic abnormalities reported are as follows: subnormal intelligence in 9%, paranoid schizophrenia in 3%, and tonic–clonic seizures in 3%. Hyperreflexia is often observed; however, the underlying pathologic lesion abnormality is unknown [17]. Neither parkinsonism nor senile dementia have been reported.

Seventy percent of the patients were the product of a consanguineous marriage, and 73% of parents in this group had married a first cousin.

Other minor findings (incidence < 10%) included liver dysfunction, hyperlipidemia, hyperuricemia, and renal dysfunction. Excessive urinary excretion of hyaluronic acid has been observed and so far "hyaluronuria" has been reported in 90% of the patients. The antinuclear antibody (speckled pattern) was detected in 30% of the patients, though the titers of serum immunoglobulins were within normal limits.

The mean age at which patients or their families recognized several characteristic manifestations of Werner's syndrome was 20 years. The earliest sign was graying of hair or alopecia, which occurred at a mean age of 20.3 years. This is followed in order by voice changes/hoarseness (22.5 years), skin changes (24 years), cataracts (29.6 years), diabetes mellitus (31.7 years), and skin ulcers (34.7 years).

Pathology

On the arms and legs, where the skin is taut, the epidermis is atrophic, hyperkeratotic, and devoid of rete ridges (Figure 25.6). The reticular dermis shows fibrosis with hyalinization of collagen, together with loss of sebaceous and eccrine glands. The subcutaneous fat is atrophic with nonspecific mild perivascular and periadnexal inflammatory cell infiltration.

Diagnosis

Since there are no generally accepted criteria for the diagnosis of Werner's syndrome, a tentative list of diagnostic criteria has been proposed [13]. Patients having at least three of the four major signs and symptoms described under clinical features are probably suffering from Werner's syndrome. Hyaluronuria and the diminished replicative life span of the fibroblast are the hallmarks of Werner's syndrome. However, the reduced replicative ability of the cultured fibroblasts was observed even in the patients with progressive systemic scleroderma. Hyaluronic aciduria is found in some patients with mucopolysaccharidosis or Wilms' tumors.

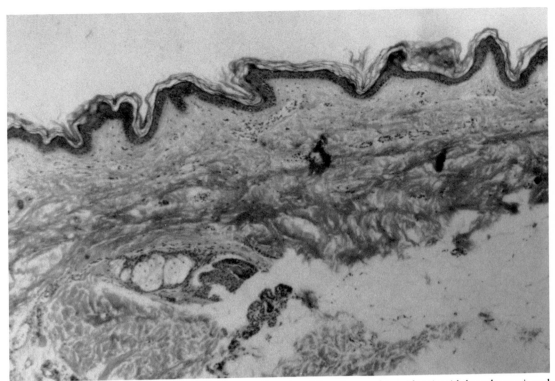

Figure 25.6. Skin biopsy of the lower leg of a 39-year-old patient. Note the atrophic epidermis with hyperkeratosis and loss of rete ridges (H & E stain × 100). The reticular dermis is also atrophic, and subcutaneous fat tissues are easily noted beneath the epidermis. The collagen bundles are eosinophilic and slightly hyalinized. Sebaceous and eccrine glands are decreased in size and number. Nonspecific mild perivascular and periadnexal inflammatory cell infiltration is noted in the mid-dermis. (Courtesy of Dr. M. Furue.)

Treatment and Prognosis

At present, since nothing is known about the pathogenesis of Werner's syndrome, most therapeutic efforts have been directed toward specific management of the cataracts, skin ulcers, and the diabetes mellitus. More general treatment, including steroid hormones, vitamins, growth hormones, and blood transfusions, have been largely ineffective.

Cataracts in Werner's syndrome are always bilateral. For surgery to be successful a skillful technique is necessary to avoid keratopathy and postoperative glaucoma. Skin ulcers are very difficult to manage, and may lead to gangrene and resultant amputation. In some cases intravenous injection of prostaglandin E and autologous skin grafting have been effective. Most diabetic patients are easily managed by administering small doses of sulfonylurea or biguanide.

The average life span of patients with Werner's syndrome has been 43.5 years. The two principal causes of death are malignancies and arteriosclerosis (myocardial and cerebrovascular accidents). However, a thorough understanding of the disease and a careful watch for and treatment of malignant tumors, diabetes mellitus, and cardiovascular and cerebrovascular diseases may prolong the life of patients with this syndrome.

References

1. Goto M, Horiuchi Y, Okumura K, et al. Immunological abnormalities of aging: an analysis of T-lymphocyte subpopulations of Werner's syndrome. J Clin Invest 1979;64:695–699.
2. Goto M, Tanimoto K, Horiuchi Y. Reduced natural killer cell activity of lymphocytes from patients with Werner's syndrome and recovery of its activity by purified human leukocyte interferon. Scand J Immunol 1982;15:389–397.
3. Goto M, Tanimoto K, Horiuchi Y. Age-related changes in auto- and natural antibody in the Werner's syndrome. Am J Med 1982;72:607–614.
4. Werner CWO. Über Kataract in Verbindung mit Sklerodermie. Inaugural dissertation. Kiel: Schmidt und Klauning, 1904.

5. Oppenheimer BS, Kugel VH. Werner's syndrome—a heredofamilial disorder with scleroderma, bilateral cataract, precocious graying of hair, and endocrine stigmatization. Trans Assoc Am Physicians 1934; 49:358–370.

6. Oppenheimer BS, Kugel VH. Werner's syndrome: report of the first necropsy and of findings in a new case. Am J Med Sci 1941;202:629–642.

7. Thannhauser SJ. Werner's syndrome (progeria of the adult) and Rothmund's syndrome: two types of closely related heredofamilial atrophic dermatoses with juvenile cataracts and endocrine features: a critical study with five new cases. Ann Intern Med 1945;23:559–626.

8. Martin GM, Gartler SM, Epstein CJ, et al. Diminished lifespan of cultured cells in Werner's syndrome. Fed Proc 1965;24:678.

9. Epstein CJ, Martin GM, Schultz AL, et al. Werner's syndrome: a review of its symptomatology, natural history, pathologic features, genetics and relationship to the natural aging process. Medicine 1966;45:177–221.

10. Zucker-Franklin D, Rifkin H, Jacobson HG. Werner's syndrome: an analysis of ten cases. Geriatrics 1968; 23:123–135.

11. Tokunaga M, Futami T, Wakamatsu E. Werner's syndrome as "hyaluronuria." Clin Chim Acta 1975;62:89–96.

12. Goto M, Murata K. Urinary excretion of macromolecular acidic glycosaminoglycans in Werner's syndrome. Clin Chim Acta 1978;85:101–106.

13. Goto M, Tanimoto K, Horiuchi Y, et al. Family analysis of Werner's syndrome: a survey of 42 Japanese families with a review of the literature. Clin Genet 1981;19:8–15.

14. Salk D. Werner's syndrome: a review of recent research with an analysis of connective tissue metabolism, growth control of cultured cells and chromosomal aberrations. Human Genet 1982;327:1–15.

15. Rabbiosi G, Borroni G. Werner's syndrome: seven cases in one family. Dermatologica 1979;158:355–360.

16. Cerimele D, Cottoni F, Scappaficci S, et al. High prevalence of Werner's syndrome in Sardinia. Description of six patients and estimate of the gene frequency. Hum Genet 1982;62:25–30.

17. Goto M, Tanimoto K, Horiuchi Y. Werner's syndrome: an analysis of 15 cases with a review of the Japanese literature. J Am Geriatr Soc 1978;26:341–347.

Chapter 26
Progeria

HANS-RUDOLF WIEDEMANN

Progeria is a rare syndrome characterized by a combination of infantilism and premature senility that is associated with alopecia, atrophy of subcutaneous fat and muscle, skeletal hypoplasia, dwarfism, and a propensity to fatal atherosclerotic complications during the first two or three decades of life [1,2].

In 1886, Hutchinson [3] described the first case. Later, Gilford [4] studied the same boy as well as a case of his own and termed the condition progeria, from a Greek word meaning "premature aging." Synonyms include Hutchinson–Gilford syndrome, pedogeria, progeronanism, and senile nanism.

Progeria has been reported in over 100 patients. Both sexes and all ethnic groups are affected. The frequency in the United States seems to be about 1 in 250,000 live births.

Clinical Features

The onset of disease manifestations is usually stated as 1 to 2 years. But there may be indicators of abnormal condition within the first year: birth weight is usually about 2,600 gm; slightly prominent eyes, absence of ear lobules, a thin nose, and the beginning of alopecia may suggest the existence of the syndrome in the first months of life. During the second or third half year of life a profound and progressive retardation in weight gain and growth becomes apparent. The facial bones are involved in this growth failure and thus the child has a hydrocephalic look, although in fact head circumference is somewhat smaller than normal. Scalp veins are prominent, and there is frontal and parietal bossing. The orbits are small with prominent eyes. The nose is thin and rather beaked. Micrognathia, a marked delay in dentition, and crowding of teeth is present. Scalp hair is lost during the second year of life, and eyebrows and eyelashes may disappear at about the same time; the result is total or nearly total alopecia (Figure 26.1). Gradual disappearance of subcutaneous and muscular fat (last areas of adipose atrophy are cheeks and pubic area) results in spindly limbs with prominent joints, especially the knees (Figure 26.2). Periarticular fibrosis leads to stiffness and partial flexion of the joints and, therefore, to a wide-based "horse-riding" stance and shuffling gait. Skin is atrophic, thin, dry, and taut or wrinkled, with prominent superficial veins; there may be brownish pigmentations and, occasionally, scleroderma. The fingers show flexion deformities and shortened terminal phalanges; the nails may be dystrophic, small, dry, and brittle (Figure 26.3).

By the tenth year, the height of the patient is approximately that of a 3- to 4-year-old, and the ultimate height achieved is often only that of a 5-year-old child. Only rarely does an adult exceed 115 cm in height or 15 kg in weight (weight always distinctly low for height). The anterior fontanelle remains open. Hypoplastic clavicles [3,4] are associated with narrow shoulders (Figure 26.2) and a pyriform-shaped thorax. The abdomen often protrudes. The external genitalia are small, and there is failure to complete sexual maturation. Intelligence is within the normal range. The voice is high pitched. The patients show a tendency to fatigue easily. Generalized atherosclerosis is early and severe; anginal attacks may begin by the age of 7 years. The patients may manifest cardiac murmur, hypertension, and left ventricular hypertrophy [5].

Many discordances exist between progeria and normal aging. Features associated with ordinary aging such as presbycusis, presbyopia, arcus senilis, senile cataracts, or senile personality changes are missing, and there is no evidence of accelerated normal aging within the CNS [1,2,6–8]. Progeria, therefore, is no simple premature senescence but a severe disorder that mimics senile aging.

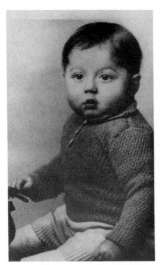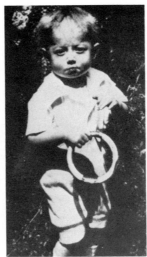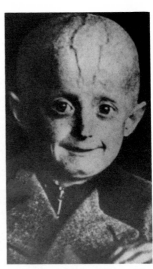

Figure 26.1. Progeria: same patient at 10 months, at 18 months, and at 8 years. Weight at birth, 2 kg, at 10 months, 8 kg, and at 8 years, 13 kg; height age, at 8 years, of 4 years. Note alopecia, thinning of skin with prominent superficial scalp veins, prominent eyes, micrognathia. (From Wiedemann [2] and Wiedemann H-R, Grosse F-R, Dibbern H. Syndrom der Progerie. In: Das charakteristische Syndrom. Stuttgart: Schattauer, 1982:194.)

Figure 26.2. Same patient as in Figure 26.1 at 14½; weight 16.8 kg; height age, 7 years. Note protruding abdomen, absence of sexual maturation, poor muscle development and loss of subcutaneous fat, protruding joints, and stooped posture. (From Wiedemann [2] and Wiedemann H-R, Grosse, F-R, Dibbern H. Syndrom der Progerie. In: Das charakteristische Syndrom. Stuttgart: Schattauer, 1982:194.)

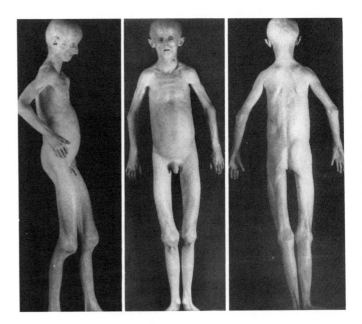

Radiographic and Laboratory Findings

Radiographic studies show marked delay in closure of the fontanelles, defective ossification of bones in the posterior cranium, gracility and porosis of long bones, shortness of clavicles, and bilateral coxa valga. Acro-osteolysis of the terminal phalanges (Figure 26.3) and loss of bone at the lateral ends of clavicles are not uncommon.

Biochemical insulin resistance [9,10], which probably results from a postreceptor defect [11,12], as well as collagen abnormalities, an increased metabolic rate, and variable anomalies of serum lipids are found. Growth hormone responses are normal. Deficient DNA repair, decreased growth capacity, and other abnormalities have been demonstrated in cultured skin fibroblasts [11,13–21].

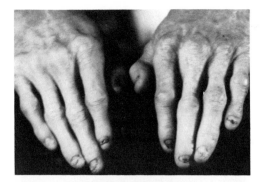

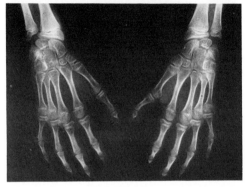

Figure 26.3. The hands of the patient shown in Figures 26.1 and 26.2. Note the inability to extend fingers fully, the somewhat knobby interphalangeal joints, short terminal phalanges with dystrophic, brittle nails, and acro-osteolysis of terminal phalanges. (From Wiedemann [2] and Wiedemann H-R, Grosse F-R, Dibbern H. Syndrom der Progerie. In: Das charakteristische Syndrom. Stuttgart: Schattauer, 1982:195.)

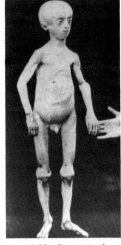

Figure 26.4. Hasting Gilford's original patient, at 17 years. (From Gilford [4].)

Diagnosis

The affected children are remarkably similar in their striking "plucked-bird appearance" (Figures 26.2, 26.4), with an angular head, the "sculptured" beaked nasal tip (Figure 26.5), the "horse-riding" stance, the protruding abdomen, and the stooped body. Therefore, progeria is easily recognizable; diagnosis is clinical and generally can be made at a glance.

Because the appearance is so characteristic, differential diagnosis is not very difficult. Nevertheless patients with Hallermann–Streiff syndrome, neonatal progeroid syndrome [22], Cockayne's syndrome, and some other syndromes have been mistakenly diagnosed as having progeria (Table 26.1).

Figure 26.5. Same patient as in Figures 26.1 and 26.2 at 14½ years. His intelligence is normal. Note small face, "sculptured" beak-like nose, absence of ear lobules, and micrognathia. The patient died from coronary occlusion at the age of 15½. (From Wiedemann [2] and Wiedemann, H-R, Grosse F-R, Dibbern H. Syndrom der Progerie. In: Das charakteristische Syndrome. Suttgart: Schattauer, 1982:195.)

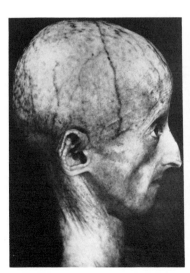

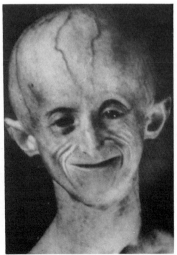

Table 26.1. Clinical Features of Neurocutaneous "Aging" Syndromes

	Progeria	Hallermann–Streiff Syndrome	Neonatal Progeroid Syndrome	De Barsy Syndrome
Manifestation	First to second year of life	Birth	Birth	First to second year of life
Mental development	Normal	Mostly normal	Mostly retarded	Mostly retarded
Stature	Dwarfish	Short	Short	Short
Neurocranium	Pseudohydrocephalic	Pseudohydrocephalic	Pseudohydrocephalic	With frontal bossing in the young child, later microcephalic
Other skeletal anomalies	Delayed closure of fontanelles; micrognathia; hypoplastic, dystrophic clavicles; coxa valga; acro-osteolysis of terminal phalanges	Delayed closure of fontanelles, small orbits, micrognathia with hypoplasia of the mandibular rami	Delayed closure of fontanelles; chin may be prominent, large hands and feet with long digits	
Scalp hair	Loss during second year of life	Sparse	Sparse to moderate	Abundant
Face	Small, bird-like, and very typical	Small, bird-like with typical appearance	Small, with a typical appearance	Narrow, with prominent nose and thin lips
Eyes	Prominent because of small orbits	Microphthalmia, cataracts	May be deep set	Corneal cloudings, may be cataracts
Dentition	Markedly delayed	Neonatal teeth and other anomalies	Neonatal teeth	Normal
Skin	Atrophic; thin, dry, and taut or wrinkled	Partly atrophic	Thin	Cutis laxa with atrophy
Subcutaneous fat tissue	Diffuse loss	Partly reduced	Diffuse deficiency with several paradoxal accumulations	Reduced
Sexual maturation		Probably reduced		
Diabetes mellitus	May be present			
Atherosclerosis	Present, early, severe			
Life span	Average of 14 years	Probably reduced	Reduced	
Inheritance	Unknown (autosomal recessive?, autosomal dominant?) (McKusick [27] 17667)	Unknown (autosomal recessive?, autosomal dominant?, or both?) (McK. 23410)	Probably autosomal recessive (McK. 26409)	Autosomal recessive

	Cockayne's Syndrome	Bloom Syndrome	Rothmund–Thomson Syndrome (Congenital Poikiloderma)	Berardinelli–Seip Syndrome (Congenital Generalized Lipodystrophy)
Manifestation	Second year of life	First year of life	Within the first years of life	Birth or shortly after
Mental development	Severely retarded	Mostly normal	Mostly normal	Often retarded
Stature	Dwarfish	Short	Mostly short	At first tall, later on normal
Neurocranium	Microcephalic	May be microcephalic	May be microcephalic	Normal
Other skeletal anomalies	Disproportionally long limbs with large hands and feet	Malar hypoplasia, micrognathia	Small hands and feet	Large hands and feet, accelerated ossification
Scalp hair	Sparse	Normal	Sparse	Abundant and curly
Face	Thin and sunken with jutten nose and chin	Small and narrow with prominent nose	Triangular with small saddle nose	Pinched with absent buccal pad of fat
Eyes	Retinal degeneration, optic atrophy	Normal	Cataracts (mostly after second year of life)	Punctate corneal opacities
Dentition	Incomplete	May be incomplete	Microdontia and other anomalies	Accelerated
Skin	Photosensitive	Photosensitive, teleangiectatic erythema about face and other regions	Poikiloderma, photosensitivity	Coarse and dry, acanthosis nigricans

Table 26.1. (continued)

	Cockayne's Syndrome	Bloom Syndrome	Rothmund–Thomson Syndrome (Congenital Poikiloderma)	Berardinelli–Seip Syndrome (Congenital Generalized Lipodystrophy)
Subcutaneous fat tissue	Diffuse loss	Not primarily affected	Not primarily affected	Diffuse loss
Sexual maturation	Reduced	Reduced	May be reduced	Normal
Diabetes mellitus	May be present			Present
Atherosclerosis	May be present			Present
Life span	Reduced	Reduced	May be reduced	Reduced
Inheritance	Autosomal recessive (McK. 21640)	Autosomal recessive (McK. 21090)	Autosomal recessive (McK. 26840)	Autosomal recessive (McK. 26970)

	SHORT Syndrome	Hypohydrotic Ectodermal Dysplasia	Yunis–Varón Syndrome	Cleidocranial Dysplasia
Manifestation	First year of life	First to second year of life	Birth	Birth
Mental development	Normal (with retarded speech)	Mostly normal	May be retarded	Normal
Stature	Short, with hyperextensibility of joints	Mostly short	Short	Mostly short, narrow shoulders
Neurocranium	Relatively large with prominent forehead	With prominent forehead	May be microcephalic	Large, brachycephalic, with frontal and parietal bossing
Other skeletal anomalies	Micrognathia, clinodactyly, shortened terminal phalanges		Delayed closure of fontanelles, micrognathia, aplasia or hypoplasia of clavicles, pelvic dysplasia, hypoplasia of fingers and thumbs, distal aphalangia	Delayed closure of fontanelles, aplasia or hypoplasia of clavicles, delayed ossification of pubic bone, tapering terminal phalanges
Scalp hair	Normal	Fine, dry, and hypochromic; sparse to absent	Sparse	Normal
Face	Thin and "senile" with wide nasal bridge and hypoplastic alae	Typical with low nasal bridge, small nose, and protruding lips and ears	Relatively small with short nasolabial distance and thin lips	Relatively small with hypertelorism and broad, flat nasal bridge
Eyes	Deep set, Rieger anomaly	Normal	Normal	Mild exophthalmos
Dentition	Delayed and irregular	Oligodontia, conical teeth	Normal	Delayed, supernumerary teeth
Skin	Soft, partly wrinkled	Soft, thin, and dry	Normal	Normal
Subcutaneous fat tissue	Widespread loss	Not primarily affected	Normal	Normal
Sexual maturation	Normal	Normal		Normal
Diabetes mellitus				
Atherosclerosis				
Life span	Normal	Mostly normal		Normal
Inheritance	Autosomal recessive (McK. 26988)	X-linked recessive (McK. 30510)	Autosomal recessive (McK. 21634)	Autosomal dominant (McK. 11960)

	Mandibuloacral Dysplasia	Acrogeria	Metageria	Werner's Syndrome
Manifestation	Second to sixth year of life	Birth or shortly after	Birth or shortly after	Second to third decade
Mental development	Normal	Normal	Normal	Mostly normal
Stature	Mostly short	Small and thin	Tall and thin	Short
Neurocranium	Normal	Normal	Normal	Normal
Other skeletal anomalies	Delayed closure of sutures, micrognathia, hypoplasia or aplasia of clavicles, acro-osteolysis of terminal phalanges	Micrognathia, small hands and feet		Porosis

Table 26.1. (continued)

	Mandibuloacral Dysplasia	Acrogeria	Metageria	Werner's Syndrome
Scalp hair	Hypotrophia or alopecia	Fine	Fine and thin	Premature graying and balding
Face	Beaked nose	Thin, pinched, with pointed nose	Thin and bird-like with beaked nose	Pinched with beaked nose
Eyes	Pseudoexophthalmos	Prominent	Prominent	Cataracts at about 25 years, retinal degeneration
Dentition	Crowding of lower teeth	Normal	Normal	Premature loss
Skin	Thin and hypotrophic	Atrophic, thin, most marked on limbs	Atrophic, most marked on limbs	Thin and dry
Subcutaneous fat tissue	Not primarily affected	Diffuse loss, most obvious on extremities	Diffuse loss	Widespread loss
Sexual maturation	May be reduced	Normal	Probably reduced	Reduced
Diabetes mellitus			Present	Present
Atherosclerosis			Present, early	Present
Life span	Normal		Reduced	Reduced
Inheritance	Autosomal recessive (McK. 24837)	Autosomal recessive (McK. 20120)	Autosomal recessive?	Autosomal recessive (McK. 27770)

Etiology and Pathogenesis

The cause and the mechanism are unknown. Most cases are sporadic. There are some few instances of affected siblings with consanguineous or not consanguineous healthy parents, suggesting autosomal recessive inheritance [23,24]. On the other hand, increased paternal age was noted in families with cases of progeria, suggesting the possibility of autosomal dominant mutation [1,25–27]. Chromosome studies have been normal. No specific endocrine disorder has been described. Perhaps there may be hypothalamic dysfunctions or, more probably, fundamental disorders in cell metabolism. The pathogenesis of atherosclerosis in progeria is obscure.

Prognosis and Treatment

The temporary general health of progeric children is good. But their life span is very much shortened by the early advent of progressive atheromatosis. Usually the cause of death is coronary occlusion during the second decade of life, less often a cerebrovascular accident. Mean age at death is about 14 years, but some patients have survived to their early or late twenties.

There is no therapy known for progeria, but symptomatic care is important. Since there is no primary effect of progeria upon the intellect, patients should be allowed as normal a social life as possible. Psychologic care may be necessary because the pa-

tients frequently have problems related to their size and to their odd appearance. The use of a wig, proper skin and dental care, and cautious physiotherapy are recommended, as is genetic counseling for the parents. As yet there is no possibility of prenatal diagnosis.

References

1. DeBusk FL. The Hutchinson–Gilford syndrome. J Pediatr 1972;80:697–724.
2. Wiedemann H-R. Syndrome mit besonderem "Altesaspekt." In: Opitz H, Schmid F, eds. Handbuch der Kinderheilkunde. Heidelberg: Springer, 1971;1:828–852.
3. Hutchinson J. Congenital absence of hair and mammary glands with atrophic condition of the skin and its appendages in a boy whose mother had been almost wholly bald from alopecia areata from the age of six. Trans Med Chir Soc (Edinburgh) 1886;69:473.
4. Gilford H. Progeria: a form of senilism. Practitioner 1904:73:188.
5. Makous N, Friedman S, Yakovac W, et al. Cardiovascular manifestations in progeria. Report of clinical and pathologic findings in a patient with severe arteriosclerotic heart disease and aortic stenosis. Am Heart J 1962;64:334–346.
6. Nelson M. Progeria: audiologic aspects. Arch Pediatr 1962;79:87–90.
7. Spence AM, Herman MM. Critical re-examination of the premature aging concept in progeria: a light and electron microscopic study. Mech Ageing Dev 1973; 2:211–227.

8. Martin GM. Genetic syndromes in man with potential relevance to the pathobiology of aging. Birth Defects Orig Art Ser 1978;14(1):5–39.

9. Villee DB, Nichols G, Jr, Talbot NB. Metabolic studies in two boys with classical progeria. Pediatrics 1969;43:207–216.

10. Rosenbloom AL, Karacan IJ, DeBusk FL. Sleep characteristics and endocrine response in progeria. J Pediatr 1970;77:692–695.

11. Rosenbloom AL, Goldstein S, Yip CC. Insulin binding to cultured human fibroblasts increases with normal and precocious aging. Science 1976;193:412–415.

12. Rosenbloom AL, Kappy MS, DeBusk FL, et al. Progeria: insulin resistance and hyperglycemia. J Pediatr 1983;102:400–402.

13. Danes BS. Progeria: a cell culture study on aging. J Clin Invest 1971;50:2000–2003.

14. Goldstein S, Moerman EJ. Heat-labile enzymes in skin fibroblasts from subjects with progeria. N Engl J Med 1975;292:1305–1309.

15. Goldstein S, Niewiarowski S. Increased precoagulant activity in cultured fibroblasts from progeria and Werner's syndromes of premature aging. Nature (London) 1976;260:711–713.

16. Brown WT, Little JB, Epstein J, et al. DNA repair defect in progeric cells. Birth Defects Orig Art Ser 1978;14(1):417–430.

17. Goldstein S, Moerman EJ. Heart-labile enzymes in circulating erythrocytes of a progeria family. Am J Hum Genet 1978;30:167–173.

18. DeFronzo RA. Glucose intolerance and aging. Evidence for tissue insensitivity to insulin. Diabetes 1979;28:1095–1101.

19. Brown WT, Darlington GJ. Thermolabile enzymes in progeria and Werner syndrome: evidence contrary to the protein error hypothesis. Am J Hum Genet 1980;32:614–619.

20. Harley CB, Goldstein S, Posner BI, et al. Decreased sensitivity of old and progeric human fibroblasts to a preparation of factors with insulin activity. J Clin Invest 1981;68:988–994.

21. Tollefsbol TO, Zaun MR, Gracy RW. Increased lability of triosephosphate isomerase in progeria and Werner's syndrome fibroblasts. Mech Ageing Dev 1982;20:93–101.

22. Devos EA, Leroy JG, Frijns J-P, et al. The Wiedemann–Rautenstrauch or neonatal progeroid syndrome. Eur J Pediatr 1981;136:245–248.

23. Mostafa AH, Gabr M. Heredity in progeria. With follow-up of two affected sisters. Arch Pediatr 1954;71:163–172.

24. Erecinski K, Bittel-Dobrzynska N, Mostowiec S. Zespol progerii u dwoch braci. Pol Tyg Lek 1961;16:806–809.

25. Jones KL, Smith DW, Harvey MAS, et al. Older paternal age and fresh gene mutation: data on additional disorders. J Pediatr 1975;86:84–88.

26. Brown WT. Human mutations affecting aging—a review. Mech Ageing Dev 1979;9:325–336.

27. McKusick VA. Mendelian inheritance in man. Catalogs of autosomal dominant, autosomal recessive and X-linked phenotypes. 6th ed. Baltimore: Johns Hopkins, 1983.

Chapter 27

Neuroectodermal Melanolysosomal Disease

B. RAFAEL ELEJALDE and
MARIA MERCEDES DE ELEJALDE

Some years ago we described a condition affecting three consanguineous families, characterized by abnormal hair color (silver-leaden), severe dysfunction of the central nervous system (profound mental, developmental, and behavioral retardation), abnormal intracytoplasmic inclusions in all tissues studied, and abnormally formed melanosomes [1]. The condition, which we called neuroectodermal melanolysosomal disease (NEMLD), affected three children, one in each family. The signs and symptoms in these children were very different from those seen in other conditions known to involve abnormal pigmentation and psychomotor developmental delay.

The three families were highly inbred. They had four common ancestors, two in the first generation and two in the second (Figure 27.1). The most likely explanation for the origin of this condition is an autosomal recessive gene, probably inherited from one of the common ancestors. Pathway analysis of the pedigree reveals either II-5 or II-6 to be the most likely carrier of the abnormal gene; this is the only pair who have complete loops to the three families.

No other family members showed any of the signs observed in the three affected children. Five members of the family (IV-4, IV-9, VII-1, VII-3, and VII-6) had hair color that differed from both the "normal" members and from those whose hair was silver-leaden. They had light brown hair, but their intellectual and developmental performance was normal.

No other individuals have been reported in the literature with this condition, but we have been informed that there may be a family in India that has a condition very similar to NEMLD (Witkop CJ: personal communication 1986).

The three families in which the condition was originally described did not reproduce any more, and we do not know of the outcome of the marriages of their children.

Clinical Features and Course

The affected children VII-5 (Figure 27.2), VII-8 (Figure 27.3), and VII-10 (Figure 27.4) were severely hypotonic and had almost complete absence of movements and no response to external stimuli. Their facies were characterized by severe hypotonia. Other features included plagiocephaly, micrognathia, crowded teeth, narrow high palate, flat chest, pectus excavatum, and cryptorchidism. One child had severe myopia and myopic changes in the retina. Their growth was within normal range for age. Cutaneous and deep tendon reflexes were hypoactive. Two of the three patients had seizures.

The syndrome is static; although the patients do not gain new developmental milestones, they do not lose the few they have acquired. They do not appear to recognize their parents, and although they occasionally smile, this is more a random activity than a response to appropriate stimuli.

Genetics

The condition appears to be caused by the pleiotropic effects of an autosomal recessive gene in its homozygous state, producing various phenotypic effects in different tissues.

The unusual hair color probably results from the melanocytes in the hair bulb producing melanin in the presence of the different substrates, as proposed

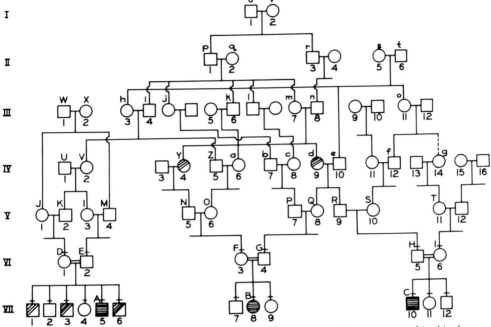

Figure 27.1. Family tree for the kindred with neuroectodermal melanolysosomal disease presented in this chapter. Note the common ancestry of the three families.

Figure 27.2. Clinical picture of patient VII-5. Note the severe hypotonia and the tanning of the distal ends of the extremities (more frequently exposed to the sunlight).

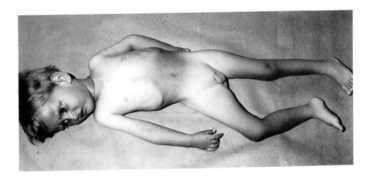

Figure 27.3. Clinical picture of patient VII-8. Note the similar hypotonic positioning seen in the previous patient.

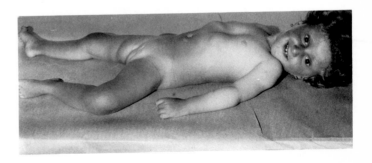

by Witkop et al. [2]. When melanosomes are transferred to the hair shaft (Figure 27.5), they clump into large, irregular granules that accumulate in the medullary zone. There are fewer but equally abnormal granules in the cortical zone.

The melanosomes are abnormal in structure (Fig-

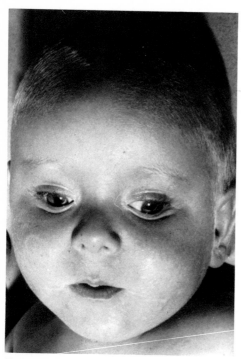

Figure 27.4. Demonstrated in this patient (VII-10) is the appearance of the face and the light-colored hair.

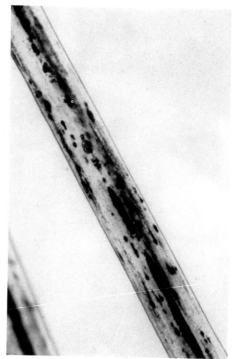

Figure 27.5. Note the characteristic pigment deposition in the hair shaft, and the large clumps of melanosomes aligned in the hair medulla.

ure 27.6) and smaller than normal, with spiral organization of the normally spindle-like matrix and abnormal deposition of the pigment.

The color of the hair is probably produced by two factors: the distribution of the melanosomes in the hair shaft, and the diffraction, refraction, and absorption of light by both the pigment granules and the hair matrix.

The color of the skin, although light, did not deviate enough from that of other members of the family to be considered abnormal. There was a good tanning response to sunlight exposure.

Severe dysfunction of the central nervous system was present in all three patients as indicated by their profound mental, social, and behavioral retardation and motor development delay, generalized hypotonia, and hyporeflexia.

Abnormal cytoplasmic granules were present in several tissues (Figures 27.7, 27.8), including but probably not limited to the epidermis, dermal fibroblasts (Figure 27.7), lymphocytes, and different cellular lines in the bone marrow (Figure 27.8). These granules are membrane bound and contain a substance of variable osmophilia. The growth of these

granules can be followed in different cells (Figure 27.8). They begin as small vesicles and progress to large rounded granules with accumulating matrix. The material they contain is homogeneous at first and takes osmium lightly. Progressively the granules stain more intensely, and at the last stage of their formation they stain deeply. At the same time that this occurs the matrix becomes fragmented until finally it is composed of smaller granules within the vesicle. Up to this time the granules are intracytoplasmic, but then they are irreversibly extruded.

Biochemistry

The granules have well-defined biochemical characteristics. The substance that they contain is not hydrolized, as indicated by its progressive accumulation, probably due to the absence of a specific hydrolytic enzyme not yet identified. Furthermore, based on the histochemical and electron microscopic characteristics of the cytoplasmic granules (Table 27.1), one can conclude that this substance is not myelin or a phospholipid. The substance appears to be a lipid

Figure 27.6. This electron micrograph demonstrates the characteristics of the melanosomes in an epithelial cell. Note their incomplete melanization, the irregular deposition of pigment, and the spiral organization exhibited by some. Many of the melanosomes are not pigmented; note the organization of their fibers (original magnification × 35,000; fixation 3% glutaraldehyde, 2% osmium tetroxide).

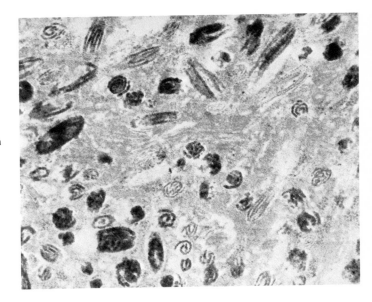

Figure 27.7. Electron micrograph of a cultured fibroblast exhibiting a prominent Golgi apparatus and the sequence in the formation and maturation of the vesicles, from the small empty ones to those (homogeneously stained) that contain the osmophilic material (original magnification × 24,000; fixation 3% glutaraldehyde, 2% osmium tetroxide).

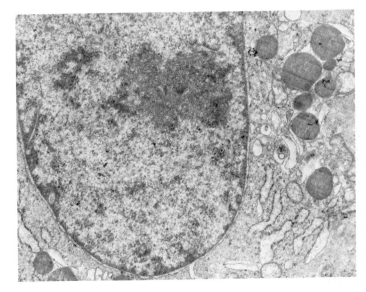

similar to the one found in granules that contain melanin, ceroid, or lipofuscin [3]. A positive Fontana stain, which is considered specific for iron-containing pigments (but is not specific for melanin), indicates that the substance present in the lysosomes of these patients is probably a lipid rich in iron, somehow related to melanin.

We have proposed two hypotheses to explain the origin of this compound. First, it may be the material that normally constitutes the melanosomal fibrils which cannot be properly assembled in this disease and consequently is accumulated in a nonfibrillar form. Alternatively, it may be a precursor of melanin, not necessarily a component of this molecule

but needed for the assembling of the melanosomes or for melanin synthesis. So far we have no evidence supporting or disproving either hypothesis.

We conclude that these granules do lack ceroid because they do not autofluoresce [4]. The compound observed in the melanosomes is not a direct precursor of melanin since fibroblasts and bone marrow cells containing the abnormal granules failed to produce melanin when incubated in the presence of tyrosine, supporting the concept that the accumulated substance is a precursor of melanin. These cells actively incorporate ³H-dopa exclusively into the granules. The significance of this observation is not known at present, but the close relationship of the

Figure 27.8. In this electron micrograph of a bone-marrow histiocyte, the variable density of the granules and their matrix is seen. Those seen inside the cytoplasm have a homogeneous matrix; both those seen in the extracellular space show an irregular matrix that becomes more granulous (original magnification × 39,000; fixation 3% glutaraldehyde, 2% osmium tetroxide).

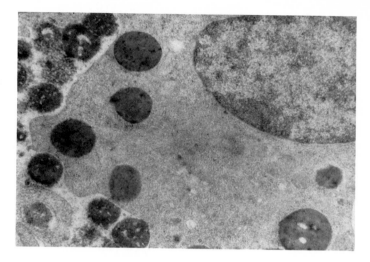

Table 27.1. Histochemical Reactions of Bone Marrow and Fibroblasts

	Bone Marrow	Fibroblasts
Periodic acid–Schiff	+ + +	+ + + +
Fontana	+ +	+ +
Autofluorescence	−	−
Luxol fast blue	−	−
Alkaline phosphatase	−	−
Peroxidase	−	−
Tyrosinase	−	−
Oil red O	+	+
Cold acetic acid extraction	−	−
Hot acetic acid extraction	−	−
Toluidine blue	−	−
Incorporation of		
^{3}H-dopa	+ + +	+ + +
^{3}H-tyrosine	+ +	+ +
^{3}H-cysteine	+ +	+ +

dopaminergic system and neuromelanin is a well-established fact. Abnormalities of the dopaminergic pathway are known to be associated with an abnormally functioning central nervous system.

The negative peroxidase reaction adds further evidence to the hypothesis that the granules and the substance contained in them are early precursors of melanin since this enzyme has been proposed to play a role in the synthesis of melanin in some tissues [5].

The absence of fibers inside the vesicles indicates that if the material contained in these vesicles is related to the melanosome, it corresponds to a very early stage, before the fibers appear and the melanin is deposited.

Pathogenesis

Some of the tissues that are altered in this condition are derived from the neuroectoderm [6]. Melanocytes are widely distributed in the central nervous system. They appear in the pia-arachnoid, the locus ceruleus, the trigeminal and other cranial sensory ganglia, the substantia nigra, the area postrema of the olfactory region, certain cells of the pineal gland [7], and throughout the pigmented column of Bazelon [8]. They are also components of the peripheral nervous system, namely in the dorsal root and sympathetic ganglia [9].

Melanocytes are not limited to the nervous system. They are also found in the retina, choroid, gall-bladder, ovary, adrenal medulla, lamina propria of the colon, rectum, and appendix [7], and in the vestibular labyrinth [8,10]. Their specific role in these tissues is not yet known. If they do have a role, abnormalities in these cells and in the pigment they produce should alter the functioning of those tissues and organs.

The pigment that melanocytes contain and transfer to other cells is suspected to play important roles in the tissues in which they are found, mostly because of the consequences of their absence, such as occurs in albinism, and of the alteration of neuromelanin found in Parkinson's disease [3].

Melanin has been classified in two major groups, neuromelanin and melanin, which are very different. Neuromelanin remains inside the cells in which it is produced, whereas melanin is transferred to the keratinocytes. Skin melanin is produced from tyrosine, dopa, or cysteine through the action of at least one enzyme, tyrosinase, which is widely distributed in the skin and hair. This enzyme is absent in the central and peripheral nervous systems, suggesting that neuromelanin is probably produced by means of a different enzyme.

The role of melanin in the central nervous system and the cells that contain it is not clearly understood at this time. Melanin is abundant in the substantia nigra, known to play an important role in maintaining normal muscular tone. Although we do not have direct evidence that neuromelanin was abnormal in these patients, we inferred that it was since they had such a pronounced central nervous system impairment. Another condition known to involve neuromelanin, Hallervorden–Spatz disease [11], has severe abnormalities of muscle tone, in this case dystonia. Parkinson's disease caused by ingestion of N-methyl-4-phenyl-1,2,3,6-tetrahydropyridine, which deposits itself preferentially in the substantia nigra, probably in the melanin-containing cells, is specially informative in the understanding of the pathogenesis of NEMLD. Many chemicals, such as paraquat and diquat, are known to attach to neuromelanin and to remain there [12,13].

Other pleiotropic effects of the same gene appear in derivatives of the mesoderm: fibroblasts, lymphocytes, and bone marrow cells. The abnormal lysosomes they display could be related to melanosomes that are formed in a very similar way. They also begin with the formation of microvesicles as a response to the interaction of melanocyte stimulating hormone with the membrane receptors. The premelanosome is one of those vesicles in which the filaments that will characterize the melanosome develop.

We believe that the vesicles seen in these cells are an indication of the activation of a gene that codes for the early events of melanosome formation, events that cannot be completed in these mesodermal cells since the other genes that code for the events that normally follow the formation of the premelanosome are not active in these cells.

In NEMLD the hypomelanized melanosomes in the skin, the lysosomal inclusions in the fibroblasts, and the lymphocytes and bone marrow cells can be considered authophenes. The severe central nervous system dysfunction could represent relational pleiotropy or a real case of cell-reactive pleiotropy [14,15]. We cannot differentiate one from the other since we do not know the basic defect that produces the condition nor its consequences in different tissues.

Differential Diagnosis

Neuroectodermal melanolysosomal disease is not the only condition in which abnormalities of pigmentation are associated with severe central nervous system dysfunction. The Beguez–Chediak–Higashi syndrome [16,17] is characterized by partial hypopigmentation involving the skin, the areolas, the genitalia, and the hair. The individuals affected by this condition have several central nervous system abnormalities, cytoplasmic inclusions in nerve cell astrocytes, epithelial and choroidal satellite cells of the dorsal spinal ganglia, irregular clumping of melanin in the substantia nigra, and lymphocytes and bone marrow cells containing inclusions different from those seen in NEMLD. The most prominent sign of this condition is the immune deficiency that affects both humans and animals who have the gene that produces the Beguez–Chediak–Higashi syndrome. These individuals have nearly normal psychomotor development and do not have the severe motor impairment seen in NEMLD.

Cross syndrome [18] is another autosomal recessive condition characterized by severe central nervous system impairment with spasticity, mental retardation, seizures, and severe hypopigmentation produced by amelanotic melanosomes. These melanosomes become pigmented if incubated in a solution containing tyrosine. This condition is also different from NEMLD.

Other syndromes with hypopigmentation and partial CNS function impairment are Woolf syndrome (congenital deafness and piebaldness) [19], Zyprowski–Margolis syndrome (albinism and congenital deaf-mutism) [20], and Waardenburg syndrome (abnormal hair pigmentation, heterochromia irides, and congenital sensorineural deafness) [21].

In conclusion, NEMLD is probably the consequence of an altered gene that codes for early events of melanosome formation, thus producing abnormal melanosomes and probably abnormal melanin and neuromelanin, altering the color of the hair and the functioning of the CNS. The condition is probably due to an autosomal recessive gene.

Treatment

No specific treatment is available for NEMLD. The infants and children require the specialized care appropriate for children with profound mental retardation and cerebral palsy. Due to their profound mental and motor retardation it is very difficult to use any type of therapy requiring the patient's cooperation; all interventions including physical therapy need to take into account the completely passive status of the patients. Consequently, passive exercises are paramount in the management of these children.

The patient's family requires understanding support to help cope with the many problems of children with profound mental and physical handicaps.

These children do not show any special propensity to suffer infectious diseases and have normal immunologic response to vaccination.

Prenatal diagnosis of this disease has not been performed but it appears it will be feasible if the abnormal cytoplasmic inclusions are found in cultured amniotic cells or fetal skin obtained by biopsy with fetoscopy.

References

1. Elejalde BR, Holguin J, Valencia A, et al. Mutations affecting pigmentation in man. I. Neuroectodermal melanolysosomal disease. Am J Med Genet 1979;3:65–80.
2. Witkop CJ, White JG, Nance WE, et al. Classification of albinism in man. BDOAS 1971;7:13–25.
3. Marsden CD. Brain melanin in pigments. In: Wolman M, ed. Pathology. New York: Academic Press, 1969:395–420.
4. Hartford WS, Porta EA. Ceroid. Am J Med Sci 1965;25:117–137.
5. Okun MR, Donnellan B, Lever WF. Peroxidase-dependent oxidation of tyrosine or dopa to melanin in neurons. Histochemie 1971;25:289–296.
6. Rawles MR. Origin of pigment cells from the neural crest in the mouse embryo. Physiol Zool 1947–1948;20:248–266.
7. Moses HL, Ganote CE, Beaver DL, et al. Light and electron microscopic studies of pigment in human and rhesus monkey nigra and locus ceruleus. Anat Rec 1966;155:167–184.
8. Bazelon M, Fenichel GM, Randall T. Studies on neuromelanin. I. A melanin system in the human adult brainstem. Neurology 1962;17:512–519.
9. De Castro F. Sensory ganglia of the cranial and spinal nerves. In: Penfield W, ed. Cytology and cellular pathology of the nervous system. New York: Paul B Hoeber, 1932:93–143.
10. La Ferriere KD, Aremberg IJ, Hawkins EJ, et al. Melanocytes of the vestibular labyrinth and their relationship to the microvasculature. Ann Otol 1974;83:685–694.
11. Elejalde BR, Elejalde MMJ, Lopez F. Hallervorden–Spatz disease. Clin Genet 1979;16:1–18.
12. Larson B, Ojkarsson A, Tjalve H. Binding of paraquat and diquat on melanin. Exp Eye Res 1977;25:353–359.
13. Lindquist NG. Accumulation of drugs on melanin. Acta Radiol 1973;(suppl)325:1–92.
14. Goldschmidt R. Theoretical genetics. Berkeley: University of California Press, 1955:393–418.
15. Rieger R, Michaelis A, Green MM. Glossary of genetics and cytogenetics. Berlin: Springer–Verlag, 1976:39,426.
16. Beguez-Cesar A. Neutropenia crónica maligna familiar con granulaciones atípicas de los leucocitos. Bol Soc Pediatr Cubana 1943;15:900–922.
17. White JG. Chediak–Higashi syndrome. Am J Pathol 1973;72:503–519.
18. Cross HE, McKusick VA, Breen W. A new oculocerebral syndrome with hypopigmentation. Pediatrics 1967;70:398–406.
19. Woolf M, Dolowitz DA, Aldow HE. Congenital deafness associated with piebaldness. Arch Otolaryngol 1965;82:244–250.
20. Ziprowski L, Krakowski A, Adam A, et al. Partial albinism and deaf mutism. Arch Dermatol 1962;86:190–198.
21. Waardenburg PJ. A new syndrome combining developmental anomalies of the eyelids, eyebrows and nose root with congenital deafness. Am J Hum Genet 1951;3:195–253.

Chapter 28
Ruvalcaba–Myhre Syndrome

DONALD ZIMMERMAN

In 1980, Ruvalcaba et al. described two unrelated men with macrocephaly, mental deficiency, hamartomatous polyps of the colon (in one patient also involving the distal ileum), and irregular pigmented macules on the glans penis [1]. While the initial report described the condition as a variant of Sotos' syndrome, one of the authors separated this condition from Sotos' syndrome in a subsequent communication [2]. More recently, a lipid storage myopathy has been described in affected individuals [3]. Other recently described abnormalities in affected patients have included ocular anomalies (both Schwalbe's lines and corneal nerves are prominent) as well as subcutaneous angiolipomas [4].

Clinical Features

Macrocephaly has been noted as early as late fetal life in one case [1] and at the time of birth in another [4]. In other cases, early measurements of head circumference have not been reported. Head circumference has generally measured three [4] to five standard deviations [1] above the mean for age. In one patient, the anterior fontanelle did not close until after age 5 years [4].

Psychomotor development varies in patients with Ruvalcaba–Myhre syndrome. Most patients appear to have delayed motor development, some in association with frank hypotonia in early childhood [3,4]. In patients manifesting weakness, muscle strength tends to improve through infancy and childhood [3].

Psychological development has also varied. One patient had severe mental retardation in addition to a seizure disorder [1,3] while another manifested mild

mental retardation [1]. Still others appear to have normal intelligence [3,4].

A mother and son with Ruvalcaba–Myhre syndrome both exhibited ocular abnormalities as well as prominent Schwalbe's lines. The son also had prominent corneal nerves.

The most characteristic skin abnormality is the presence of pigmented macules over the glans penis (Figure 28.1). In one of the affected patients, these macules were not detected until approximately 2 years of age [4]. However, a 4-year-old boy who had been reported with Ruvalcaba–Myhre syndrome had not yet developed such pigmentation [3].

A mother and son affected with Ruvalcaba–Myhre syndrome both had angiolipomas. The son also had a lipoma and several café-au-lait spots on the trunk and lower limbs. In another affected patient acanthosis nigricans was described [1,3].

Intestinal polyposis has presented with rectal bleeding [1], intussusception [4], and as an incidental finding on proctoscopic and radiologic examination of the bowel. In one patient, three polyps were also present on the dorsum of the tongue. However, another patient is reported to have Ruvalcaba–Myhre syndrome without either associated intestinal polyposis or penile pigmentation [3].

One affected patient in whom angiolipoma and hamartomatous intestinal polyps were present underwent removal of a mucoepidermoid carcinoma of the parotid gland [3,4].

Laboratory Findings

Computerized tomograms of the brain have been described both as normal [3,4] and as showing generalized brain enlargement [1]. In three of four patients

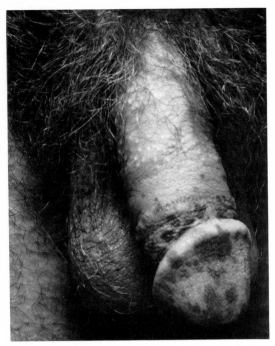

Figure 28.1. Pigmented lesion of the penis in a patient with Ruvalcaba–Myhre syndrome.

electromyography revealed an increase in short-duration polyphasic motor unit potentials, decreased recruitment, and no evidence of denervation [3]. In all four patients so studied, muscle biopsies exhibited greater variation in size of muscle fibers than normally observed. In addition, Oil Red O-stained sections of muscle showed a marked increase in the size and number of neutral lipid droplets, predominantly in type I fibers [3].

Gastrointestinal x-rays have revealed polyposis, either limited to the colon or involving the colon as well as the distal ileum [1]. The polyps have been described as hamartomatous with histology resembling that of patients with Peutz-Jegher syndrome.

Increased urinary excretion of mucopolysaccharides has been observed in one patient [4].

Genetics and Nosology

Since only five cases of Ruvalcaba–Myhre syndrome have been extensively reported [1,3,4] the genetics of the condition are presently uncertain. The presence of this condition in a mother and her child has suggested probable autosomal dominant inheritance [4]. As noted earlier, the authors who originally reported the Ruvalcaba–Myhre syndrome initially considered this condition a variant of Sotos' syndrome [1]. However, these authors subsequently came to regard the Ruvalcaba–Myhre syndrome as a distinctive entity [2,3].

Some investigators have raised the possibility that Ruvalcaba–Myhre syndrome may be the same as Bannayan–Zonana syndrome (Gorlin R: personal communication 1985). In the latter, macrocephaly is associated with mild to moderate psychomotor delay and mesodermal hamartoma—particularly lipoma and hemangioma [5]. It is noteworthy, however, that both Zonana et al. [6,7] and Ruvalcaba [3] have reported these entities to be distinct. Clearly, patients with the Bannayan–Zonana syndrome should be examined for muscle lipomas, hamartomatous intestinal polyps, and pigmented macules of the penis.

Treatment

Since malignant transformation of intestinal polyps has not been described in patients with the Ruvalcaba–Myhre syndrome, most patients have undergone polypectomy when polyps have produced symptoms. One patient underwent subtotal colectomy and ileorectal anastomosis. Subsequently, he has had recurrent benign polyps of the rectal remnant that are removed intermittently [1].

No specific treatment for muscle lipomatosis has been attempted.

References

1. Ruvalcaba RHA, Myhre S, Smith DW. Sotos syndrome with intestinal polyposis and pigmentary changes of the genitalia. Clin Genet 1980;18:413–416.
2. Smith DW, Jones KL. Recognizable patterns of human malformation: genetic embryologic and clinical aspects. 3rd ed. Philadelphia: Saunders, 1982:387.
3. DiLiberti JH, D'Hoestino AN, Ruvalcaba RHA, et al. A new lipid storage myopathy observed in individuals with the Ruvalcaba–Myhre–Smith syndrome. Am J Med Genet 1984;18:163–167.
4. DiLiberti JH, Weieber RG, Budden S. Ruvalcaba–Myhre–Smith syndrome: a case with probable autosomal-dominant inheritance and additional manifestations. Am J Med Genet 1983;15:491–495.
5. Bannayan GA. Lipomatosis, angiomatosis, and macrencephalia. Arch Pathol 1971;92:1–5.
6. Zonana J, Rimoin DL, Davis DC. Macrocephaly with multiple lipomas and hemangiomas. J Pediatr 1976;89:600–603.
7. Miles HR, Zonana J, McFarland J. Macrocephaly with hemartomas: Bannayan–Zonana syndrome. Am J Med Genet 1984;19:225–234.

PART THREE

DISEASES WITH X-LINKED INHERITANCE

Chapter 29
Fabry–Anderson Disease

MICHEL PHILIPPART

Fabry–Anderson disease (FAD) is an X-linked gly-colipid lysosomal storage disorder that is caused by an alpha-galactosidase deficiency. In two independent reports, published in 1898, Fabry and Anderson described the striking angiokeratoma that is relatively uncommon in its most florid presentation. This is the reason that there were so few reports of this disease over the years and why the recognition that FAD is inherited and multisystemic has been delayed.

The unusual array of mostly nonspecific symptoms by which FAD may express itself explains why these historical difficulties are still extant for the clinician who needs to distinguish a rare disorder under commonplace manifestations.

Pedigrees extending up to seven generations demonstrate that the gene is often transmitted by unsuspected heterozygous females. In many families, it has not been possible to perform biochemical studies or even to clinically evaluate all the males at risk. Verbal information on deceased or otherwise unavailable males likely misses those hemizygotes with mild, hidden, or delayed symptoms. With the exception of early kidney failure that will affect a male in his thirties, the clinical problems of the hemizygote are extremely nonspecific and are not likely to be thought significant by the inquiring physician. Indeed, FAD may masquerade as heart disease, stroke, joint disease, gastrointestinal disturbances, or neurosis, the most common problems in any practice.

That the symptoms have a chronic or insidious character further contributes to their apparent banality. Even the more characteristic kidney failure may not appear until the patient is in his or her late fifties. In many cases FAD is actually less disabling that might be anticipated on the basis of published reports.

History

In 1897 Anderson reported a 39-year-old man who had developed skin lesions at the age of 11. These angiectases progressively spread and he also had albuminuria, finger deformity, varicose veins, and leg edema. A skin biopsy showed capillary dilation in the papillary layer of the dermis. Anderson correctly surmised that the albuminuria was related to diseased kidney vessels [1]. In 1962, Wise et al. [2] discovered that this patient had died at the age of 54 from tuberculous enteritis and had two affected grandsons.

Fabry [3] described a 13-year-old boy with purpura hemorrhagica nodularis. This child, whose maternal grandfather had died of kidney disease, first presented with skin lesions around the knee at age 9. He later developed proteinuria and periorbital edema before dying of lung disease at the age of 42 [4]. Steiner and Voerner [5] reported a man with more characteristic symptoms since the age of 14, including anhydrosis, intolerance to hot weather, and episodes of pain and paresthesias in the extremities. The relationship between skin disease and general symptoms was suspected but the kidney disease was felt to be incidental. A genetic factor was appreciated as the patient's mother had many small angiomas. The autopsy of two patients [6,7] with vascular abnormalities throughout the body established the multisystemic character of FAD. The smooth muscles and heart had vacuoles suggesting a lipid storage disorder. In 1962, Wise et al. [2] analyzed 70 published cases and 8 new families. This report of FAD, which is one of the best, conclusively showed that the gene is X-linked with occasional expression in the heterozygous female.

Rahman and Lindenberg [8] demonstrated limited storage in the central nervous system and widespread storage in the sympathetic nervous system. Sweeley and Klionsky [9] identified ceramide trihexoside in the kidney.

In 1967, Brady et al. [10] demonstrated a specific deficiency of ceramide trihexosidase activity in intestinal mucosa. Heterozygous females had a 50% reduction of that activity. Urbain et al. [11] found ceramide trihexoside excretion in the urinary sediment of an individual without skin lesions. In 1970, Kint [12] demonstrated a deficiency of alpha-galactosidase activity in leukocytes, opening the way to simple diagnostic screening.

Clinical Presentation

Fabry–Anderson disease is a chronic malady with lifelong, mostly nonspecific manifestations. As is expected for a lysosomal storage disorder the disease is progressive but so insidious that worsening is not easily recognized.

The clinical onset often occurs between the ages of 5 and 10 years in a child who complains of pain in the hands and feet. The episode may be associated with fever and generally lasts for a few days. Similar episodes recur rather randomly for many years and may subside entirely after age 20. The angiokeratomas are either not present or not likely to be recognized in a child less than 10 years of age. Characteristic corneal opacities exist but the clinician is unlikely to search for them. Leg edema may occur, often in an asymmetrical fashion (Figure 29.1). A diagnosis of juvenile rheumatoid arthritis is often considered although joint pain is rare, and signs of inflammation are probably never present. Many children look small for their age. While the pain has a predilection for the extremities, any part of the body may be involved. Recurrent abdominal pain may lead to an erroneous diagnosis of appendicitis. Proteinuria may occur in association with a bout of pain during the late teens but kidney disease is rare before the late twenties. Kidney failure is the leading problem in the thirties and forties, although in a few cases heart or brain disease predominates.

Attempts to describe a typical course are artificial. Resemblances between family members may be apparent but differences are often more striking. The diagnosis is likely to be difficult or erroneous unless the angiokeratomas and genetic character of the condition are recognized. The combination of symptoms is endless, and they are often milder and less conspicuous than reports biased toward the most severe complications indicate.

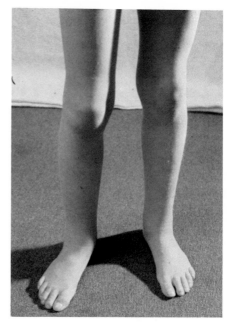

Figure 29.1. Ten-year-old boy with asymmetric leg edema. The left ankle is only slightly swollen. Both the right ankle and knee are moderately swollen.

Skin

The angiokeratoma is the hallmark of this disease. Identified in most published cases, it is inconspicuous or even absent in the majority of patients, which explains why additional reports were so slow to appear after the disease was originally described. The angiokeratoma is a small, round or oblong, dark red or violet lesion, generally less than 2 mm in diameter, isolated or in irregular clusters. The skin is dry and slightly hyperkeratotic and unevenly raised over the lesions, feeling like sandpaper when brushed lightly with the fingers. Striking dense lesions in the bathing trunk area are exceptional. The elective location of angiokeratoma in the folds of the umbilicus and over the genital organs (Figure 29.2) contributes to its difficult detection. Pressure points such as the anterior iliac crest and buttocks are often involved.

A large pedigree [13] illustrates well the range and type of expression in a single family. Enzyme determinations identified 21 affected males, 18 of whom, aged 3 to 47 years, were examined. In 4 subjects no angiokeratoma could be found, and in 5 others they would have been easily missed if the biochemical diagnosis had not been made. More than 200 relatives were normal or of uncertain status. Only one of the affected males had lost significant time from work

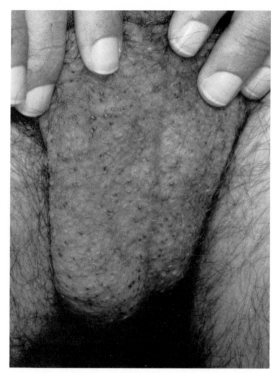

Figure 29.2. Pinhead-shaped, dark or glistening angiokeratomas are scattered over the scrotum of a 27-year-old male.

due to his disease, pointing out the generally mild character of the clinical manifestations.

Pain

The first symptom of FAD is generally a bout of excruciating burning pain in the extremities. About 90% of males but less than 10% of females experience this problem [14]. The attack may be precipitated by hot or cold weather but a triggering factor often cannot be identified. Fever in the absence of infection is often associated with these episodes. Anhydrosis or hypohydrosis decreases the ability of the body to lower its temperature and causes intolerance to hot weather. Juvenile rheumatoid arthritis or rheumatic fever is often suspected, and acetylsalicylic acid or even steroids are given. The negative laboratory investigations and the lack of response to medications distress the child and parents, and may lead the clinician to raise the issue of neurosis or hysteria. Wise et al. [2] first pointed out the causalgic character of the pain, which can be felt in the abdomen and, less frequently, in the chest in addition to the extremities. Recurrent headaches are common.

Many adults feel a chronic discomfort, difficult to describe or localize. Unless questioned they are not likely to mention this problem that has been present since childhood.

Gastrointestinal Tract

Symptoms are frequent but generally not severe. Episodic diarrhea and abdominal pain are more frequent than indigestion, nausea, and vomiting. Fever may occur. A study of 30 cases in four families revealed symptoms in 5 of 13 males and 5 of 17 females [15]. No evidence of malabsorption or celiac disease was found. Radiologic abnormalities consisted of thickened folds, mild dilation throughout, granular appearance of the ileum, and loss of haustral markings in the distal colonic segments [15,16]. One male had a thickened wall of the mid small bowel, which was attributed to an ischemic process [16]. Ulcerative colitis may be suggested by barium enema [17].

Eye

Whorl-like corneal opacities had been described in a family that many years later was proven to have FAD [18]. These opacities are found in 80 [19] to 95% [20] of patients of both sexes after age 10 years. They are more likely to be absent in young children but have also been absent in a few middle-aged patients [19,20]. Similar opacities have been described in individuals exposed to prolonged treatment with antimalarials or chlorpromazine [20]. A lenticular opacity with spoke-like deposits, found in 37% of hemizygotes and 14% of heterozygotes, may be specific for FAD [20]. The lens is abnormal in 79% of hemizygotes and 54% of heterozygotes [19].

Vascular lesions are of special interest because they focus the attention on a tissue electively involved by the storage. The veins of the conjunctiva and retina present with corkscrew tortuosity, beading, and aneurysmal dilations in 50 to 78% of hemizygotes and 44 to 48% of heterozygotes over the age of 10 [19,20]. None of these abnormalities leads to visual impairment. Central retinal artery occlusion is rare [20].

Heart and Vessels

Cardiac abnormalities have been reported incidentally, perhaps because they are generally not predominant or even symptomatic [21]. An infiltrative cardiomyopathy with storage of glycolipid in the myocardium, conducting tissues, valves, and endocardium, is found in nearly all cases. An electrocardiogram commonly reveals a short P-R interval. Primary cardiac involvement is often combined with the effects of renal failure or hypertension in leading to congestive heart failure [21]. Myocardial infarction is rare [22]. Cardiac problems are mentioned in 30% of published cases [22]. Angina is uncommon and probably overdiagnosed.

Vasomotor disturbances in the extremities are often falsely diagnosed as Raynaud's disease. Peripheral hemodynamics have been studied in a small series of patients (2 hemizygotes, 6 heterozygotes, 9 to 46 years of age) [23]. The abnormalities, remarkably consistent and independent of age or sex, included increased forearm vascular resistance with decreased venous capacitance, and decreased blood flow and pulse volume in toes and fingers with abnormal response to vasodilation procedures. These studies indicated an early vasoconstrictive process in cutaneous and skeletal muscular beds.

Lungs

Pulmonary parenchyma and vessels are involved. Pulmonary arterial obstruction and hemoptysis may occur. These abnormalities have little clinical or functional impact [24]. In seven patients, including one heterozygote, the five who smoked had shortness of breath and episodic pulmonary infections. Three had bullous disease and multiple ventilation and perfusion defects. All had some functional airway obstruction; five had reduced diffusing capacity; four had inclusion bodies in ciliated epithelial and goblet cells [25]. Lung involvement may be disabling in patients with renal and cardiac disease.

Central Nervous System

Cerebral vascular accidents [8,26] with ischemia, infarction, thrombosis, or less frequently, hemorrhage, occur at an untimely age, though seldom as early as in the late teens. They become more frequent with advancing age. Recurrent episodes of hemiparesis or hemianesthesia may mistakenly suggest multiple sclerosis. Confusion and focal or generalized seizures may occur. The asymmetrical presentation of the neurologic deficit belies the generalized alterations of the cerebral vessels. Angiograms are generally normal. Permanent deficits, less common, are often

slowly progressive. Death in the early thirties from neurologic involvement has been reported [27].

Peripheral Nervous System

Clinical signs of peripheral neuropathy are not a feature of FAD. In a serial study [28] of ulnar and peroneal nerves in 35 subjects, abnormalities, mostly slight, were found in 66% of the males and 15% of the females. Ulnar nerve conduction velocities were slightly decreased (34 to 40 m/sec) in 4 males and 1 female, age 4 to 13 years. Peroneal nerve conduction velocities were markedly slow (8 to 25 m/sec) in 2 males, aged 41 and 45, and in 1 female, age 39. In no subject were both nerves impaired. There was no correlation between abnormal nerve conduction velocity and complaint of pain in the extremities.

Autonomic dysfunction impairs the ability to sweat, to vasoconstrict, and to vasodilate [29]. In 10 males age 16 to 57 years [30], impaired sweating was uniform; saliva and tear formation and pupillary response to pilocarpine were abnormal in half the cases. Responses to scratch and to intradermic histamine injection were diminished; pruritus was not experienced. Heart rate, blood pressure, and blood norepinephrine concentration responded normally to changing from supine to erect position.

Kidney and Urogenital Systems

Abnormal urinary glycolipids may be detected from birth [31]. Glycolipid excretion as such is not a sign of kidney dysfunction but rather of the tubular storage that leads to it. Proteinuria does not generally occur until the third decade and may still be absent at the age of 29 [32]. Diagnostic renal studies are generally negative at this stage. Kidney failure, developing within a few years, is a major cause of death in hemizygotes—only exceptionally in heterozygotes—in their thirties and forties. Inability to concentrate urine, urinary frequency, nocturia, polyuria, and a variety of renal tubular disorders have been reported [33]. Voiding difficulties have not been specifically investigated. Priapism is a rare complication, which in one case was prompted by the use of phenoxybenzamine [34].

Joints

Acute rheumatic fever or arthritis is often diagnosed when pain in the extremities, shoulders, or hips is present. Radiologic or blood abnormalities have not generally supported such diagnoses. Mild deformities of the interphalangeal joints (Figure 29.3) are frequent but are not associated with Heberden's nodes. The rare occurrence of avascular necrosis of the femoral capital epiphysis [35] is probably indicative of the vascular disorder at this level.

Reticuloendothelial System

Since globoside, the major erythrocyte glycolipid, is an important source of ceramide trihexoside during the degradation of aging cells, one would expect that the reticuloendothelial system is heavily involved, as is the rule in the multisystemic storage disorders. However, this is not the case. Periportal macrophages are affected and hepatocytes contain lipid inclusions, but hepatic architecture is not significantly altered [36].

Bone marrow examination only occasionally shows lipid-laden macrophages. The spleen and the lymph nodes, especially abdominal ones, may be enlarged [37].

Personality

Many patients have vague complaints, suggesting a neurosis or even a psychoneurosis [2,38]. Frank psychosis [39] or mild mental deficiency [17] is quite uncommon. While many complaints are related to FAD and are compounded by frustration when the physicians fail to identify the underlying etiology, some patients exhibit chronic invalidism or inability to hold a steady job, suggesting psychological abnormalities that still need to be properly investigated. These patients lack drive, procrastinate, do not comply with recommendations for regular checkups or additional evaluations, and are negativistic.

Biochemistry

Enzyme: Alpha-Galactosidase

Fabry–Anderson disease results from a mutation of the alpha-galactosidase gene situated on the X chromosome. Several different variants have already been identified [40]. Two main groups, A and B, of molecular forms of alpha-galactosidase can be separated by electrophoresis. The B group, which depends on a gene located on chromosome 22, is an alpha-galactosaminidase that does not act on the natural substrates accumulating in FAD. The B enzyme, reacting with artificial substrates commonly used in screening, accounts for the residual activity found in FAD tissues and body fluids. In most FAD hemizygotes the deficiency of alpha-galactosidase activity is profound.

Exceptional cases of unknown etiology may mimic FAD. One patient had normal alpha-galactosidase activity despite suggestive clinical problems. He had a normal glycolipid excretion and thus could not have had FAD [41]. A personal unpublished case presented angiokeratomas and unilateral congenital leg edema without evidence of lysosomal storage or alpha-galactosidase deficiency.

Glycolipid Storage

Ceramide trihexoside is the main natural substrate cleaved by alpha-galactosidase A. It is also the major

Figure 29.3. Ten-year-old boy with interphalangeal joints that are slightly deformed. Excess soft tissue can be clearly seen above the thumbnails. Fingers cannot be fully extended and the pale domed nails are characteristic of the disease.

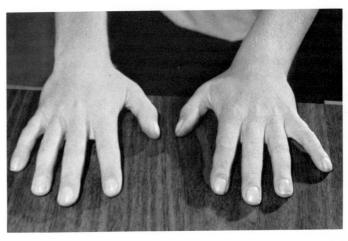

glycolipid synthesized in fibroblasts and thus accounts for the glycolipid storage in FAD connective tissues. Globoside, a tetrahexoside that is its major precursor, is found in erythrocytes, blood vessels, and the kidney. The storage site that leads to most clinical manifestations is the blood vessel. A secondary metabolite, ceramide galactosyl-alpha-galactose, found mostly in the kidney, is excreted in urine of individuals with FAD. Their plasma contains greatly elevated levels of ceramide trihexoside.

Pathology

The skin [42] and conjunctiva [43] are easily accessible sites for biopsies. Light microscopy reveals dilated blood-filled vessels in the upper dermis but the associated lipid inclusions can be easily overlooked. Lamellar inclusions can be demonstrated by electron microscopy in endothelial and perithelial cells, macrophages, smooth muscle cells of sweat glands and larger vessels, even in areas devoid of angiokeratomas [42,44,45]. Unmyelinated axons and Schwann cells are seldom affected.

Some inclusions organized in stacks or hexagonal arrangements [44], also demonstrated in cultured fibroblasts [46], are fairly distinctive and possibly specific for FAD.

Kidney biopsies in 12 patients without renal disease [32] showed diffuse glycolipid accumulation in every glomerular, vascular, and interstitial cell; with irregular tubular involvement, predominantly of distal convoluted tubules and Henle's loop in males; similar but patchy involvement in 2 females; and no anomaly in 1 female. Age-related changes were necrosis of smooth muscle cells, intimal thickening, and degenerative glomerular and tubular changes, suggesting ischemic damage.

In the central nervous system elective involvement of its autonomic component has been confirmed [8,47]. Other affected structures include the amygdala, the hippocampus, and the inferior temporal gyrus, which may have relevance to the still poorly defined mental changes. Peripheral nerves contain lipid inclusions in the perineurium and occasionally in the axons, and loss of unmyelinated, small myelinated, and, infrequently, large myelinated fibers [44,45,48]. Alterations of the spinal root ganglia [47] are probably responsible for the painful Fabry crises.

Genetics

The rules of transmission by the X chromosome apply. Heterozygotes have two cell populations [49].

While the inactivation of the X chromosome is random, wide differences are encountered between heterozygotes, and perhaps between distinct tissues of the same individual, which accounts for the varied clinical manifestations and the difficult detection of heterozygotes.

Pathophysiology

Deficiency in alpha-galactosidase activity leads to ceramide trihexoside storage, mostly in blood vessels and connective tissue. The resulting storage, present from birth, is tolerated for decades before damage to the kidneys, heart, or brain leads to death. The wide variations in phenotypic expression cannot be explained and do not correlate with residual enzyme activity or urinary glycolipid excretion [50]. The storage process within the endothelial cells causes ischemia, which seems to be the main factor of tissue damage throughout the body. The recurrent crises of pain in the extremities or abdomen are quite intriguing, and probably result from a combination of factors rather than a single one. The failure of vessels to dilate or constrict normally may result from rigidity secondary to the storage process and impaired contractility due to damaged smooth muscle cells and autonomic neurons. The beneficial action of phenytoin and carbamazepine points to a primary neuronal factor—the effectiveness of phenoxybenzamine suggests the involvement of peripheral and possibly central [39] alpha-adrenergic receptors. Ischemia, at a central as well as peripheral level, may be the common final pathway.

Diagnosis

Fluorometric determination of alpha-galactosidase activity in plasma and leukocytes is the most widely available screening technique [49]. Hair follicles, tears, urine, fibroblast culture, and a variety of biopsied tissues are also suitable. Amniotic cells, and presumably chorionic villi, can be used for prenatal diagnosis. Except for rare variants, the diagnosis of hemizygotes offers no problem. The detection of heterozygotes may be uncertain in about 15% of cases [49].

Glycolipid analysis in urine, plasma, or tissues provides an important confirmation of the diagnosis in hemizygotes. As expected by the wide variation in enzyme activities, difficulties may arise in detecting heterozygotes, although high performance liquid chromatography may improve the yield [51].

Whenever possible, an ultrastructural study of the

skin or conjunctiva should be obtained to demonstrate the characteristic glycolipid inclusions. Uncertainty in establishing the heterozygote status of females at risk can never be entirely eliminated and should be remembered when giving genetic counsel. Careful clinical examination, including a search for corneal opacities, should always be conducted. Since the definite proof of heterozygosity is the birth of a hemizygote, prenatal diagnosis may be a reasonable alternative to resolve the issue.

Enzyme screening of all individuals at risk in the family of a proband is essential. Comprehensive evaluation of all the suspected individuals is desirable.

Treatment

Fabry–Anderson disease is compatible with a long productive life. Patients are often unnecessarily frightened by a description of the worst complications. Reassurance and regular checkups should be provided. Painful crises respond well to low doses of phenoxybenzamine (generally 10 to 40 mg daily) in heterozygotes. Phenytoin [52] should be used first in hemizygotes because of the potential risk of priapism secondary to phenoxybenzamine [34]. The lowest effective dosage should be established by trial and error. As little as 50 to 100 mg daily is often sufficient. If the crises are infrequent and last several days or weeks, intermittent administration might be considered during the episodes. Patients may do well on low or even undetectable blood levels. Carbamazepine is also effective.

Plasma exchange is an expensive treatment, the value of which has not been proven. The difficulties of evaluating the treatment of an episodic problem and the association of a strong placebo effect have been discussed [53].

Acetylsalicylic acid and dipyridamole can be used in patients with transient ischemic accidents but their efficacy has not been demonstrated.

Kidney insufficiency can be monitored with blood urea nitrogen and creatinine determinations. Kidney transplantation has permitted survival of 10 to 15 years in several patients who had reached the stage of kidney failure [54,55]. Early evidence of improvement beyond the complications of kidney disease [54,56] has not been confirmed. The rate of complications, especially fatal sepsis, has been unacceptably high [57]. Splenectomy may have increased the risk of sepsis. This may account for long survival in several patients in whom this procedure has not been performed. Transplantation remains the only life-saving procedure in cases of kidney failure, although it can no longer be recommended without reservation.

References

1. Anderson W. A case of "Angeio-Keratoma." Br J Dermatol 1898;10:113–117.
2. Wise D, Wallace JH, Jellinek EH. Angiokeratoma corporis diffusum. Q J Med 1962;31:177–206.
3. Fabry J. Ein Beitrag zur Kenntniss der Purpura haemorrhagica nodularis (Purpura papulosa haemorrhagica Haebrae). Arch Dermatol Syph 1898;43:187–200.
4. Fabry J. Weiter Beitrag zur Klinik des Angiokeratoma naeviforme (Naevus angiokeratosus). Dermatol Wochenschr 1930;90:334–341.
5. Steiner L, Voerner H. Angiomatosis miliaris: eine idiopathische Gefässerkrankung. Dtsch Arch Klin Med 1909;96:105–116.
6. Ruiter M, Pompen AWM, Wyers JJG. Über interne und pathologisch-anatomische Befunde bei Angiokeratoma corporis diffusum (Fabry). Dermatologica (Basel) 1947;94:1–12.
7. Pompen AWM, Ruiter M, Wyers JJG. Angiokeratoma corporis diffusum (universale) Fabry, as a sign of an unknown internal disease; two autopsy reports. Acta Med Scand 1947;128:234–255.
8. Rahman AN, Lindenberg R. The neuropathology of hereditary dystopic lipidosis. Arch Neurol 1962;9:373–385.
9. Sweeley CC, Klionsky B. Fabry's disease: classification as a sphingolipidosis and partial characterization of a novel glycolipid. J Biol Chem 1963;238:3148–3150.
10. Brady RO, Gal AE, Bradley RM, et al. Enzymatic defect in Fabry's disease. N Engl J Med 1967;276:1163–1167.
11. Urbain G, Peremans J, Philippart M. Fabry's disease without skin lesions? Lancet 1967;1:1111.
12. Kint JA. Fabry's disease: alpha-galactosidase deficiency. Science 1970;167:1268–1269.
13. Spence MW, Clarke JTR, D'Entremont DM, et al. Angiokeratoma corporis diffusum (Anderson–Fabry disease) in a single large family in Nova Scotia. J Med Genet 1978;15:428–434.
14. Wallace HJ. Anderson–Fabry disease. Br Med J 1973;88:1–23.
15. Sheth KJ, Werlin SL, Freeman ME, et al. Gastrointestinal structure and function in Fabry's disease. Am J Gastroenterol 1981;76:246–251.
16. Rowe JW, Gilliam JI, Warthin TA. Intestinal manifestations of Fabry's disease. Ann Intern Med 1974;81:628–631.
17. Flynn DM, Lake BD, Boothby CB, et al. Gut lesions in Fabry's disease without a rash. Arch Dis Child 1972;47:26–33.
18. Franceschetti AT, Philippart M, Franceschetti A. A study of Fabry's disease. Dermatologica 1969;138:209–221.
19. Franceschetti A Th. The eye and inborn errors of metabolism. In: Bergsma D, Bron AH, Cotlier E, eds. Birth Defects 1976;12:195–208.
20. Sher NA, Letson RD, Desnick RJ. The ocular manifestations in Fabry's disease. Arch Ophthalmol 1979;97:671–676.

21. Colucci WS, Lorell BH, Schoen FJ, et al. Hypertrophic obstructive cardiomyopathy due to Fabry's disease. N Engl J Med 1982;307:926–928.

22. Mossard JM, Jossot G, Wolfe LS. Le cœur dans la maladie de Fabry. Arch Mal Coeur 1972;65:495–503.

23. Seino Y, Vyden JK, Philippart M, et al. Peripheral hemodynamics in patients with Fabry's disease. Am Heart J 1983;105:783–787.

24. Bartimmo EE, Guisan M, Moser KM. Pulmonary involvement in Fabry's disease: a reappraisal. Am J Med 1972;53:755–764.

25. Rosenberg DM, Ferrans VJ, Fulmer JD, et al. Chronic airflow obstruction in Fabry's disease. Am J Med 1980;68:898–905.

26. Lou JOC, Reske–Nielsen E. The central nervous system in Fabry's disease. Arch Neurol 1971;25:351–359.

27. Jensen E. On the pathology of angiokeratoma corporis diffusum (Fabry). Acta Pathol Microbiol Scand (A) 1966;68:313–331.

28. Sheth KJ, Swick HM. Peripheral nerve conduction in Fabry disease. Ann Neurol 1980;7:319–323.

29. Rahman AN, Simeone FA, Hackel DB, et al. Angiokeratoma corporis diffusum universale (hereditary dystopic lipidosis). Trans Assoc Am Physicians 1961; 74:366–377.

30. Cable WJL, Kolodny EH, Adams RD. Fabry disease: impaired autonomic function. Neurology (NY) 1982;32:498–502.

31. Philippart M, Franceschetti A Th. Early detection of Fabry's disease. Lancet 1967;2:1368.

32. Gubler MC, Lenoir G, Grunfeld JP, et al. Early renal changes in hemizygous and heterozygous patients with Fabry's disease. Kidney Int 1978;13:223–235.

33. Pabico RC, Atanacio BC, McKenna BA, et al. Renal pathologic lesions and functional alterations in a man with Fabry's disease. Am J Med 1973;55:415–425.

34. Funderburk SJ, Philippart M, Dale G, et al. Priapism after phenoxybenzamine in a patient with Fabry's disease. N Engl J Med 1974;290:630–631.

35. Pittelkow RB, Kierland RR, Montgomery J. Angiokeratoma corporis diffusum. Arch Dermatol 1955; 72:556–561.

36. Meuwissen SGM, Dingemans KP, Strijland A, et al. Ultrastructural and biochemical liver analyses in Fabry's disease. Hepatology 1982;2:263–268.

37. Urbain G, Philippart M, Peremans J. Fabry's disease with hypogammaglobulinemia and without angiokeratomas. Arch Intern Med 1969;124:72–76.

38. Pilz H, Volles E, Paul HA, et al. Neurologische Symptome bei Fabryscher Krankheit (Angiokeratoma corporis diffusum). Z Neurol 1972;202:307–322.

39. Liston EH, Levine MD, Philippart M. Psychosis in Fabry disease and treatment with phenoxybenzamine. Arch Gen Psychiatry 1973;29:402–403.

40. Abreo K, Oberley TD, Gilbert EF, et al. Clinicopathological conference: a 29-year-old man with recurrent episodes of fever, abdominal pain and vomiting. Am J Med Genet 1984;18:249–264.

41. Peltier A, Herbeuval E, Brondeau MT, et al. Pseudoclinical Fabry's disease without alpha galactosidase deficiency. Biomedicine 1977;26:194–201.

42. Sagebiel RW, Parker F. Cutaneous lesions of Fabry's disease: glycolipid lipidosis. J Invest Dermatol 1968; 50:208–213.

43. Libert J. Diagnosis of lysosomal storage diseases by the ultrastructural study of conjunctival biopsies. Pathol Annu 1980;15:37–66.

44. Perrelet A, Forssmann WG, Franceschetti A Th, et al. A study of Fabry's disease. Dermatologica 1969; 138:222–237.

45. Dvorak AM, Cable WJL, Osage JE, et al. Diagnostic electron microscopy. Fabry's disease: use of biopsies from uninvolved skin. Acute and chronic changes involving the microvasculature and small unmyelinated nerves. Pathol Annu 1981;16(pt 1):139–158.

46. Kamensky E, Philippart M, Cancilla P, et al. Cultured skin fibroblasts in storage disorders. Am J Pathol 1973;73:59–72.

47. Tabira R, Goto I, Kuroiwa Y, et al. Neuropathological and biochemical studies in Fabry's disease. Acta Neuropathol 1974;30:345–354.

48. Sima AAF, Robertson DM. Involvement of peripheral nerve and muscle in Fabry's disease. Arch Neurol 1978;35:291–301.

49. Spence MW, Goldbloom AL, Burgess JK, et al. Heterozygote detection in angiokeratoma corporis diffusum (Anderson–Fabry disease). J Med Genet 1977;14:91–99.

50. Hamers MN, Wise D, Ejiofor A, et al. Relationship between biochemical and clinical features in an English Anderson–Fabry family. Acta Med Scand 1979;206:5–10.

51. Cable JHL, McCluer RH, Kolodny EH, et al. Fabry disease: detection of heterozygotes by examination of glycolipids in urinary sediment. Neurology (NY) 1982;32:1139–1145.

52. Lockman LA, Hunninghake DB, Krivit W, et al. Relief of pain of Fabry's disease by diphenylhydantoin. Neurology (NY) 1973;23:871–875.

53. Braine HG, Pyeritz RD, Folstein MF, et al. A prospective double-blind study of plasma exchange therapy for the acroparesthesia of Fabry's disease. Transfusion 1981;21:686–689.

54. Philippart M, Franklin SS, Gordon A, et al. Studies on the metabolic control of Fabry's disease through kidney transplantation. Adv Exp Biol Med 1972;19:641–649.

55. Ahlmen J, Hultberg B, Brynger H, et al. Clinical and diagnostic considerations in Fabry's disease. Acta Med Scand 1982;211:309–312.

56. Desnick RJ, Simmons RL, Allen KY, et al. Correction of enzymatic deficiencies by renal transplantation: Fabry's disease. Surgery 1972;72:203–211.

57. Maizel SE, Simmons RL, Kjellstrand C, et al. Ten-year experience in renal transplantation for Fabry's disease. Transplant Proc 1981;13:57–59.

Chapter 30
Adrenoleukodystrophy

BRIAN P. O'NEILL

Adrenoleukodystrophy (ALD) is a genetically determined disorder associated with progressive demyelination and adrenal cortical insufficiency. In its fullest form, there is dementia associated with paralysis, cortical blindness, deafness, and Addison's disease. All forms so far studied conform to an X-linked pattern of inheritance, and the disorder encloses several specific subtypes. All affected persons show increased levels of saturated, unbranched, very long chain fatty acids due to an impaired capacity to degrade them. This degradation normally takes place in a subcellular organelle called the peroxisome. Adrenoleukodystrophy, along with the related disorders of Zellweger cerebro-hepato-renal syndrome and hyperpipecolic acidemia, belong to a newly formulated category of peroxisomal disorders. Biochemical assays designed to detect such elevations of very long chain fatty acids are the basis of tests for prenatal diagnosis, carrier detection, kindred analysis, and identification of homozygotes.

History

"Bronzekrankheit und sklerosierende Encephalomyelitis" (bronzed sclerosing encephalomyelitis) was first described by Siemerling and Creutzfeldt in 1923 [1]. During the next 40 years, clinical reports established this disorder as a clearly defined syndrome with an X-linked mode of inheritance and described an adult form [2–5]. In 1970, Blaw assigned the now generally used name of adrenoleukodystrophy [6].

In the past decade, ALD was determined to be a specific lipidosis, having distinctive genetic, clinical, pathologic, and biochemical features. In 1974, Powers and Schaumburg made the crucial observation that adrenal cortical cells and Schwann cells of ALD patients contained characteristic lamellar cytoplasmic inclusions [7]. These inclusions were subsequently shown to consist of cholesterol esterified with abnormally long, saturated fatty acids in the cholesterol ester and ganglioside fractions of the brain white matter and adrenal cortex [8]. In 1975, Schaumburg's group presented the first detailed clinical and pathologic analysis of a large series of ALD patients [9]. More recently, Moser et al. extended these biochemical findings into the development of clinically useful very long chain fatty acid assays [10–12]. Values from such assays correlate with clinical features and have been used for carrier and prenatal detection and to discover previously unrecognized clinical forms [13–17].

Clinical Features

Adrenoleukodystrophy is expressed clinically by varying combinations of dysfunction in the central and peripheral nervous systems and in the endocrine system. Table 30.1 summarizes the currently recognized ALD phenotypes. Most cases fall into one of two categories: typical childhood ALD and the adult-onset adrenomyeloneuropathy (AMN) variant. Childhood ALD and AMN are X-linked, occur in the same kindred, and are considered variant forms of the same illness.

Signs and symptoms of typical childhood ALD begin most commonly between the ages of 4 and 8 years and consist of progressive dementia, paralysis, visual or hearing disturbances, and adrenal cortical insufficiency [9]. The adult form (AMN) begins in young adulthood and progresses slowly with spastic paraparesis, sensory and urinary disturbances, and endocrinopathy [18]. A connatal [19] and neonatal [20] form of ALD has been described. This form appears to be distinct from childhood ALD and AMN and shows more similarity with the cerebro-hepato-renal syndrome of Zellweger (Table 30.2). In addi-

Table 30.1. Adrenoleukodystrophy Phenotypes

	Childhood ALD	Adrenomyelo-neuropathy	Mixed Form	Addison's Disease	Symptomatic Heterozygote
Sex	Male	Male	Male	Male	Female
Age at onset	4–8 years	20–30 years	10–30 years	5–10 years	20–30 years
Duration	1–5 years	Chronic; probably greater than 2 decades	Incomplete data; probably greater than 1 decade	Incomplete data; probably greater than 2 decades	Incomplete data; probably normal life span
Predominant neurologic symptoms	Cortical blindness, deafness, dementia, quadriparesis	Spastic paraparesis, polyneuropathy	Variety reported: frontal lobe syndrome, Klüver–Bucy syndrome, cerebrospinal syndrome, spinocerebellar syndrome	None	Spastic paraparesis
Predominant endocrine symptoms	Addison's disease	Addison's disease, hypogonadism	Incomplete data; some with Addison's disease, hypogonadism	Addison's disease, ? hypogonadism	None

Table 30.2. Pathophysiologic Features of Peroxisomal Disorders

	Zellweger Syndrome	Neonatal Adrenoleukodystrophy	Childhood Adrenoleukodystrophy	Adrenomyeloneuropathy
Atrophy of adrenal cortex	0[a]	+ +	+ +	+ +
Cytoplasmic inclusions in adrenal cells	+ +	+ +	+ +	+ +
Abnormal neuronal migration	+ +	+	0	0
Enlarged liver	+ +	+	0	0
Retinopathy	+ +	+	0	0
Dysmorphic features	+ +	+	0	0
Renal cortical cysts	+ +	–	0	0
Chondrodystrophia calcificans	+ +	–	0	0
Elevated very long chain fatty acids in plasma	+ +	+ +	+ +	+ +
Elevated plasma pipecolic acid	+ +	+ +	0	0
Decreased plasmalogen levels	+ +	+ +	0	0

Source: modified from Moser et al. [22].

Abbreviations: + + = always present; + = often present; 0 = not present; − = non reported

[a]Adrenal insufficiency, evidenced by failure to respond to ACTH stimulation, has been detected in Zellweger patients by L. Govaerts and her collaborators in Nijmegen, the Netherlands.

tion to exhibiting phenotypic differences, these patients also have a different inheritance pattern (this form never occurs in the same kindreds with childhood ALD or AMN) and have biochemical and pathologic dissimilarities [see references 19–22 for more details].

A recent analysis of 303 ALD patients and 33 significantly symptomatic heterozygotes is summarized in Table 30.3 [13]. Childhood ALD was the most common form. In nearly 75% of the cases neurologic symptoms typically preceded clinical signs of adrenal insufficiency. At the time of onset of neurologic symptoms, 22% had clinically evident Addison's disease and another 19% had a subnormal cortisol response to adrenocorticotropic hormone (ACTH) or cosyntropin stimulation. Behavioral disorders and dementia were the most common first symptoms, followed by impaired vision and hearing and motor disturbances. Adrenomyeloneuropathy was the next most common form of ALD. In almost all cases, symptoms of spastic paraparesis began after the age of 21, with 30% occurring after the age of

Table 30.3. Clinical Manifestations of Adrenoleukodystrophy among Cases Verified by Biochemical Assays at the Kennedy Institute

Manifestation	No. of Cases
Neurologic symptoms resulting from brain disorder	
Onset before age 21	153
Onset after age 21	5
Total	158
Spinal cord symptoms (adrenomyeloneuropathy)	
Onset before age 21	4
Onset after age 21	46
Total	50
Adrenal insufficiency only	22
Presymptomatic	23
Asymptomatic	16
Total	39
Childhood adrenoleukodystrophy– adrenomyeloneuropathy; incomplete clinical data	14
All X-linked cases	283
Neonatal adrenoleukodystrophy (autosomal recessive)	20
All hemizygotes and homozygotes	303
Significantly symptomatic heterozygotes for X-linked adrenoleukodystrophy	33

Source: Moser et al. [13]. With permission.

35. Most men with AMN have signs of hypoadrenalism at initial neurologic diagnosis; some also have hypogonadism with azoospermia and hypotestosteronemia [23]. Unlike childhood ALD, in which the duration of the illness is short, AMN patients usually do not have a shortened survival.

Addison's disease without neurologic symptoms can be observed in kindreds that have more typical forms; some of these patients will very likely develop neurologic symptoms later. However, a few kindreds, spanning several generations, are composed of males with Addison's disease alone [24]. Thus, biochemical testing for ALD seems appropriate for all newly diagnosed males with Addison's disease to discover those that may be manifestations of ALD.

In addition to these common clinical manifestations, diagnostic biochemical testing has shown that (a) presymptomatic and asymptomatic forms exist [13]; (b) adolescent and adult-onset cerebral syndromes can occur albeit with some clinical differences, such as frontal-temporal demyelination [25,26]; and (c) cases of familial spastic paraparesis, progressive spinal cerebellar degeneration, and olivopontocerebellar atrophy may be variants of ALD

[27–29]. A fluctuating course more consistent with a diagnosis of multiple sclerosis has been recently described as an ALD variant on the basis of abnormal very long chain fatty acid accumulation [30]. Therefore, biochemical testing is appropriate in obscure neurologic illnesses that conform to an X-linked inheritance pattern or have some features of ALD or both.

Approximately 10% of female heterozygotes will have significant neurologic disability [13,15]; a greater number may have mild or asymptomatic disease. In almost all instances, this disability consists of a spastic paraparesis without other neurologic signs [15]. No heterozygote has yet been found to have clinical or laboratory evidence of hypoadrenalism. For unknown reasons such affected carriers may be more common in certain kindreds. In general, the presence of neurologic signs, particularly a spastic paraparesis, in a woman at risk in an ALD kindred presupposes carrier status until biochemical testing can be done.

Laboratory Investigations

Radiology

Routine x-rays of the skull are normal. Computed tomographic scanning is often pathognomonic, demonstrating a distinctive picture of decreased attenuation of cerebral white matter that begins in the occipital pole and then advances forward. Contrast enhancement at the edge of these lesions may be seen in the early phases of the illness [31] (Figure 30.1). Although this enhancement may be seen in acquired white matter diseases such as multiple sclerosis, it does not occur in any other leukodystrophy [32]. Thus, the CT scan may be diagnostic when obtained in a patient with indeterminate neurologic symptoms.

Computed tomography may also aid diagnosis by demonstrating bilateral white matter disease in those unusual cases that have had an asymmetric or even focal onset [26]. The CT scan in AMN is normal or nonspecifically abnormal, consistent with the predominant spinal and peripheral white matter involvement [33]. In the variant form, frontal lobe demyelination, often with an enhancing rim that proceeds posteriorly, correlates with the clinically observed frontal lobe syndrome [28]. The CT scan of symptomatic heterozygotes has been normal in all women so far studied [33].

Magnetic resonance imaging (MRI) may be more useful than CT in white matter diseases [34]. Typically, the T_2 spin-echo relaxation of white matter is prolonged. In ALD, it is now known that the disease

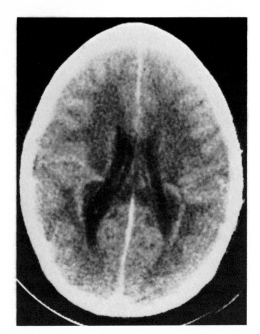

Figure 30.1. Computed tomography scan of young male patient with typical childhood ALD. Note the decreased white matter attenuation through the centrum semiovale and the rim of contrast enhancement adjacent to the posterior horns of the lateral ventricles.

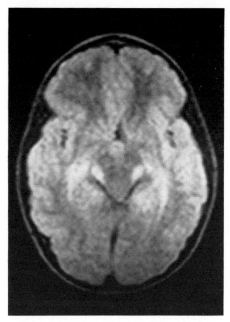

Figure 30.2. Magnetic resonance imaging (MRI) of a young male patient with early childhood ALD. CT scan was normal. MRI displays prolonged T_2 signal in deep parietal white matter and adjacent midbrain.

can be apparent on MRI when CT is normal and that when CT is abnormal greater evidence of disease will be apparent by MRI [35] (Figure 30.2).

Electrophysiology

Electroencephalograms demonstrate frequency slowing and amplitude reduction maximal in the parieto-occipital region in typical childhood ALD. These changes are usually symmetric and become more extensive as the disease advances. Focal epileptiform changes in the forms of spikes or sharp waves are uncommon. The EEG may even be disproportionally normal and is typically normal in AMN and symptomatic heterozygotes [Westmoreland BF, O'Neill BP: unpublished data 1984].

Nerve conduction velocities may be normal to slightly low and usually fail to parallel the pathologic evidence of peripheral nerve involvement. The sensory latency of the sural nerve may also be decreased. Patients with abnormal nerve conduction velocities in the lower extremities usually have normal values in the upper extremities. Similarly, electromyograms may be normal or mildly abnormal; abnormalities, when described, have consisted of fibrillation potentials, diminished recruitment, and

prolonged high-amplitude polyphasic potentials [Stevens JC, Litchy WJ, O'Neill BP: unpublished data 1983].

Evoked potential studies may demonstrate early involvement in fiber tract systems and highlight the topography of the illness. Visual evoked responses (VER) are normal early in the course of typical ALD. They become abnormal later in the course of the illness and fail to correlate with the prominent early visual symptoms, which suggests that they are on a cortical rather than on an optic nerve basis [36]. In AMN and in heterozygotes, VERs are normal and remain normal throughout the illness. In general, brain stem auditory evoked responses (BAER) in ALD demonstrate a similar pattern: they may become abnormal as the disease progresses [36]. Like the visual responses, the late abnormalities in the BAER do not always correlate with the early auditory complaints, suggesting that these too are on a cortical rather than a nerve or brain stem basis. Some patients with AMN without auditory complaints and some carriers, both symptomatic and asymptomatic, have had abnormal BAERs [37]. It is likely, however, that BAERs are infrequently abnormal in carriers and when present do not correlate with the presence and degree of neurologic disease or with the level of very long chain fatty acid accumulation [38].

Clinical Laboratory

Serum electrolyte levels, except during crises, are normal or mildly abnormal. This lack of significant hyponatremia and hyperkalemia typical of other forms of Addison's disease is not adequately explained. Aldosterone is present and may rise with ACTH infusion, although subnormally, and this may explain why salt craving and crises are absent in many patients. Baseline ACTH values are elevated and may be reliably abnormal even when plasma cortisol values are normal. Provocative clinical testing, in the form of cosyntropin or ACTH stimulation, is usually required to demonstrate the diminished adrenal reserve.

Testicular signs and symptoms are conspicuous in adult-onset disease and consist of diminished libido, impotence, and infertility [23]. In some patients, serum testosterone levels are low even when adrenal function is normal [27]. Adrenoleukodystrophy males can reproduce, however, and can produce female carriers. In fact, in a recent review 18 kindreds were traced back to male carriers [13].

Pathology

The gross appearance of the brain and spinal cord are usually normal, but the cut section of the brain is granular and gray (Figure 30.3). There is contiguous and hemispheric demyelination often asymmetric and predominant in the posterior quadrant of the brain. The gray matter and subcortical fibers are usually normal. Deposits of demyelination occasionally are seen in the frontal lobes and in rare individuals the frontal lobe may bear the brunt of damage [25]. Secondary tract degeneration occurs, producing demyelination in the corpus callosum, internal capsule, and cerebral peduncles and tracts from the brain stem to the spinal cord [9]. In AMN, the cut appearance of the cord may demonstrate contracted fiber tracts throughout its length; the spinal roots and peripheral nerves usually appear grossly normal [39].

In the white matter of the cerebral hemispheres, the distribution of the microscopic lesions corresponds to the gross changes. Three histopathologic zones have been described by Schaumburg: (a) the peripheral zone containing scattered macrophages and axons that are demyelinated to various degrees; (b) a large rim containing a vigorous perivascular mononuclear cell response, usually at the leading edge of the lesion; and (c) an inner zone of dense gliosis [9]. Similar changes probably occur at the spinal level as well although the data are less complete.

The rapid progression of the typical childhood form, the frequent asymmetric distribution, and the striking accumulations of lymphocytes in active brain lesions suggest involvement of immunologic mechanisms. However, decisive evidence is lacking. Increased levels of free IgG and IgA in ALD brain tissues, comparable to those in multiple sclerosis brain tissues and 2 to 10 times higher than in controls, have been demonstrated. Furthermore, there is an accumulation of lymphoid cells staining for IgG, IgA, and IgM in the areas of recent demyelination [40]. Unlike multiple sclerosis, bound immunoglobulins are not detected, and the free immunoglobulins in ALD

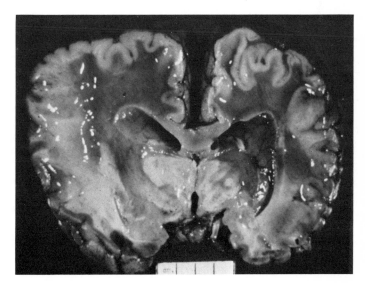

Figure 30.3. Cut section of a young male patient with typical childhood ALD. Note the widespread demyelination sparing cortex and immediate subcortical areas.

brain tissue may represent soluble immune complexes or exudative serum protein secondary to the inflammatory compromise of the blood–brain barrier.

The nervous system macrophages contain membrane-bound inclusions composed of characteristic trilaminar structures called lamellar lipid profiles [41]. Their presence in macrophages is thought to represent a debris-removal phenomenon with the intensity of its response related to rapid primary demyelination. Similar lamellar lipid profiles are found unbound in the cytoplasm of adrenal cortical cells and in the Leydig cells of the testes [42,43]. These lamellar cytoplasmic inclusions are the pathologic benchmarks of ALD and are the morphological link between the endocrine and nervous system diseases. Although originally thought to be composed of defective membranes, more recent work suggests that they may be the morphologic counterparts of the accumulated cholesterol-esterified very long chain fatty acids [8,44].

The adrenal glands are usually atrophic and are sometimes difficult to locate in the perinephric fat. Microscopic studies of the adrenal gland will often reveal a preserved outer zone, or zona glomerulosa, with more significant disruption of the fascicularis and reticularis zones. In some cases, the pathologic disruption is such that differentiation into zones is not possible. There are usually greatly enlarged cells with granular or hyaline eosinophilic cytoplasm; these ballooned cells may contain abundant lamellar lipid profiles [45].

The neurologic presentation and progression appears to closely parallel the neuropathology. The endocrine pathology correlates with the severity of the endocrine disease but bears no relation to the extent or severity of the neurologic disease [46]. Adrenocorticosteroid treatment although capable of compensating for the hypoadrenalism has no effect on the course of the neurologic illness [47]. In one series, a variable mixture of ballooned striated cells, macrovacuoles, and atrophic adrenal cortices were present in childhood-, juvenile-, and adult-onset cases, and the age of onset correlated with the histologic appearance [48].

In studies done on aborted fetuses, the adrenal cortex has been found to be grossly normal early in the disease. The earliest adrenal lesions are birefringent, cytoplasmic striations in the inner zone of the cortex. This striated material gradually accumulates, impairing cell function, and produces death of the adrenal cortical cells [49]. Testicular interstitial cells have the same intracytoplasmic lamellae as those seen in the adrenal cortical cells, but the adrenal pathol-

ogy and the testicular pathology may not be congruent [43].

To date, no carrier has been studied pathologically. Despite the lack of clinically apparent endocrine symptoms and signs on clinical testing, it is not certain whether subclinical adrenal disease may be present in such patients. One might suppose that mild neurologic disease is more easily detected clinically than a similar degree of endocrine (that is, adrenal) disturbance.

Biochemistry

The accumulation of saturated unbranched very long chain fatty acids, particularly hexacosanoate (C26:0), has been demonstrated in all ALD patients and is nearly unique for this disorder (it has also been reported in the Zellweger cerebro-hepato-renal syndrome and in the closely related disorder, hyperpipecolic acidemia). These fatty acids may account for up to 40% of the total fatty acid content of the cholesterol ester and of the ganglioside fractions of brain white matter and adrenal cortex.

Similar accumulations of these very long chain fatty acids have been demonstrated in nearly all lipid moieties, tissues, and body fluids of ALD patients, including muscle [50], skin fibroblasts [10], and plasma [11]. These observations suggest that ALD is due to a metabolic defect involving all cells, but which is expressed clinically in only some organ systems.

The precise enzyme defect in ALD has not been identified. Initial studies were geared toward conventional degradation pathways. However, the activity of mitochondrial-, microsomal-, and myelin-associated cholesterol esterases in ALD brain tissues are normal, as is cholesterol lignocerate hydrolysis in fibroblasts [51]. The very long chain fatty acid accumulation in all lipid classes argues for a defect that involves the metabolism of the acids themselves; the accumulation would then be a secondary phenomenon with the lamellar lipid profiles as their morphological counterpart.

There is now strong evidence that the defect causing ALD is a specific impairment of the degradation of very long chain fatty acid. When [^{14}C]-labeled fatty acids of varying chain lengths were incubated with homogenates of white blood cells, cultured skin fibroblasts, and amniocytes, ALD and control homogenates did not differ in CO_2 release from 16- and 18-carbon length acids, but ALD homogenates produced CO_2 release from 24- and 26-carbon length fatty acids at 10 to 20% of controls [52]. Furthermore, when intact skin fibroblasts were incubated with radiolabeled C24:0 fatty acid, those from ALD patients produced less CO_2 than did control cell lines [53]. This impaired capacity to form CO_2 or water-soluble intermediates from 24- and 26-carbon length fatty acids has been a consistent finding in those ALD and AMN patients studied. Thus, there may be an impaired capacity to oxidize very long chain fatty acids while the capacity to degrade the more common acids remains intact.

Fatty acid oxidation may occur through several pathways. A specific oxidation system particularly active in the handling of very long chain fatty acids resides in a subcellular organelle, the peroxisome. In fact, recent evidence suggests that a group of peroxisomal disorders exists analogous to the well-established lysosomal disorders [22,54]. However, the evidence that ALD represents a disease of the peroxisome is so far inferential. The C24:O oxidation shown to be impaired in ALD (and the related disorders) takes place mainly in the peroxisome [55]. Although present in ALD patients, peroxisomes are absent in the liver and kidney of patients with the Zellweger syndrome [56]. Thus, there may be a deficiency of a specific peroxisomal enzyme in ALD.

Diagnostic assays exploit the expression of the metabolic defect in accessible tissues such as plasma [11], red [57] and white blood cells [58], and skin fibroblasts [10]. The most convenient and widely used assay is the measurement of total plasma lipids, followed under special circumstances by studies of cultured skin fibroblasts. In affected men, the results of plasma and fibroblasts have always been congruent. In women heterozygous for ALD, the two may not be congruent; depending on their clinical situation, a normal plasma assay may be followed up by study of cultured fibroblasts.

Table 30.4 shows the results of a recent study on diagnostic assays in ALD. Of the patients studied, 268 were classified as ALD heterozygotes. Strikingly increased levels were also observed in the Zellweger syndrome and in the related disorder hyperpipecolic acidemia. ALD differs from these latter two disorders in respect to the patterns of very long chain fatty acid accumulation (see Table 30.2). The levels in these two disorders is significantly higher than in ALD, and there are increases in both mono-unsaturated and saturated very long chain fatty acids, while in ALD the increase is confined to the saturated very long chain fatty acids. Normal levels of very long chain fatty acids were observed in almost 2,000 subjects; most samples were obtained from subjects with other neurologic diseases including other types of leukodystrophy and lipidoses, multiple sclerosis, other types of Addison's disease, various types of peripheral neuropathy, spinocerebellar degeneration, familial spastic paraparesis, and other neurologic and degenerative disorders.

Table 30.4. Experience at Kennedy Institute with Assays for Very Long Chain Fatty Acids in Plasma and/or Cultured Skin Fibroblasts[a]

Diagnostic Category	Plasma			Cultured Skin Fibroblasts	
	C26:0 (µg/ml plasma)	C24:0/ C22:0 Ratio	C26:0/C22:0 Ratio	C26:0 (µg/ml protein)	C26:0/C22:0 Ratio
Childhood adrenoleukodystrophy– adrenomyeloneuropathy hemizygotes (n = 282)	1.6 ± 0.84	1.6 ± 0.17	0.075 ± 0.02	0.42 ± 0.15	0.67 ± 0.21
Heterozygotes for X-linked ALD (n = 268)	0.81 ± 0.33	1.3 ± 0.20	0.039 ± 0.017	0.26 ± 0.16	0.41 ± 0.25
Neonatal ALD (n = 20)	2.4 ± 0.73	1.8 ± 0.35	0.30 ± 0.14	0.37 ± 0.14	0.80 ± 0.43
Zellweger syndrome (n = 36)	2.5 ± 0.85	2.0 ± 0.24	0.49 ± 0.03	0.78 ± 0.24	2.0 ± 1.2
Hyperpipecolic acidemia (n = 4)	1.7	1.4	0.16	0.42 ± 0.06	0.90 ± 0.11
Normal controls (n = 65)	0.33 ± 0.15	0.83 ± 0.15	0.014 ± 0.076	0.079 ± 0.066	0.080 ± 0.029
Other diseases (n = 1,858)	0.24 ± 0.16	0.81 ± 0.09	0.014 ± 0.056	0.066 ± 0.035	0.093 ± 0.062

Source: Moser et al. [13]. With permission.

[a]Most studies involved plasma. Cultured skin fibroblasts were included in about one-fourth of the cases. Fatty acid levels show mean ± SD. The number of cases included in each category is smaller than the total number, especially for cultured skin fibroblasts. C26:1 levels are increased above normal in Zellweger syndrome but not in childhood adrenoleukodystrophy or adrenomyeloneuropathy (data not shown).

Most women heterozygous for ALD can be detected by study of very long chain fatty acids. Using a classification function that takes into account the levels of fatty acids as well as their ratios in plasma, 88% of obligate heterozygotes can be identified [16]. Plasma assay, followed by fibroblast assay when plasma is normal, identifies a total of 93% of obligate heterozygotes [13,16]. Adrenoleukodystrophy can also be diagnosed prenatally. Amniocytes obtained by amniocentesis are cultured, and measurements are made of the very long chain fatty acids and their ratios. So far, no false-negative or false-positive results have been documented [17]. Unfortunately, while the prenatal assays are capable of identifying male fetuses with a biochemical defect of ALD, they cannot determine whether the disease would manifest severely in childhood or as one of the somewhat milder forms.

Genetics

All reported pedigrees have shown a pattern of inheritance consistent with X-linked recessive inheritance. There does not appear to be any racial or geographic predilection, nor does there appear to be a distinct environmental influence [13]. The full syndrome of neurologic and endocrine failure has only been seen in men hemizygous for ALD. The women heterozygous for ALD who have neurologic disease typically display spastic paraparesis and no endocrine symptoms.

There may be striking variability within a given kindred. Table 30.5 shows results of the investigation of 176 pedigrees in which there were sufficient data for kindred analysis. In some kindreds as many as four different phenotypes have been observed. The co-occurence of ALD and AMN within a single kindred is almost as common as the occurrence of either alone. Individuals without neurologic or endocrine symptoms but with elevated levels of very long chain fatty acid are seen in some kindreds; these individuals are of particular interest since they may reproduce and transmit ALD to another generation.

There is no correlation between the age of the patient, the presence or extent of disease, and the amount of very long chain fatty acid accumulation. Some asymptomatic heterozygotes have had levels higher than their offspring, and some asymptomatic hemizygotes have had levels higher than their severely affected sibs [14]. Thus, the degree of very long chain fatty acid elevation on diagnostic testing has no prognostic significance. Also, there so far seems to be no correlation between the presence or

Table 30.5. Clinical Presentation of X-Linked Adrenoleukodystrophy Kindreds (ALD, AMN, Addison's Disease)

Presentation	No. of Kindreds
Single cases per kindred	
Classic ALD	65
Late ALD	3
AMN	15
Addison's disease	3
Total	86
Multiple cases per kindred	
ALD only	34
AMN only	8
Addison's disease only	2
ALD–AMN	28
ALD–Addison's disease	6
AMN–Addison's disease	1
AMN or ALD—asymptomatics	11
Total	90
Insufficient pedigree data	41
All X-linked kindreds	217
Kindreds with affected male ancestor	18
Kindreds with significantly disabled heterozygotes	17

Source: Moser et al. [13]. With permission.

degree of neurologic disease in the affected parent and the phenotype of the affected child.

Studies with cultured fibroblasts from skin biopsies of heterozygotes have provided proof of X-linkage. Fibroblast clones were of two types: one with normal levels of very long chain fatty acids, the other with levels similar to those of ALD patients [24]. Furthermore, the great majority of clones were of the ALD type, suggesting a proliferative advantage of clones expressing the abnormal gene. In studies conducted in a large kindred where women were heterozygous for both ALD and G6PD deficiency, there was a close linkage between the G6PD locus and the putative ALD locus [59]. Again, there was no correlation between these findings and the presence of disease in the carriers studied or in the phenotype of their offspring.

Since the enzyme (or group of enzymes) defect responsible for ALD is still unknown, the various hemizygote manifestations, and the restricted heterozygote expression are not yet fully understood. There has been speculation that these phenomena represent work and environmental factors, modified gene variation, or multiple allelism, or a combination of these. Current research strategies are involved in developing DNA probes for the ALD locus on the X-chromosome and in identifying the peroxisomal enzyme responsible for catalyzing the oxidation of very long chain fatty acids. In addition, a major effort is being directed at studying the possibility that at least one component of ALD is immunologically determined [60].

Treatment

The devastating effects of this disease have led to several treatment trials. These have included immunosuppression, plasma exchange, bone marrow transplantation, and the administration of carnitine and clofibrate [13,61]. None of them proved successful.

Since the observation of Kishimoto et al. [62] that the $C_{26:0}$ which accumulates in ALD brain is, at least in part, of dietary origin, attempts are being made to use diets restricted in $C_{26:0}$. Initial trials, however, failed to lower plasma VLCFA levels or cause clinical improvement [61,63].

The failure of $C_{26:0}$ restrictions to lower VLCFA may be due to the fact that the $C_{26:0}$ that accumulates in tissues is derived from both diet and endogenous synthesis. In fact, synthesis may have been stimulated by such restriction. Current treatment strategies involve an approach that restricts dietary intake of $C_{26:0}$ and administers a glycerol trioleate oil to maintain total fat content. The rationale for such an approach is based on Rizzo's observations that the additions of oleic acid to culture medium reduced $C_{26:0}$ synthesis in ALD cultured fibroblasts by 58% [64]. Preliminary evidence suggests a consistent decline in VLCFA. Clinical studies are under way to determine if clinical stabilization or reversal also occurs.

References

1. Siemerling E, Creutzfeldt HC. Bronzekrankheit und sklerosierende Encephalomyelitis (diffuse Sclerose). Arch Psychiatr 1923;68:217–244.
2. Fanconi A, Prader A, Isler W, et al. Morbus Addison mit Hirnsklerose im Kindesalter. Ein hereditäres Syndrome mit X-chromasomaler Vererbung? Helv Paediatr Acta 1963;18:480–501.
3. Gagnon J, Leblanc R. Sclérose cérébrale diffuse avec mélanodermie et atrophie surrénale. Union Med Can 1959;88:392–412.
4. Hoefnagel D, van den Noort S, Ingbar SH. Diffuse cerebral sclerosis with endocrine abnormalities in young males. Brain 1962;85:553–568.
5. Harris-Jones JM, Nixon PGF. Familial Addison's disease with spastic paraplegia. J Clin Endocrinol 1955; 15:739–744.
6. Blaw ME. Melanodermic type leukodystrophy (adreno-leukodystrophy). In: Vinken PJ, Bruyn GW, eds. Handbook of clinical neurology. New York: American Elsevier, 1970;10:1128–1133.
7. Powers JM, Schaumburg HH. Adrenoleukodystrophy: similar ultrastructural changes in adrenal cortical cells and Schwann cells. Arch Neurol 1974;30:406–408.
8. Igarashi M, Schaumburg HH, Powers J, et al. Fatty acid abnormality in adrenoleukodystrophy. J Neurochem 1976;26:851–860.
9. Schaumburg HH, Powers JH, Raine CS, et al. Adrenoleukodystrophy: a clinical and pathological study of 17 cases. Arch Neurol 1975;32:577–591.
10. Moser HW, Moser AB, Kawamura N, et al. Adrenoleukodystrophy: elevated C26 fatty acid in cultured skin fibroblasts. Ann Neurol 1980;7:542–549.
11. Moser HW, Moser AB, Frayer KK, et al. Adrenoleukodystrophy: increased plasma content of saturated very long chain fatty acids. Neurology (NY) 1981;31:1241–1249.
12. Yahara S, Moser HW, Kolodny EH, et al. Reverse phase high performance liquid chromatography of cerebrosides, sulfatides and ceramides: microanalysis of homolog composition without hydrolysis and application to cerebroside analysis in peripheral nerves of adrenoleukodystrophy patients. J Neurochem 1980; 34:694–699.
13. Moser HW, Moser AE, Singh I, et al. Adrenoleukodystrophy: survey of 303 cases: biochemistry, diagnosis and therapy. Ann Neurol 1984;16:628–641.
14. O'Neill BP, Moser HW, Marmion LC. Adrenoleukodystrophy: elevated C26 fatty acid in cultured skin fibroblasts and correlation with disease expression in three generations of a kindred. Neurology (NY) 1982;32:540–542.
15. O'Neill BP, Moser HW, Saxena KM, et al. Adrenoleukodystrophy. Clinical and biochemical manifestations in carriers. Neurology (Cleveland) 1984;34:798–801.
16. Moser HW, Moser AE, Trojak JE, et al. Identification of female carriers for adrenoleukodystrophy. J Pediatr 1983;103:54–59.
17. Moser HW, Moser AB, Powers JM, et al. The prenatal diagnosis of adrenoleukodystrophy: demonstration of increased hexacosanoic acid in cultured amniocytes and fetal adrenal gland. Pediatr Res 1982;16:172–175.
18. Griffin JW, Goren E, Schaumburg H, et al. Adreno-myeloneuropathy: a probable variant of adrenoleukodystrophy. Neurology (NY) 1977;27:1107–1113.
19. Ulrich J, Herschkowitz N, Heitz P, et al. Adrenoleukodystrophy: preliminary report of a connatal case. Acta Neuropathol 1978;43:77–83.
20. Haas JE, Johnson ES, Farrell DL. Neonatal-onset adrenoleukodystrophy in a girl. Ann Neurol 1982;12:449–457.
21. Moser AE, Singh I, Brown FR III, et al. The cerebro-hepato-renal (Zellweger) syndrome: increased levels and impaired degradation of very long fatty acid and prenatal diagnosis. N Engl J Med 1984;310:1141–1146.

22. Moser HW, Goldfischer SL. The peroxisomal disorders. Hosp Pract 1985;20:61–70.

23. Powers JM, Schaumburg HH. A fatal cause of sexual inadequacy in men: adrenoleukodystrophy. J Urol 1980;124:583–585.

24. O'Neill BP, Moser HW, Saxena KM. Familial X-linked Addison's disease as an expression of adrenoleukodystrophy (ALD): elevated C26 fatty acid in cultured skin fibroblasts. Neurology (NY) 1982;32:543–547.

25. Marler JR, O'Neill BP, Forbes GS, et al. Adrenoleukodystrophy (ALD): clinical and CT features of a childhood variant. Neurology (Cleveland) 1983;33:1203–1205.

26. Powers JM, Schaumburg HH, Gaffney CL. Kluver–Bucy syndrome caused by adrenoleukodystrophy. Neurology (NY) 1980;30:1131–1132.

27. O'Neill BP, Swanson JW, Brown FW, et al. Familial spastic paraparesis as an expression of adrenoleukodystrophy. Neurology (Cleveland) 1985;35:1233–1236.

28. Marsden CD, Obeso JA, Lang AE. Adrenomyeloneuropathy presenting as spino-cerebellar degeneration. Neurology (NY) 1982;32:1031–1032.

29. Ohno T, Tsuchiya H, Fukuhara N, et al. Adrenoleukodystrophy: new clinical variant presenting as olivopontocerebellar atrophy. Ann Neurol 1983;14:147–148.

30. Walsh PJ. Adrenoleukodystrophy: report of two cases with relapsing and remitting courses. Arch Neurol 1980;37:448–450.

31. O'Neill BP, Forbes GS. Computed tomography and adrenoleukodystrophy: differential appearance in disease subtypes. Arch Neurol 1981;38:293–298.

32. Lane B, Carroll BA, Pedley TA. Computerized cranial tomography in cerebral diseases of white matter. Neurology 1978;28:534–544.

33. Greenberg HS, Halverson D, Lane B. CT scanning and diagnosis of adrenoleukodystrophy. Neurology 1977;27:884–886.

34. Frytak S, Earnest F, O'Neill BP, et al. Magnetic resonance imaging for neurotoxicity in long-term survivors of carcinoma. Mayo Clin Proc 1985;60:803–812.

35. O'Neill BP, Forbes GS, Gomez MR, et al. A comparison of magnetic resonance imaging and computed tomography in adrenoleukodystrophy. Neurology (Cleveland) 1985;35:83.

36. Markand ON, Garg BP, De Myer WE, et al. Brainstem auditory, visual and somatosensory evoked potentials in leukodystrophies. Electroencephalogr Clin Neurophysiol 1982;54:39–48.

37. Garg BP, Markand ON, De Myer WE, et al. Evoked response studies in patients with adrenoleukodystrophy and heterozygous relatives. Arch Neurol 1983;40:356–359.

38. O'Neill BP, Westmoreland BF, Tiffany C, et al. Brainstem auditory evoked potentials in adrenoleukodystrophy carriers. Neurology (Cleveland) 1984;34:164.

39. Schaumburg HH, Powers JM, Raine CS, et al. Adrenomyeloneuropathy—a probable variant of adrenoleukodystrophy. Part 2. General pathologic, neuropathologic and biochemical aspects. Neurology (NY) 1977;27:1114–1119.

40. Bernheimer H, Budka H, Muller P. Brain tissue immunoglobulins in adrenoleukodystrophy: a comparison with multiple sclerosis and systemic lupus erythematosus. Acta Neuropathol (Berl) 1983;59:95–102.

41. Schaumburg HH, Powers JM, Suzuki K, et al. Adrenoleukodystrophy (sex-linked Schilder disease): ultrastructural demonstration of specific cytoplasmic inclusions in the central nervous system. Arch Neurol 1974;31:210–213.

42. Powers JM, Schaumburg HW. Adreno-leukodystrophy (sex-linked Schilder's disease): a pathogenetic hypothesis based on ultrastructural lesions in adrenal cortex, peripheral nerve and testes. Am J Pathol 1974;76:481–500.

43. Powers JM, Schaumburg HH. The testis in adrenoleukodystrophy. Am J Pathol 1981;102:90–98.

44. Johnson AB, Schaumburg HH, Powers JM. Histochemical characteristics of the striated inclusions of adrenoleukodystrophy. J Histochem Cytochem 1976;24:725–730.

45. Weiss GM, Nelson RL, O'Neill BP, et al. Use of adrenal biopsy in diagnosing adrenoleukomyeloneuropathy. Arch Neurol 1980;37:634–636.

46. de Weerd AW, van Huffelen AC, Resser HM. Progression of endocrinological and neurological dysfunction in adrenoleukodystrophy. Eur Neurol 1982;21:117–123.

47. Stumpf DA, Hayward A, Haas R, et al. Adrenoleukodystrophy: failure of immunosuppression to prevent neurological progression. Arch Neurol 1981;38:48–49.

48. Powers JM, Schaumburg HH, Johnson AB, et al. A correlative study of the adrenal cortex in adrenoleukodystrophy: evidence for a fatal intoxication with very long chain saturated fatty acids. Invest Cell Pathol 1980;3:353–376.

49. Powers JM, Moser HW, Moser AB, et al. Fetal adrenoleukodystrophy: the significance of pathologic lesions in adrenal glands and testis. Hum Pathol 1982;13:1013–1019.

50. Askanas V, McLaughlin J, Engel KW, et al. Abnormalities in cultured muscle and peripheral nerve of a patient with adrenomyeloneuropathy. N Engl J Med 1979;301:588–590.

51. O'Neill BP, Moser HW. Adrenoleukodystrophy. Can J Neurol Sci 1982;9:449–452.

52. Singh I, Moser HW, Moser AB, et al. Adrenoleukodystrophy: impaired oxidation of long chain fatty acids in cultured skin fibroblasts and adrenal cortex. Biochem Biophys Res Commun 1981;102:1223–1229.

53. Rizzo, Avigan J, Chemke J, et al. Adrenoleukodystrophy: very long chain fatty acid metabolism in fibroblasts. Neurology (Cleveland) 1984;34:163–169.

54. Goldfischer S. Peroxisomes and human metabolic disease: the cerebro-hepato-renal syndrome (CHRS), ce-

rebrotendinous xanthomatosis and Schilder's disease (adrenoleukodystrophy). Ann NY Acad Sci. 1982; 386:526–529.

55. Rolbert E. Metabolic pathways in peroxisomes and glyoxysomes. Annu Rev Biochem 1981;50:133–157.

56. Brown FR III, McAdams AJ, Cummins JW, et al. Cerebro-hepato-renal (Zellweger) syndrome and neonatal adrenoleukodystrophy: similarities in phenotype and accumulation of very long chain fatty acids. Johns Hopkins Med J 1982;144:344–351.

57. Tsuji S, Suzuki M, Ariga T, et al. Abnormality of long chain fatty acids in erythrocyte membrane sphingomyelin from patients with adrenoleukodystrophy. J Neurochem 1981;36:1046–1049.

58. Molzer B, Bernheimer H, Heller R, et al. Detection of adrenoleukodystrophy by increased C26:0 fatty acid levels in leukocytes. Clin Chim Acta 1982;125:299–305.

59. Migeon BR, Moser HW, Moser AB, et al. Adrenoleukodystrophy: evidence of X-linkage, inactivation, and selection favoring the mutant allele in heterozygous cells. Proc Natl Acad Sci USA 1981;78:5066–5070.

60. Griffin DE, Moser HW, Mendoza Q, et al. Identification of the inflammatory cells in the central nervous system of patients with adrenoleukodystrophy. Ann Neurol 1985;18:660–664.

61. Brown FR III, Van Duyn MA, Moser AB, et al. Adrenoleukodystrophy: effects of dietary restriction of very long chain fatty acids and of the administration of carnitine and cleofibrate on clinical status and plasma fatty acids. Johns Hopkins Med J 1982;151:164–172.

62. Kishimoto Y, Moser HW, Kawamura N, et al. Adrenoleukodystrophy: evidence that abnormal very long chain fatty acids of brain diolesterol esters are of exogenous origin. Biochem Biophys Res Commun 1980;96:69–76.

63. Van Duyn MA, Moser AB, Brown FR III, et al. The design of a diet restricted in saturated very long chain fatty acids: therapeutic application in adrenoleukodystrophy. Am J Clin Nutr 1984;40:277–282.

64. Rizzo WB, Watkins PA, Phillips MW, et al. Adrenoleukodystrophy: oleic acid lowers fibroblast C_{22-26} fatty acids. Neurology 1986;36:357–361.

Chapter 31
Kinky Hair Disease

JOHN H. MENKES

Kinky hair disease, also known as Menkes' kinky hair disease or trichopoliodystrophy, is a focal degenerative disorder of gray matter first described in 1962 by Menkes et al. [1]. Some ten years after the disease was first described, Danks et al. found serum copper and ceruloplasmin levels to be reduced and suggested that the primary defect involved copper metabolism [2]. Since this has now been proven, it is appropriate to review briefly our present knowledge of the field [3,4].

Biochemistry

The daily dietary intake of copper ranges between 1 and 5 mg. Healthy children receiving a free diet absorb 150 to 900 μg/day or about 40% of dietary copper. The absorption site is probably in the proximal portion of the gastrointestinal tract. Metallothionein, a low-molecular-weight metal protein, is involved in regulating copper absorption at high copper intakes and in the intestinal transport of the metal, and probably also in its initial hepatic uptake. There are two major isoforms of the protein, MT–I and MT–II, with closely related, but distinct, amino acid sequences. At least three forms of MT–I are demonstrable in man by protein sequencing. The metallothioneins are encoded by multiple genes, of which one cluster is localized in chromosome 16; the others are dispersed to at least four other autosomes [5]. The transcription of each of these genes is induced by copper, cadmium, and other heavy metals [6].

Following its intestinal uptake, copper enters plasma, where it is bound to albumin in the form of the cupric ion. Within 2 hours, the absorbed copper becomes incorporated into liver. The concentration of the metal in normal liver ranges from 30 to 50 μg/gm of dry weight. In liver, copper is either excreted into bile, stored in liver lysosomes in what is probably a polymeric form of metallothionein, or combines with apoceruloplasmin to form ceruloplasmin, which then enters the circulation. More than 95% of serum copper is in this form. Ceruloplasmin is an alpha globulin with a single, continuous polypeptide chain and a molecular weight of 132,000; it has six copper atoms per molecule. This protein has multiple functions, and although it is not involved in copper transport from the intestine, it may be the major vehicle for the transport of the metal from the liver and may function as a copper donor in the formation of a variety of copper-containing enzymes. It controls the release of iron into plasma from the cells, in which the metal is stored as ferritin. Ceruloplasmin is also the most prominent serum antioxidant, and as such, catalyzes the oxidation of ferrous ion to ferric ion and prevents the oxidation of polyunsaturated fatty acids and other similar substances. Finally, it modulates the inflammatory response and may regulate the concentration of various serum biogenic amines.

The concentration of ceruloplasmin in plasma is normally between 30 and 40 mg/dl. It is elevated under a variety of circumstances, including pregnancy and other conditions with high estrogen concentrations, infections, cirrhosis, malignancies, hyperthyroidism, and myocardial infarction. The concentration is low in children suffering from a combined iron and copper deficiency anemia and in normal infants up to approximately 2 months of age. In the nephrotic syndrome, low levels are due to the vast renal losses of ceruloplasmin.

Several other copper-containing enzymes have been isolated from mammalian tissues. These enzymes are outlined in Table 31.1, together with the manifes-

284

Table 31.1. Cuproenzymes Affected in Kinky Hair Disease

Affected Enzyme	Manifestation
Tyrosinase	Depigmentation of hair Skin pallor
Lysyl oxidase	Frayed and split arterial intima (defect in elastin and collagen cross-linking)
Monoamine oxidase	Kinky hair
Cytochrome c oxidase	Hypothermia
Dopamine-β-hydroxylase	??
Ascorbate oxidase	Skeletal demineralization

Note: The activity of superoxide dismutase, a soluble copper enzyme, is normal in cultured fibroblasts derived from the mottled mouse, an animal model for kinky hair disease [49].

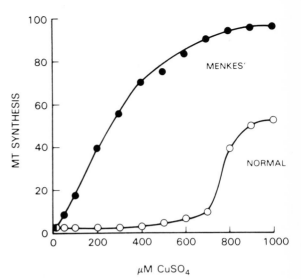

Figure 31.1. Copper induction curves in fibroblasts from a patient with kinky hair disease. Kinky hair disease cells (●) or normal cells (○) were preincubated for 12 hours in Eagle's minimal essential medium with 20% chelated fetal calf serum and were then treated with the indicated concentration of copper sulfate for 9 hours. The cells were labeled with ^{35}S-cysteine in a medium containing 20% chelated serum during the final hour of induction and then were analyzed for metallothionein synthesis. The gel autoradiograms were scanned in a densitometer to estimate metallothionein synthesis and the results were normalized to give a value of 100 for kinky hair disease cells at 1,000 μM copper sulfate. (From Leone et al. [11] with permission of the authors.)

tations resulting from their deficiency in kinky hair disease.

The basic cellular defect for kinky hair disease is still not clarified. The characteristic feature of the disease is a maldistribution of body copper, so that it accumulates to abnormal levels in a form or location rendering it inaccessible for the synthesis of copper enzymes [2]. Patients absorb little or no orally administered copper but when the metal is given intravenously, they experience a prompt rise in serum copper and ceruloplasmin [7]. Levels are low in liver and brain but are elevated in several other tissues, notably intestinal mucosa, muscle, spleen, and kidney. The copper content of cultured fibroblasts derived from patients with kinky hair disease is four to six times greater than that of control cells, with excess copper accumulating in metallothionein [8–10]. Synthesis of metallothionein protein in fibroblast cells derived from infants with kinky hair disease is inducible at lower copper levels than it is in normal cells [11] (Figure. 31.1), an effect due to an increase in metallothionein mRNA levels. The increased expression of the metallothionein gene in mutant cells is due, in part at least, to an abnormality in a diffusible factor, a product of the X-linked gene. In addition to metallothionein at least two other proteins are abnormally induced. Their role in the pathogenesis of the disease is as yet unknown.

It is likely that the excessive amounts of metallothionein prevent copper from becoming accessible for the synthesis of ceruloplasmin, superoxide dismutase [12], cytochrome oxidase [13], and the other copper-containing enzymes listed in Table 31.1. The finding that metallothionein, as isolated from the livers of infants with kinky hair disease, has a lower than normal copper and cadmium content and ap-

pears to have a reduced affinity for these metals [14] has yet to be confirmed.

Pathology

Because of these metalloenzymes' defective activity, a variety of pathologic changes are set into motion. Arteries both systemically and within the brain are tortuous with irregular lumen and a frayed and split intimal lining (Figure 31.2). These abnormalities indicate the failure in elastin and collagen cross-linking that is caused by dysfunction of the key enzyme for this process: copper-dependent lysyl oxidase [15].

Changes within the brain may result from vascular lesions, copper deficiency, or a combination of the two. Extensive focal degeneration of gray matter with neuronal loss and gliosis and an associated axonal degeneration in white matter is present. Cellular loss is prominent in the cerebellum, where Purkinje cells are hard hit; many are lost, and others show

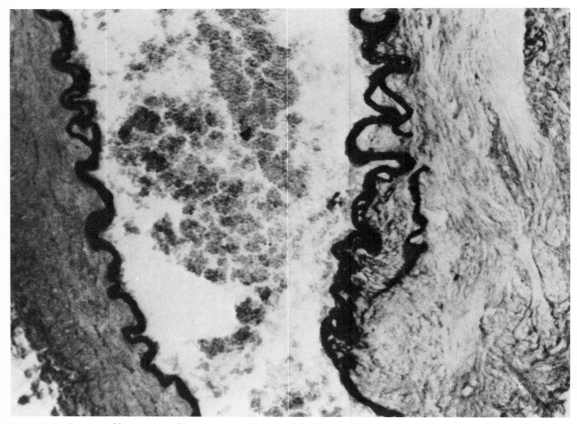

Figure 31.2. Section of large artery from patient with kinky hair disease. Note frayed and split internal elastic lamina.

abnormal dendritic arborization ("weeping willow") and perisomatic processes. Focal axonal swellings (torpedoes) are also observed [1,16] (Figures 31.3, 31.4). In the thalamus there is a primary cellular degeneration which spares the smaller, inhibitory neurons [16a]. On electron microscopy there is a marked increase in the number of mitochondria in the perikaryon of Purkinje cells and, to a lesser extent, in the neurons of cerebral cortex and the basal ganglia [17] (Figure 31.5). Mitochondria are enlarged and there are intramitochrondrial electron-dense bodies. The pathogenesis of these changes is a matter of controversy, but they may be caused by the reduced activity of the mitochondrial, copper-containing enzymes [18].

Clinical Manifestations

Kinky hair disease is transmitted as an X-linked trait (Figure 31.6). Linkage studies, using restriction frag-

ment length polymorphisms, suggest that the gene locus is close to the centromere of the chromosome, probably on the proximal portion of its long arm [19,20]. It is not too rare a disorder; its frequency has been estimated at 2 per 100,000 male live births [21].

Symptoms appear during the neonatal period. Most commonly, hypothermia, poor feeding, and impaired weight gain are noted. Seizures soon become apparent. There is marked hypotonia, poor head control, and progressive deterioration of all neurologic function. The facies have a cherubic appearance with a depressed nasal bridge and reduced movements [22] (Figure 31.7). Optic discs are pale, and there are microcysts of the pigment epithelium and the iris [23]. The urinary tract is not spared. Hydronephrosis, hydroureter, and bladder diverticuli are common [24,25]. The most striking finding is the appearance of hair. It is colorless and friable. On examination under microscope, a variety of abnormalities are evident, most often pili torti (twisted

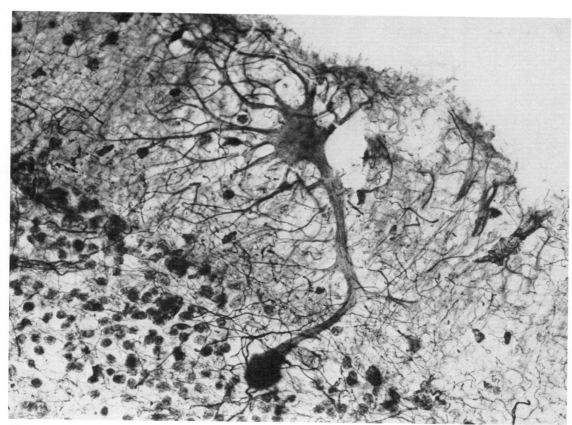

Figure 31.3. Cerebellum in kinky hair disease. Purkinje cell with "Medusa head" formation (Bodian × 500). (Courtesy of Dr. D. Troost, Department of Neuropathology, University of Utrecht, Utrecht, the Netherlands.)

hair) and trichorhexis nodosa (fractures of the hair shaft at regular intervals [1] (Figure 31.8).

Radiographs of long bones show a variety of abnormalities, which include osteoporosis, metaphyseal spurring, a diaphyseal periosteal reaction, and scalloping of the posterior aspects of the vertebral bodies [26,27]. Skull radiographs may reveal the presence of Wormian bones. On arteriography, the cerebral vessels are markedly elongated and tortuous (Figure 31.9). Similar changes are seen in the systemic vasculature [28]. Computed tomography and NMR scans may reveal the presence of cerebral atrophy, cortical areas of low density, and tortuous and enlarged intracranial vessels [29,30 Menkes J:personal observations]. Subdural effusions are not unusual [29,31].

The EEG is generally severely abnormal and demonstrates diffuse, multifocal spike activity. The course is inexorably downhill but the rate of neurologic deterioration varies. The mean age at death in the cases reviewed by French [32] was 19 months, but survival to 12 years of age has been reported.

Diagnosis

In many instances the diagnosis is suggested by the clinical history of unexplained hypothermia and hypotonia, and the appearance of the infant's hair. However, in some cases the primary fetal hair is normal, and the hair abnormalities are not evident for a few weeks. Inasmuch as serum ceruloplasmin and copper levels are normally low in the neonatal period and do not reach adult levels until the age of 1 month these determinations are not diagnostic during the first few weeks of life [33]. These determinations must therefore be performed serially to demonstrate a failure in the expected rise. Oral loading tests with radioactively labeled copper will result in a flat curve. Intravenous loading shows the syn-

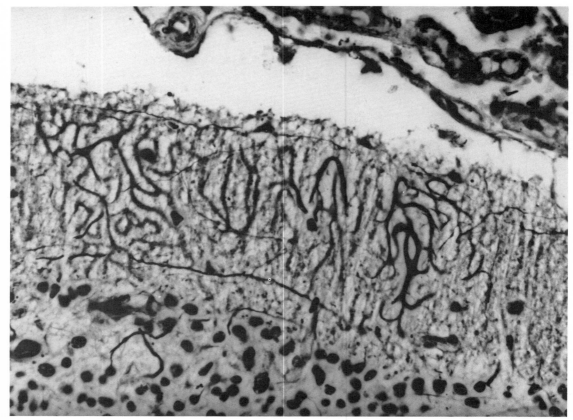

Figure 31.4. Cerebellum in kinky hair disease. Note "weeping willow" formation of cerebellar molecular layer (Bodian × 500). (Courtesy of Dr. D. Troost, Department of Neuropathology, University of Utrecht, Utrecht, the Netherlands.)

thesis of labeled ceruloplasmin [34]. The increased copper content of fibroblasts and the increased uptake of labeled copper in cultured cells [35] permit an intrauterine diagnosis of the disease [36]. Chorionic villi of affected fetuses also show an increased copper content during the first trimester of gestation [37].

Heterozygotes may have areas of pili torti comprising between 30 and 50% of their hair [38]. Less commonly, there is skin depigmentation. The full neurodegenerative disease has been encountered in two girls [39,39a]. In one instance this was accompanied by a chromosome X/2 reciprocal translocation with the X break at Xg13 [39a].

Several variants of kinky hair disease have been recognized by low serum copper concentrations. These may present with ataxia and mild mental retardation [40] or with extrapyramidal symptoms [41].

Low copper and ceruloplasmin concentrations have also been reported in a variant of Ehlers–Danlos syndrome in which the brain appears to remain spared [42].

Trichorrhexis nodosa may also be seen in arginosuccinicaciduria (see Chapter 16), biotin deficiency, and Pollitt's syndrome. The last is an autosomal recessive condition with additional manifestations of nonprogressive mental retardation, seizures, and spasticity [34,43–45].

Treatment

Treatment appears to be ineffective in arresting the progressive cerebral degeneration, even though in some cases parenterally administered copper may

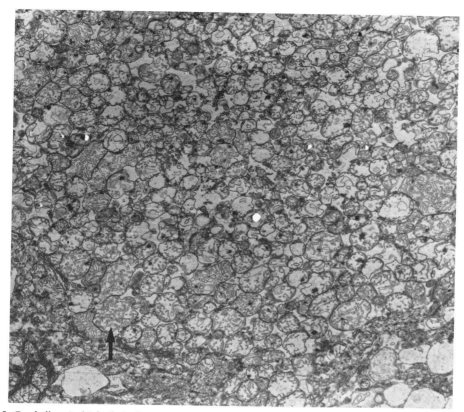

Figure 31.5. Cerebellum in kinky hair disease—Purkinje cell dendrite. The expanded dendrite is replaced by mitochondria greatly increased in number; most have undergone both enlargement and swelling. Note enlarged mitochondria having prominent tubulo-vesiculated cristae *(arrows)* (original magnification × 6500). (Courtesy of Dr. N. Yoshimura, Brain Research Institute, Hirosaki University School of Medicine, Hirosaki, Japan.)

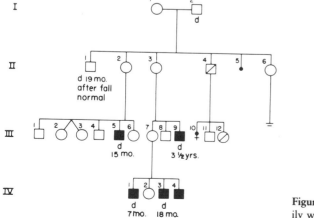

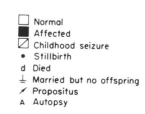

□ Normal
■ Affected
▨ Childhood seizure
• Stillbirth
d Died
⊥ Married but no offspring
↗ Propositus
A Autopsy

Figure 31.6. Pedigree of the "G" family, the original family with kinky hair disease.

correct the hepatic copper deficiency and restore serum copper and ceruloplasmin levels to normal [46]. Failure to improve brain function may be due to an inability of the central nervous system to utilize the administered copper. Since the rate of deterioration is so variable, and since it is not unlikely that milder forms of the disease may respond to copper infusions, the author does however advise treatment until it becomes evident that it does not arrest neurologic deterioration.

Grover and Scrutton [47] have suggested the following protocol to raise serum copper and ceruloplasmin: copper infusions (550 to 850 μg/kg cupric acetate) given daily until both values have returned to normal: thereafter, copper acetate once or twice a week (190 to 220 μg/kg) to maintain a normal serum copper level (about 100 μg/dl).

The effectiveness of ceruloplasmin infusions is still under investigation [48].

Figure 31.7. Typical facies of one of the original subjects with kinky hair disease.

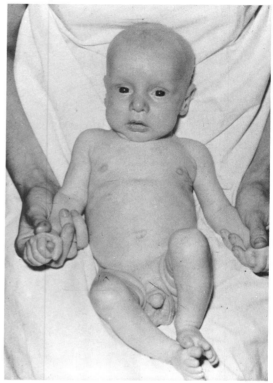

Figure 31.8. Kinky hair disease. Hair of scalp. Pt = characteristic twisting of pili torti. M = monilethrix with varying diameter of hair shaft. Tn = fractures of shafts at regular intervals (trichorrhexis nodosa).

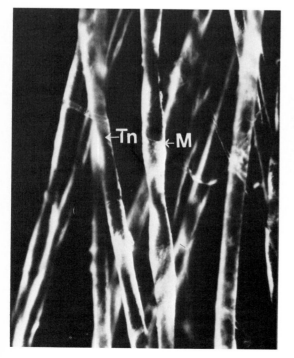

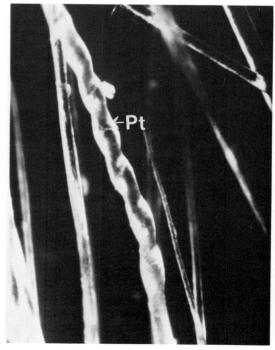

Figure 31.9. Right carotid angiogram of a 5-month-old infant with kinky hair disease showing tortuous and anomalous middle cerebral artery vessels. In addition, there was marked tortuosity of the superior aspect of the cervical portion of the internal carotid artery in the early arterial phase. Lateral projection at 3 seconds. (Courtesy of Dr. John L. Gwinn, Department of Radiology, Children's Hospital of Los Angeles.)

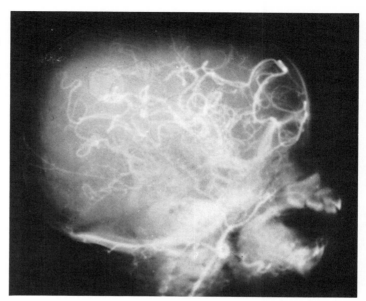

References

1. Menkes JH, et al. A sex-linked recessive disorder with growth retardation, peculiar hair, and focal cerebral and cerebellar degeneration. Pediatrics 1962;29:764–779.
2. Danks DM, et al. Menkes's kinky hair syndrome. An inherited defect in copper absorption with widespread effects. Pediatrics 1972;50:188–201.
3. Solomons NW. Biochemical, metabolic and clinical role of copper in human nutrition. J Am Coll Nutr 1985;4:83–105.
4. Bremmer I. Absorption, transport and distribution of copper. In: Biological roles of copper. Amsterdam: Ciba Found Symp 1980;79:23–48.
5. Schmidt CJ, Hamer DH, McBride OW. Chromosomal location of human metallothionein genes: implication for Menkes' disease. Science 1984;224:1104–1106.
6. Richards RI, Heguy A, Karin M. Structural and functional analysis of the human metallothionein-la gene: differential induction by metal ions and glucocorticoids. Cell 1984;37:263–272.
7. Bucknall WE, Haslam RHA, Holtzman NA. Kinky hair syndrome: response to copper therapy. Pediatrics 1973;52:653–657.
8. Goka TJ, et al. Menkes' disease: a biochemical abnormality in cultured human fibroblasts. Proc Natl Acad Sci USA 1976;73:604–606.
9. Labadie GU, et al. Increased copper metallothionein in Menkes cultured fibroblasts. Pediatr Res 1981;15:257–261.
10. Yazaki M, et al. Copper-binding proteins in the liver and kidney from the patients with Menkes' kinky hair disease. Tohoku J Exp Med 1983;139:97–102.
11. Leone A, Pavlakis GN, Hamer DH. Menkes' disease: abnormal metallothionein gene regulation in response to copper. Cell 1985;40:301–309.
12. Onishi T, et al. Nature of copper and zinc compounds in tissues from a patient with Menkes kinky hair syndrome. Eur J Pediatr 1981;137:17–21.
13. Maehara M, et al. Cytochrome c oxidase deficiency in Menkes kinky hair disease. Brain Dev 1983;5:533–540.
14. Chan WY, Garnica AD, Rennert OM. Metal-binding studies of metallothioneins in Menkes kinky hair disease. Clin Chim Acta 1978;88:221–228.
15. O'Dell BL. Roles for iron and copper in connective tissue biosynthesis. Philos Trans R Soc Lond [Biol] 1981;294:91–104.
16. Hirano A, et al. Fine structure of the cerebellar cortex in Menkes kinky-hair disease. Arch Neurol 1977;34:52–56.
16a. Martin JJ, Leroy JG. Thalamic lesions in a patient with Menkes kinky-hair disease. Clinical Neuropathology 1985;4:206–209.
17. Yoshimura N, Kudo H. Mitochondrial abnormalities in Menkes' kinky hair disease (MKHD). Acta Neuropathol (Berl) 1983;59:295–303.
18. Yamano T, Paldino AM, Suzuki K. Ultrastructural and morphometric studies of Purkinje cells of brindled mouse after administration of cupric chloride. J Neuropathol Exp Neurol 1985;44:97–107.
19. Wieacker P, et al. Menkes kinky hair disease: a search for closely linked restriction fragment length polymorphism. Hum Genet 1983;64:139–142.
20. Horn N, et al. Linkage studies in Menkes disease. The Xg blood group system and C-banding of the X chromosome. Ann Hum Genet 1984;48:161–172.

21. Horn N, Morton NE. Genetic epidemiology of Menkes disease. Genetic Epidemiol 1986;3:225–230.

22. Grover WD, Johnson WC, Henkin RI. Clinical and biochemical aspects of trichopoliodystrophy. Ann Neurol 1979;5:65–71.

23. Seelenfreund MH, Gartner S, Vinger PF. The ocular pathology of Menkes' disease. Arch Ophthalmol 1968;80:718–720.

24. Wheeler EM, Roberts PF. Menkes's steely hair syndrome. Arch Dis Child 1976;51:269–274.

25. Daly WJ, Rabinovitch HH. Urologic abnormalities in Menkes' syndrome. J Urol 1981;126:262–264.

26. Wesenberg RL, Gwinn JL, Barnes GR. Radiological findings in the kinky hair syndrome. Radiology 1968;92:500–506.

27. Stanley P, Gwinn JL, Sutcliffe J. The osseous abnormalities in Menkes' syndrome. Ann Radiol 1976; 19:167–172.

28. Ahlgren P, Vestermark S. Menkes' kinky hair disease. Neuroradiology 1977;13:159–163.

29. Seay AR, et al. CT scans in Menkes disease. Neurology 1979;29:304–312.

30. Farelly C, et al. CT manifestations of Menkes' kinky hair syndrome (trichopoliodystrophy). J Can Assoc Radiol 1984;35:406–408.

31. Adams PC, et al. Serial study of radiological findings with emphasis on similarity to the battered child syndrome. Radiology 1974;112:401–407.

32. French JH. X-chromosome-linked copper malabsorption (X-cLCL). In: Vinken PJ, Bruyn GW, eds. Handbook of clinical neurology. vol. 29. Amsterdam: North–Holland 1977;50:188–201.

33. Gunn TR, Macfarlane S, Phillips LI. Difficulties in the neonatal diagnosis of Menkes' kinky hair syndrome—trichopoliodystrophy. Clin Pediatr 1984;23:514–516.

34. Willemse J, et al. Menkes' kinky hair disease. I. Comparison of classical and unusual clinical and biochemical features in two patients. Brain Dev 1982;4:105–114.

35. Horn N. Menkes' X-linked disease: prenatal diagnosis and carrier detection. J Inher Metab Dis 1983; (suppl 1)6:59–62.

36. Camakaris J, et al. Altered copper metabolism in cultured cells from human Menkes' syndrome and mottled mouse mutants. Biochem Genet 1980;18:117–131.

37. Tonneson T, et al. Measurement of copper in chorionic villi for first-trimester diagnosis of Menkes' disease. Lancet 1985;1:1038–1039.

38. Collie WR, et al. Pili torti as marker for carriers of Menkes disease. Lancet 1978;1:607–608.

39. Iwakawa Y, et al. Menkes' kinky hair syndrome: report on an autopsy case and his female sibling with similar clinical manifestations. Brain Dev (Domestic Ed) 1979;11:260–266.

39a. Kapur S, et al. Menkes syndrome in a girl with X-autosome translocation. Am J Human Genet 1987; 26:503–510.

40. Procopis P. A mild form of Menkes steely hair syndrome. J Pediatr 1981;98:97–99.

41. Haas RH, et al. An X-linked disease of the nervous system with disordered copper metabolism and features differing from Menkes' disease. Neurology 1981;31:852–859.

42. Peltonen L, et al. Alterations in copper and collagen metabolism in the Menkes syndrome and a new subtype of the Ehlers–Danlos syndrome. Biochemistry 1983;22:6156–6163.

43. Pollitt RJ, Jenner FA, Davies M. Sibs with mental and physical retardation and trichorrhexis nodosa with abnormal amino acid composition of the hair. Arch Dis Child 1968;43:211–216.

44. Coulter DL, Beals TF, Allen RJ. Neurotrichosis: hairshaft abnormalities associated with neurological diseases. Dev Med Child Neurol 1982;24:634–644.

45. Ullmo A. Un nouveau type d'agénesie et de dystrophie pilaire familiale et héréditaire. Dermatologica 1944;90:75–79.

46. Garnica AD. The failure of parenteral copper therapy in Menkes kinky hair syndrome. Eur J Pediatr 1984;142:98–102.

47. Grover WD, Scrutton MC. Copper infusion therapy in trichopoliodystrophy. J Pediatr 1975;86:216–220.

48. Garnica A, Chan WY, Rennert OM. Ceruloplasmin infusion in Menkes syndrome. Pediatr Res 1986;20:264A.

49. Packman S, Chin P, O'Toole C. Copper utilization in cultured fibroblasts of the mottled mouse, an animal model for Menkes' kinky hair syndrome. J Inher Metab Dis 1984;7:168–170.

Chapter 32
Incontinentia Pigmenti

N. PAUL ROSMAN

Incontinentia pigmenti is a rare inherited disorder, seen mostly in girls, which affects a variety of tissues derived from ectoderm and mesoderm. The earliest and most clinically distinctive manifestations are the dermatologic ones, and it is from these that the disease derives its name. Other organ systems are frequently involved, however, and can be quite disabling to the child. Particularly important in that regard is involvement of the central nervous system.

History

The first description of this disorder was by Garrod, who in 1905 described a 2½-year-old girl with "peculiar pigmentation of the skin" [1]. She reportedly had always been very backward, had never sat or talked, had a brachycephalic head and spastic legs, and was said to have shown "some of the characteristics of the 'Mongolian' variety of idiocy." The most remarkable feature of the case was a peculiar pigmentation of the skin, of gray-brown tint, which had a linear distribution and in places was arranged in whorls. A photograph of the child accompanied the report which appeared in *Transactions of the Clinical Society of London* in 1906. The second case description was by Adamson in 1908 who reported on a case of "congenital pigmentation with atrophic scarring associated with other congenital anomalies" [2]. He described a 19-year-old girl, small and of feeble intellect, whose skin showed a generalized retiform red-brown pigmentation with areas of scarring. The girl also had absent earlobes, facial asymmetry, patchy alopecia, absence of two fingers on one hand, only four toes on each foot, and two nipples on the right breast. The next report was by Bardach who reported in 1925 on the disorder in identical twins said to have "systematized nevi" [3]. The fifth case was reported by Bloch, who in 1926

described a 1½-year-old girl with "splashed pigmented skin lesions" and proposed the name "incontinentia pigmenti" [4]. The same patient was reported again in 1928 by Sulzberger [5] and once again, in adult life, by Franceschetti and Jadassohn in 1954 [6], by which time the skin lesions had cleared completely. Though Bloch's patient was said to have been neurologically intact, one of her eyes had been surgically removed at 1 month of age because of glioma or pseudoglioma. By 1976, a total of 653 cases of incontinentia pigmenti had been reported in the literature [7].

Dermatologic Features

The skin manifestations of incontinentia pigmenti usually pass through three distinctive but somewhat overlapping stages [7–13]. Lesions characteristic of the first stage are erythematous, macular, papular, vesicular, bullous, and sometimes pustular. They appear within the first 2 weeks of life in 90% of cases; in half of these, the abnormalities are present at birth. During this first stage the lesions are located primarily over the limbs and trunk and to a lesser extent on the scalp. On the limbs, they are linear in distribution, mainly proximal, and affect primarily the flexor surfaces. The infants usually have a blood leukocytosis with an accompanying eosinophilia at this time, but they are not systemically ill. Eosinophils are also found in the vesicular and bullous skin lesions and in the underlying dermis. Lesions of the first phase can last from several days to several months.

The second stage is characterized by lesions that are variously pustular, lichenoid, verrucous, keratotic, and dyskeratotic. The peak age for this phase is between the second and sixth weeks. The lesions are most prominent over the limbs, particularly distally, and affect primarily their dorsal aspects. Lesions of this stage usually persist for several months. They may disappear without sequelae or may be followed by areas of hypopigmentation or atrophy of the skin.

The third phase is the one characterized by development of pigmentation. This occurs over a period of weeks, with a peak occurrence between the twelfth and twenty-sixth weeks. The coloration can be tan, chocolate brown, or slate gray, with lesions of varying configurations: stellate macules, streaks, whorls, and flecks. They are most prominent over the trunk, particularly laterally, and on the limbs, especially proximally (Figure 32.1). In a sizable minority of children, only stage 3 (pigmentary) skin lesions are seen; in such circumstance, it is possible that erythematous, vesicular, or verrucous lesions could have appeared in utero. Although the areas of pigmentation may be a residuum of the earlier inflammatory lesions, the pigmentary changes are often located in regions removed from the sites of the earlier lesions. In such circumstances, however, the pigment may have traveled via perivascular spaces or lymphatics from original sites of deposition to new locations. The pigmentation usually persists for many years, usually disappearing in the second or third decade. As with lesions of the second stage, areas of skin hypopigmentation or atrophy may follow. Streaked hypomelanotic macules of the calves may be the only dermatologic indication of incontinentia pigmenti in adult life [12]. An additional dermatologic finding in incontinentia pigmenti is alopecia of the scalp, seen in more than one-third of patients [7].

Dermatologically, the term incontinentia pigmenti refers to a decrease or absence of melanin in the basal cells of the epidermis with an accompanying increase in the dermis (Figure 32.2). This redistribution of melanin suggests that the basal epidermal cells may have become "incontinent" of

melanin, allowing it to drop into the dermis [14]. The melanin that accumulates in dermal macrophages later undergoes degradation and dispersal, and regions that were once darkly pigmented now become leukodermic. This skin histopathology though distinctive, is not pathognomonic of incontinentia pigmenti. Nonetheless, the occurrence of such pigmentary skin lesions in an infant girl with earlier bullous and verrucous skin lesions and a high eosinophil count is indicative of no other disorder [13].

Nondermatologic Features

Extradermatologic manifestations are found in 50 to 80% of incontinentia pigmenti cases. These include abnormalities of the eyes, bony skeleton, teeth, other organ systems, and the central nervous system [10,13].

Eye Abnormalities

Ophthalmic abnormalities are found in about one-third of patients with incontinentia pigmenti [9,10,14,15]. In more than half of these, they are severe [7]. Literally dozens of abnormalities have been described. The most typical ocular abnormality is said to be a retrolental mass with detachment of a dysplastic retina; this mass has variously been called a persistent hyperplastic primary vitreous, a pseudoglioma, or retrolental fibroplasia [9]. Other ophthalmic findings have included strabismus, cataract, optic atrophy, pigmentary retinopathy, microphthalmos, corneal clouding, uveitis, myopia, blue sclera, nystagmus, vascular and proliferative changes in the fundus, phthisis bulbi, ptosis, pigmentary changes in the conjunctiva and iris, seclusion of the pupil, absence of the anterior chamber, ciliary body atrophy, vitreous hemorrhage, persistence of the hy-

Figure 32.1. Infant with incontinentia pigmenti. Note the pigmentary lesions (stage 3) prominently involving both lower limbs and to a lesser extent the trunk.

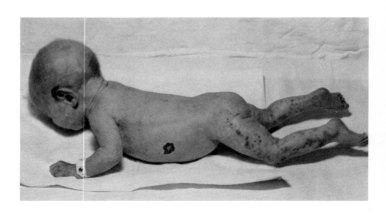

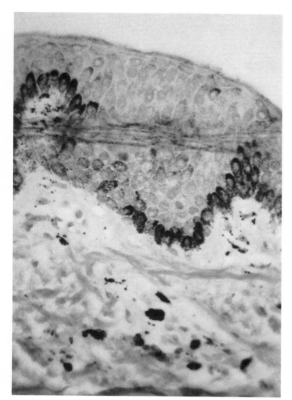

Figure 32.2. Skin biopsy from a child with incontinentia pigmenti. Melanin deposits (black) are seen normally located in the basal epidermis and abnormally located in the underlying dermis.

aloid artery, papillitis, chorioretinitis, metastatic ophthalmia, retinitis proliferans, glial retinal strands, microaneurysms, telangiectasia, and hemorrhagic retinitis [9].

Bony Abnormalities

These occur in more than 20% of cases [9]. They include skull deformities, seen in about 10% [16], small stature, curvature of the spine, hemivertebrae and spina bifida, extra ribs, hip dislocation, syndactyly, club foot, cleft palate, and chondrodystrophy [10].

Dental Abnormalities

These have been found in one-third [9] to two-thirds [10] of patients. Both deciduous and permanent teeth can be affected. The abnormalities include partial and occasionally complete anodontia, conical crown deformities, and delayed dentition.

Other Somatic Abnormalities

These include dystrophy of the nails, seen in about 7% of cases [6,10,17], ear deformities, cleft lip, and genitourinary and cardiovascular anomalies [13].

Neurologic Abnormalities

Central nervous system involvement is common in incontinentia pigmenti, with frequencies varying from 30 to 50% in different series [7,8,10,16,18,19]. The most common neurologic findings have been psychomotor retardation (8 to 16% of cases), generalized and focal seizures (9 to 13%), spastic paralyses (10 to 12%), and microcephaly (5%). Additional neurologic abnormalities, mentioned frequently in individual case reports, include hypertonia, cerebellar ataxia, reduced motor activity in the newborn, and visual impairment (from a variety of ophthalmic pathologies).

Clearly, many children with incontinentia pigmenti exhibit more than one neurologic abnormality: for example, most children with microcephaly would be expected to be retarded, and seizures and spastic paralyses frequently coexist. The degree of retardation varies considerably, however. In general, the development of seizures early in life portends unfavorable neurologic development [20]. There are exceptions, however; in one personally studied case in whom left-sided seizures began on the third day of life, with later development of a left hemiparesis, cognitive functioning at 3 years of age was only mildly delayed.

Radiology

Radiologic studies of the head in incontinentia pigmenti have revealed no distinctive findings in the brain. The most frequent finding on pneumoencephalography [8,21,22] or more recently, on cranial CT scanning [8,23], has been a general reduction in brain size, reflecting either shrinkage (cerebral atrophy) or underdevelopment (cerebral hypoplasia).

Pathology

There have been few postmortem studies of the brain in incontinentia pigmenti. The first was by O'Doherty and Norman who in 1968 described findings in the brain of a girl with incontinentia pigmenti who died at 7 weeks of age [24]. She had been observed at birth to have eosinophil-containing bullae on the limbs and a blood eosinophilia. On examination, she fisted excessively and showed a general reduction in motor activity. By the fifth day of life, she was no longer able to suck or swallow and required tube feeding. Her skin lesions went through the "classical cycle of evolution," and her peripheral eosinophilia disappeared by 6 weeks. She died following a pneumonia with a supervening hemorrhagic gastroenteritis.

The brain showed few sulci in the frontal and parietal regions with mild lateral ventricular enlargement, particularly on the left, and polymicrogyria in the left frontal parietal, superior temporal, and lateral occipital regions. The cerebral gray matter was unduly thick, lacked normal lamination, and had multiple superficial small folds. In addition, the left cerebral hemisphere showed a number of necrotic foci in the white matter and cortex (that had probably developed at or around the time of birth). The cerebellar cortex showed multiple demarcated areas of neuronal loss, resembling minor dysplasias.

In their paper, O'Doherty and Norman referred to abnormalities that had been reported by van Bogaert (1957) in the brain of one of three sisters said to have incontinentia pigmenti. The findings in that case were very different, however, with cerebellar Purkinje cell and myelin loss in the corticospinal tracts and posterior columns of the spinal cord. Furthermore, the cases were very atypical from a clinical standpoint for incontinentia pigmenti, for the daughters were children of a consanguineous Jewish marriage and in addition to a congenital pigmentation, they had a macular degeneration and a progressive cerebellar ataxia. It seems likely that they had a different disorder.

In 1977 Hauw et al. [25] reported a very different neuropathology in a child with incontinentia pigmenti who died at age 3 months. Her brain showed a destructive encephalopathy, apparently of perinatal onset, with cerebral ulegyria, white matter cavitation, and scarring of the cerebellar cortex. Additionally, there was a diffuse inflammatory cell infiltration of the pia-arachnoid and brain parenchyma. No brain malformations were seen.

The following year, Siemes et al. [26] reported on cases of incontinentia pigmenti occurring in three generations of one family and described the neuropathologic findings in one of three affected sisters. The first girl was noted at birth to have pigmented skin lesions of the trunk and legs. Her subsequent growth and development were normal. At 21 months, she received an injection of vaccinia antigen, followed 25 days later by vaccination with vaccinia vi-

rus. Three days after that she became irritable, and the next day she had a grand mal convulsion. She was admitted to hospital unconscious with meningeal signs. Cerebrospinal fluid contained 1 lymphocyte/mm^3, a normal amount of glucose, and an elevated CSF protein of 102 mg/100 ml. She was treated with diazepam and dexamethasone, improved, and was discharged home in 2 weeks, free of neurologic abnormalities. Neurologic examination 3½ months later was again normal. Two weeks after that, however, she again became irritable, and the following day she had another grand mal seizure. She was again treated with diazepam but remained comatose. Repeat CSF examination showed 5 lymphocytes/mm^3, a normal amount of glucose, and an elevated protein of 270 mg/100 ml. Trepanation of the skull to show the right cerebral hemisphere, done because of suspected tumor, disclosed edematous necrotic tissue; the girl continued to deteriorate and died the next day.

Neuropathologically, there was marked brain edema with early right temporal lobe and marked cerebellar tonsillar herniation. Both cerebral hemispheres showed hemorrhagic necrosis of the white matter, the insular and parasagittal cortex of the parietal lobe, the corpus striatum, and the thalamus. Histopathologically, there was evidence of perivenous encephalitis in the telencephalic white matter with residual lesions of differing ages.

A second sister had been noted from the second week of life to have brownish pigmentation of the trunk and proximal limbs. Her subsequent growth and development were normal. At 7 months, she was given her first injection of diphtheria tetanus toxoid and 3 weeks later she developed a one-sided convulsion unaccompanied by fever. She was treated with phenobarbital for a year. At 27 months, following an upper respiratory infection, she developed a generalized convulsion; thereafter she remained stuporous with bilateral papilledema. Cerebrospinal fluid examination showed 9 lymphocytes/mm^3 with a normal sugar and increased protein. Several additional grand mal seizures developed. Cranial CT scan showed a mild diffuse decrease in the density of the white matter, in keeping with an encephalitis. Repeat CSF examination disclosed 1 lymphocyte/mm^3 and a normal protein content. She improved and was discharged home after 9 weeks. Several months later, she showed normal mentation but a spastic diplegia. Investigation of this girl's immune status failed to show any defect of humoral or cellular mechanisms.

The third sister with incontinentia pigmenti had an afebrile seizure at 5 months of age with a normal CSF examination. At 1 year of age, pigmentation developed without prior inflammatory change. Growth and development were normal except for delayed dentition.

The authors suggested on the basis of these cases that inflammatory processes of encephalitic type (postvaccinal or postinfectious) may play an important role in triggering the neurologic disorders seen frequently with incontinentia pigmenti.

More recently, Avrahami et al. [8] in 1985 reported brain changes on cranial CT scan in two children with incontinentia pigmenti. One child was born with characteristic stage-1 lesions of the upper limbs; trunkal lesions developed 2 weeks later, and 2 months after that, pigmentation typical of stage 3 appeared. The child's psychomotor development was delayed. A cranial CT scan done at age 2 months showed low-density areas in the right frontal and parietal regions, with normal lateral ventricular size and pontine and cerebellar atrophy. The child's subsequent development showed severe retardation. Follow-up cranial CT scan at age 2 years showed diffuse brain atrophy, lateral ventricles that were now enlarged, and again, pontine and cerebellar atrophy. The authors suggested that the brain changes seen on CT scan at age 2 months, at which time the child had vesiculoerythematous skin lesions, were compatible with an acute encephalitis, as described earlier by Siemes et al. [26].

In the second case, characteristic skin lesions were present at birth with development of hyperpigmentation a few months later. Generalized seizures appeared at 5 years, at which time the girl showed microcephaly, a spastic left hemiparesis, cerebellar ataxia, and a borderline low IQ. Computed tomography scan showed diffuse brain atrophy with enlarged ventricles. Unfortunately, there is no mention of a cranial CT scan earlier in life.

Genetics

Of the 653 cases of typical incontinentia pigmenti reported by 1976, 593 or 91% had been in females [7]. Subsequent series have disclosed as great or an even greater predilection for females. Three possible patterns of inheritance have been suggested: (a) an autosomal-dominant gene with female sex limitation; (b) an autosomal-dominant gene, prenatally lethal in males; and (c) an X-linked dominant gene, prenatally lethal in males. Of these possibilities, the last seems much the most likely [7,10]. In that circumstance, of two male and two female offspring born to an affected woman, one of the males would be expected to be an affected hemizygote and to die

in utero, the other would be expected to be a healthy boy; one of the girls would be expected to have incontinentia pigmenti (usually clinically more severe than in the mother [16]), and the other would be expected to be a healthy girl. Those expectations are supported by the statistics observed in this disorder [7,10]. Although isolated cases in families most likely arise by mutation, familial occurrence should be excluded only after careful examination of other family members, looking for microsymptoms of incontinentia pigmenti in the mother of an affected child [10]. The frequency with which incontinentia pigmenti has affected two or more members of the same family has varied in different reports from 15 to 55% [9].

In those infrequent cases in which a male is affected with the disorder, chromosomal analysis should be carried out to determine whether an XXY or another abnormal karyotype is present. Though some authors have found an increased frequency of chromosomal instability (breaks, gaps) in incontinentia pigmenti, the frequency of malignancy is not increased [10]. This contrasts with the increased incidence of malignancies in chromosomal instability syndromes such as ataxia-telangiectasia, Bloom syndrome, Fanconi anemia, and xeroderma pigmentosum, suggesting that any chromosomal abnormalities found in cases of incontinentia pigmenti are probably nonspecific [23].

Differential Diagnosis

Franceschetti and Jadassohn [6] have divided the syndrome of incontinentia pigmenti into two basic subtypes: the Bloch (1926)–Sulzberger (1928) variety and the Naegeli (1927) variety [14]. In the Bloch–Sulzberger type, the great majority of patients are female, there are usually early inflammatory lesions of the skin (with later pigmentation), eye abnormalities are frequent, the teeth are often absent or malformed, and neurologic abnormalities are common. In the Naegeli variant, males and females are affected with equal frequency, and skin pigmentation is not preceded by an inflammatory stage, is more reticular and widespread, and usually does not appear until the second or third year; also, the skin tends to be hypohidrotic with hyperkeratosis of the palms and soles. In addition, eye and neurologic abnormalities are not features of the Naegeli variant, and dental abnormalities are less prominent than in the Bloch–Sulzberger type [10,14].

Some authors do not regard the disorder described by Naegeli [27] as a subtype of incontinentia pigmenti but rather as a disorder to be differentiated from it and call the disorder chromatophore naevus of Naegeli, a term used synonymously with France-schetti–Jadassohn syndrome [10].

Another condition to be distinguished from incontinentia pigmenti is incontinentia pigmenti achromians (hypomelanosis of Ito) [28]. That disorder shows bilateral linear depigmentation and a variety of associated abnormalities of the eyes and central nervous and musculoskeletal systems. Unlike the Bloch–Sulzberger disorder, incontinentia pigmenti achromians shows no inflammatory or hyperkeratotic stage, no pigmentary incontinence histologically, and like the Naegeli variant, its inheritance appears to be autosomal dominant [10,29].

Pathogenesis

Though the pathogenesis of incontinentia pigmenti remains uncertain, a number of inferences and speculations can be made. The spotty distribution of the pigmentary deposits suggests that the pigmentation occurs after melanoblasts have reached their final position in the skin, which is between the third and fourth gestational months. This, and the known appearance of precursors of teeth and hair during the fourth to sixth gestational months, suggests that incontinentia pigmenti has its beginnings during the second trimester of pregnancy [30]. The pathogenesis of the pigment deposition in the dermis—not the initial dermatologic change but the one from which the disorder derives its name—is uncertain. It has been suggested that there is damage to the basal layer of the epidermis, rendering it incapable of holding pigment that then leaks into the dermis, that is, epidermal incontinence. Alternatively, it has been thought that the basal epidermal melanocytes may be overactive (rather than incontinent) and that it is this that causes them to release pigment to the underlying dermal layer [21].

What then is the inciting stimulus? The eosinophils found in the vesiculo-bullous skin lesions, in the underlying dermis, and in the blood, suggest a possible allergic or autoimmune basis for this disorder, but studies of immunoglobulins have not supported that thesis [23,26]. Others have stressed the potential importance of immunization or infection (viral or other) as possible triggering events [26]. While no one infectious agent has been implicated in the evolution of lesions of incontinentia pigmenti [31], it is known that all of the cutaneous stages of incontinentia pigmenti can be mimicked by viral infections of the skin [26]. Also, on occasion, herpes simplex and other viruses have been isolated from skin lesions of incontinentia pigmenti. In addition, it is known that a wide variety of dermatotropic viruses are capable of causing fetal deformities [32]. Although most mothers who give birth to a child with incontinentia pigmenti have had apparently uncomplicated pregnancies [7], it is widely recognized that viral and other infections often occur during pregnancy without accompanying symptoms or signs.

Inflammatory encephalopathies have been seen in cases of incontinentia pigmenti coming to autopsy [25,26]. In the two sisters reported by Siemes et al. [26], neurologic deterioration occurred after immunization in one and after immunization followed by infection in the other. This suggested that both girls may have been genetically predisposed to developing an encephalopathic reaction to an antecedent immunization or infection. Researchers from Japan have postulated a congenital dysfunction of the autonomic nervous system in incontinentia pigmenti which, when exposed to infections or other environmental stimuli, could result in inflammatory eruptions [33].

Finally, the cerebral dysgenesis (polymicrogyria) found in the brain of the child with incontinentia pigmenti reported by O'Doherty and Norman [24] merits additional comment. It may be that the association was simply by chance, since similar brain malformations have not been reported in other cases of incontinentia pigmenti. It should be noted, however, that very few children with incontinentia pigmenti have come to autopsy, and that polymicrogyria has been observed to result from a variety of maldevelopmental and destructive brain pathologies. Among these are hypoxic–ischemic encephalopathy that may be triggered by an inflammatory disorder [34]. Thus, as additional cases of incontinentia pigmenti are examined neuropathologically, other instances of cerebral maldevelopment may be found.

Treatment and Prognosis

The management of incontinentia pigmenti is fundamentally symptomatic and should include attention to treatable components of the disorder. The skin lesions usually do not need specific treatment unless secondary infection (particularly of vesiculo-bullous lesions) should develop. A number of ophthalmologic interventions may be indicated, their nature depending on the kind of eye abnormality present. Thus, corrective lenses may be required for a refractive error, patching for a strabismus, or surgery for a cataract or detached retina. Abnormalities of the musculoskeletal system, such as dislocation of the hip or scoliosis, can be expected to respond well to conventional therapies. Anticonvulsants should be used for seizure management. Physiotherapy, bracing, or selective surgeries may be needed for spastic paralyses. A variety of remedial services can be offered to the child with specific learning disabilities or a more generalized developmental delay, while accompanying behavioral and emotional disorders may call for psychotherapeutic input.

Genetic counseling should be offered to mothers with incontinentia pigmenti who wish to have children as well as to any affected females as they approach childbearing age.

Clearly, the outlook for persons with incontinentia pigmenti depends on the extent to which nondermatologic structures are involved, the severity of such involvement, and its potential for treatment. More research is needed before the pathogenesis of incontinentia pigmenti can be more fully understood. Once this is achieved, the complications of the disorder can be better anticipated and the most effective interventions provided.

References

1. Garrod AE. Peculiar pigmentation of the skin in an infant. Trans Clin Soc Lond 1906;39:216–217.
2. Adamson HG. Congenital pigmentation with atrophic scarring associated with other congenital abnormalities. Proc R Soc Med 1908;1:9–10.
3. Bardach M. Systematisierte Nävusbildungen bei einem eineiigen Zwillingspaar. Ein Beitrag zur Nävusätiologie. Z Kinderheilkd 1925;39:542–550.
4. Bloch B. Eigentümliche, bisher nicht beschriebene Pigmentaffektion (incontinentia pigmenti). Schweiz Med Wochenschr 1926;7:404–405.
5. Sulzberger MB. Über eine bisher nicht beschriebene congenitale Pigmentanomalie (incontinentia pigmenti). Arch Dermatol Syph (Berlin) 1928;154:19–32.
6. Franceschetti A, Jadassohn W. À propos de l'incontinentia pigmenti: délimitation de deux syndromes différents figurant sous le même terme. Dermatologica 1954;108:1–28.
7. Carney RG. Incontinentia pigmenti. A world statistical analysis. Arch Dermatol 1976;112:535–542.
8. Avrahami E, Harel S, Jurgenson U, et al. Computed tomographic demonstration of brain changes in incontinentia pigmenti. Am J Dis Child 1985;139:372–374.
9. Francois J. Incontinentia pigmenti (Bloch–Sulzberger syndrome). Br J Ophthalmol 1984;68:19–25.
10. Wettke–Schafer R, Kantner G. X-linked dominant inherited diseases with lethality in hemizygous males. Hum Genet 1983;64:1–23.
11. Guerrier CJW, Wong CK. Ultrastructural evolution of the skin in incontinentia pigmenti (Bloch–Sulzberger): study of six cases. Dermatologica 1974;149:10–22.
12. Wiley HE, Frias JL. Depigmented lesions in incontinentia pigmenti: a useful diagnostic sign. Am J Dis Child 1974;128:546–547.
13. Morgan JD. Incontinentia pigmenti (Bloch–Sulzberger syndrome): a report of four additional cases. Am J Dis Child 1971;122:294–300.
14. Rosenfeld SI, Smith ME. Ocular findings in incontinentia pigmenti. Ophthalmology 1985;92:543–546.
15. Raab EL. Ocular lesions in incontinentia pigmenti. J Pediatr Ophthalmol Strabismus 1983;20:42–48.
16. Pfeiffer RA. Das Syndrom der Incontinentia pigmenti (Bloch–Siemens). Münch Med Wochenschr 1959;101:2312–2316.
17. Simmons DA, Kegel MF, Scher RK, et al. Subungual tumors in incontinentia pigmenti. Arch Dermatol 1986;122:1431–1434.
18. Simonsson H. Incontinentia pigmenti: Bloch–Sulzbergers syndrome associated with infantile spasms. Acta Paediatr Scand 1972;61:612–614.
19. O'Doherty N. Bloch–Sulzberger syndrome. Incontinentia pigmenti. In: Vinken PJ, Bruyn GW, eds. Handbook of clinical neurology. New York: American Elsevier, 1972:213–222.
20. O'Brien JE, Feingold M. Incontinentia pigmenti: a longitudinal study. Am J Dis Child 1985;139:711–712.
21. McPherson A, Auth TL. Bloch–Sulzberger syndrome (incontinentia pigmenti). Arch Neurol 1963;8:332–339.
22. Kauste O, Paatela M. Incontinentia pigmenti (Bloch–Sulzberger syndrome): report of two cases. Ann Paediatr Fenn 1961;7:79–84.
23. Kurczynski TW, Berns JS, Johnson WE. Studies of a family with incontinentia pigmenti variably expressed in both sexes. J Med Genet 1982;19:447–451.
24. O'Doherty NJ, Norman RM. Incontinentia pigmenti (Bloch–Sulzberger syndrome) with cerebral malformation. Dev Med Child Neurol 1968;10;168–174.
25. Hauw J-J, Perie G, Bonnette J, et al. Les lésions cérébrales de l'incontinentia pigmenti. À propos d'un cas anatomique. Acta Neuropathol (Berl) 1977;38:159–162.
26. Siemes H, Schneider H, Dening D, et al. Encephalitis in two members of a family with incontinentia pigmenti (Bloch–Sulzberger syndrome): the possible role of inflammation in the pathogenesis of CNS involvement. Eur J Pediatr 1978;129:103–115.
27. Naegeli O. Familiarer Chromatophorennavus. Schweiz Med Wochenschr 1927;8:48.
28. Ito M. Incontinentia pigmenti achromians: a singular case of nevus depigmentosus systematicus bilateralis. Tohoku J Exp Med 1952;(suppl 1)55:57–59.
29. Rubin MB. Incontinentia pigmenti achromians. Multiple cases within a family. Arch Derm 1972;105:424–425.
30. Epstein S, Vedder JS, Pinkus H. Bullous variety of incontinentia pigmenti (Bloch–Sulzberger). Arch Dermatol Syph 1952;65:557–567.
31. Schmalstieg FC, Jorizzo JL, Tschen J, et al. Basophils in incontinentia pigmenti. J Am Acad Dermatol 1984;10:362–364.
32. Miller OB, Arbesman C, Baer RL. Disseminated cutaneous herpes simplex (Kaposi's varicelliform erup-

tion): report of a case complicated by pregnancy and herpetic keratitis and review of the literature of congenital malformations due to dermatotropic virus infections in the pregnant mother. Arch Dermatol Syph 1950;62:477–490.

33. Kitamura K, Fukushiro R, Miyabayashi T. Incontinentia pigmenti in Japan: introduction of twenty-one observed cases. Arch Dermatol Syph 1954;69:667–673.

34. McBride MC, Kemper TL. Pathogenesis of four-layered microgyric cortex in man. Acta Neuropathol (Berl) 1982;57:93–98.

Chapter 33

A Syndrome of Anosmia, Ichthyosis, and Hypogonadism with Steroid Sulfatase and Arylsulfatase C Deficiencies

NOBUHIKO SUNOHARA and
EIJIRO SATOYOSHI

We reported on three male patients in a family [1] with congenital anosmia, ichthyosis, and hypogonadotropic hypogonadism. In addition, all three patients had borderline IQs, mirror movements of the hands and feet, and ocular manifestations that included congenital nystagmus, strabismus, hypoplastic optic discs with decreased visual acuity, and hypopigmentation of the irides. Two patients had unilateral renal agenesis or hypogenesis, and one patient had preauricular pits (Table 33.1). Enzymatic study of the leukocytes and skin fibroblasts revealed steroid sulfatase and arylsulfatase c deficiencies.

Maurer and Sotos [2] described patients who closely resemble ours. Their patients exhibited mild mental retardation, decreased adrenocorticotropic hormone secretion, and a hypoplastic kidney in addition to anosmia, hypogonadotropic hypogonadism, and ichthyosis. Ocular manifestations or mirror movements were not described. No enzymatic study of steroid sulfatase and arylsulfatase c was performed. However, Maurer and Sotos' patients and ours shared many common features, including an X-linked recessive inheritance and the three cardinal manifestations (anosmia, ichthyosis, and hypogonadism). The pathogenesis of this syndrome remains unknown.

Clinical Features and Laboratory Findings

Ichthyosis

Ichthyosis was generalized with large dark scales present over the surface of the skin except on the palms and soles. It was noted during the first week of life, increased with age, and worsened in winter. Skin pathology disclosed marked hyperkeratosis and an increased granular layer. The stratum spinosum showed definite acanthosis, and the rete ridges were prominent and well developed. Perivascular cell infiltrations were frequently encountered. Corneal opacities of the eyes were seen in the deep layer. These findings are compatible with those of X-linked ichthyosis.

Levels of serum cholesterol sulfate were high in our patients (Figure 33.1). Steroid sulfatase and arylsulfatase c activity in leukocytes and in skin fibroblasts was extremely low, although the activity of arylsulfatases a and b was normal (Table 33.2). Patients with X-linked ichthyosis are well known to have a deficiency of steroid sulfatase, the gene of which resides on the distal portion of Xp, as well as a deficiency of arylsulfatase c [3–5]. These deficiencies, of steroid sulfatase and arylsulfatase c, and the

Table 33.1. Summary of Clinical Features

	Case 1	Case 2	Case 3
Age and sex	54, M	47, M	17, M
Anosmia	+	+	+
Ichthyosis	+	+	+
Hypogonadism	+	+	+
Ocular manifestations			
Hypoplastic papillae	+	+	+
Congenital nystagmus	+	+	+
Hypopigmentation of iris	+	+	+
Strabismus	+	+	+
Limitation of extraocular movements (EOM)	−	+	+
Mirror movement	+	+	+
High-arched palate	+	−	−
Periauricular pits	+	−	−
Pes cavus	+	−	−
Unilateral renal agenesis or hypogenesis	−	+	+

+ = present, − = absent

increased serum cholesterol sulfate we observed in our patients, are considered to be deeply related to the X-linked ichthyosis.

Hypogonadism

The penis was thin, and the testes were either small or absent. The scrotum was also small and hypopigmented. There was no axillary or pubic hair. Gynecomastia was present, and the voice was high pitched. Pubertal changes in the adult were not recognized. Serum levels of pregnenolone, testosterone, 5-alpha-dehydrotestosterone, and estradiol were extremely low and serum levels of progesterone, 17-alpha-hydroprogesterone, 17-alpha-hydroxypregnenolone, dehydroepiandrosterone, dehydroepiandrosterone sulfate, androstenodione, and estrone were within normal limits (Figure 33.1) as were urinary testosterone and estrogen levels. A human chorionic gonadotropin (HCG) loading test disclosed markedly diminished responses of serum testosterone levels. A luteinizing hormone releasing factor (LH-RH) infusion test after 5 days of treatment with this hormone became normal. It suggests that the hypogonadism is primarily from hypothalamic involvement [6,7].

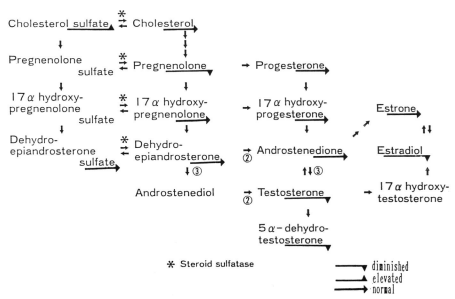

Figure 33.1. Steroids and steroid sulfates.

Table 33.2. Enzyme Activities in Leukocytes and Skin Fibroblasts

	Case 1	Case 2	Normal Adults
In leukocytes			
Arylsulfatase a	133	108	68–133 n mol/mg protein/hr
Arylsulfatase b	37.8	40.0	35.5–57.7 n mol/mg protein/hr
Arylsulfatase c	12.8	11.8	75.0 ± 27.2 p mol/mg protein/hr
Steroid sulfatase	1.9	1.2	63–101 × 10^{-3} p mol/mg protein/hr
In skin fibroblasts			
Arylsulfatase a	1,246	937	746–1,553 n mol/mg protein/hr
Arylsulfatase b	430	299	143–250 n mol/mg protein/hr
Arylsulfatase c	116	32	848–1,022 p mol/mg protein/hr
Steroid sulfatase	ND	0.68	133–310 × 10^{-3} p mol/mg protein/hr

ND = not detected

We did not perform testicular biopsies in our patients; however, a testicular biopsy of Maurer and Sotos' [2] 30-year-old patient revealed an absence of Leydig cells and immature tubules. Other endocrine function studies, including those of hypothalamic, pituitary, thyroid, parathyroid, and adrenal hormones were all normal except for a partial defect of ADH secretion in our patients and a decreased ACTH secretion in Maurer and Sotos' patients. The chromosome karyotype was 46 XY in all patients.

Anosmia

The patients were confirmed to be anosmic by a minute olfactory function test. Family members without hypogonadism or ichthyosis revealed no abnormality in olfactory function test. Autopsy of those cases of Kallmann syndrome, in which anosmia and hypogonadotropic hypogonadism is present, showed hypoplasia or agenesis of the olfactory system. In addition, some of our patients with Kallmann syndrome have a unilateral kidney defect. These facts indicate that one of the defects of Kallmann syndrome derives from lateral parasagittal dysplasias [8,9]. Kallmann [10] and Conrad et al. [11] reported on several patients in which Kallmann syndrome was associated with mirror movements, which were recognized in our patients. These commonalities between Kallmann syndrome and our patients suggest that the disorder in our patients may have a similar pathogenesis to that of Kallmann syndrome.

Treatment

We treated one of our patients (case 3) with testosterone propionate and gonadotropin from age 11. At the age of 17, his penis and scrotum developed to the Tanner stage III, and axillary and pubic hair appeared.

One of Maurer and Sotos' patients (a 16-year-old male) showed adequate androgen effects and testicular enlargement after 12 weeks of HCG administration. After treatment, Leydig cells and arrested spermatogenesis were observed in the biopsied testes.

Differential Diagnosis

Congenital ichthyosis, hypogonadism, and anosmia have been seen as a part of various syndromes as shown in Table 33.3. As mentioned above, symptoms of Kallmann syndrome closely resemble those of our patients. However, there is no ichthyosis in that syndrome. Patients with Rud's [12,13], Sjögren–Larsson [14], De Sanctis–Cacchione [15], or Netherton's [16] syndrome may exhibit both ichthyosis and hypogonadism. Some patients [17,18] have hypogonadism associated with a syndrome of ichthyosis and renal disorder. These patients do not have anosmia and do not show an X-linked recessive inheritance. Lynch et al. [19] described a family in which, over three generations, five males had con-

Table 33.3. Anosmia, Ichthyosis, and hypogonadism

Syndromes of anosmia and hypogonadism:
Kallmann syndrome [10]
Syndromes of ichthyosis and hypogonadism:
Rud's syndrome [12, 13]
Sjögren–Larsson syndrome [14]
Netherton's syndrome [16]
De Sanctis–Cacchione syndrome [15]
A syndrome of X-linked ichthyosis and hypogonadism [19]
A syndrome of ichthyosis and renal disorders [17, 18]
Syndromes of anosmia and ichthyosis:
Refsum's syndrome [21]
Syndromes of anosmia, ichthyosis, and hypogonadism:
A syndrome of anosmia, ichthyosis, and hypogonadism with X-linked recessive inheritance [1, 2]

genital ichthyosis and secondary hypogonadism, and Abe et al. [20] reported on two brothers who showed ichthyosis, bilateral cryptorchidism, hypogenitalism, and mental retardation. This syndrome is transmitted in X-linked recessive fashion. However, it does not involve anosmia, which is one of the cardinal manifestations in our patients. Refsum's syndrome is characterized by pigmentary retinal degeneration, chronic polyneuritis, an elevated cerebrospinal fluid protein, ataxia, and other cerebellar signs. In some cases [21,22], hearing loss, cardiopathy, pupillary abnormalities, lens opacities, anosmia, and skin changes resembling ichthyosis were present. Hypogonadism, which we saw in our patients, is not observed in Refsum's syndrome and the main clinical features of Refsum's syndrome were not recognized in our patients. Patients with multiple sulfatase deficiency are frequently associated with ichthyosis. However, our patients did not show deficiencies of arylsulfatases a and b.

References

1. Sunohara N, Sakuragawa N, Satoyoshi E, et al. A new syndrome of anosmia, ichthyosis, hypogonadism and various neurological manifestations with deficiency of steroid sulfatase and arylsulfatase c. Ann Neurol 1986;19:174–181.

2. Maurer WF, Sotos JF. Sex-linked familial hypogonadism and ichthyosis. Proceedings of the 39th annual meeting of the society for pediatric research. Baltimore: William & Wilkins, 1969:181.

3. Shapiro LJ, Weiss R, Buxman MM, et al. Enzymatic basis of typical X-linked ichthyosis. Lancet 1978;2:756–757.

4. Meyer JCh, Weiss H, Grundmann HP, et al. Deficiency of arylsulfatase c in cultured skin fibroblasts of X-linked ichthyosis. Hum Genet 1979;53:115–116.

5. Tiepolo L, Zuffardi O, Fraccaro M, et al. Assignment by deletion mapping of the steroid sulfatase X-linked ichthyosis locus to Xp 223. Hum Genet 1980;54:205–206.

6. Hashimoto T, Miyai K, Uozumi T, et al. Effect of prolonged LH-releasing hormone administration on gonadotropin response in patients with hypothalamic and pituitary tumors. J Clin Endocrinol Metab 1975;41:712–716.

7. Yoshimoto Y, Moridera K, Imura H. Restoration of normal pituitary gonadotropin reserve by administration of luteinizing hormone–releasing hormone in patients with hypogonadotropic hypogonadism. N Engl J Med 1975;292:242–245.

8. de Morsier G. Etudes sur les dysraphies crânio-encêphaliques. I. Agénésie des lobes olfactifs (télencéphaloschiziz latéral) et des commissures calleuse et antérieure (télencéphaloschizis médian). La dysplasie olfacto-génitale. Schweiz Arch Neurol Neurochir Psychiatr 1955;74:309–361.

9. de Morsier G. Median cranioencephalic dysraphias and olfactogenital dysplasia. World Neurol 1962;3:485–506.

10. Kallmann FJ, Schoenfeld WA, Barrere SE. The genetic aspects of primary eunuchoidism. Am J Ment Defic 1944;48:203–236.

11. Conrad B, Kriebel J, Hetzel WD. Hereditary bimanual synkinesis combined with hypogonadotropic hypogonadism and anosmia in four brothers. J Neurol 1978;218:263–274.

12. Rud E. Et Tilfaelde af Infantilisme med Tetani, Epilepsi, Polyneuritis, ichthyosis og Anaemi af perniciøs Type. Hospitalstidende 1927;70:525–538.

13. Rud E. Et Tilfaelde af Hypogenitalisme (Eunuchoidismus feminicus) med partiel Gigantisme og Ichthyosis. Hospitalstidende 1929;72:426–433.

14. Sjögren T, Larsson T. Oligophrenia in combination with congenital ichthyosis and spastic disorders. A clinical and genetic study. Acta Psychiatr Neurol Scand Suppl 1957;32:1–113.

15. de Sanctis C, Cacchione A. L'idiozia xerodermica. Riv Sper Freniat 1932;56:269–292.

16. Netherton EW. A unique case of trichorrhexis nodosa, "bamboo hair." Arch Dermatol 1958;78:483–487.

17. Passwell J, Zipperkowski L, Katznelson D, et al. A syndrome characterized by congenital ichthyosis with atrophy, mental retardation, dwarfism and generalized aminoaciduria. J Pediatr 1973;82:466–471.

18. Rayner A, Lampert RP, Rennert OM. Familial ichthyosis, dwarfism, mental retardation and renal disease. J Pediatr 1978;92:766–768.

19. Lynch HT, Ozer F, McNutt CW, et al. Secondary male hypogonadism and congenital ichthyosis. Association of two rare genetic diseases. Am J Hum Genet 1960;12:440–447.

20. Abe K, Matsuda I, Matsuda N, et al. X-linked ichthyosis, bilateral cryptorchidism, hypogonadism and mental retardation in two siblings. Clin Genet 1976; 9:341–345.

21. Refsum S. Heredoataxia hemeralopia polyneuritiformis, et tidligere ikka beskrevet familiaert syndrome? Nord Med 1945;28:2682–2685.

22. Refsum S. Heredopathia atactica polyneuritiformis. A familial syndrome not hitherto described. A contribution to the clinical study of the hereditary diseases of the nervous system. Acta Psychiatr Scand Suppl 1946;38:1–303.

PART FOUR

DISEASES WITH UNKNOWN OR MULTIPLE INHERITANCE

Chapter 34
Coffin–Siris Syndrome

WILLIAM A. DE BASSIO

The Coffin–Siris syndrome is characterized by defects in the skin, hair, brain, cerebellum, brain stem nuclei, and the nails and skeleton of fifth digits.

Coffin and Siris originally described this disorder in 1970 when they reported three females with mental retardation, lax joints, postnatal growth retardation, and brachydactyly of the fifth digits with absent nails. Subsequent reports focused on these features and also included hypotonia, body hypertrichosis, and abnormal facies [1–13]. Although the cause is unclear, reported cases support an autosomal recessive [2,3] or a dominant inheritance with variable expressivity [4]. The 21:4 female to male ratio (Table 34.1) suggests that the disorder is often lethal to males.

Clinical Features

The clinical features are shown in Table 34.1. Consistent features include developmental delay, abnormal facies, absent fifth distal phalanx, hypoplastic nails, hypotonia, and body hypertrichosis. Very common features are postnatal growth deficiency, feeding difficulties, microcephaly, and scalp hypotrichosis. There is some confusion in the literature about what constitutes the Coffin–Siris syndrome. Part of this relates to a report in 1966 by Coffin et al. [14] in which two unrelated male patients, small in stature with osteocartilaginous anomalies, were described. Lowry et al. [15] described a similar series, and others called this the Coffin–Lowry syndrome [16]. These patients were retarded and had coarse facial features, large hands, and tapering fingers. Males were much more severely affected than females. Mattei et al. [10] clearly described two females with Coffin–Siris syndrome, but suggested that the two syndromes were the same. Others have reviewed the distinctiveness of the Coffin–Siris syndrome [17] with the consensus clearly indicating it to be a distinct clinical entity [13,18]. In addition to its distinguishing clinical features, neuropathologic similarities help to define the Coffin–Siris syndrome.

Pathology

The neuropathologic features of the three cases described are summarized in Table 34.2. Two cases showed Dandy–Walker (D–W) malformation on gross inspection. One of these two also showed partial agenesis of the corpus callosum and agenesis of

Table 34.1. General Features of Coffin–Siris Syndrome

	Incidence[a]
Developmental abnormalities	
Postnatal growth deficiency	20/24 (83)[b]
Developmental delay	24/24 (100)
Feeding problems	17/19 (89)
Craniofacial abnormalities	
Microcephaly	15/23 (65)
Abnormal facies	25/25 (100)
Scalp hypotrichosis	16/22 (78)
Limb abnormalities	
Absent fifth distal phalanx	25/25 (100)
Hypoplastic nails	25/25 (100)
Other abnormalities	
Hypotonia (lax joints)	21/21 (100)
Congenital heart disease	8/25 (32)
Body hypertrichosis	25/25 (100)
Sex–Female	21/25 (84)

Source: adapted from DeBassio and Kemper [13]. With permission of the publisher. Copyright © 1985, the American Medical Association.

[a]References 1 through 13.

[b]Numbers in parentheses are percents. Not all reports commented on each problem. A total of 25 cases are reported here.

Table 34.2. Neuropathologic Features of the Coffin–Siris Syndrome

	Coffin and Siris [1]	Tunnessen et al. [5]	DeBassio and Kemper [13]
Dandy–Walker malformation	+	+	−
Hypoplasia or partial agenesis of corpus callosum	−	+	+
Agenesis of anterior commissure	−	+	+
Abnormal olives	ND	ND	+
Abnormal arcuate nuclei	ND	ND	+
Ectopic cerebellar nuclei	ND	ND	+

ND = not described; + = present; − = absent

Source: Adapted from DeBassio and Kemper [13]. With permission of the publisher. Copyright © 1985, the American Medical Association.

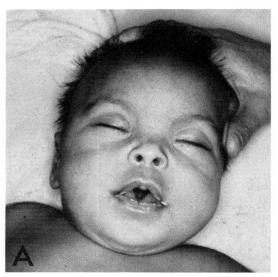
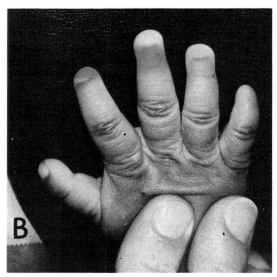

Figure 34.1. Photographs of patient at age 3 months. *(A)* Face shows coarse features, and there is sparse head hair. *(B)* Hand shows abnormal nail development and absent distal fifth phalanx. (From DeBassio and Kemper [13]. With permission. Copyright © 1985, the American Medical Association.)

the anterior commissure. The third case included extensive microscopic studies using sections with both the Nissl and Golgi stains. Findings included hypoplasia of the corpus callosum, abnormal lamination of the lateral geniculate nuclei, abnormal olivary and arcuate nuclei, and ectopic cerebellar nuclei (heterotopias). Neuropathologically, the consistently abnormal findings involved the cerebellum, the brain stem, and the corpus callosum. A fourth brain was examined and considered normal [2], but no microscopic sections were described.

The relationship of the brain abnormalities is best understood if one briefly reviews experimental studies of the D–W malformation. In animals, maldevelopment of the anterior roofing membrane of the fourth ventricle leads to the classic D–W triad: malformed cerebellar vermis, membranous cyst of the fourth ventricle, and elevation of the torcula herophili [19]. In addition, the lateral border of the anterior and posterior roofing membrane forms a secondary germinal zone, the rhombic lip [20,21]. The anterior part generates cells for deep nuclei and for the external granular layer of the cerebellum [22,23]; the posterior portion for the inferior olive, raphe nucleus, basis pontis, and arcuate nucleus [24]. In human studies, D–W malformation is frequently associated with abnormal cerebellar nuclei [25], and careful microscopic investigation suggests that abnormalities of the inferior olive [26] may be an integral part of the malformation. Other clinical studies

Figure 34.2. *(A)* Brain stem at level of inferior olive. Note the abnormal layering of cells in the inferior olive (1), large medial accessory olive (2), large arcuate nucleus (3), and small heterotopic olivary nuclei (4) (original magnification × 12; Nissl's stain). *(B)* Cerebellum shows normal folia and ectopic neurons (1) in white matter (original magnification × 4.5; Nissl's stain). (From DeBassio and Kemper [13]. With permission. Copyright © 1985, the American Medical Association.)

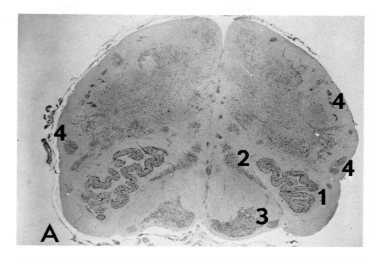

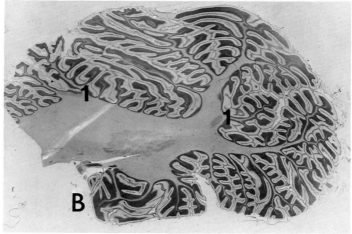

indicate frequent abnormalities of the corpus callosum [27]. This information suggests that all three cases are neuropathologically related by abnormalities of the roofing membrane and of the rhombic lip derivatives in the cerebellum and brain stem.

Genetics

The genetics of the Coffin–Siris syndrome continue to be of major interest. One phenotypically similar patient has been described with partial trisomy 9 [28]. Similar neuropathologic abnormalities have been reported with trisomy 18 [29]. In cases of Coffin–Siris syndrome, no chromosomal abnormalities have been described [13] despite the suggestions about its inheritance patterns [2–4]. Only with careful clinical descriptions correlated with well-documented neu-

ropathologic material and genetic studies can this syndrome be better understood.

Treatment

At the current time there is no specific therapy, and management is only symptomatic.

References

1. Coffin GS, Siris E. Mental retardation with absent fifth fingernail and terminal phalanx. Am J Dis Child 1970;119:433–439.
2. Carey JC, Hall BD. The Coffin–Siris syndrome. Am J Dis Child 1978;132:667–671.
3. Franceschini P, Cirillo SM, Bianco R, et al. The Cof-

fin–Siris syndrome in two siblings. Pediatr Radiol 1986;16:330–333.

4. Haspeslagh M, Fryns JP, Van den Berghe H. The Coffin–Siris syndrome: report of a family and further delineation. Clin Genet 1984;26:374–378.

5. Tunnessen WW, McMillan JA, Levin MB. The Coffin–Siris syndrome. Am J Dis Child 1978;132:393–395.

6. Bartsocas CS, Tsiantos AK. Mental retardation with absent fifth fingernail and terminal phalanx. Am J Dis Child 1970;120:493–494.

7. Weiswasser WH, Hall BD, Delavan GW, et al. Coffin–Siris syndrome. Am J Dis Child 1973;125:838–840.

8. Schinzel A. The Coffin–Siris syndrome. Acta Paediatr Scand 1979;68:449–452.

9. Ueda K, Saito A, Nakano H, et al. The Coffin–Siris syndrome: a case report. Helv Paediatr Acta 1980;35:385–390.

10. Mattei JF, Laframboise R, Rouault F, et al. Brief clinical report: Coffin–Lowry syndrome in sibs. Am J Med Genet 1981;8:315–319.

11. Lucaya J, Garcia-Conesa JA, Bosch-Banyeras JM, et al. The Coffin–Siris syndrome: a report of four cases and review of the literature. Pediatr Radiol 1981;11:35–38.

12. Foasso MF, Hermier M, Descos B, et al. Le syndrome de Coffin–Siris. Etude critique de la littérature à propos d'un cas. Pediatrie 1983;38:111–117.

13. DeBassio WA, Kemper TL, Knoefel JE. Coffin–Siris syndrome: neuropathologic findings. Arch Neurol 1985;42:350–353.

14. Coffin GS, Siris E, Wegienka LC. Mental retardation with osteocartilaginous anomalies. Am J Dis Child 1966;112:205–213.

15. Lowry B, Miller JR, Fraser C. A new dominant gene mental retardation syndrome. Am J Dis Child 1971;121:496–500.

16. Temtamy SA, Miller JD, Hussels-Maumenee J. The Coffin–Lowry syndrome: an inherited faciodigital mental retardation syndrome. J Pediatr 1975;86:724–731.

17. Feingold M. The Coffin–Siris syndrome. Am J Dis Child 1978;132:660–661.

18. Gorlin RJ. Lapsus-caveat emptor: Coffin–Lowry syndrome vs Coffin–Siris syndrome—an example of confusion compounded. Am J Med Genet 1981;10:103–104.

19. Brodal A, Hauglie-Hanssen E. Congenital hydrocephalus with defective development of the cerebellar vermis (Dandy–Walker syndrome). J Neurol Neurosurg Psychiatry 1959;22:99–108.

20. Ellenberger C, Hanaway J, Netsky MG. Embryogenesis of the inferior olivary nucleus in the rat: a radioautographic study and a reevaluation of the rhombic lip. J Comp Neurol 1969;137:71–88.

21. Sidman RL, Rakic P. Neuronal migration with special reference to developing human brain: a review. Brain Res 1973;62:1–35.

22. Rakic P, Sidman RL. Histogenesis of cortical layers in human cerebellum, particularly the lamina dissecans. J Comp Neurol 1970;139:473–500.

23. Zecevic Z, Rakic P. Differentiation of Purkinje cells and their relationship to other components of developing cerebellar cortex in man. J Comp Neurol 1976;167:27–48.

24. Essick CR. The development of the nucleus pontis and the nucleus arcuatus in man. Am J Anat 1912;13:25–54.

25. Hart MN, Malamud N, Ellis WG. The Dandy–Walker syndrome: a clinicopathological study based on 28 cases. Neurology 1972;22:771–780.

26. Hanaway J, Netsky MG. Heterotopias of the inferior olive: relation to Dandy–Walker malformation and correlation with experimental data. J Neuropathol Exp Neurol 1971;30:380–389.

27. Sawaya R, McLaurin RL. Dandy–Walker syndrome: clinical analysis of 23 cases. J Neurosurg 1981;55:89–98.

28. Kushnick T, Adessa GM. Partial trisomy 9 with resemblance to Coffin–Siris syndrome. J Med Genet 1976;13:237–239.

29. Sumi SM. Brain malformations in the trisomy 18 syndrome. Brain 1970;93:821–830.

Chapter 35
Albinism

RICHARD A. KING

Albinism refers to a group of inherited disorders of the pigment system in which there is a reduction or an absence of melanin formation. The abnormality in the formation in melanin can involve the melanocytes in the skin, in the hair follicles, and in the eyes, resulting in oculocutaneous albinism (OCA). Or the abnormality can be localized to the melanocyte in the eyes, resulting in ocular albinism (OA). There are several types of OCA and OA, each presumed to represent a different mutation involving the melanin synthesis pathway. The clinical features and consequences of these mutations appear to be the result of the reduction or absence of melanin. All are autosomal recessive in inheritance except for one type of OA. The characteristics of the different types of OCA and OA are given in Table 35.1. It is important to note that in many types of albinism minimal to moderate amounts of melanin form in the skin, in the hair, and in the iris, and in only one type of OCA, type IA, is there total absence of pigment. In none of the types of OA does this total absence of pigment exist.

History

Because of its visibility, this history of albinism is primarily that of OCA. Variations of melanin pigmentation have long been intriguing, and descriptions of individuals with unusual patterns date to the writings of antiquity. The classical historians, including Pliny and Ptolemy, referred to lightly pigmented people of Africa (Leucaethiopes), and Pliny described the albino phenotype in quoting from the Greek writer Isogonus of Nicaea ". . . with eyes like owls, where of the sight is fire-red: who from their childhood are gray-haired and can see better by night than by day" [1].

The term albino, derived from the Latin *albus*, meaning white, was first used by Balthazar Tellez in the 1600s to describe albino blacks who were seen by traders along the African coast [2]. Cortés, in 1519, described men and women with white hair who were kept in the palace for the pleasure of Montezuma, and Salcedo in 1640 described the San Blas albinos along the Panamanian coast. Popular interest in albinism increased greatly in the eighteenth century with the slave trade and the return of albino blacks to Europe and America. The first published autopsy on an albino was in 1783. Garrod [3] provided the first insight into the pathogenesis of albinism, describing it as an inborn error of metabolism that was most likely the result of an enzymatic defect in the pigment pathway.

Through most of recorded history, the term albino (or oculocutaneous albino) referred to an individual with white hair, white skin, and blue eyes, with a marked red reflex, photophobia, and poor vision. This describes the classic complete or perfect albino. Other individuals were referred to as partial, incomplete, or imperfect albinos because of the formation of some melanin in the hair, skin, or eyes, but the biologic basis for separating complete from partial forms was unknown. The description of "perfect albino" was first made by Saint Hilaire in 1832 who also distinguished this type from partial or incomplete albinism. Trevor-Roper [4] provided the first genetic evidence of genetic heterogeneity with a description of a husband and wife, both with OCA, who had normally pigmented children (genetic complementation). In 1961, Kugelman and Van Scott [5] provided histochemical evidence for genetic heterogeneity by separating individuals with OCA into those who had residual tyrosinase activity in melanocytes and those who did not. The biochemical demonstration of a lack of tyrosinase activity in the melanocyte of the classic albino, as predicted by Garrod, was made in 1976 [6]. The use of the terms incomplete,

Table 35.1. Characteristics of Oculocutaneous and Ocular Albinism

Type		Inheritance	Color			Tyrosinase Activity[b]
			Hair Color[a]	Iris Color[a]	Skin Color	
Oculocutaneous albinism						
IA	Tyrosinase negative	AR	White	Blue	No pigment	Absent
IB	Yellow	AR	White→yellow→blond	Blue→hazel→brown	No generalized pigment, pigmented nevi, lentigines, slight tanning	Low–absent
II	Tyrosinase positive	AR	White→yellow→blond	Blue→hazel→brown	No generalized pigment, pigmented nevi, lentigines	Normal–high
III	Minimal pigment	AR	White	Blue→pigment ring	No generalized pigment	Absent
IV	Brown	AR	Light brown	Blue→brown	Light generalized pigment	Normal
V	Red	AR	Auburn→red	Brown	Light generalized pigment	?
VI	Hermansky–Pudlak syndrome	AR	White→yellow→blond →brown	Blue→hazel→brown	No generalized pigment, pigmented nevi, lentigines	Absent–normal
VII	Autosomal dominant	AD	Blond→light brown	Blue→hazel	Light generalized pigment	?
Ocular albinism						
I	Nettleship–Falls	XR	Normal	Blue→hazel→brown	Normal (light)	Normal
II	Forsius–Eriksson, Åland eye disease	XR	Normal	Normal	Normal	?
III	Autosomal recessive	AR	Normal	Blue→hazel→brown	Normal (light)	Normal

AR = autosomal recessive; AD = autosomal dominant; XR = X-linked recessive.
[a]Arrows indicate change with age.
[b]Tyrosinase activity determined by tritiated tyrosine assay [5,71].

partial, complete, or classic have now been replaced by the name for the specific type.

Clinical Symptoms

The clinical symptoms of albinism are related to eye and skin involvement, and few symptoms are unrelated to involvement of these two systems. The ocular features are common to both OCA and OA whereas the cutaneous features are prominent only in OCA. The separation of OCA and OA by skin involvement is not as clear as was once thought, however, and there are minor cutaneous features in some cases of OA.

Ocular Symptoms

Nystagmus, photophobia, strabismus, and reduced visual acuity are found in most cases of OCA and OA, with nystagmus and reduced acuity the most common features.

Nystagmus

Pendular nystagmus is characteristic of OCA and OA [7]. The parents often notice this at birth or within the first few days of life although many parents are not aware of nystagmus until the child is 2 to 3 months of age. The nystagmus is usually horizontal but a rotatory component may be present and may be the most prominent motion. Nystagmus is most pronounced when the patient is young and tends to decrease in severity with age. In older individuals nystagmus may not be obvious, revealed only by careful examination. Stress and fatigue increase the nystagmus.

Many individuals with nystagmus will find a head position in which the eye motion is less marked or suppressed (the null position), often with an apparent improvement in vision, particularly for close vision with reading or watching television. Because of this, individuals with albinism often hold books off to one side while reading or sit with their head tilted back while watching television.

Nystagmus has been considered a requirement for diagnosis of OCA and OA but rare individuals have been reported without nystagmus [7,8]. Collewijn et al. [8] have categorized individuals with OCA and OA into three classes: class I—vigorous spontaneous pendular unidirectional or bidirectional nystagmus; class II—vigorous unidirectional nystagmus that reverses in direction spontaneously or as a result of visual stimulation; and class III—little or no spontaneous nystagmus. The pathophysiologic reason for an absence of nystagmus in albinism is unknown. Because of the rarity of this finding, nystagmus should be considered important in the diagnosis of most cases of albinism.

Photophobia

Photophobia results from translucency of the iris and globe and hypopigmentation of the retina. It is most pronounced in the young and becomes less severe with age. The severity of the photophobia is related to the amount of ocular pigment that forms. Newborn babies often have severe photophobia and can hardly open their eyes, particularly in bright light. Photophobia can be so severe that a child will stay inside and not play outside in the sun or even in the shade. Severe photophobia may be lifelong for individuals with type IA OCA who develop no ocular pigment. For other types of OCA and OA, photophobia becomes less of a problem as the amount of iris pigment increases.

Strabismus

Strabismus is common in OCA and OA and appears to be related to changes in the formation of the optic system (see Visual Acuity, below) [7,9]. Parents often will not be aware of strabismus until the child is 2 or 3 years of age. Esotropia or exotropia may be present, and the strabismus usually appears to alternate between the right and left eye. Stress and fatigue make the strabismus more pronounced. Many individuals with albinism will appear at times to have no strabismus and prominent strabismus at other times.

Visual Acuity

The most constant and debilitating symptom of albinism is the reduction in visual acuity. All individuals with albinism have reduced visual acuity which, because of the foveal hypoplasia, cannot be fully corrected. Vision is usually in the 20/100 to 20/400 range but may be as good as 20/30 or better on occasion [7,10–13]. Near vision is better than distance vision, and most individuals with albinism function quite well in the range of 2 to 6 feet. Books are held close to the face for reading and the television is often viewed by sitting directly in front of the screen (to the consternation of the rest of the family).

Visual acuity is also reduced because of astigmatic errors, which are often associated with hyperopia or myopia [11,12]. High refractory errors (greater than 8 diopters) are common, and many individuals with albinism will find their useful vision substantially improved by glasses.

The question of improved acuity with age has not been settled. There are anecdotal reports of an increase in visual acuity as the amount of pigment in the iris increases with age but these are poorly documented [7]. In a recent study, the visual acuity of an infant with uncharacterized OCA was studied from 15 weeks to 3 years of age and was estimated to be normal through the first 15 to 16 months, particularly when tested under subdued lighting conditions [14]. Subsequent testing showed the expected reduction in acuity by 3 years of age. Many individuals with albinism feel that their useful vision improves as they learn to use visual cues more effectively. In general, individuals with albinism do not drive and are unable to obtain a driver's license.

Cutaneous Symptoms

Symptoms involving the skin and hair are related to the degree of hypopigmentation present at birth and later in life. Some pigment forms in the skin and hair in all types of OCA except for type IA, and the ethnic background and type of OCA are major factors in determining the extent of hypopigmentation. Children with OCA from Caucasian families with light or fair coloration will have snow white hair and milky white skin at birth. For type IA OCA, this will also be true for all other ethnic groups, while children with other types of OCA in darker ethnic groups may have light yellow, blond, or light brown hair at birth. Except for type IA OCA, hair color may darken with age.

Generalized pigment in the skin does not develop in OCA except in type IV. The skin is milky or creamy white at birth and remains so throughout life. As a result of the lack of melanin, the skin is sensitive to the sun's ultraviolet radiation and repeatedly burns when exposed. Many individuals with albinism will note an increased tolerance to the sun with age, thought to be the result of ultraviolet screening changes in the skin from the chronic irritation rather than from an accumulation of melanin. A tan line will occasionally be described but this is the result of chronic skin irritation. Localized pigment may develop as freckles or pigmented nevi, most prominently in sun-exposed areas.

The skin is normal in all other aspects. Sweating and healing are normal, and there is no increase in the propensity to infection. When properly protected, the texture and suppleness of the skin remain normal.

Physical Findings

The clinical history is often similar for many types of OCA and OA, and the diagnosis of a specific type is based on the physical examination and the laboratory studies.

Physical Findings Common to All Types of Oculocutaneous and Ocular Albinism

The amount of retinal pigment is markedly reduced or absent in all types of albinism [7]. The choroidal vessels are visible through the retina, but often cannot be seen in the macular region. Retinal pigment does not have to be absent for the diagnosis of albinism, and several types of OCA are characterized by moderate accumulation of retinal pigment with age (see Type II, III, and VI OCA).

The fovea is hypoplastic in albinism, and a normal foveal light reflex is absent [7,9,15,16]. Normal hyperpigmentation of the macular region is absent.

Iris pigment is reduced, and the iris will show translucency on globe illumination. Iris color ranges from blue to gray to hazel to light brown, depending on the type of albinism. A simple flashlight with an extension tube on the end or a narrow fiberoptic light, held against the lower lid, will transilluminate the globe and reveal gross iris translucency in most children and adults with albinism. Retroillumination with a slit-lamp will reveal more subtle translucent patterns of the iris, particularly of the peripheral iris [17,18]. When there is no iris stromal or posterior surface pigment present, the iris is diaphanous. Pigment may be present in a diffuse pattern, with a general reduction in translucency, in a cartwheel pattern with a ring of pigment at the pupillary border and the periphery, with connecting spokes of pigment columns, or in a blotchy pattern with irregular clumps of pigment in different parts of the iris.

A marked red reflex, present in many albinos, results from the increased amount of light reflected through the translucent iris. It is a misconception that albinos have red or pink eyes.

Nystagmus is a constant feature of albinism, and its presence has often been considered necessary for diagnosis. There is a rough correlation between the amount of melanin that forms in the eye and the severity of the nystagmus, although there are many exceptions to this generalization. Individuals with type IA OCA, having no retinal or iris pigment, often have severe nystagmus which persists throughout life. For other types of OCA and OA, the nystagmus becomes less noticeable as the amount of iris pigment increases. As previously stated, there have been reported, on rare occasions, cases of albinism with no nystagmus [1,8].

Strabismus is usually alternating and not fixed. Because of the misrouting of the optic fibers (see Pathology: Eyes), most individuals with albinism do not have binocular vision and use one eye at a time with suppression of vision in the other eye. The exotropia or esotropia develops in the suppressed eye, and may shift to the opposite eye with different visual settings or may disappear completely.

Color vision is generally intact when tested with the standard Ishihara test. More sensitive testing has demonstrated minor variations in color vision, but these do not appear to be clinically significant [9,19,20].

Characteristic Features of Specific Types of Oculocutaneous Albinism

Type IA (Tyrosinase-Negative) Oculocutaneous Albinism

Type IA is a common type of OCA and is the most depigmented of all types. The prevalence in the United States is estimated to be 1 in 39,000 in the Caucasian population and 1 in 20,000 in the black population [12]. No pigment forms in the skin, hair, or eyes, and the phenotype is similar in all ethnic groups. At birth the hair is snow white, the skin pink or milky white, and the irides blue; these features change little with age [1,9,12]. The hair may develop a very faint yellow tint that results from protein denaturation of the hair shaft. No pigmented nevi or freckles develop, but amelanotic nevi can be found.

The irides are blue to light gray, develop no pigment, and are markedly translucent throughout life. No retinal pigment develops, and photophobia and nystagmus are severe.

Type IB (Yellow) Oculocutaneous Albinism

Yellow OCA was first described in the Amish population and has now been recognized as an uncommon type that occurs in most populations [12,21]. The phenotype varies by ethnic group. At birth, Caucasian individuals with type IB have a phenotype similar to that of type IA with white hair and skin and blue irides [21]. The hair turns bright yellow in the first few years and golden blond to light brown

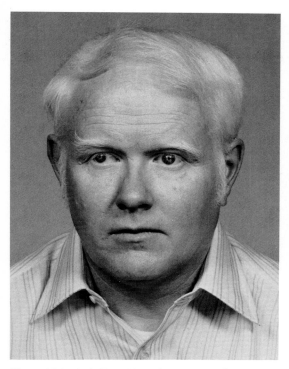 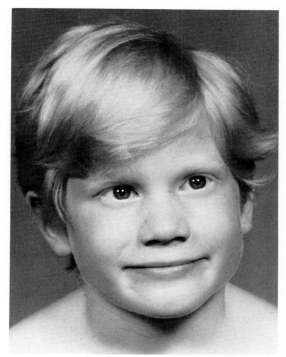

Figure 35.1. *(Left)* Type IA oculocutaneous albinism in a 38-year-old man. *(Right)* Type II oculocutaneous albinism in a 9-year-old boy.

by the end of the second decade. Simultaneously the skin darkens to a more creamy color, and sun exposure produces a minimal tan. The irides turn dark blue-gray but show little accumulation of pigment with age. Globe transillumination demonstrates persistent iris translucency and a minimal cartwheel pigment pattern [12].

Blacks with type IB OCA generally have more pigment. The hair turns bright yellow in the first year, eventually turning dark yellow to reddish-brown. The skin develops a darker creamy color. Pigmented nevi may develop. The irides are blue to blue-gray at birth and develop pigment in the first decade. By the age of 3, there is usually a well-developed cartwheel pigment pattern in the iris with globe transillumination but the iris remains translucent. Retinal pigment is absent at birth and slowly accumulates to a moderate degree, but is never normal. Photophobia, nystagmus, strabismus, and reduced visual acuity are present but often are much less severe than that which are seen in type IA or type II OCA.

Yellow OCA is listed as a subclass of type I because it is thought to be allelic to type IA [22].

Type II (Tyrosinase-Positive) Oculocutaneous Albinism

This is the most common type of OCA [9,12]. The prevalence in the United States is estimated to be 1 in 37,000 in the Caucasian population and 1 in 15,000 in the black population [12]. The phenotype varies by ethnic group. In general, over their lifetime, pigment slowly accumulates in the skin, hair, and eyes of an individual with type II OCA; this is more marked in those from darker ethnic groups [1,9,12,23–25]. Caucasian individuals with type II OCA resemble those with type IA at birth, with white hair, blue to blue-gray irides, and milky white skin. The hair slowly turns yellow to light blond over the first two decades. The skin remains milky white and does not tan. Pigmented nevi, freckles, and irregularly shaped lentigines develop in sun-exposed skin with age [25]. The irides are blue-gray, hazel, or occasionally, light brown and are translucent with a minimal to moderate cartwheel pigment pattern on globe transillumination. Little retinal pigment develops.

Black individuals with type II OCA have white or

light yellow hair, creamy white skin, and gray irides at birth. The hair turns yellow to light blond to light brown over the first two decades. The skin remains creamy white and does not tan. The irides accumulate pigment and turn hazel or brown. Iris translucency is reduced, and there is a prominent cartwheel pigment pattern on globe transillumination. Retinal pigment is absent in most individuals but small amounts develop in some.

In general, the reduction in visual acuity is less severe in type II OCA than in type IA, and the nystagmus and photophobia become less of a problem as the amount of iris pigment increases.

Type III (Minimal Pigment) Oculocutaneous Albinism

Type III OCA has only been described in a small number of Caucasian families, and the phenotype in other ethnic groups is unknown [26]. Its frequency is unknown. At birth, individuals with type III OCA have no skin, hair, or eye pigment and appear to have type IA OCA. However, during the first decade of life, minimal amounts of pigment develop in the iris as a ring of pigment near the pupillary border and in small clumps at the periphery of the iris. The hair may turn light yellow but no other pigment develops in the skin or eyes. The irides remain blue-gray with marked translucency.

Hairbulb tyrosinase studies (see Laboratory Findings) suggest that the individuals with type III OCA may be genetic compounds [26].

Type IV (Brown) Oculocutaneous Albinism

Type IV OCA has only been described in blacks; the phenotype in other racial groups is unknown [25,27] as is its frequency [28]. At birth, the skin and hair are light brown, and the irides gray to tan; there is some increase in hair and iris pigment with age. The skin remains light brown. A slight tan develops when the skin is exposed to the sun, but the skin is resistant to the acute effects of sun exposure. Pigmented freckles, nevi, or lentigines are uncommon. The diagnosis of albinism is made because of the presence of the characteristic nystagmus, strabismus, and reduced visual acuity. Retinal pigment is present but in reduced amounts. The iris is moderately translucent on globe transillumination.

Type V (Red) Oculocutaneous Albinism

A red type of OCA has been described in the older accounts of explorations of West Africa and in the natives of New Guinea [1,29–31]. There is no description of an individual with type V OCA in the U.S. population, and it is not known if this type of OCA exists in Caucasian populations. In those cases described, the hair color is dark reddish-brown to sandy red, and the skin color is dark reddish-brown. The irides are red-brown to brown, and transillumination of the globe shows little iris translucency. Retinal pigment is present.

Type VI (Hermansky–Pudlak Syndrome) Oculocutaneous Albinism

Type VI, an uncommon type of OCA, presents with albinism, a bleeding diathesis secondary to storage-pool deficient platelets, and an accumulation of a ceroid-like material in epithelial cells and in the reticuloendothelial system [12,32–36]. More than 300 cases are known, and the prevalence in Puerto Rico is unusually high, where it is estimated to be approximately 1 in 2,000 by Witkop [37]. The albino phenotype is quite variable, extending from severe congenital hypopigmentation similar to type IA OCA to minimal cutaneous hypopigmentation that suggests OA. Individuals with type VI OCA from England and Northern Europe will usually appear to have type IA or II OCA. Those from Puerto Rico and India will usually appear to have type IB or II OCA or to have OA with pigmented skin and hair. Most individuals note a slow accumulation of pigment with age. The eye changes of nystagmus, photophobia, strabismus, and reduced visual acuity are the most consistent indicators of albinism, particularly when the individual is well pigmented. Globe transillumination will usually demonstrate iris translucency with a cartwheel pattern developing as iris pigment accumulates.

The platelet storage-pool deficiency is associated with a mild bleeding diathesis [32,33,36,38,39]. Easy bruising with ecchymoses, epistaxis, gingival bleeding, menorrhagia, and extended mild bleeding after dental extraction and surgery are common, but the bleeding is usually not severe. Aspirin or aspirin-like drugs will make the bleeding diathesis more severe because they inhibit cyclooxygenase which results in a reduction in synthesis of endoperoxide and thromboxane. These drugs should be avoided in individuals with albinism until the specific diagnosis of type VI OCA is established.

A ceroid-like material accumulates in the tissues and is excreted in the urine with age [9,39]. In the urine it appears as a yellow granular urinary sediment. Tissue involvement includes the reticuloendothelial system; the lungs, heart, and kidneys; and the oral mucosa and gastrointestinal tract [9,39–43]. This accumulation appears to be associated with the development of diffuse interstitial pulmonary fibrosis [41,42] and granulomatous colitis [43], both of which can be severe and life threatening. Renal involvement may also be associated with renal insufficiency [37,44].

Type VII Oculocutaneous Albinism

Type VII OCA is characterized by autosomal dominant inheritance and mild hypopigmentation [45]. Only a few families have been reported, and the mild phenotype may go unrecognized. Hair is blond to light brown. Skin is creamy white with some generalized pigment, and some tanning occurs with sun exposure. The irides are blue-gray to hazel, and globe transillumination shows translucency in a diffuse, fine punctate or cartwheel pattern. Mild nystagmus, photophobia, and reduced visual acuity are present, but vision can be corrected to near normal (20/30 or 20/40) levels. Frenk and Calame have described a family in which four members in three generations had OCA associated with small melanosomes [46]. The albino phenotype in this family, although of dominant inheritance, was similar to type IA or type II OCA. One family member had OCA and Prader–Willi syndrome.

Other Types of Oculocutaneous Albinism

Several very rare conditions have hypopigmentation as a minor part of the phenotype or have oculocutaneous hypopigmentation associated with other, severe manifestations. Chediak–Higashi syndrome, discussed in Chapter 20, is associated with hypopigmentation of the skin, hair, and eyes with nystagmus and photophobia. Retinal pigment is reduced. The hypopigmentation is thought to result from an inability of the melanocyte to pass abnormal, giant melanosomes to the keratinocyte. Individuals with Cross syndrome have blond hair, milky white skin, and microphthalmos with corneal opacities [9,12,47]. Progressive neurologic deterioration develops with marked developmental delay, spasticity, and athetoid movements. Oculocutaneous albinism with black (patches) locks and congenital sensorineural deafness (BADS syndrome) has been described in one family [37]. The albino phenotype is similar to type IA OCA except for patches (locks) of pigmented scalp hairs and brown macules in the skin. Profound congenital hearing loss is present.

Characteristic Features of Specific Types of Ocular Albinism

Type I (X-linked Recessive) Ocular Albinism

Type I OA is the classical type, presenting with males affected in families that demonstrate a pattern of X-linked recessive inheritance [48–51]. Affected males have nystagmus, strabismus, and reduced visual acuity. In some males, the iris appears normally pigmented, and there is little translucency, while in most, the iris is gray to hazel and there is moderate to marked translucency and photophobia [49,52,53]. The lack of pigment in the peripheral retina with visualization of the choroidal vessels and foveal hypoplasia are typical of other types of albinism. Some pigment may be present at the central part of the posterior pole, obscuring the choroid in this area.

Obligate heterozygous females have normally pigmented irides that often demonstrate some translucency on globe transillumination [50–53]. Funduscopic examination in obligate heterozygotes demonstrates a characteristic mosaic pattern of pigment that is thought to result from random X-inactivation [49–52]. Irregular clumps of pigment are distributed throughout the fundus in an irregular pattern. An occasional heterozygous female will have nystagmus and reduced visual acuity similar to that of the male [53–55]. Obligate heterozygotes have been described with normal retinal pigment [51,53].

The skin and hair pigment of affected males is usually thought to be normal. Several authors have suggested that the skin color is lighter than that of unaffected siblings, but this is unsubstantiated. O'Donnell has described hypopigmented macules and patches in the skin of affected males [56]. Microscopic examination of normally pigmented skin from affected males and obligate heterozygous females demonstrates large pigment granules, called macromelanosomes or melanin macroglobules, in the melanocytes [57]. These have also been demonstrated in the eye [58]. Clearly, type I OA is an oculocutaneous process with minimal clinical changes in the skin or hair.

Type II (Forsius–Eriksson Syndrome) Ocular Albinism

Forsius and Eriksson described a rare form of OA affecting males in the Åland Islands [59,60]. All changes are ocular with no cutaneous manifestations. Affected males have nystagmus, retinal hypopigmentation, and foveal hypoplasia, but the iris is normally pigmented with little or no translucency. Astigmatism and myopia are present and visual acuity is poor. The retinal hypopigmentation is not typical of OA in that pigmented areas are often found in the periphery as well as at the posterior pole. Obligate heterozygous females do not have a mosaic retinal pigment pattern. Macromelanosomes are not found in this type of OA [59]. Recent visual evoked potential studies show that there is no optic misrouting in Åland eye disease, suggesting that this is not a true form of OA [9,61].

Type III (Autosomal Recessive) Ocular Albinism

Females with OA have occasionally been noted and thought to be the expression of unusual X-inactivation of the gene for type I OA, but in 1978, an autosomal recessive type of OA was described [62]. Males and females with type III OA have nystagmus, photophobia, strabismus, and reduced visual acuity. Iris color is blue to light brown, and the iris is translucent on globe transillumination. Some pigment is present at the posterior pole of the fundus, but the peripheral retina has no pigment and the choroidal vessels are easily seen. Foveal hypoplasia is present. The skin and hair are light at birth and slowly accumulate pigment with age. Tanning of the skin is minimal. Although not proven, it has been suggested that type III OA in a Caucasian is the same as type-IV OCA in a black person [27].

Laboratory Findings

Three tests are useful in the evaluation of an individual with albinism: hairbulb incubation, hairbulb tyrosinase assay, and electron microscopy of a melanocyte.

For the hairbulb incubation test, 8 to 10 freshly plucked anagen hairbulbs are incubated in a solution containing 80 mg L-tyrosine in 100 ml of 0.1 M phosphate buffer, pH 6.8, at 37°C for 12 to 24 hours and are observed with a dissecting microscope for pigment formation in the melanocytes at the base of the hairbulb [5,12,37]. Variable amounts of pigment form in type II OCA hairbulbs, and this is somewhat dependent on the familial pigment pattern. Hairbulbs from individuals with type II OCA from lightly pigmented families form little pigment while those from more darkly pigmented families form more pigment.

The tyrosine hyroxylase activity of tyrosinase in the hairbulb is determined with a tritiated tyrosine assay [6,63,64]. Assay results for normal and OCA types are given in Table 35.2. The hairbulb tyrosinase assay is the preferred method for the evaluation of an individual and family with albinism. In OA the hairbulb tyrosinase activity is normal. It should be noted that normal and albino hairbulbs often have little tyrosinase activity until the age of 4 or 5 years in Caucasian and 2 or 3 years in Negro children, thus the tyrosinase assay and the hairbulb incubation tests are unreliable before this.

Heterozygotes for type IA OCA can be detected with the hairbulb tyrosinase assay. This will often help in the evaluation of a family with an albino newborn at which time the parents can be tested before the child's hairbulbs are adequate for testing.

The melanocyte can be observed on electron microscopy in a biopsy specimen from the skin and in a hair follicle. The basic structure of the melanocyte is normal in all types of OCA and OA [9,12,22,23,26,27,34,53,56,59,62]. The melanosomes were found to have an abnormal structure (macromelanosomes) in type I OA [56] in the one family with autosomal dominant OCA and Prader–Willi syndrome [46] and in the Chediak–Higashi syndrome. The demonstration of macromelanosomes in the skin of affected males and carrier females in type I OA is very helpful in differentiating this type of OA from type III OA and can provide important information for genetic counseling. In all other types of OCA the melanosomes have a normal structure but exhibit varying degrees of hypomelanization. No pigment is present in type IA OCA melanosomes. Minimal to normal amounts of pigment are present in the other types of OCA and in OA, and the amount of melanization correlates with the pigment phenotype. Except for type I OA, the microscopic evaluation of the melanocyte does not provide specific diagnostic information but does support the clinical and biochemical findings.

Biochemistry

Melanin is synthesized in the melanocyte, a dendritic cell found in the skin at the dermal–epidermal junction, in the hair follicle, and in the iris, retina, and choroid of the eye [65]. Melanocytes in the skin, hair follicles, and iris stroma and choroid are derived from cells that migrate from the neural crest while those in the retina pigment epithelium and the ciliary body are neuroectodermal in origin. The average cell density in the skin is estimated to be 1,000 to 1,500 melanocytes per mm², with each cell in contact with its surrounding keratinocyte through the dendritic

Table 35.2. Hairbulb Tyrosinase Activity

| | No. | pmol Tyrosine Oxidized/120 Min/Hairbulb | |
		Mean ± SD	Range
Normal controls			
Hair color			
Brown	22	1.49 ± 0.79	0.27–3.31
Black	10	1.68 ± 0.67	0.94–3.06
Blond	13	1.50 ± 0.85	0.19–2.66
Red	12	2.72 ± 1.26	0.78–4.99
Albino and heterozygotes			
Type			
IA (Tyrosinase negative)	32	0.01 ± 0.02	0–0.08
IA Heterozygotes	23	0.08 ± 0.10	0–0.34
IB (Yellow)	5	0.13 ± 0.19	0–0.50
IB Heterozygotes	3	0.03	0–0.09
II (Tyrosinase positive)	22	1.53 ± 1.01	0.11–3.87
Type II appears to separate into three groups:			
High	4	3.13 ± 0.51	2.81–3.87
Intermediate	9	1.78 ± 0.35	1.43–2.56
Low	9	0.57 ± 0.28	0.11–0.95
II Heterozygotes	24	1.04 ± 0.72	0.44–3.90
III (Minimal pigment)	3	0.01	0–0.02
III Heterozygotes			
High	3	1.15	0.98–1.35
Low	3	0.16	0.10–0.18
IV (Brown)	1	1.75	
VI (Hermansky–Pudlak syndrome)	10	0.37 ± 0.45	0–1.18
Type VI appears to separate into two groups:			
High	5	0.71 ± 0.35	0.37–1.18
Low	5	0.03 ± 0.03	0–0.07
VI Heterozygotes	6	1.03 ± 0.64	0.17–1.80

processes forming the epidermal melanin unit [66]. The melanin forms in the granular intracellular organelle, the melanosome, and is distributed to the adjacent cells by melanosomal transfer.

The melanin pathway is shown in Figure 35.2. Tyrosine is the initial substrate for the pathway and two types of melanin can form: black-brown eumelanin and reddish brown-yellow pheomelanin [67]. The enzyme tyrosinase catalyzes the oxidation of tyrosine to dopa (3,4-dihydroxyphenylalanine) and the dehydrogenation of dopa to dopaquinone. Dopaquinone is a very reactive compound that quickly enters the pheomelanin or eumelanin pathway. The classic concept of eumelanin synthesis has been that all of the steps in the eumelanin pathway are spontaneous and have no enzyme requirement, but recent work suggests that this may not be true. A factor (dopachrome conversion factor) has been described to promote the conversion of dopachrome to 5,6-dihydroxyindole, and analysis of a crude preparation of this factor shows that it has the characteristics of an enzyme (tentatively called dopachrome oxidoreductase) [68,69]. Tyrosinase will catalyze the conversion of 5,6-dihydroxyindole to indole-5,6-quinone but the biologic significance of this action of tyrosinase is unknown [65,70,71].

In pheomelanin synthesis, dopaquinone reacts with sulfhydryl compounds such as cysteine or glutathione to form cysteinyl-dopa intermediate compounds that undergo oxidative cyclization and polymerization to pheomelanin. No enzyme control of pheomelanin synthesis has been described, but the ability of glutathione to form glutathione-dopa and cysteinyl-dopa suggests that enzymatic regulation of these compounds could influence melanin synthesis [67,72]. Natural melanin includes pure eumelanin, pure

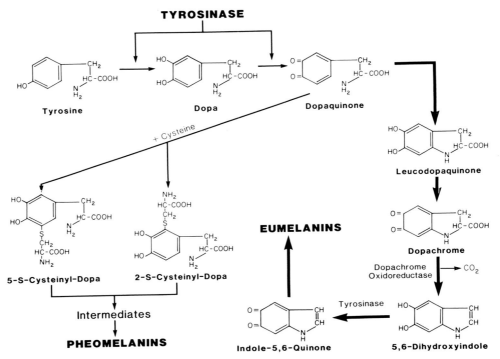

Figure 35.2. The melanin synthesis pathway.

pheomelanin, and a mixed reddish-brown melanin derived from components of both pathways [67]. All types of melanin will form within the same melanocyte but the melanosomal structure differs [73]. The earliest stage (stage 1) of the developing eumelanosome is a Golgi-derived spherical vacuole that elongates into an ellipsoidal granule with an internal lamellar matrix (stage 2). Tyrosinase (and possibly other enzymes) are transported from the Golgi complex to the developing melanosome through vesiculoglobular bodies, and melanin begins to form on the internal matrix (stage 3). Melanin eventually fills the ellipsoidal eumelanosomes and obliterates all internal architecture except for the residual vesiculoglobular bodies that stay unmelanized around the periphery (stage 4). The early spherical vacuole (stage 1) of the developing pheomelanosome is the same. Multiple vesiculoglobular bodies accumulate in the round granule (stage 2) and form granular melanin that aggregates (stage 3) and eventually fills the round pheomelanosome (stage 4).

Tyrosinase is a copper-containing enzyme requiring dopa as a cofactor in the oxidation of tyrosine and the dehydrogenation of 5,6-dihydroxyindole. The characteristic electrophoretic pattern of tyrosinase is the result of post-translational glycosylation [74]. Native soluble tyrosinase, isozyme T_3, has a molecular weight of 54,000. T_3 is glycosylated to soluble isozyme T_1, with a molecular weight of 72,000, and this is incorporated into the melanosome becoming membrane bound, insoluble isozyme T_4. The glycosylation is important for melanin synthesis, and inhibition of glycosylation blocks melanin formation in cultured melanocytes [75].

In human tissue, tyrosinase can be studied in melanocytes contained in a skin biopsy or in a plucked hair follicle. The plucked anagen hairbulb is an excellent and easily available source of melanocytes, and methods have been developed to study the activity of hairbulb tyrosinase (see Laboratory Findings) [63,64]. Methods are now being developed to measure other components of the pathway, including the activity of dopachrome oxidoreductase, but these determinations are not in general use at the present time.

Pathology

Albinism results from the reduction or absence of melanin in the melanocytes and in the cells, such as in the keratinocyte, which receive melanin from the melanocyte. The structure of the melanocyte is normal. The reduction in melanin is associated with the production of melanosomes that are structurally normal but do not complete the melanization phase of development. This has no detrimental effect on the melanocyte or on the cells that receive the hypopigmented premelanosomes. All of the pathologic changes of albinism are the result of secondary changes that develop because of the lack of melanin in the involved tissues.

Skin and Hair

The hair is hypopigmented but otherwise normal. Individuals with type IA OCA often appear to have fine hair, and their hairbulbs are more difficult to obtain. However, these changes have not been quantitated, and their biologic basis is unknown. Hypopigmented skin is sensitive to ultraviolet radiation from the sun, and individuals with albinism often have chronic sun irritation with erythema and thickening (pachydermia) of exposed skin. Individuals with type II OCA develop large pigmented lentigines on exposed areas of the skin after prolonged sun exposure [25], and pigmented nevi develop in most types of OCA in which pigment develops (types IB to VII) [1,9,12,25,27].

The most serious secondary pathologic change in the skin is the development of skin cancer. Squamous cell and basal cell carcinoma have been reported, and the frequency varies between populations [1,25,76–79]. Skin cancer in individuals with OCA in the U.S. population is very uncommon. In contrast to this, the majority of individuals with OCA (mostly type II) in the Nigerian population develop squamous cell carcinoma, one of the most common causes of death for albinos in this population [25,77]. Basal cell carcinoma is infrequent in this population. The frequency of skin cancer in individuals with type VI OCA in Puerto Rico is also increased [12]. Of note is the fact that melanoma is an infrequent tumor in individuals with albinism [80–82]. Most likely the skin protection offered by the latitude as well as the life and clothing styles are important in keeping the frequency of skin cancer low in albino individuals in the U.S. population.

Eyes

There are two major changes in the optic system that appear to be related to the reduction of melanin in the eye during development. The first is foveal hypoplasia, which is responsible for much of the reduced visual acuity [15,83,84]. The second is the abnormal development of the optic nerve routing from the eye to the lateral geniculate and optic cortex [12,85–88]. In individuals with all types of OCA and OA, the optic fibers from the temporal side of the retina cross abnormally at the chiasm to the contralateral geniculate rather than project normally to the ipsilateral geniculate. The structure of the lateral geniculate is abnormal, as is the optic radiation [88,89]. This misrouting can be detected by visual evoked potential analysis [85,87]. The nystagmus and strabismus associated with albinism are due in part to these changes in the routing of the optic fibers and the structure of the lateral geniculate. Similar changes were recently described in hypopigmented but non-albino individuals with Prader–Willi syndrome [90], and in normally pigmented cats who were heterozygous for type IA OCA [91], suggesting that optic system abnormalities may be more widespread than originally thought and could account for some optic system problems such as strabismus in the normally pigmented population.

Pathogenesis

All types of OCA and OA are recessive in inheritance, except for type VII OCA, which suggests that the primary defect for each type is an abnormality of enzyme function. To date, no gene for albinism has been isolated. Each type of OCA is thought to represent a different mutation, and several types of OCA are thought to result from allelic mutations.

Hairbulb tyrosinase activity has been determined in most types of OCA, and these results, along with the phenotype, suggest possible mechanisms for the abnormal pigment formation [64]. Type IA and IB OCA result from reduced tyrosinase activity, and most likely are due to allelic mutations that affect the structure of tyrosinase [22,64]. The melanin pathway is blocked completely in type IA OCA, with no pigment formation, and there is no residual tyrosinase activity [64]. Heterozygotes for type IA OCA have markedly reduced activity and can be detected with this assay [64,92]. The pathway block is incomplete in type IB OCA, perhaps from a partially active tyrosinase, and the dopaquinone product of the initial steps rapidly enters the high-affinity pheomelanin pathway, which produces the yellow or blond phenotype (see Figure 35.2). Type III OCA may also be due to changes in tyrosinase activity [26]. Individuals with this type have no hairbulb tyrosinase activity. Most importantly, parental studies show that one parent has normal activity and the other has low activity, suggesting that each parent carries a different mutant tyrosinase allele. If this is true, then individuals with type III OCA are genetic compounds.

Tyrosinase is normal in type II OCA. This type of OCA is the result of an abnormality in another, presently undescribed enzyme of the pathway [64,93,94]. The block in this type of OCA appears to be in the distal eumelanin pathway. Tyrosinase generates dopaquinone, which enters the high-affinity pheomelanin pathway, resulting in the yellow-blond phenotype. The eumelanin pathway is not blocked completely, however, as some eumelanin is formed as the individual ages. It is possible that the block involves the steps controlled by the partially characterized dopachrome oxidoreductase but this has not yet been demonstrated. Type IV OCA appears to be a partial block in the eumelanin pathway and could be allelic to type II OCA, similar to that proposed for type IA and IB OCA [27,64]. The defects in type VI and VII OCA are unknown.

The biochemical defects responsible for the different types of OA are unknown, and no biochemical studies on melanocytes from the eye in OA are available. Type I OA has an X-linked recessive inheritance, and the gene is located on the short arm of the X chromosome [95,96]. Recent molecular studies using restriction fragment length polymorphism analysis have located three restriction length polymorphisms that are tightly linked to the OA locus, and which should facilitate isolation of the OA gene [97].

Prognosis

Limitation of vision and sensitivity of the skin to sunlight are the major complications of albinism. In the United States and in Europe, the visual limitations are the most significant, and the skin changes are not a significant problem, except for the cosmetic effect of the hypopigmentation. In more sun-intense areas such as equatorial regions, the skin sensitivity is serious, and skin cancer is common.

Most individuals with albinism require regular ophthalmologic evaluation and care, and may require the use of low-vision programs. With the proper use of glasses and reading aids, almost all individuals with albinism can attend regular school and participate in most of the regular school and social activities.

Treatment

Individuals with OCA must learn to protect their skin from the ultraviolet radiation of the sun. Long sleeve shirts and hats that cover the ears and face are helpful. Sun screens that block the ultraviolet rays are effective and should be used for any prolonged exposure. Sun screens with a rating of 15 are generally effective.

No lens correction will provide normal vision for an individual with albinism; however, the majority of individuals with albinism have improved their vision with appropriate corrections for their astigmatism, myopia, or hyperopia. It is important that all individuals with albinism undergo a complete ophthalmologic evaluation and establish a regular follow-up program for their vision. Rose-tinted lenses or lenses that darken on sun exposure help reduce the photophobia, but dark glasses often are not comfortable because they further reduce vision. Low-vision aids, including large-print books and light-intensifying magnifying lenses can help with reading. Close vision is usually good and appropriate use of space and seating in the classroom is important. The child with albinism does not have to sit in the seat with the best lighting and should be allowed to hold a book close to the face for reading.

Strabismus is common in albinism and is related to the misrouted optic nerves. The strabismus is alternating and unfixed in most cases and is not associated with the development of amblyopia. Corrective surgery is not necessary for the majority of individuals with albinism and usually does not completely correct the strabismus. When performed, however, the nystagmus may be reduced along with the strabismus [9].

The diagnosis of type VII OCA must be considered in any individual with OCA and a history of bleeding. Aspirin and aspirin-like drugs should not be given to individuals with type VII OCA.

References

1. Pearson K, Nettleship E, Usher CH. Early notices of the occurrence of albinism. In: A monograph on albinism in man. Draper's Company research memoirs, biometric series VI, part I. London: Dulan and Co, 1911:11–26.
2. Froggatt P. The legend of a white native race. Med Hist 1960;4:228–235.
3. Garrod AE. Inborn errors of metabolism. First Croonian lecture. Lancet 1908;2:1–7.
4. Trevor-Roper PD. Marriage of two complete albinos with normally pigmented offspring. Br J Ophthalmol 1952;36:107–108.
5. Kugelman TP, Van Scott EJ. Tyrosinase activity in melanocytes of human albinos. J Invest Dermatol 1961;37:73–76.

6. King RA, Witkop CJ. Hairbulb tyrosinase activity in oculocutaneous albinism. Nature 1976;263:69–71.

7. Krill AE. Albinism. In: Krill AE, Archer DB, eds. Krill's hereditary retinal and choroidal diseases. New York: Harper & Row, 1977:645–663.

8. Collewijn H, Apkarian P, Spekreijse H. The oculomotor behavior of human albinos. Brain 1985;108:1–28.

9. Kinnear PE, Jay B, Witkop CJ. Albinism. Survey Ophthalmol 1985;30:75–101.

10. Fonda G. Characteristics and low-vision corrections in albinos. Arch Ophthalmol 1962;68:754–761.

11. Fonda G, Thomas H, Gore GV. Educational and vocational placement and low-vision corrections in albinism. Sight Sav Rev 1971;41:29–36.

12. Witkop CJ, Jr, Quevedo WC, Jr, Fitzpatrick TB. Albinism and other disorders of pigment metabolism. In: Stanbury JB, Wyngaarden JB, Fredrickson DS, et al., eds. The metabolic basis of inherited disease. 5th ed. New York: McGraw–Hill, 1983:301–346.

13. Taylor WOG. Visual disabilities of oculocutaneous albinism and their alleviation. The 1978 Edgridge–Green lecture. Trans Ophthalmol Soc UK 1978;98:423–445.

14. Jacobson SG, Mohindra I, Held R, et al. Visual acuity development in tyrosinase negative oculocutaneous albinism. Doc Ophthalmol 1984;56:337–344.

15. Fulton AB, Albert DW, Craft JL. Human albinism: light and electron microscopy study. Arch Ophthalmol 1978;96:305–310.

16. Froggatt P. Albinism in Northern Ireland. Ann Hum Genet 1960;24:213–237.

17. Abrams JD. Transillumination of the iris during routine slit-lamp examination. Br J Ophthalmol 1964; 48:42–44.

18. Wirtschafter JD, Denslow GT, Shine IB. Quantification of iris translucency in albinism. Arch Ophthalmol 1973;90:274–277.

19. Pickford RW, Taylor WOG. Color vision of two albinos. Br J Ophthalmol 1968;52:640–641.

20. Lourenco PE, Fishman GA, Anderson RJ. Color vision in albino subjects. Doc Ophthalmol 1983;55:341–350.

21. Nance WE, Jackson CE, Witkop CJ, Jr. Amish albinism: a distinctive autosomal recessive phenotype. Am J Hum Genet 1970;22:579–586.

22. Fu H, Hanifin JM, Prescott GH, et al. Yellow mutant albinism: cytochemical, ultrastructural, and genetic characterization suggesting multiple allelism. Am J Hum Genet 1980;32:387–395.

23. Witkop CJ, Jr, Nance WE, Rawls RF, et al. Autosomal recessive oculocutaneous albinism in man: evidence for genetic heterogeneity. Am J Hum Genet 1970;22:55–74.

24. Okoro AN. Albinism in Nigeria: a clinical and social study. Br J Dermatol 1975;92:485–492.

25. King RA, Creel D, Cervenka J, et al. Albinism in Nigeria with delineation of new recessive oculocutaneous type. Clin Genet 1980;17:259–270.

26. King RA, Wirtschafter JD, Olds DP, et al. Minimal pigment: a new type of oculocutaneous albinism. Clin Genet 1986;29:42–50.

27. King RA, Lewis RA, Townsend D, et al. Brown oculocutaneous albinism: clinical, ophthalmological, and biochemical characterization. Ophthalmology 1985; 92:1496–1505.

28. King RA, Rich SS. Segregation analysis of brown oculocutaneous albinism. Clin Genet 1986;29:1496–501.

29. Walsh RJ. A distinctive pigment in the skin in New Guinea indigenes. Ann Hum Genet 1971;34:379–388.

30. Stannus HS. Anomalies of pigmentation among natives of Nyasaland: a contribution to the study of albinism. Biometrika 1913;9:333–365.

31. Hornabrook RW, McDonald WI, Carroll RL. Congenital nystagmus among the red-skins of the highlands of Papua, New Guinea. Br J Ophthalmol 1980; 64:375–380.

32. Hermansky F, Pudlak P. Albinism associated with hemorrhagic diathesis and unusual pigmented reticular cells in the bone marrow: report of two cases with histochemical studies. Blood 1959;14:162–169.

33. Simon JW, Adams RJ, Calhoun JH, et al. Ophthalmic manifestations of the Hermansky–Pudlak syndrome (oculocutaneous albinism and hemorrhagic diathesis). Am J Ophthalmol 1982;93:71–77.

34. Frenk E, Lattion F. The melanin pigmentary disorder in a family with Hermansky–Pudlak syndrome. J Invest Dermatol 1982;78:141–143.

35. Takahashi A, Yokoyama T. Hermansky–Pudlak syndrome with special reference to lysosomal dysfunction. A case report and review of the literature. Virchows Arch (Pathol Anat) 1984;402:247–258.

36. Depinho RA, Kaplan KL. The Hermansky–Pudlak syndrome: report of three cases and review of pathophysiology and management considerations. Medicine 1985;64:192–202.

37. Witkop CJ, Jr. Inherited disorders of pigmentation. Clin Dermatol 1985;3:70–134.

38. Logan LJ, Rapaport SI, Maher I. Albinism and abnormal platelet function. N Engl J Med 1971;284:1340–1346.

39. Witkop CJ, Jr, White JG, Gerritsen SM, et al. Hermansky–Pudlak syndrome (HPS): a proposed block in glutathione peroxidase. Oral Surg Oral Med Oral Pathol 1973;35:790–806.

40. White JG, Witkop CJ, Jr, Gerritsen SM. The Hermansky–Pudlak syndrome. Ultrastructure of bone marrow macrophages. Am J Pathol 1973;70:329–338.

41. Davies BH, Tuddenham EGD. Familial pulmonary fibrosis associated with oculocutaneous albinism and platelet function defect. Q J Med 1976;178:219–232.

42. Garay SM, Gardella JE, Fazzini EP, et al. Hermansky–Pudlak syndrome: pulmonary manifestation of a ceroid storage disease. Am J Med 1979;66:737–747.

43. Schinella RA, Greco MA, Cobert BL, et al. Hermansky–Pudlak syndrome with granulomatous colitis. Ann Intern Med 1980;92:20–23.

44. Bomalaski JS, Green D, Carone F. Oculocutaneous albinism, platelet storage pool disease, and progressive lupus nephritis. Arch Intern Med 1983;143:809–811.

45. Bergsma DR, Kaiser–Kupfer M. A new form of albinism. Am J Ophthalmol 1974;77:837–844.

46. Frenk E, Calame A. Hypopigmentation oculo-cutanée familiale à transmission dominante due à un trouble de la formation des mélanosomes. Schweiz Med Wochenschr 1977;107;1964–1968.

47. Cross HE, McKusick VA, Breen W. A new oculocerebral syndrome with hypopigmentation. J Pediatr 1967;70:398–406.

48. Nettleship E. On some hereditary diseases of the eye. Trans Ophthalmol Soc UK 1909;29:57–198.

49. Falls HF. Sex-linked ocular albinism displaying typical fundus changes in the female heterozygote. Am J Ophthalmol 1951;34(part II):41–50.

50. Gillespie FD. Ocular albinism with report of a family with female carriers. Arch Ophthalmol 1961;66:774–777.

51. Gillespie FD, Covelli B. Carriers of ocular albinism with and without ocular changes. Arch Ophthalmol 1963;70:209–213.

52. Waardenburg PJ, Van den Bosch J. X-chromosomal ocular albinism in a Dutch family. Ann Hum Genet 1956;21:101–122.

53. Cortin P, Tremblay M, Lemagne JM. X-linked ocular albinism: relative value of skin biopsy, iris transillumination, and funduscopy in identifying affected males and carriers. Can J Ophthalmol 1981;16:121–123.

54. Pearce WG, Johnson GJ, Gillan JG. Nystagmus in a female carrier of ocular albinism. J Med Genet 1972;9:126–129.

55. Jaeger C, Jay B. X-linked ocular albinism: a family containing a manifestating heterozygote, and an affected male married to a female with autosomal recessive ocular albinism. Hum Genet 1981;56:299–304.

56. O'Donnell FE, Hambrick GW, Green R, et al. X-linked ocular albinism: an oculocutaneous macromelanosomal disorder. Arch Ophthalmol 1976;94:1883–1892.

57. Nakagawa H, Hori Y, Sato S, et al. The nature and origin of the melanin macroglobule. J Invest Dermatol 1984;83:134–139.

58. O'Donnell FE, Green R, Fleischman JA, et al. X-linked ocular albinism in blacks: ocular albinism cum pigmento. Arch Ophthalmol 1978;96:1189–1192.

59. O'Donnell FE, Green WR, McKusick VA, et al. Forsius–Eriksson syndrome: its relation to the Nettleship–Falls X-linked ocular albinism. Clin Genet 1980;17:403–408.

60. Waardenburg PJ, Eriksson AW, Forsius H. Åland eye disease (syndroma Forsius-Eriksson). Prog Neuro Ophthalmol 1969;2:336–339.

61. van Dorp DB, Eriksson AW, Delleman JW, et al. Åland eye disease: no albino misrouting. Clin Genet 1985;28:526–531.

62. O'Donnell FE, King RA, Green WR, et al. Autosomal recessively inherited ocular albinism. Arch Ophthalmol 1978;96:1621–1625.

63. King RA, Olds DP, Witkop CJ, Jr. Characterization of human hairbulb tyrosinase: properties of normal and albino enzyme. J Invest Dermatol 1978;71:136–139.

64. King RA, Olds DP. Hairbulb tyrosinase activity in oculocutaneous albinism: suggestions for pathway control

65. Jimbow K, Quevedo WC, Jr, Fitzpatrick TB, et al. Some aspects of melanin biology: 1950–1975. J Invest Dermatol 1976;67:72–89.

66. Rosdahl I, Rorsman H. An estimate of the melanocyte mass in humans. J Invest Dermatol 1983;81:278–281.

67. Prota G. Recent advances in the chemistry of melanogenesis in mammals. J Invest Dermatol 1980;75:122–127.

68. Pawelek J, Korner A, Bergstrom A, et al. New regulators of melanin biosynthesis and the auto destruction of melanoma cells. Nature 1980;286:617–619.

69. Barber JI, Townsend D, Olds DP, et al. Dopachrome oxidoreductase: a new enzyme in the pigment pathway. J Invest Dermatol 1984;83:145–149.

70. Korner A, Pawelek J. Mammalian tyrosinase catalyzes three reactions in the biosynthesis of melanin. Science 1982;217:1163–1165.

71. Miranda M, Botti D, Bonfigli A, et al. 5,6-dihydroxyindole oxidation by mammalian, mushroom and amphibian tyrosinase preparations. Biochim Biophys Acta 1985;841:159–165.

72. Benedetto JP, Ortonne JP, Voulet C, et al. Role of thio compounds in mammalian melanin pigmentation. II. Glutathione and related enzymatic activities. J Invest Dermatol 1982;79:422–424.

73. Jimbow K, Oikawa O, Sugiyama S, et al. Comparison of eumelanogenesis and pheomelanogenesis in retinal and follicular melanocytes: role of vesiculo-globular bodies in melanosome differentiation. J Invest Dermatol 1979;73:278–284.

74. Hearing VJ, Nicholson JM, Montague PM, et al. Mammalian tyrosinase: structural and functional interrelationships of isozymes. Biochim Biophys Acta 1978;522:327–339.

75. Imokawa G, Mishima Y. Functional analysis of tyrosinase isozymes of cultured malignant melanoma cells during recovery period following interrupted melanogenesis induced by glycosylation inhibitors. J Invest Dermatol 1984;83:196–201.

76. Witkop CJ, Jr. Epidemiology of skin cancer in man. B. Genetic factors. In: Laerum OD, Iverson OH, eds. Biology of skin cancer (excluding melanoma). Union Internationale Coutre le Cancer, Technical Report Series 1981:69:67–85.

77. Okoro AN. Albinism in Nigeria. Br J Dermatol 1975;92:485–492.

78. Claudy AL, Ortonne JP. Tyrosinase-negative albinism with congenital malformations and squamous cell carcinoma of the genitalia. Acta Dermatol 1982;62:260–262.

79. Freire–Maia N, Cavalli IJ. Albinism, skin carcinoma and chromosome aberrations (letter to the editor). Clin Genet 1980;17:46–47.

80. Pehamberger H, Honigsmann H, Wolff K. Dysplastic nevus syndrome with multiple primary melanomas in oculocutaneous albinism. J Am Acad Dermatol 1984;11:731–735.

81. Wood C, Graham D, Willsen J, et al. Albinism and amelanotic melanoma: occurrence in a child with positive test results for tyrosinase. Arch Dermatol 1982; 118:283–284.

82. Kennedy BJ, Zelickson AS. Melanoma in an albino. JAMA 1963;186:839–841.

83. Adler JE, McIntosh J. Histological examination of a case of albinism. Biometrika 1910;7:237–247.

84. Usher CH. Histological examination of an adult human albino's eyeball, with a note on mesoblastic pigmentation in the foetal eyes. Biometrika 1920;13: 46–56.

85. Creel D, Witkop CJ, King RA. Asymmetric visually evoked potentials in human albinos: evidence for visual system anomalies. J Invest Ophthalmol 1974; 13:430–440.

86. Carroll WM, Jay BS, McDonald WI, et al. Pattern evoked potentials in human albinos: evidence of two different topographical asymmetries reflecting abnormal retino-cortical projections. J Neurol Sci 1980; 48:265–287.

87. Creel D, Spekreijse H, Reits D. Evoked potentials in albinos: efficacy of pattern stimuli in detecting misrouted optic fibers. Electroencephalogr Clin Neurophysiol 1981;52:595–603.

88. Guillery RW, Okoro AN, Witkop CJ, Jr. Abnormal visual pathways in the brain of a human albino. Brain Res 1975;96:373–377.

89. Guillery RW. Visual pathways in albinos. Sci Am 1974;230:44–54.

90. Creel DJ, Bendel CM, Wiesner GL, et al. Abnormalities of the central visual pathways in Prader–Willi syndrome associated with hypopigmentation. N Engl J Med 1986;314:1606–1609.

91. Leventhal AG, Vitek DJ, Creel DJ. Abnormal visual pathways in normally pigmented cats that are heterozygous for albinism. Science 1985;229:1395–1397.

92. King RA, Witkop CJ, Jr. Detection of tyrosinase-negative oculocutaneous albino heterozygote by hairbulb tyrosinase assay. Am J Hum Genet 1977;29:164–168.

93. King RA, Olds DP, Witkop CJ, Jr. Characterization of human hairbulb tyrosinase: properties of normal and albino enzyme. J Invest Dermatol 1978;71:136–139.

94. King RA, Olds DP. Electrophoretic pattern of human hairbulb tyrosinase. J Invest Dermatol 1981;77:201–204.

95. Fialkow PJ, Giblett ER, Motulsky AG. Measureable linkage between ocular albinism and Xg. Am J Hum Genet 1967;19:63–69.

96. Drayna D, White R. The genetic linkage map of the human X chromosome. Science 1985;230:753–758.

97. Kidd JR, Castiglione CM, Davies KE, et al. Mapping the locus for X-linked ocular albinism. Am J Hum Genet 1985;37:A161.

PART FIVE

CONGENITAL AND VASCULAR ANOMALIES

Chapter 36

Neurocutaneous Melanosis

IGNACIO PASCUAL-CASTROVIEJO

In 1861 Rokitansky [1] reported on a 14-year-old mentally retarded and hydrocephalic girl with many large pigmented skin nevi who at postmortem was found to have leptomeningeal infiltration with pigmented cells but no cerebral involvement. This is probably the first description of neurocutaneous melanosis (NCM) although the name was first used by van Bogaert in 1948 [2] for a heredofamilial disorder that he described.

NCM, believed to result from a congenital dysplasia of the melanocytes, cells of neuroectodermal origin, is characterized by hairy pigmented nevi located in any skin region with infiltration of the meninges and the CNS by melanin-containing cells. Fox [3] in 1972 proposed the following differentiating characteristics for NCM: (a) presence of a nevus or diffuse melanotic pigmentation on an area of skin occupying more than 20 cm in diameter, (b) the pigmented area does not demonstrate malignant transformation to melanoma, and (c) no evidence of a primary malignant melanoma outside the CNS. For a definitive diagnosis of NCM it is essential to do a thorough examination of extensive pathologic specimens or a complete postmortem examination.

The disease is more frequent than estimated if one includes the incomplete forms, benign meningeal melanosis without associated skin lesions and primary meningeal melanoma without the skin nevus. The number of patients reported in the medical literature before 1986 is less than 100, including the 8 cases reported by Fanconi [4] in 1956 and the 3 cases reported by Fox et al. [5]. We have followed over a period of 20 years 6 patients with skin lesions, none of whom thus far has developed neurologic symptoms.

Clinical Features

The disease affects males and females with the same frequency. It is not hereditary and occurs almost exclusively in whites; only rarely is it found in blacks [6,7]. The nevi are dense skin spots with abundant hair (Figure 36.1). The color of the skin and hair in the nevi is similar and varies between very dark and light brown, being darker in the blacks. The nevi are often very abundant but generally there is only one giant nevus, usually located in the trunk, extending to the gluteal–perineal–genital region, thus occupying the area covered by swimming trunks. Occasionally this giant nevus covers the lower extremities giving the appearance of stockings or high boots, or the upper extremities in the shape of long gloves. It may be on the head. One may find just one single giant nevus which may contain several shades of pigmentation (Figure 36.2).

Some, but not all, individuals with large or numerous hairy pigmented skin nevi develop intracranial or spinal melanomas. Although the cutaneous nevi themselves are benign, the melanin-containing cells in the pia mater have a great potential for malignancy.

Hydrocephalus, and consequently macrocephaly, is the most common manifestation of NCM, although it is not present in all patients with a congenital giant hairy pigmented nevus. The proportion of patients with the congenital pigmented nevus who develop intracranial symptomatology is not known. Approximately 50% of reported cases have developed CNS involvement during the first year of life but only 12 to 15% have done so as adults [8].

The pathogenesis of the hydrocephalus is obscure.

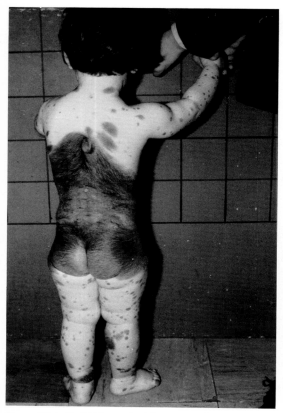 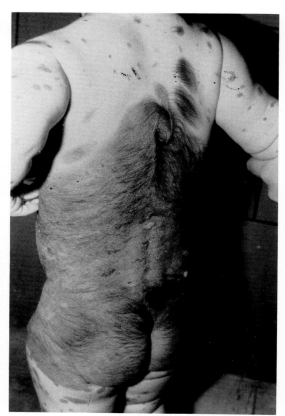

Figure 36.1. *(Left)* Shown in this young girl is a giant hairy pigmented nevus over her trunk and numerous small nevi over her extremities and upper trunk. *(Right)* Detail of the giant nevus on the back and gluteal regions shown at left. Observe the abundant hair and rough skin with small nodules.

It has been attributed to failure of CSF reabsorption due to infiltration of the arachnoid villi by melanocytes or obstruction at the cisterna magna also by arachnoid infiltration. However, such pathology was not found in many cases examined. Obstructive hydrocephalus due to aqueductal stenosis has been rarely described in isolation [9] or associated with arachnoid cysts of the posterior fossa [10].

Many patients have generalized or partial seizures beginning early in life, often before hydrocephalus develops. The seizures are often refractory to anticonvulsant therapy.

Other findings associated with NCM are intellectual deterioration and motor deficit. The mental disorder may appear at any time, and it is not unusual that a patient has been under psychiatric care for years before other signs or symptoms of CNS disease reveal themselves [11]. When the melanosis predominates at the base of the brain, the clinical picture may resemble that of tuberculous meningitis, with

the combination of increased intracranial pressure and cranial nerve deficit. Occasionally the melanotic infiltration is in the spinal meninges, thus simulating chronic spinal arachnoiditis, which may progress to spinal block and extend along spinal roots to include the cauda equina [12].

Laboratory Findings

Findings from examination of the CSF are usually negative but occasionally disclose increased protein and decreased glucose concentrations without an elevation in the number of cells. Rarely, the CSF contains malignant epithelial cells loaded with melanin [7,12]. Consequently, a careful cytologic CSF examination may be rewarding. Patients with meningeal melanomatosis are rarely asymptomatic.

Electroencephalographic studies, which may be useful in localizing a tumor mass [12], often dem-

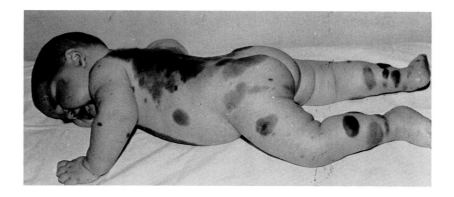

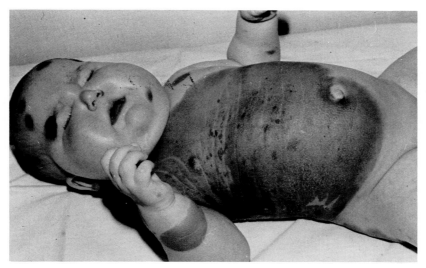

Figure 36.2. Note the giant nevus on the right side of the trunk and numerous nevi on the head, trunk, and extremities. Not all parts of the infant's nevi are hairy.

onstrate focal or generalized abnormalities in keeping with the clinical picture.

Hydrocephalus, usually of the communicating type, formerly demonstrable with air encephalography, is now better shown by ultrasound or computed tomography imaging. The hydrocephalus may be caused by obstruction of the aqueduct or the outlet of the fourth ventricle. The latter may be associated with a posterior fossa cyst and cerebellar hypoplasia [10]. Cerebral angiography may demonstrate profuse vascularization corresponding to a well-localized cerebral lesion [8]. Localization within the spinal canal is demonstrable with myelography [7,13], CT scanning [12], and probably with magnetic resonance imaging (MRI).

Pathology

In his review of 40 patients, Fox [3] noted that approximately 85% had marked leptomeningeal pigmentation in all regions at the base of the brain, the cerebellum, and the brain stem, particularly over the medulla, pons, midbrain, and interpeduncular fossa. Melanin is rarely found in the cerebral cortex but is found in the cerebellum in 25% of patients and in the spinal cord in 20% of patients. It is indeed rare in NCM to find a solid tumor or nodule within the cerebral parenchyma.

Faillace et al. [12] reported a patient with a 3-cm nodule in the parietal cortex and numerous 3- to 8-mm pigmented nodules throughout the cerebral hemisphere, an anatomic distribution quite different from what has been previously reported. A second patient reported by Faillace et al. [12] had "total spinal cord leptomeningeal infiltration resulting in a myelopathy." No CSF could be obtained by lumbar puncture, thus myelography was impossible. There was an increase of the interpedicular distance in the spine radiographs. This patient also had communicating hydrocephalus. The first case reported by Fox et al. [5] had a seminecrotic black tumor mass, replacing the right occipital lobe and posterior portion of the right temporal lobe formed by spindle cells with considerable pleomorphism and many mitotic figures, giving the appearance of a malignant melanoma.

Melanoblastic infiltration of the leptomeninges, although diffuse, is always most marked at the base of the brain, the interpeduncular fossa, and over the pons, medulla, and cerebellum. Gross pigmentation of the cerebral cortex is uncommon. However, cerebellar pigmentation is always most marked in the cortex. Sometimes one or both dentate nuclei are affected. Pontine pigmentation is invariably confined to the gray matter of the reticular formation. The thalamic nuclei may also be pigmented [5].

Melanoblasts infiltrating the meninges tend to arrange themselves in sheaths or nests. There is much variation in the amount of pigment in melanoblasts. These infiltrate into the Virchow–Robin spaces and penetrate with the vessels to form perivascular cuffs. Cellular pleomorphism and increased mitotic activity of melanoblasts are evidence of malignancy.

Pigmentation seen on gross inspection of the brain is by itself insufficient evidence of malignant cell invasion. Such pigmentation often results from melanin-containing histiocytes and is not necessarily due to infiltrating melanoblasts. These pigment-laden macrophages or melanophores must be distinguished from infiltrating malignant cells. Cerebral pigmentation without pigmentation of the overlying meninges is rare [5].

A malignant tumor within the meninges that covered a cerebral hemisphere was present in Björnboe's case (cited by Fox et al. [5]). In other instances the tumor mass was in the cerebellum, as in the case reported by Obendurfer [5] or in the pons as in Berblinger's case [5]. In all instances there was multifocal cerebral invasion or localized tumor formation; the melanoblasts infiltrating the meninges were spindle-shaped, pleomorphic, and arranged in sheets. In other areas, however, there were melanoblasts that displayed little pleomorphism and were arranged in clusters or nests [5]. Invasion of the brain from the

meninges seems to occur when the melanoblasts are spindle-shaped and pleomorphic.

Certain authors believe that the giant congenital pigmented nevus, the multiple pigmented nevi of the head, and the pigmented nevus of the occipitocervical region are the lesions that most frequently associate with leptomeningeal melanomatosis [6]. It has been said that statistically there is a greater incidence of malignancy in leptomeningeal melanosis than in cutaneous melanosis [3,6,14–16].

Pathogenesis

The pathogenesis of NCM is not at all clear. Cases of benign melanosis of the meninges without skin lesions have been found incidentally at postmortem examination [17]; and malignant melanomas of the meninges not associated with skin lesions have been reported many times since the original description by Virchow in 1859 [18].

The normal leptomeninges have melanin-containing cells that are more abundant over the superior cervical and ventral surfaces of the lumbosacral spinal cord. These melanin-containing cells in the pia mater and the rest of the pial cells derive from the neural crest [19]. The skin melanoblasts originate from neural crest cells [20], in at least amphibians, birds, and some mammals. During embryogenesis they migrate toward the basal epidermal layer. Subsequently the skin melanoblasts differentiate into melanin-producing melanocytes. After birth, the melanin is distributed to melanophores. It is believed that the superficially localized nevi derive from the epidermic melanocytes. The cells of congenital melanocytic nevi have three characteristics that differentiate them from acquired melanocytic nevi: (a) they are in the deeper two-thirds of the dermis; (b) they are arranged in Indian file or scattered between collagen fibers; (c) they usually affect dermal zones, nerves, and vessels in the deeper two-thirds of the reticular dermis [21].

Differential Diagnosis

Melanoma, the neoplasm with the highest incidence of CNS metastasis [22], should be differentiated from NCM. Other entities to be differentiated from NCM are [8]:

1. Hederofamilial melanosis, a disorder de-

scribed by Van Bogaert in 1948 [2], is a benign melanosis affecting the skin and leptomeninges with autosomal dominant inheritance. The hyperpigmented areas, although containing an abnormal amount of melanocytes, are benign cells.

2. Primary malignant melanoma of the leptomeninges, described by Virchow in 1859 [18], may be diffuse or localized and is relatively frequent. Savitz and Anderson [23] collected from the literature 82 patients reported before 1974 with intracranial localization and 69 with intervertebral localization. Melanomas are occasionally found in rare locations such as in the pituitary gland or the choroid plexus. Melanotic components also may be found in tumors of different histopathology such as meningiomas, neurofibromas, acoustic neuromas, and gliomas. In these cases, diffuse dissemination of melanotic cells through the subarachnoid space and infiltration through the Virchow spaces and cranial nerves occurs without associated cutaneous melanosis. In addition, the above-mentioned tumors may be associated with the nevus fuscoceruleus of Ota or oculocutaneous melanosis.

3. Metastatic melanoma or intracranial dissemination of a malignant melanoma of the skin, which may be observed at any age of life.

4. Progonoma, a rare benign tumor with different tissue components (dermoid or epidermoid, lipoma) in addition to melanotic cells [24]. It appears in the cranial bone and in neighboring areas of the meninges and more frequently in the anterior fontanelle and temporal regions. It is also known as the melanotic neuroectodermal tumor and is most common in infancy and young children. The tumor displaces the brain but does not infiltrate it. The skin is not involved, and it can be surgically removed from the dural and adjacent bone. The prognosis is excellent after complete excision. Radiotherapy is effective in partially resected lesions.

5. Melanotic nerve sheath tumor is a solitary melanin-bearing slow growing plexiform neurofibroma of young adults that causes no metastasis. In almost all reported cases it is in the subcutaneous tissue [25]. It has been found in association with meningeal melanomatosis, and in one case there was spinal cord compression at T7, vertebral body erosion, and incomplete spinal block by myelography [13].

Treatment

When there is cerebral or spinal infiltration by the melanoma there is a poor prognosis regardless of the treatment used, including radiation therapy and chemotherapy. Death occurs within a few months. Leptomeningeal infiltration and involvement of cranial or spinal nerve roots also carries a poor prognosis.

Hydrocephalus should be treated with a shunt to control, at least temporarily, the increased intracranial pressure. However, this may serve to disseminate the melanoma through the blood stream or over the peritoneum [12,15]. It has been recommended that a filter be used to prevent dissemination of malignant cells [12] but this form of treatment has not been tested as yet. For the rare association of NCM with syringomyelia [26] the syrinx may need to be catheterized and drained.

Seizures that appear during the course of the disease should be treated with anticonvulsant medications. The radicular pain secondary to infiltration of the roots should be treated with antalgic medication and, if necessary, narcotics.

Prognosis

Patients with leptomeningeal, cerebral, or spinal cord infiltration by malignant melanotic cells rarely live past the age of 20 years. Many have been stillborn or have died in the first year of life. There are rare cases with years of evolution from the time the clinical symptoms appear [13] but these are not those who presented with the giant dermal nevi. Patients with malignant NCM rarely have lived past the age of 25 years. On the other hand, there are cases of NCM who have had a benign course because the cells involved, being nonmalignant, cause no symptoms. We know about the existence of such cases only from postmortem examination as an incidental finding. Hydrocephalus can be temporarily controlled with a shunt but the time of evolution is usually short and rarely measured in years. The progression is dictated by the leptomeningeal infiltration with malignant cells and metastasis to other anatomic sites directly or through a shunt. Involvement of abdominal viscera is uncommon. One of the patients reported by Fox et al. [5] was found to have "nevus cells" in the testes and bladder wall, and the patient reported by Kaplan et al. [7] had metastasis in the liver and ribs.

References

1. Rokitansky J. Ein ausgezeichneter Fall von Pigment-Mal mit ausgebreiteter Pigmentierung der inneren Hirn und Rückenmarkshaute. Allg Wien Med Z 1861; 6:113–116.

2. Van Bogaert LC. La mélanose neurocutanée diffuse hérédofamiliale. Bull Acad R Med Belg 1948;3:397–427.

3. Fox H. Neurocutaneous melanosis. In: Vinken PJ, Bruyn GW, eds. The phakomatoses. Handbook of clinical neurology. Amsterdam: Elsevier, 1972;14:414–428.

4. Fanconi A. Neurocutane Melanoblastose mit Hydrocephalus comunicans bei zwei Säuglingen. Helv Paediatr Acta 1956;11:376–402.

5. Fox H, Emery JL, Goodbody RA, et al. Neurocutaneous melanosis. Arch Dis Childh 1964;39:508–516.

6. Reed WB, Becker WS, Sr, Becker WS, Jr, et al. Giant pigmented nevi, melanoma and leptomeningeal melanocytosis. Arch Dermatol 1965;91:100–119.

7. Kaplan AM, Itabashi HH, Hanelin LG, et al. Neurocutaneous melanosis with malignant leptomeningeal melanoma. A case with metastases outside the nervous system. Arch Neurol 1975;32:669–671.

8. Lamas E, Diez Lobato R, Sotelo T. et al. Neurocutaneous melanosis. Report of a case and review of the literature. Acta Neurochir 1977;36:93–105.

9. Harper CG, Thomas DGT. Neurocutaneous melanosis. J Neurol Neurosurg Psychiatry 1974;37:760–763.

10. Humes RA, Roskamp J, Eisenbrey AB. Melanosis and hydrocephalus. Report of four cases. J Neurosurg 1984;61:365–368.

11. Dailly R, Forthomme J, Samson M, et al. Mélanose neurocutanée à évolution tumorale. Presse Med 1965;73:2867–2972.

12. Faillace WJ, Okawara S-H, McDonald JV. Neurocutaneous melanosis with extensive intracerebral and spinal cord involvement. Report of two cases. J Neurosurg 1984;61:782–785.

13. Mandybur TI. Melanotic nerve sheath tumors. J Neurosurg 1974;41:187–192.

14. Hoffman HJ, Freeman A. Primary malignant leptomeningeal melanoma in association with giant hairy nevi. Report of two cases. J Neurosurg 1967;26:62–71.

15. Russell JL, Reyes RG. Giant pigmented nevi. JAMA 1959;171:141–144.

16. Morris LL, Danta G. Malignant cerebral melanoma complicating giant pigmented naevus: a case report. J Neurol Neurosurg Psychiatry 1968;31:628–632.

17. Kessler, M. Melanoblastosis and melanoblastoma: primary and secondary involvement of the brain. Am J Cancer 1937;30:19–31.

18. Virchow R. Pigment und diffuse Melanose der Arachnoides. Virchows Arch Path Anat Physiol 1859;16:180–182.

19. Newth DR. A remarkable embryonic tissue. Br Med J 1951;2:96–99.

20. Rawles ME. Origin of melanophores and their role in development of color patterns in vertebrates. Physiol Rev 1948;28:383–408.

21. Mark GJ, Mihn MC, Liteplo MG, et al. Congenital melanocytic nevi of the small and garment type. Clinical, histologic and ultrastructural studies. Hum Pathol 1973;4:395–418.

22. Dasgupta TK, Brasfield RD, Paglia MA. Primary melanomas in unusual site. Surg Gynecol Obstet 1969;128:841–848.

23. Savitz MH, Anderson PJ. Primary melanoma of the leptomeninges: a review. Mount Sinai J Med 1974;41:774–791.

24. Gilmor RL, Mealey J, Jr. Melanotic neuroectodermal tumor involving the cranium in infancy. J Neurosurg 1972;36:507–511.

25. Bird CC, Willis RA. The histogenesis of pigmented neurofibromas. J Pathol 1969;97:631–637.

26. Leaney BJ, Rowe PW, Klug GL. Neurocutaneous melanosis with hydrocephalus and syringomyelia J Neurosurg 1986;62:148–152.

Chapter 37

Linear Sebaceous Nevus

ARTHUR L. PRENSKY

Linear sebaceous nevus was first described as a dermatologic entity by Jadassohn [1] in 1895. Robinson [2] originally described the lesion in the English literature. Feuerstein and Mims [3] appreciated that the linear sebaceous nevus could be associated with neurologic lesions and was thus a neurocutaneous syndrome. Synonyms for linear sebaceous nevus include the term nevus linearis sebaceus, sebaceous nevus of Jadassohn, and the organoid nevus syndrome. However, organoid nevi are not limited to the linear sebaceous nevus; they also include other epidermal nevi syndromes.

The Skin Lesion

The diagnosis of a linear sebaceous nevus can often be made by observation. The typical lesion is visible in infancy, often at birth. It is a raised, smooth, linear plaque whose color is usually orange-yellow or orange-pink. The typical plaque is located at or near the midline and extends linearly from the forehead to the bridge of the nose (Figure 37.1), although it can also involve the upper lip and the midline mental region. The lesion usually does not straddle the midline but abuts it, being located predominantly to the right or left. In the series of Serpas-de-Lopez and Hernandez-Perez [4] only 41.3% of the lesions involved the face while a slightly greater number involved the scalp. Scalp nevi can be small nonlinear plaques as well as linear or curvilinear lesions. The overlying area is usually devoid of hair or at best covered with lanugo. This calls attention to the skin disorder early in life. Unilateral, elevated plaques can occur on the cheek and less often over the trunk or extremities. Even when they are extensive, the lesions are usually confined to one side of the body although bilateral lesions occur rarely [5,6].

Both Mehregan [6] and Morioka [7] published large series of patients who have had no neurologic deficits. They noted that the skin lesion evolved with age. The first stage is the smooth yellow-orange plaque seen in infancy. By the latter part of the first decade or during adolescence, the lesions enter a second stage in which they assume a verrucous quality (although the verrucous nature of some lesions can be seen at their margins even in the first years of life). Hyperkeratosis becomes more obvious (Figure 37.2). The third stage occurs in late adolescence or early adult life. The verrucous nature of the lesions is further emphasized, and skin tumors occur in as many as 20 to 30% of patients. Most of these tumors are benign, and include basal cell epitheliomas, sebaceous adenomas and epitheliomas, trichilemmomas, and apocrine tumors. Basal cell carcinomas are unusual, and squamous cell carcinomas are very rare.

The histologic character of the lesions also changes with age [6]. Early in life the epidermis is acanthotic, but pigment is only slightly increased. Hair follicles may be present but they are usually small and poorly formed. They are often represented only by cords of basaloid cells. Sebaceous glands may not be very prominent though they can be increased in number. Apocrine glands may not have developed. In the second stage of the disorder the hair follicles remain primordial but sebaceous glands proliferate and in many patients the apocrine glands dilate. In the third stage, large clumps of sebaceous glands occur in the dermis, and apocrine glands may be located aberrantly throughout the thickness of the skin. The hair follicles remain primordial strands.

Patients who have a linear sebaceous nevus may have other types of skin lesions (Table 37.1). The most common of these are small nonlinear, hyperpigmented nevi that usually occur over the trunk.

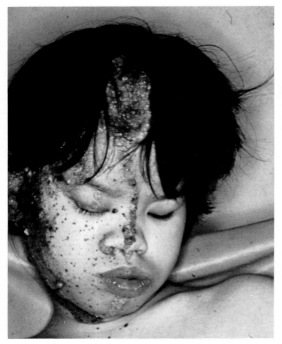

Figure 37.1. Patient with linear sebaceous nevus. (From Sugarman and Reed [12]. With permission. Copyright © 1969, the American Medical Association.)

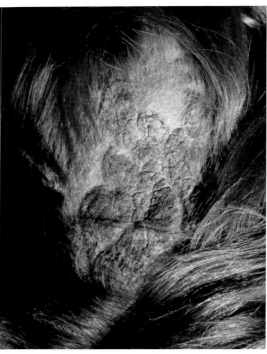

Figure 37.2. Verrucous stages of a nevus sebaceus on the scalp of a patient with the linner sebaceous nevus syndrome.

Table 37.1. Linear Sebaceous Nevus: Neurological Studies and Disease of Other Organ Systems

	Electroencephalogram	Special Neurologic Studies	Central Nervous System	Eye	Oral Cavity	Other Organs	Other Skin Lesions
Feuerstein and Mims, 1962 [3]							
Case 1	Spikes right hemisphere	—	—	None	—	None	None
Case 2	Right frontotemporal spike focus	—	—	None	—	None	None
Marden and Venters, 1966 [8]	Decreased voltage left; right frontotemporal spikes	Pneumoencephalogram; large left lateral ventricle	—	Chorioretinal colobomas; retinal degeneration; lipodermoids, conjunctiva	Hypoplastic dentition	Coarctation, aorta; facial anomalies	Multiple small nevi, trunk
Moynahan and Wolff, 1967 [9]	Generalized and multifocal paroxysmal discharges	Right frontal transillumination increased	—	Bilateral lipodermoids, conjunctiva	None	Cyst of left humerus; failure to thrive	Multiple small nevi

Table 37.1. (continued)

	Electroencephalogram	Special Neurologic Studies	Central Nervous System	Eye	Oral Cavity	Other Organs	Other Skin Lesions
Solomon and Fretzin, 1967 [10]	—	—	—	Coloboma, iris	High arched palate; hypoplastic dentition; papilloma, tongue	Scoliosis; pes cavus	Focal dermal hypoplasia; strawberry hemangioma, abdomen
Lantis et al., 1968 [11]							
Case 1	—	—	—	Dermoid of conjunctiva and cornea	—	None	None
Case 2	—	—	—	Dermoid of conjunctiva and cornea	—	None	None
Sugarman and Reed, 1969 [12]	Diffuse, severe abnormalities	Pneumoencephalogram: ventricular dilatation and cerebral atrophy	—	Dermoid of cornea of right eye	None	Osteomalacia; lytic lesions, ribs; deformed clavicles	Pigmented and blue nevi; mongolian spots
Bianchine, 1970 [13]	Grossly abnormal, epileptiform	—	—	Alternating esotropia	Irregular dentition	None	Pinhead nevi, trunk
Herbst and Cohen, 1971 [14]	Hypsarrhythmia	—	—	None	None	None	None
Lansky et al., 1972 [15]							
Case 1	Focal right parieto-occipital spikes	—	—	None	None	Hypoplasia, right renal artery; nephroblastoma; sclerosis, distal radius	Hyperpigmented nevi, trunk
Case 2	Multifocal spikes and spike waves	—	—	None	None	Wandering pacemaker	None
		—	—	None	None	Ventricular septal defect	None
Case 3	Normal	—	—	—	—	—	—
Haslam and Wirtschafter, 1972 [16]	Normal	—	—	Left third nerve palsy; aberrant lacrimal glands	None	None	Areas of hypopigmentation
Holden and Dekaban, 1972 [17]							
Case 1	Diffuse spike waves from left hemisphere	Pneumoencephalogram: enlarged left lateral ventricle	Left frontal arachnoidal cyst over area; cortical dysgenesis	Hemangioma, sclera and conjunctiva, left eye; chorioretinal coloboma, left eye	None	Double urinary collecting system	None

Table 37.1. (continued)

	Electroenceph-alogram	Special Neurologic Studies	Central Nervous System	Eye	Oral Cavity	Other Organs	Other Skin Lesions
Case 2	Left focal spikes	Pneumoen-cephalo-gram: enlarged left lateral ven-tricle	Left cortical atrophy	Conjunctival vascularity, left eye	None	None	Hemangioma of the penis
Lovejoy and Boyle, 1973 [18]							
Case 1	Bursts, sharp waves, and spikes, right hemisphere	Normal scans	—	None	Papules, right buccal mu-cosa	None	None
Case 2	Normal	—	—	—	Ameloblas-toma, right mandible	None	Verrucous nevi, trunk
Mollica et al., 1974 [19]	—	—	Leptomen-ingeal he-mangioma	Lipodermoid, conjunctiva	None	Patent ductus; cyst, liver; horseshoe kidneys	Angiomas, scalp
Challub et al., 1975 [20]	Diffuse spike wave, right-sided em-phasis	CT: poren-cephaly on right; angio-gram: blocked venous si-nuses	—	None	None	None	Hemangioma, scalp
Campbell et al., 1978 [21]	Left temporal slowing and sharp waves	CT and arteri-ogram: vas-cular anomaly left hemisphere	—	Left ptosis; conjunctival telangiecta-sia	None	None	None
Clancy et al., 1985 [22]							
Case 3	Disorganized on right with multi-focal spikes; Lennox–Gastaut	CT: right hemimeg-alencephaly; low densi-ties in white matter; dys-myeliniza-tion	—	None	None	None	None
Case 4	Left temporal slow and sharp	CT: left hemi-sphere atro-phy and ventricular dilatation; low densi-ties, left temporal, right frontal regions; left lesion en-larged over time	Left temporal vascular ha-martoma with dys-plastic cor-tex	Lipodermoid cyst, left eye; colo-boma, left optic nerve	None	None	None
Case 6	Normal	CT: bilateral macroen-cephaly	—	Bilateral exo-tropia; hy-pertelorism	Anomalous dentition	Pulmonary stenosis; midfacial hypoplasia	—

Capillary hemangiomas have also been described in several patients. Other lesions include areas of hypopigmentation and focal dermal hypoplasia.

The Nervous System

Table 37.2 summarizes the neurologic findings in 22 children who have been reported in the English literature as having the neuroectodermal form of the disorder. Sixteen of the 22 had seizures, which in all cases began prior to the first 8 months of life. In 5 patients, the seizures began within the first week of life. The epileptic manifestations of the disorder were variable. Eight children had generalized tonic or tonic–clonic seizures; 4 had focal motor seizures; 3 had infantile spasms; and 2 had recurrent apneic attacks that were considered to be a manifestation of epilepsy. Four children had prominent changes in their activity level, notably lethargy.

Thirteen of the 22 children were considered to be retarded. Most were severely or profoundly retarded but at least 3 had IQs of 50 or above. Many children were not formally tested. One child was considered to have multiple learning deficits, including impaired visual perception and perceptual motor skills. Six of the children had hemiparesis; 2 of those 6 had paralysis of facial movement on the side contralateral to the weak extremities. One child had a spastic quadriparesis while another was described as diffusely hypertonic and a third as diffusely hypotonic. Two children had hemianopias, and 1 was cortically blind.

With the exception of the electroencephalogram, laboratory tests were relatively benign. Of the 11 children who had their cerebrospinal fluid analyzed, only 1 had a definite abnormality, an increased protein level on two occasions. No reason for this abnormality could be discovered. Eighteen children had skull radiographs. In 2 patients, one orbit was enlarged when compared to the other. Two other children had hemicranial enlargement. One child had a widened sella, and 1 child had a small sella. The remaining patients had normal skull radiographs. Twenty children had electroencephalograms described although only 18 had neurologic deficits. Three had normal electroencephalograms. The remainder had epileptiform abnormalities or sharp waves that were either localized or that recurred as diffuse or multifocal bursts. Hypsarrhythmia was noted in 1 child. In 10 of the 11 children who had focal paroxysmal electroencephalographic abnormalities, the epileptiform focus was ipsilateral to the major skin lesions.

In only about half of the patients who had neurologic symptoms or signs was the cerebral morphology evaluated either radiographically or anatomically. With the exception of an enlarged ipsilateral lateral ventricle or an ipsilateral porencephaly that was present in 6 of the 11 cases evaluated by pneumoencephalography or by computed tomography, the lesions have been multiple and nonspecific, including bilateral cerebral atrophy, focal cortical atrophy, hypodense white matter, bilateral macrencephaly, and hamartomas [22,23]. One patient also had a left frontal arachnoidal cyst that overlaid an area of cortical dysgenesis. Four patients had some type of intracranial vascular abnormality. The patient of Challub et al. [20] who had a porencephaly also had evidence of multiple blocked venous sinuses on angiography. A second patient had a vascular anomaly of the left hemisphere [21]. A third had a left temporal vascular hamartoma that overlaid a dysplastic cortex [22]. A fourth patient had a leptomeningeal hemangioma at autopsy [19].

The entire group of radiographic and pathologic abnormalities appears to reflect disordered growth in some instances and disordered replication and migration in others.

Involvement of Other Organs

In those patients who have central nervous system disease with a midline linear sebaceous nevus, the eye is the other most commonly involved organ.

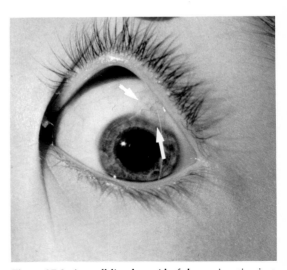

Figure 37.3. A small lipodermoid of the conjunctiva just above the iris of the eye opposite to the side in which there is a linear sebaceous nevus.

Many different abnormalities affect the eye, and as is the case in the brain, these reflect either abnormalities in cell migration or problems of growth. Thus, the two most common eye lesions are dermoid or lipodermoid lesions of the conjunctiva (Figure 37.3) or cornea, or colobomas that may involve the iris, choroid, retina, optic nerve, or a combination thereof. Excessive conjunctival vascularity has been described in several cases, and in one case [17] there was a hemangioma of the sclera and conjunctiva of the left eye. Several children have had eye movement abnormalities of uncertain origin. Bilateral or alternating esotropias or exotropias have been noted that may be unrelated to the disorder. One patient [16] had a total left third nerve palsy of unknown cause.

Organs derived from the mesoderm are involved in many patients who have a linear sebaceous nevus. In this group of children 10 of 22 had some type of

Table 37.2. Linear Sebaceous Nevus: Disease of Skin and Nervous System

	Lesion Biopsy Proven	Sex	Family History	Side of Major Lesions	Neurologic Symptoms	Neurologic Signs	Skull X-rays	Cerebrospinal Fluid
Feuerstein and Mims, 1962 [3]								
Case 1	Yes	M	Negative	Right	Generalized seizures at 7 weeks	Developmental retardation	Normal	Normal
Case 2	Yes	M	Negative	Left	Generalized seizures at 4 months	Developmental retardation	Normal	Normal
Marden and Venters, 1966 [8]	Yes	F	None	Bilateral	Apneic spells week 1 of life; generalized seizures at 3 months	Severe retardation	Widened sella	—
Moynahan and Wolff, 1967 [9]	—	M	None	Right	Infantile spasms at 5 months	Severe retardation	Left hemicranium smaller than right; small sella	—
Solomon and Fretzin, 1967 [10]	Yes	M	None	Left	None	Left hemiparesis and hemiatrophy; right facial paresis	Normal	—
Lantis et al., 1968 [11]								
Case 1	Yes	F	None	Left	None at age < 1 month	None	Left orbit > right	—
Case 2	Yes	F	None	Left	None at age < 1 month	None	—	—
Sugarman and Reed, 1969 [12]	Yes	F	Seizures in sister	Right	Generalized seizures at age < 2 years	Profound retardation; spastic quadriparesis	—	—
Bianchine, 1970 [13]	Yes	M	Convulsions and retardation in 3 of 4 sibs and father	Right	Generalized seizures; hyperactive	Verbal IQ: 66	Normal	Normal
Herbst and Cohen, 1971 [14]	Yes	F	None	Right	Extensor spasms at 5 months	Developmental retardation	Normal	Normal
Lansky et al., 1972 [15]								
Case 1	No	F	None	Right	Generalized seizures at 5 months; lethargy	None	Normal	Normal

Table 37.2. (continued)

	Lesion Biopsy Proven	Sex	Family History	Side of Major Lesions	Neurologic Symptoms	Neurologic Signs	Skull X-rays	Cerebrospinal Fluid
Case 2	No	M	None	Right	Generalized seizures at 8 months	Cortically blind; severe retardation	Normal	Normal
Case 3	No	F	None	Bilateral	Lethargy	None	Normal	Normal
Haslam and Wirtschafter, 1972 [16]	No	F	Ptosis in left eye of sib	Left	None	30 dB hearing loss in left ear	Right orbit > left; left sphenoid smaller than right	—
Holden and Dekaban, 1972 [17]								
Case 1	Yes	M	None	Left	Right focal seizures on day 2 of life	Severe retardation; right hemiparesis; hemisensory loss; inattention, right field	Normal	Normal
Case 2	Yes	M	None	Left	Right focal seizures at 3 months	Right field defect; increased DTR on right; severe retardation	Normal	Normal
Lovejoy and Boyle, 1973 [18]								
Case 1	Yes	M	None	Right	Recurrent-apnea at < 2 months	Severe retardation	Normal	Normal
Case 2	Yes	M	"Moles" on paternal side of family	Left	None	None	Normal	Increased protein
Mollica et al., 1974 [19]	Yes	F	None	Right	Lethargy	Hypertonic	—	—
Challub et al., 1975 [20]	Yes	F	Probably none	Right	Generalized seizures from birth	Hypotonic; hypoactive	Larger right hemicranium	White cells increased
Campbell et al., 1978 [21]	Yes	F	None	Left	Right focal seizures at 7 months	Right hemiparesis	—	—
Clancy et al., 1985 [22]								
Case 3	Yes	M	None	Right	Focal motor seizures on day 2 of life; infantile spasms at 5 months	Left hemiparesis and hemiatrophy; moderate retardation; IQ 50	—	Normal
Case 4	Yes	M	None	Left	Seizures on day 3 of life	Right hemiparesis; left facial atrophy; IQ 75	—	—
Case 6	No	F	None	Right	None	Impaired auditory and visual perception and perceptual–motor skills; clumsy	Macrocephaly	—

mesodermal abnormality. This percentage (41%) is similar to that seen for mesodermal involvement in other phakomatoses. Mesodermally derived organs also contain a variety of lesions that are not consistent from patient to patient and involve bone, the heart, the kidneys, and the face, and in one instance, the liver. The cardiac disorders described include pulmonary stenosis, patent ductus arteriosus, ventricular septal defect, wandering pacemaker, and coarctation of the aorta. Another patient had hypoplasia of the right renal artery reminiscent of the vascular narrowing noted occasionally in neurofibromatosis. Among the renal lesions were horseshoe kidneys, a double urinary collecting system, and nephroblastoma. Scoliosis, osteosclerosis, osteomalacia, and bone cysts have been seen. Mesodermal involvement does not seem directly related to the type or severity of the neurologic involvement or to the location or extent of the skin lesions.

Differential Diagnosis

The typical case of linear sebaceous nevus syndrome can usually be diagnosed by the appearance of the skin lesion. A slightly elevated, yellow-orange, smooth linear plaque that abuts the midline of the anterior scalp, forehead, distal nose, upper lip, or mental region can rarely be confused with other hamartomas of the skin. In the second decade of life the diagnosis can almost always be confirmed by biopsy because of the proliferation of sebaceous glands [6,7]. However, in the first decade of life in Morioka's series [7], excessive development of sebaceous glands was found in only 8 of 21 cases although one of those was age 3 months. In the remaining 13 cases sebaceous glands either were underdeveloped or were not found on histologic examination. Therefore, lesions that are more plaque-like than linear and do not occur at the midline of the anterior scalp or the face, but are located laterally on the scalp, the cheek, or the trunk may be confused with other varieties of organoid nevi that are also pigmented and hyperkeratotic.

Clancy et al. [22] question whether there is a real difference in the subclassification of organoid nevi into the epidermal nevus syndrome, the nevus unius lateris, linear verrucous epidermal nevus, and the linear sebaceous nevus. All of these lesions can be associated with neurologic abnormalities. The nevus unius lateris and epidermoid nevi tend to be composed of more discrete, darker papules with a less linear organization. These lesions are less often seen on the scalp and face than are those of the linear sebaceous nevus. Histologic abnormalities are generally limited to the epidermis and consist of hyperkeratosis and acanthosis along with epidermal papillomas. The dermis appears normal. In the linear sebaceous nevus, the dermis is abnormal, even in the first decade although the sebaceous glands may be normal or even slightly decreased in number and size. Hair follicles are always absent or underdeveloped and are replaced by strands of basaloid cells in the linear sebaceous nevus [6,7].

Later in life, as the lesions become more verrucous, juvenile melanomas, xanthoendotheliomas, xanthomas, and verruca vulgaris have to be thought of as part of the differential diagnosis [24].

Occasionally, early in life, if superficial eye involvement is the most prominent feature, a distinctly different neurocutaneous syndrome, encephalocraniocutaneous lipomatosis must be considered. These patients also have severe mental retardation and epilepsy associated with unilateral eye and skin lesions and ipsilateral cerebral malformations [25].

Pathophysiology

The cause of the linear sebaceous nevus syndrome is not known. While it has been postulated that it may be inherited as a dominant trait with highly variable penetrance, the great majority of patients have no known family history of similar skin lesions or of neurologic disease. Out of the 22 cases with neurologic symptoms or signs summarized in Table 37.1, 1 patient had a sister who had epilepsy [12], and a second patient had a strong family history of seizures and mental retardation which involved his father and 3 of his 4 sibs [13]. In no instance was there an immediate family member who also had a linear sebaceous nevus. The skin lesions are congenital hamartomas, present at birth, and Jadassohn felt that they were representative of abnormal embryonic development. Levin et al. [26] have interpreted dilatation of the lateral ventricle or widening of the subarachnoid space as consistent with hypoplasia due to defective neuronal migration rather than atrophy. This analysis was based upon the lack of history of an intrauterine insult in most of these patients. In their cases ventricular dilatation was usually ipsilateral to the skin lesion and was often associated with areas of low attenuation in the same hemisphere that they felt were consistent with heterotopic or dysplastic gray matter in other disorders such as tuberous sclerosis. While Levin et al. [26] had no pathologic confirmation of this interpretation, Clancy et al. [22] did have a single patient in whom such finding proved to be due to a hamartoma. Mesodermal lesions involving the heart, kidney, and bone also suggest problems in cellular organization early in development.

In many neurocutaneous diseases abnormalities of migration and cellular organization are associated with a propensity to form tumors. At least 20% of patients with the linear sebaceous nevus syndrome develop tumors of the skin. Levin et al. [26] felt that 3 of their 11 cases of linear sebaceous nevus had a brain tumor, either at surgery or by the image on CT scan. Levin et al. also remark on the increased tendency toward intracranial vascular proliferation that appears to be a reduction in growth restraint.

We are unaware of biochemical studies of growth factors in the linear sebaceous nevus syndrome or in related disorders. However, it seems to us that it must be more than a coincidence that many of the disorders associated under the rubric of the phakomatoses are neurocutaneous syndromes that couple disordered ectodermal and mesodermal migration and organization with an increased propensity to develop tumors. This suggests they share some related pathophysiologic mechanisms.

Prognosis and Management

The prognosis and treatment of this disorder depends upon whether the patient has neurologic involvement. The incidence of involvement of the nervous system in patients who have these skin lesions is not known, but is certainly under 50%. Most who have involvement of the CNS have lesions of the face and/or scalp [3]. However, muscle weakness due to vitamin D resistant rickets has recently been reported which suggests that in a small number of patients neuromuscular symptoms may be the result of endocrine or metabolic changes seen in this syndrome [27].

If there is no neurologic involvement, in many patients the skin lesions can be removed surgically. This is advisable when the lesions are circumscribed because of the tendency toward tumor formation later in life. The only neurologic symptoms amenable to treatment are the seizures, although they are often refractory to the antiepileptic drugs currently available. Mental retardation is usually severe, but it is static or there is no significant loss of function later in childhood or in adult life.

References

1. Jadassohn J. Bemerkungen zeis Histologie der systematisierten Naevi und über "Talgdrusen-Naevi." Arch Dermatol Syph 1895;33:355–394.

2. Robinson SS. Naevus sebaceus (Jadassohn). Arch Dermatol Syph 1932;26:663–670.

3. Feuerstein RC, Mims LC. Linear nevus sebaceus with convulsions and mental retardation. Am J Dis Child 1962;104:675–679.

4. Serpas-de-Lopez RM, Hernandez-Perez E. Jadassohn's sebaceous nevus. J Dermatol Surg Oncol 1985;11:68–72.

5. Lentz CL, Altman J, Mopper C. Nevus sebaceus of Jadassohn: report of a case with multiple and extensive lesions and an unusual linear distribution. Arch Dermatol 1968;97:294–296.

6. Mehregan AH. Sebaceous tumors of the skin. J Cutan Pathol 1984;12:196–199.

7. Morioka S. The natural history of nevus sebaceus. J Cutan Pathol 1985;12:200–213.

8. Marden PM, Venters HD. A new neurocutaneous syndrome. Am J Dis Child 1966;112:79–81.

9. Moynahan EJ, Wolff OH. A new neurocutaneous syndrome (skin, eye and brain) consisting of linear naevus, bilateral lipodermoid of the conjunctivae, cranial thickening, cerebral cortical atrophy and mental retardation. Br J Dermatol 1967;79:651–652.

10. Solomon LM, Fretzin DF. An unusual neurocutaneous syndrome. Arch Dermatol 1967;96:732–773.

11. Lantis S, Leyden J, Thew M, et al. Nevus sebaceus of Jadassohn: part of a new neurocutaneous syndrome? Arch Dermatol 1968;98:117–123.

12. Sugarman GI, Reed WB. Two unusual neurocutaneous disorders with facial cutaneous signs. Arch Neurol 1969;21:242–247.

13. Bianchine JW. The nevus sebaceous of Jadassohn, a neurocutaneous syndrome and a potentially premalignant lesion. Am J Dis Child 1970;120:223–228.

14. Herbst BA, Cohen ME. Linear nevus sebaceus: a neurocutaneous syndrome associated with infantile spasms. Arch Neurol 1971;24:317–322.

15. Lansky LL, Finderbunk S, et al. Linear sebaceous nevus syndrome. Am J Dis Child 1972;123:587–590.

16. Haslam RHA, Wirtschafter JD. Unilateral external oculomotor nerve palsy and nevus sebaceous of Jadassohn. Arch Opthalmol 1972;87:293–300.

17. Holden KR, Dekaban AS. Neurological involvement in nevus unis lateris and nevus linearis sebaceus. Neurology (Minneap) 1972;22:879–887.

18. Lovejoy FH, Jr, Boyle WE, Jr. Linear nevus sebaceous syndrome: report of two cases and a review of the literature. Pediatrics 1973;52:382–387.

19. Mollica F, Pavone L, Nuciforo G. Linear sebaceous nevus syndrome in a newborn. Am J Dis Child 1974;128:868–871.

20. Challub EG, Volpe JJ, Gado MJ. Linear nevus sebaceous syndrome associated with porencephaly and nonfunctioning major cerebral venous sinus. Neurology (Minneap) 1975;25:857–860.

21. Campbell WW, Buda FB, Sorensen G. Linear nevus sebaceous syndrome: neurological aspects documented by brain scans correlated with developmental history and radiographic studies. Milit Med 1978;143:175–178.

22. Clancy RR, Kurtz MB, Baker D, et al. Neurologic manifestations of the organoid nevus syndrome. Arch Neurol 1985;42:236–240.

23. Moskowitz R, Honig PJ. Nevus sebaceus in association with an intracranial mass. J Am Acad Dermatol 1982;6:1078–1080.

24. Fitzpatrick TB, Eisen AZ, Wolff K, et al. Dermatology in general medicine. 2nd ed. New York: McGraw–Hill, 1979:501–502.

25. Fishman MA, Chang CSC, Miller JE. Encephalocraniocutaneous lipomatosis. Pediatrics 1978;61:580–582.

26. Levin S, Robinson RO, Aicardi J, et al. Computed tomography appearances in the linear sebaceous naevus syndrome. Neuroradiology 1984;26:469–472.

27. Carey DE, Drezner MK, Hamden JA, et al. Hypophosphatemic rickets/osteomalacia in linear sebaceous nevus syndrome: a variant of tumor-induced osteomalacia. J Pediatr 1986;109:994–1000.

Chapter 38
Cerebello-Trigemino-Dermal Dysplasia

MANUEL R. GOMEZ

A congenital anomaly involving the cerebellum, the trigeminal nerves, and the scalp is apparently an uncommon nonhereditary central nervous system malformation. Four patients with cerebello-trigemino-dermal dysplasia have been described since 1979 [1–3]. There are few cases in the earlier literature: In 1921 Kayser [4] reported a boy with bilateral congenital corneal anesthesia and difficulty swallowing and chewing who was unable to stand or walk and who died of pneumonia at the age of 3½ years; Pillat [5] in 1949 reported a patient with congenital trigeminal anesthesia and symmetrical hypoplasia of the hair and part of the temporal muscles but did not mention ataxia.

In a recent review of congenital trigeminal anesthesia Rosenberg [6] cataloged patients with this entity with other patients having in common a congenital sensory deficit of the skin innervated by the first division of the trigeminal nerves. The group thus formed includes patients with disorders as different from each other as Goldenhar's syndrome (oculo-auriculo-vertebral dysplasia), Möbius syndrome (congenital facial paralysis, horizontal gaze disturbance, and possible deficit of other cranial nerve nuclei), anophthalmia, and occipital encephalocele. These disorders seldom are accompanied by sensory deficit. We prefer to separate the disorder described here from other congenital anomalies involving the eyes, the skeleton, and other parts of the central nervous system at least until more is known about the etiology and pathogenesis of these malformations.

Clinical Symptoms

At birth all four recently reported patients [1–3] had an area of alopecia on the scalp, and in three of these the alopecia involved the parieto-occipital regions symmetrically (Figure 38.1). The cranial vault had a tower-like appearance due to occipital flattening. Hypertelorism was present. The patients kept their mouths open and had difficulty chewing due to weak masseter and temporal muscles. Their ability to smile and to sit and stand alone came late, and they did not walk independently until after 5 years of age. They all had facial analgesia in all three divisions of the trigeminal nerves. Being unprotected from accidental or self-induced facial and corneal injuries they had been left with scars. The patient reported by Gomez [1] had intentionally burned her forehead above the nasal bridge with an incandescent light bulb (Figure 38.1). Other patients had scarring of their nasal vestibules and nostrils from self-inflicted injuries.

Other significant findings were related to cerebellar hypoplasia. They had severe truncal ataxia so that at age 3 or 4 years they stood only if supported and at 5 years of age walked only with assistance. When the patients finally started walking independently, they often stumbled and fell.

All reported patients were mentally dull or frankly subnormal and had generalized hypotonia, tendon hyperreflexia, absent corneal reflexes, and a cloudy cornea from repeated trauma. Two patients were microcephalic [2], and one had bilateral upgoing toe signs [1]. Vision was greatly reduced in all patients due to the corneal scarring. One patient had alopecia predominantly in the frontal region where the skin was rough early in life but subsequently, as the child became older, it became smooth and remained alopecic.

Laboratory Findings

Pneumoencephalography and CT of the head have demonstrated cerebellar hypoplasia [2]. In addition, on two occasions the CT scan demonstrated fusion

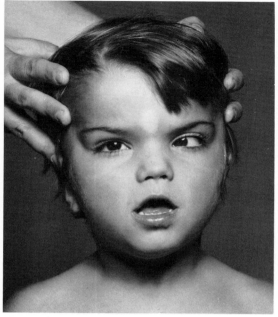
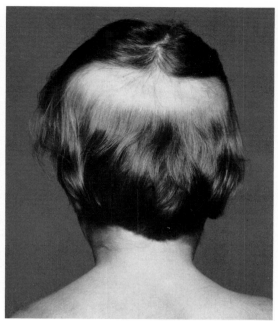

Figure 38.1. Patient with cerebello-trigemino-dermal dysplasia. Note the round scar above nose caused by an incandescent light bulb she placed against her forehead. Also note bilateral band-like area of alopecia in parietal region of scalp. (From Gomez [1]. With permission.)

of the vermis and pons [2]. Head radiographs demonstrate a tower skull as well as a flattened occiput caused by reduced posterior fossa volume. As expected, the cranial sutures closed prematurely in the microcephalic patients. In two patients histologic examination of the biopsied affected area of the scalp demonstrated a decreased number of hair follicles [2].

Differential Diagnosis

Congenital cerebellar ataxia may be the result of cerebellar hypoplasia that may or may not be associated with other disorders. The following entities have been described in patients with congenital cerebral ataxia:

- Nonprogressive cerebral ataxia, either sporadic or familial [7]
- Ataxia associated with moderate [7] or severe mental retardation [8]
- Ataxia associated with posterior fossa malformation and hydrocephalus (Dandy–Walker syndrome)
- Ataxia with mental retardation and partial aniridia [9,10]
- Ataxia with episodic hyperpnea, abnormal eye

movements, and mental retardation [11] or Joubert syndrome
- Ataxia with spastic diplegia, retinal coloboma, and mental retardation [12]
- Autosomal recessive cerebellar ataxia with cataracts and mental retardation [13,14] or Marinesco–Sjögren syndrome
- X-linked recessive ataxia with spasticity and mental retardation [15]
- Familial cerebellar ataxia with macular dystrophy and congenital pigmentation of the skin [16]
- Hereditary cerebellar ataxia, mental deficiency, pyramidal tract involvement, and macular pigmentation [17,18]
- Dysequilibrium syndrome [19,20]

Congenital corneal anesthesia is a rare disorder that has been reported unilaterally or bilaterally as an isolated finding, usually appearing in the first or second year of life. The patients are usually referred to ophthalmologists because of a corneal opacity or ulcer. When the sensation has been tested by corneal stimulation with a cotton wisp, it has been absent and remained so after the ulcer healed. In the pure form of congenital corneal anesthesia patients exhibit no other clinical evidence of autonomic dysfunction, congenital anhidrotic ectodermal dysplasia, or vitamin A deficiency. Interstitial keratitis due to congenital syphilis does not appear this early in life, and although it causes clouding of the cornea there is no sensory deficit.

Although it has been suggested that this loss of corneal sensation is secondary to its desiccation or that it has contributed to the development of analgesia and anesthesia, the evidence is against such statements; nevertheless, healing of the ulcers and improvement of the keratitis with appropriate treatment has led to improvement of vision [21].

Congenital trigeminal anesthesia is often found in families with other neurologic lesions [22–24]. In a review and classification of congenital trigeminal anesthesia, Rosenberg [6] divided the 43 cases he had collected from the literature and from his own experience into three groups: In the first are 10 patients with isolated congenital trigeminal anesthesia, all of whom had bilaterally absent corneal sensation except for 3 who had absent sensation in one eye and decreased sensation in the other. Facial sensation was normal in 4 patients, decreased in 4, and absent in 2. The second group, formed by 21 patients, includes 3 of the 4 described in this chapter under the label cerebello-trigemino-dermal dysplasia. These 3 patients differ from the rest in this group in that all had ataxia, complete bilateral involvement of all three divisions of the trigeminal nerves, hypoplasia of the maxilla, and symmetrical focal alopecia of the parieto-occipital region of the scalp. The other 17 patients in this group had a variety of anomalies such as bilateral facial weakness, torticollis, anophthalmia, Duane's syndrome, sensorineural hearing loss, micrognathia, imperforate anus, bilateral club feet, hemifacial hypoplasia, harelip, cleft palate, and occipital meningoencephalocele. Ten of these patients were diagnosed with oculo-auriculo-vertebral dysplasia (Goldenhar's syndrome). Finally, the third group is made by 2 patients with unilaterally absent ocular sensation, diminished sensation in the same side of the face, and either weakness of the ipsilateral facial and ocular abducens muscles or ipsilateral gaze palsy and internuclear ophthalmoplegia.

Pathogenesis

The cerebellum develops late in the human embryo and first appears as the rhombic lip, a swelling of the rhombencephalon on each side of the rostral portion of the membranous roof of the fourth ventricle. At 4 months of gestation these swellings have fused in the midline producing the vermis. At this age the semilunar ganglion of the trigeminal nerve has already been formed from migrating neural crest cells and thickened epidermis on each side of the head that formed placodes. Experimental studies have proven that the semilunar ganglion is formed by both neural crest cells and placodal cells [25]. The placodes (Figure 38.2) are formed by thickening of the epidermis, and their cells are the origin of the purely somatic sensory ophthalmic and maxillary divisions and the somatic sensory fibers of the mandibular division of the trigeminal nerve. The latter division also has visceral motor fibers, derived from ganglion cells, that are located in the metencephalic wall.

It thus appears that three neighboring structures in the embryo, the primordial cerebellar hemispheres, the placodes that give origin to the trigeminal nerve, and the epidermis of the occipito-parietal region that must originate from contiguous cells of the ectoderm, are affected in this dysplasia. Thus one can propose that failure of local epidermal development and of migration and multiplication of specific cells from a selective region in the ectoderm could cause hypoplasia or dysplasia of the cerebel-

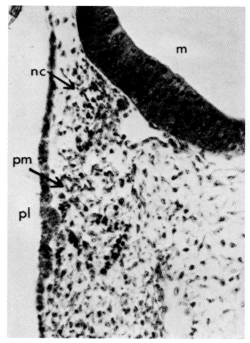

Figure 38.2. Cells of origin of the semilunar ganglion in the chick embryo. Abbreviations: m = medulla oblongata; nc = neural crest mesenchyme; pm = mesenchyme derived from placode; pl = trigeminal epidermal placode. (From Hamburger V. Specificity in neurogenesis. J Cell Physiol 1962;(suppl 1)60:81–92. With permission.)

lum, trigeminal nerves, and a parieto-occipital segment of the scalp.

Genetics

All four recently reported cases of cerebello-trigemino-dermal dysplasia belong to different families and only two are from the same country. It affects both sexes. There is insufficient data from so few cases to catalog their disease as hereditary. Chromosomal studies were normal in the two patients from Mexico [2].

Treatment

To prevent self-induced abrasions, treatment of congenital trigeminal anesthesia should be instituted as soon as anesthesia of the cornea is detected. Unfortunately, corneal anesthesia is seldom recognized before self-induced trauma and scarring have occurred. Gloves, hand bandages, or arm restraints may be necessary. The children need gait training, protection from frequent falls, and special education at school. Accidental burns and cuts constitute a serious hazard in these patients who have a double handicap: corneal–facial anesthesia and mental subnormality.

References

1. Gomez MR. Cerebello-trigeminal and focal dermal dysplasia: a newly recognized neurocutaneous syndrome. Brain Dev 1979;1:253–256.
2. López-Hernández A. Craniosynostosis, ataxia, trigeminal anesthesia and parietal alopecia with pons-vermis fusion anomaly (atresia of the fourth ventricle). Neuropediatrics 1982;13:99–102.
3. Pascual-Castroviejo I. Displasia cerebelotrigeminal. Neurologia Infantil. Barcelona: Editorial Cientifico–Medica, 1983;1:680.
4. Kayser B. Ein Fall von angeborener Trigeminuslähmung und angeborenem totalem Tränenmangel. Klin Mbl Augenheilkd 1921;66:652–654.
5. Pillat A. Wiener Ophthalmologische Gesellschaft. Epithelschädigung der Hornhaut bei angeborener Trigeminushypoplasie. Wien Klin Wochenschr 1949;61:605.
6. Rosenberg ML. Congenital trigeminal anesthesia: review and classification. Brain 1984;107:1073–1082.
7. Schutt W. Congenital cerebellar ataxia. In: Walsh G, ed. Little club clinics in developmental medicine. London: Heinemann, 1963;8:83–90.
8. DeHaene A. Agénésie partialle du vermis du cervelet à caractère familial. Neurol Belg 1955;55:622–628.
9. Gillespie FD. Aniridia, cerebellar ataxia and oligophrenia in siblings. Arch Ophthalmol 1965;73:338–341.
10. Sarsfield JK. The syndrome of congenital cerebellar ataxia, aniridia and mental retardation. Dev Med Child Neurol 1971;13:508–511.
11. Joubert M, Eisenring JJ, Robb JP, et al. Familial agenesis of the cerebellar vermis: a syndrome of episodic hyperpnea, abnormal eye movements, ataxia and retardation. Neurology 1969;19:813–825.
12. Pfeiffer RA, Palm D, Junemanr G, et al. Nosology of congenital non-progressive cerebellar ataxia. Neuropaediatrie 1974;5:91–102.
13. Marinesco G, Dragonesco S, Vasiliu D. Nouvelle maladie familiale caracterisée par une cataracte congénitale et un arrêt du développement somato-neuropsychique. Encephale 1931;26:97–109.
14. Sjögren T. Hereditary congenital spinocerebellar ataxia accompanied by congenital cataract and oligophrenia. Conf Neurol 1950;10:293–308.
15. Seemanova E, Lesńy I, Hyánek J, et al. X-chromosomal recessive microcephaly with epilepsy, spastic tetraplegia and absent abdominal reflexes, new variety of Paine syndrome? Humangenetik 1973;20:113–117.
16. Ledic H, van Bogaert L. Hérédodégénérescence cérébelleuse et spastique avec dégénérescence maculaire. J Genet Hum 1960;9:140–157.
17. Singh SD, Husain S. Hereditary cerebellar ataxia, mental deficiency, pyramidal involvement and macular pigmentation. Ind Med J 1964;31:355–358.
18. Stewart RM. Amentia, familial cerebellar diplegia and retinitis pigmentosa. Proc R Soc Med 1937;30:849–850.
19. Hagberg B, Sanner G, Steen M. The dysequilibrium syndrome in cerebral palsy. Acta Paediatr Scand 1972;(suppl) 226:63.
20. Sanner G. The dysequilibrium syndrome. Neuropaediatrie 1973;4:403–413.
21. Carpel EF. Congenital corneal anesthesia. Am J Ophthalmol 1978;85:357–359.
22. Segall W. Congenital neuroparalytic keratitis. Am J Ophthalmol 1955;39:334–335.
23. Schenk H. Hornhautbefunde bei idiopathischer Anästhesie der Hornhaut. Klin Mbl Augenheilkd 1958;133:506–518.
24. Verrey A, Jéquier M. Kératites neuroparalytiques familiales. Bull Soc Trans Ophthalmol 1949;62:171–178.
25. Hamburger V. Experimental analysis of the dual origin of the trigeminal ganglia in the chick embryo. J Exp Zool 1961;148:91–124.

Chapter 39
Encephalo-Cranio-Cutaneous Lipomatosis

MARVIN A. FISHMAN

Haberland and Perou [1], in 1970, reported the clinical and necropsy findings of a 5½-year-old epileptic, mentally retarded boy. They suggested that the patient had a previously unreported neurocutaneous syndrome, which they called encephalo-cranio-cutaneous lipomatosis. The salient features included unilateral cutaneous abnormalities of the face, eye, and scalp accompanied by ipsilateral malformations of the brain. Fishman et al. [2] subsequently reported two additional cases with similar cutaneous, ophthalmologic, and cerebral malformations who were not as mentally retarded as the original patient. A fourth youngster has been studied, and one of the previously reported patients has now been followed for 14 years during which time additional clinical features have been observed.

Clinical Features

The following information summarizes the experience with the current series of three cases, two males and one female. All cases have been sporadic, and there have been no family histories of similar or other neurocutaneous disorders.

All three patients had epilepsy. The onset of seizures occurred during the neonatal period or early infancy. In two patients, the seizures were focal or unilateral and occurred on the side contralateral to the cerebral malformation. In one patient, the seizures were generalized. Occasionally, the convulsions were precipitated by minor head trauma. The epilepsy was relatively well controlled with antiepileptic drugs in all patients but persisted even though there were periods of years during which no seizures occurred.

Testing of intellectual function revealed IQ scores between 65 and 75.

The cutaneous abnormalities involved only the head and face and were unilateral (Figure 39.1). All patients had fleshy pterygium-like lesions on the sclera, which in two patients invaded the cornea. One patient had persistent posterior hyaloid vessels in the involved eye. One of the other patients had a dysplastic iris. Both of these patients had markedly impaired vision in the affected eye, related in part to scarring and corneal involvement. All patients had large, slightly protuberant, soft tissue masses of the scalp. They were located on one side of the cranium and did not cross the midline. The skin over the masses was devoid of hair. Multiple small papular lesions and skin tags were present on the face and eyelid in a unilateral distribution on the same side as the scalp lesions. One patient had a small pigmented nevus on the foot, ipsilateral to the other cutaneous malformations, and a second patient had five small (four of which were less than 1 cm) brown pigmented nevi located on both sides of the body. The pigmented lesions were not characteristic of neurofibromatosis and did not appear to be part of this syndrome.

Ill-defined bony protuberances were present on the skull, and were associated with the scalp lesions. All three patients had head circumferences at or greater than the 98th percentile. Two of the three had hemiparesis contralateral to the involved hemisphere and cutaneous lesions.

Radiology

The most striking and unique feature has been the appearance of the brain malformation which has been similar in all three patients (Figures 39.2 to 39.5). Computed tomography of the head revealed the hemisphere ipsilateral to the cutaneous lesions to be

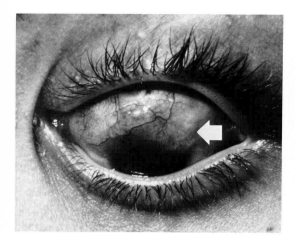

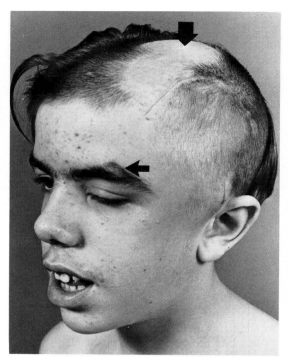

Figure 39.1. *(Left)* Fleshy pterygium-like lesion *(arrow)* on the sclera extending onto the cornea. A portion of the lesion has been surgically removed. *(Right)* Protuberant soft tissue scalp mass devoid of hair *(large arrow)*. Note raised skin lesion in area of eyebrow *(small arrow)*. The patient has recently had a craniotomy, and the short hair is in the process of growing back. It is usually long and of normal consistency and color.

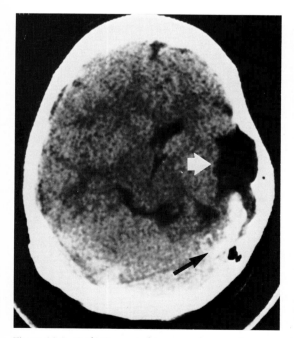

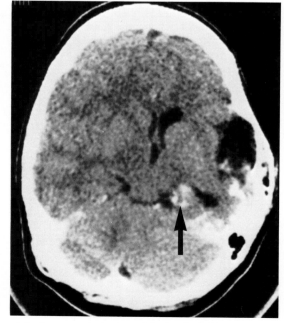

Figure 39.2. *(Left)* Computed tomography scan demonstrating defective opercularization of the insula *(white arrow)*, cortical calcification *(black arrow)*, and atrophy of the affected hemisphere. *(Right)* Contrast enhancing lesion (arrow) in the region of the cerebellopontine angle.

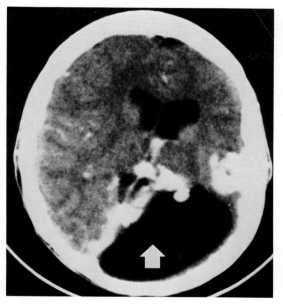

Figure 39.3. Computed tomography scan demonstrating a porencephalic cyst *(arrow)* occupying the posterior hemicranium, calcifications of the adjacent brain tissue, and atrophy of the hemisphere.

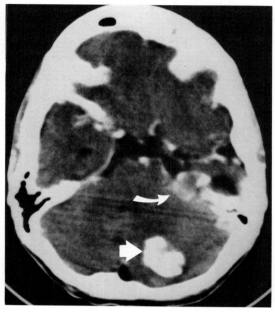

Figure 39.4. Computed tomography scan *(enhanced)* demonstrating a large calcification in the cerebellum *(large arrow)* and an enhancing lesion *(curved arrow)* in the region of the petrous ridge.

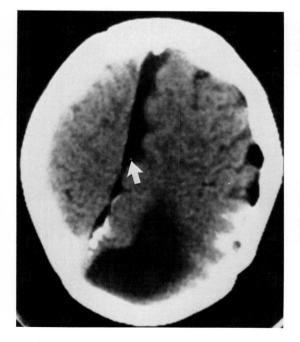

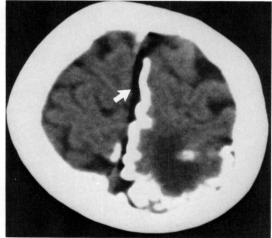

Figure 39.5. Computed tomography scans of two different patients demonstrating similar findings of calcifications of the cerebral hemispheres, the superior aspect of a porencephalic cyst, and a low-density area in the interhemispheric fissure *(arrows)* compatible with adipose tissue. In one patient *(left)* slight calcification of the medial aspect of the contralateral hemisphere is noted.

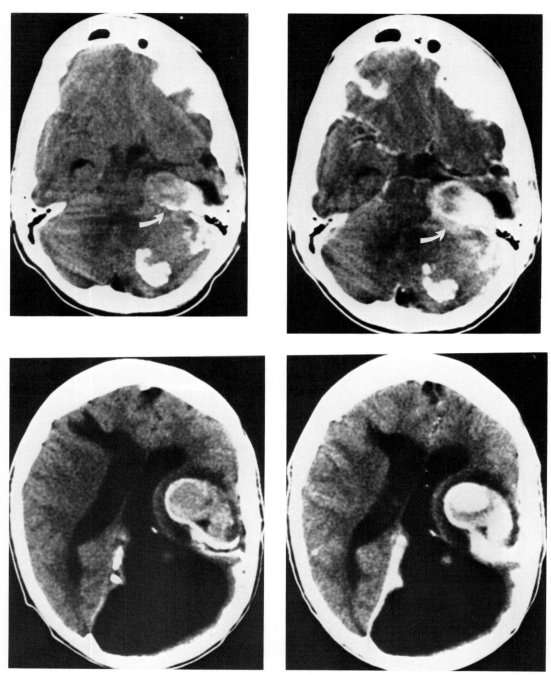

Figure 39.6. *(Top: left unenhanced, right enhanced)* Computed tomography scans demonstrating progression of the lesions *(curved arrows)* seen on prior scan (see Figure 39.4) performed 13 months earlier. *(Bottom: left unenhanced, right enhanced)* Computed tomography scans demonstrating a large lesion anterior to the porencephalic cyst. Both of these enhancing lesions were the partially thrombosed vascular malformations demonstrated in Figure 39.7.

atrophic. A large porencephalic cyst occupied the posterior aspect of the involved hemicranium. Enlargement of the extra-axial cerebrospinal fluid spaces over the involved hemisphere and defective opercularization of the insula were present. Localized widening of the diploic space of the skull was also noted. Progressive abnormalities occurred during serial studies. Striking calcifications involving the ipsilateral cerebral and cerebellar hemispheres developed. Some of these have followed the contour of the hemisphere. In one case, calcifications were noted in the cortices adjacent to the interhemispheric fissure. This has been the only involvement of the contralateral cerebral hemisphere. Areas of extremely low density, consistent with adipose tissue, were demonstrated in the subarachnoid space. A contrast-enhancing lesion near the base of the brain has been noted in two of the older patients.

In one patient significant increases in the size of that lesion and a calcified hemisphere lesion occurred over a 13-month period. Both lesions enhanced significantly after the administration of contrast material (Figure 39.6). Cerebral angiography revealed both lesions to be partially thrombosed saccular-type vascular malformations (Figure 39.7). These lesions were not seen during an angiogram performed in the neonatal period.

Pathology

Biopsy of the scleral lesion revealed the presence of a choristoma composed of lipoid and dermoid tissues and cartilage. The scalp lesion consisted of adipose tissue intermixed with large blood vessels. The overlying epidermis lacked rete ridges, and the underlying dermis did not contain epidermal appendages and consisted of prominent fibrous tissue and increased numbers of large blood vessels. Excisional biopsy of a lesion in the region of the eyebrow revealed a neurofibroma. Biopsies of the papular lesions and skin tags have revealed papillomas and connective tissue nevi.

The only postmortem examination performed was reported by Haberland and Perou [1]. Examination of the skull revealed hyperostosis in the frontal and orbital regions and enlargement of the diploic space by a mixture of fat and hematopoietic tissue. Examination of the nervous system revealed extra-axial lipomas on the side of the atrophic hemisphere. These were attached to the skull and the cranial nerve roots and one extended above and below the foramen magnum from the level of the medulla oblongata to the cervical cord. There was lipoangiomatosis of the meninges, that is, thick, gelatinous, and highly vascularized membranes, containing islands of fatty tissue. Microscopic examination revealed an increase in connective tissue, fibroblasts, embryonic mesenchymal cells, capillaries, thin-walled veins, and thickened arteries. The ipsilateral cerebral hemisphere contained polymicrogyria. An oval-shaped defect occupied the anterior temporal lobe. It extended through the entire thickness of the cerebral wall and communicated with the temporal horn. The frontal operculum was absent, the white matter hy-

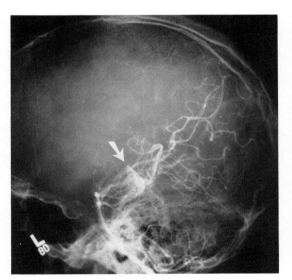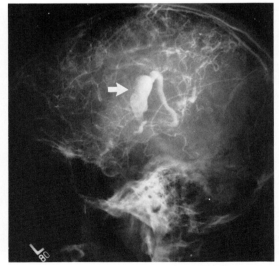

Figure 39.7. *(Left)* partially thrombosed vascular malformation *(arrow)* seen in Figure 39.6 top. *(Right)* Partially thrombosed vascular malformation *(arrow)* seen in Figure 39.6 bottom.

poplastic, and the lateral ventricle enlarged. The contralateral cerebral hemisphere was normal. Histologic examination revealed a four-layered cortical lamination. There was a well-developed external molecular layer and a broad pyramidal layer that was divided into two sublayers by an acellular strip. Glial heterotopias were present, and these were also found in the ipsilateral cerebellum and contralateral medulla. Calcifications ranging in size from small granules to large concretions were noted in the outer cortical lamina and the subcortical white matter.

The only other organ involved, the heart, had subepicardial fat, lipomatous infiltration in the atrial myocardium, and perivascular fat in the ventricular myocardium.

Pathogenesis

Although there are defects in tissues of mesodermic and ectodermic origin, the mechanism responsible for the malformations is unknown. Haberland and Perou [1] speculated as to whether the ectodermal malformations are manifestations of the same basic defect responsible for the mesenchymal malformations or whether they were secondary to the mesodermal dysgenesis. In the fourth to fifth week of gestation the mesoderm covers the brain and spinal part of the neural tube with mesenchymal cells that give rise to connective tissue, blood vessels, cartilage, bone, and adipose tissue. If the cerebral malformation is considered a part of the failure of the neural tube to develop and differentiate, then the timing when this event occurred is the same as that of the mesenchymal abnormality and would perhaps be related in origin. However, if the hemispheric defect is secondary to impaired blood supply, the time when the insult occurred would have been after the second month of embryonic life and be secondary to the mesenchymal defect.

Course

The oldest patient is now 16½ years old. The intellectual impairment has remained static. The epilepsy, as previously mentioned, has been relatively easy to control. Hyperactivity and attention deficit have been common complaints. Two patients have developed unilateral throbbing headaches ipsilateral to the cerebral malformation. In one patient, the headaches were accompanied by numbness of the tongue, face, and limbs, resembling migraine.

Two patients have experienced recurrent episodes of transient hemiparesis and in one patient it was accompanied occasionally by transient aphasia. The deficits have improved over hours to days except in one patient whose hemiparesis became gradually worse. Repeat CT scans at the time of the deficits revealed no new changes. Examination of the cerebrospinal fluid in one patient revealed no evidence of bleeding. However, when the oldest patient experienced an acute severe unilateral headache, more severe than any previous one, accompanied by exacerbation of the hemiparesis and meningismus, the cerebrospinal fluid was xanthochromic, and cerebral angiography revealed vascular malformations (Figure 39.7). In another patient cerebral angiography did not disclose occlusive vascular disease, arteritis, or vascular malformation but mild irregularities in the caliber of some of the arteries. Thus no anatomic lesion was found to explain the patient's recurrent symptoms. Nevertheless, intermittent deficits suggest a vascular mechanism that remains to be determined.

Differential Diagnosis

The presence of unilateral lesions of the eye, scalp, and face combined with the striking unilateral cerebral malformation appears to characterize this unique syndrome, which is unlike any other neurocutaneous disorder. There is superficial resemblance to other neurocutaneous syndromes, such as the Sturge–Weber syndrome, the linear sebaceous nevus syndrome, and neurofibromatosis.

The Sturge–Weber syndrome is characterized by epilepsy, intracranial calcifications, hemianopia, glaucoma, mental retardation, hemiplegia, and cutaneous vascular nevi affecting the upper part of the face [3]. All of these features may not be present in every patient. The present syndrome differs in the cutaneous manifestations, which do not include vascular nevi. The intracranial pathology is also different. The pattern of intracranial calcifications, which may appear superficially similar, is different. Both conditions have a gyriform pattern of calcifications in the cerebral cortex but the double line of calcification along cerebral sulci seen in Sturge–Weber syndrome has not yet been described in encephalo-cranio-cutaneous lipomatosis. The isolated large calcifications noted in the cerebellar hemisphere in this syndrome have not been described in Sturge–Weber syndrome. The characteristic porencephaly, the lack of opercularization of the insula, and the lipomatosis noted in all of the present patients do not occur in the Sturge–Weber syndrome.

Choristomas, epilepsy, and mental retardation,

present in these patients, also occurs in the linear sebaceous nevus syndrome. The cutaneous lesions involve the face, most often in the midline, and are composed of hyperplastic sebaceous glands, atypical apocrine glands, and immature hair follicles. The cerebral malformations may include unilateral ventricular enlargement, hydrocephalus ex vacuo, arachnoid cyst, leptomeningeal hemangioma, porencephaly, and nonfunctioning of the major dural venous sinuses [4–8]. Thus the two syndromes share some common features but the cutaneous signs and the neuropathologic findings are different.

Several other clinical entities involving the skin, eyes, and brain have been described [9,10] that, although they may resemble the linear sebaceous nevus syndrome, are unlike the present syndrome because they have bilateral findings and different central nervous system lesions. Although occasional small pigmented skin nevi and a neurofibroma were noted in one of the patients with encephalo-craniocutaneous lipomatosis, there were no other features in common with neurofibromatosis.

Treatment

One patient initially thought to have hydrocephalus was treated with a ventriculoperitoneal shunt from the lateral ventricle of the unaffected cerebral hemisphere. Subsequent CT examinations revealed a small ventricular system but the persistence of a large porencephalic cyst. Her head circumference remained above the 98th percentile. Treatment of the headaches with analgesics, beta-adrenergic receptor blocking agents, antidepressants, and calcium channel blockers resulted in only a transient symptomatic improvement. The patient with the vascular malformation underwent clipping of the vessels feeding the anomaly, which produced only transient aggravation of his hemiparesis.

References

1. Haberland C, Perou M. Encephalocraniocutaneous lipomatosis. Arch Neurol 1970;22:144–155.
2. Fishman MA, Chang CSC, Miller JE. Encephalocraniocutaneous lipomatosis. Pediatrics 1978;61:580–582.
3. Alexander GL. Sturge–Weber syndrome. In Vinken PJ, Bruyn GW, eds. Handbook of clinical neurology. vol. 14. New York: American Elsevier 1972:223–240.
4. Feuerstein RC, Mims LC. Linear nevus sebaceous with convulsions and mental retardation. Am J Dis Child 1962;104:675–679.
5. Sugarman GI, Reed WB. Two unusual neurocutaneous disorders with facial cutaneous signs. Arch Neurol 1969;21:242–247.
6. Holden KR, Dekaban AS. Neurological involvement in nevus unilateris and nevus linearis sebaceous. Neurology 1972;22:879–887.
7. Mollica F, Pavone L, Nuciforo G. Linear sebaceous nevus syndrome in a newborn. Am J Dis Child 1974;128:868–871.
8. Chalub EG, Volpe JJ, Gado MH. Linear nevus sebaceous syndrome associated with porencephaly and nonfunctioning major cerebral venous sinuses. Neurology 1975;25:857–860.
9. Monahan RH, Hill CW, Venters HD. Multiple choristomas, convulsions and mental retardation as a new neurocutaneous syndrome. Am J Ophthalmol 1967; 64:529–532.
10. Moynahan EJ, Wolff OH. A new neurocutaneous syndrome consisting of linear nevus, bilateral lipodermoids of the conjunctivae, cranial thickening, cerebral cortical atrophy and mental retardation. Br J Dermatol 1967;79:651–652.

Chapter 40
Sturge–Weber Syndrome

MANUEL R. GOMEZ and
ELIZABETH M. BEBIN

The Sturge–Weber syndrome (SWS), also known as encephalotrigeminal angiomatosis, encephalofacial angiomatosis, angio-encephalo-cutaneous syndrome, vascular neuro-oculo-cutaneous syndrome, or Sturge–Kalischer–Weber syndrome, is a congenital malformation of cephalic venous microvasculature. It more commonly occurs on one side of the head than on both, at least in its full and typical expression.

History

Schirmer in 1860 [1] described the association of bilateral facial nevus angiomatosus and unilateral buphthalmos. The credit, however, belongs to Sturge [2] who gave also in 1879 a clear clinical description of this condition and predicted its cerebral pathology. The patient, a 6½-year-old girl, had a deep purple "mother's mark" on the right side of the head and face including the lips, gums, tongue, floor of mouth, palate, uvula, pharynx, and back of neck extending "as low as the third and fourth dorsal vertebrae behind and the second costal cartilage in front." The right eye was larger than the left. The patient had "attacks of twitching in her left side affecting the face, arm and leg," lasting 10 or 12 minutes since the age of 6 months. As she grew older the seizures became stronger and were followed by temporary weakness. By age 5 years she had loss of consciousness with the attacks. Sturge cleverly deduced that an underlying flat vascular nevus over the cerebral cortex gave rise to the partial seizures.

Kalischer [3] was the first to confirm pathologically what Sturge had predicted. Weber [4] reported the radiographic intracranial calcifications, Dimitri [5] described the characteristic double-contoured lines, and Krabbe [6] correctly interpreted these lines as calcifications of the cerebral cortex, not of the

walls of cerebral vessels. Van der Hoeve [7] classified SWS as another phakomatosis thus muddling a concept he had introduced earlier to encompass tuberous sclerosis, neurofibromatosis, and von Hippel–Lindau disease.

Choroidal angioma, first reported by Jennings Milles in 1884 [8], was extensively described by Rosen [9]. Cerebral hemisphere hypoplasia, reported in 1901 by Kalischer in his second paper on the subject [10], and focal microgyria [11] are uncommon.

Definition

The complete SWS consists of cerebral, ocular, and facial symptoms and signs. In the complete form it consists of a telangiectatic venous angioma of the leptomeninges overlying the occipital, the parieto-occipital regions, or the entire cerebral hemisphere; ipsilateral facial angiomatous nevus; and choroidal angioma. The facial cutaneous angioma, nevus flammeus, or port-wine stain occupies at least the upper part of the face, that is, the forehead, eyelids, and conjunctiva, and may extend to contiguous areas of the face and even the neck, trunk, and extremities on either side of the cerebral lesion (Figure 40.1). Partial or generalized seizures, hemiparesis, hemianopsia, or hemiatrophy all contralateral to the cortical lesion, and ipsilateral choroidal angioma, with or without buphthalmos or glaucoma, complete the clinical picture.

The incomplete SWS may consist of one of the following combinations:

- Facial and leptomeningeal angioma and cerebral symptoms but no glaucoma (not even choroidal angioma)
- Clinical/radiologic evidence of cerebral and lep-

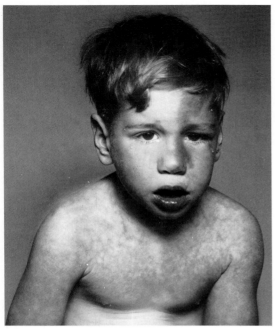

Figure 40.1. In this patient nevus flammeus occupies the left side of the face, including the forehead and upper eyelid, the left side of the nose and mucosa of the lips, as well as both the upper extremities and the upper part of the chest.

tomeningeal nevus and choroidal angioma but no facial nevus [12]

- Facial nevus and choroidal angioma without clinical but with radiologic evidence of cerebral angiomatosis
- Cerebral and leptomeningeal angiomatosis alone [12]

The lack of cerebral or ocular symptoms in patients with the facial nevus does not preclude future cerebral or ocular symptomatology.

It does not seem appropriate to use the name SWS when neither cerebral nor ocular symptoms have appeared, or for choroidal angioma with buphthalmos but without facial nevus and cerebral involvement. The head radiograph of a young patient with leptomeningeal angiomatosis is often normal and only computed tomography, magnetic resonance imaging, or cerebral angiography will demonstrate the characteristic findings of SWS.

Epidemiology

The syndrome affects both sexes and all races. There is a slight male predominance [13,14]. There is no known racial or geographical preference. The prevalence is unknown but judging from reported clinical observations it is less common than either neurofibromatosis or tuberous sclerosis.

Clinical Features

Facial Nevus Angiomatosus

The skin lesion is first seen at birth as a purplish-red flat facial angiomatous nevus, the so-called port-wine stain (Figure 40.2) or nevus flammeus. This is the most recognizable feature of SWS. Its absence does not exclude the diagnosis of leptomeningeal angiomatosis and cerebral involvement as seen in SWS. Thanks to technological advances in imaging methods, the diagnosis of this type of angiomatosis can be made in patients who lack the facial nevus. It may be argued that the facial nevus is an integral part of the syndrome Sturge described [3]. This is historically correct but from a practical point of view patients with leptomeningeal nevus and no facial nevus [12,14–16] are not clinically different from those with the complete syndrome.

It has been noted that when the facial nevus flammeus is present, it always involves that part of skin

Figure 40.2. Nevus flammeus of the left side of the face in addition to parts of the trunk, the left upper extremities, and both lower extremities.

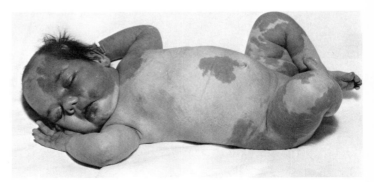

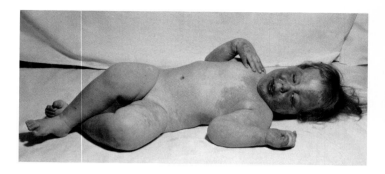

Figure 40.3. Nevus flammeus that involves both sides of the face, the upper trunk, and the upper extremities. Note that the left-sided lesion but not the right-sided lesion comes to the midline on the forehead.

innervated by the first division of the trigeminal nerve [14,15,17]. The nevus besides occupying the area of skin innervated by the first division of a trigeminal nerve, may, and often does, involve areas of skin innervated by the other two ipsilateral divisions and even contralateral regions of the face (Figure 40.3). Also the neck, trunk, and extremities on one or both sides may be involved (Figures 40.1 to 40.3). The lower extremities are more often involved than the upper [18]. The nevus may be on the lips, mucosa of the palate, tongue, gums, cheeks, pharynx, or larynx. Occasionally there is hypertrophy of the underlying soft tissues of the face (Figure 40.4), trunk, or extremities.

In a study done at the Mayo Clinic 30 years ago [19], 5 of 35 patients (14%) with SWS had no facial nevus although clinical and radiographic findings were characteristic of the disease. At present the number of patients without nevus seen in this institution has increased to 13 of the total 101 patients with SWS (13%). A large number of patients have bilateral facial nevi but this does not necessarily mean bilateral cerebral involvement and vice versa [14].

Seizures

The first cerebral symptoms appear, usually as partial motor seizures, in the first weeks or months of life, often with a jacksonian march. There may be unilateral or generalized seizures from onset. Seizures occur in 75 to 90% of all patients [14,18–20]. Partial motor seizures most often have their onset in the first months of life. As the patient gets older, the seizures may become more frequent and severe, progress with a jacksonian march, spread to the opposite side, and sometimes become generalized. Clinically, they may be generalized from onset even before 6 months of age. Myoclonic, tonic, or atonic seizures or infantile spasms are rarely the initial seizure type [20]. Postictal transient hemiparesis lasting minutes or hours is common and may be later replaced by a permanent hemiparesis or hemiplegia. Partial motor seizures with a jacksonian march may not begin until childhood or adult life. The frequency and severity of the seizures vary from one patient to another and probably depend on the extent of the cerebral lesion.

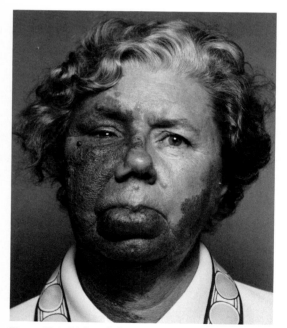

Figure 40.4. Right-sided nevus flammeus with additional involvement of parts of the left side of the face and neck. Note the hypertrophy of the lower lip, and to a lesser extent the right cheek, both upper and lower eyelids, and the right ala nasi.

Neurologic Deficit

The following findings are detected as the child grows older, and motor and sensory functions can be examined: spastic hemiparesis or hemiplegia, hemianopsia or cortical hemisensory deficit (astereognosis) contralateral to the cerebral lesion. At an early stage a hemiparesis or hemiplegia may be only transient postictally and then in the course of the disease may become permanent. Hemiparesis ipsilateral to the facial nevus but with hemispheric atrophy contralateral to the hemiparesis has been reported [18] and is probably indicative of bihemispheric disease even when the facial nevus is unilateral [11].

Either hemiplegia or hemiparesis is reported in 26% of patients of all ages [19] and in 18% of patients less than 14 years old, the majority of whom were less than 7 years old [18]. Hemiatrophy has been found in 31% of patients of all ages [19]. Spastic quadriplegia or quadriparesis, in reality a double hemiplegia or hemiparesis, is often found in patients with bilateral facial nevus but this is not necessary. Sensory deficit is difficult to estimate in those with hemiplegia, with severe mental handicaps, or in the very young patients. It is almost always associated with hemiatrophy after the first years of life. Hemianopia is almost always associated with seizures in patients younger than 3 months. Bilateral hemianopia or cortical blindness was present in 3 of the 12 patients with bihemispheric SWS who had bilateral or generalized seizures [14]. The association of hemiatrophy, hemianopia, and hemiplegia is uncommon in the first years of life. To our knowledge no seizure-free patient with SWS has been found to have mental deficit.

Mental Subnormality

There is much variation in the proportion of mental subnormality among patients with SWS. In the Mayo Clinic series published in 1958, 19 of 35 patients (54%) were mentally handicapped [19]. In a more recent and larger group of patients from the same place [14], 101 patients were grouped according to the involvement of one or both cerebral hemispheres and the occurrence or not of seizures. Of the 63 patients with unilateral lesions who had had seizures, only 21 (33%) had average intelligence, 13 (21%) had a severe mental handicap, and 23 (36%) were educable. The remainder were lost to follow-up. Of the 25 patients with unilateral lesions who never had seizures none is known to be mentally subnormal. Of the 13 patients with bihemispheric lesions only 1 never had seizures, and he was of normal intelligence. The intelligence of 12 patients who had had seizures ranged between borderline and severely subnormal, the majority being severely retarded [14].

This finding and the common clinical observation of regressed mental capacity that occurs in children with SWS after seizures begin, or when they increase in frequency, have practical value when planning therapy. Since the most devastating consequence of SWS is severe mental subnormality, and since this is always associated with generalized seizures that start early in life and continue without control for months or years, if anticonvulsant drug treatment fails, surgical treatment should be considered at an early stage for those patients with clinical, radiologic, and electrographic evidence of unilateral cerebral involvement [21,22].

Increased Intracranial Pressure

Macrocephaly has been recognized in patients with SWS alone or in association with Klippel—Trenaunay—Weber syndrome [23,24].

A 26-month-old infant with a variant of SWS reported by Fishman and Baram [24] had facial and truncal angiomatous nevi, unilateral glaucoma, seizures, hemiparesis, cerebral calcifications by CT scan, progressive macrocephaly, and bilateral periorbital venous distention from the age of 2 months. Serial CT scans revealed a large brain and slowly progressive dilatation of the cerebral ventricles and subarachnoid channels. Cerebral angiography showed dilated superficial cortical veins and absence of the deep galenic venous system. The encephalic venous drainage was through the cavernous sinus, and the ophthalmic, periorbital, and facial veins. The progressive hydrocephalus was corrected with a ventriculoperitoneal shunt. In this patient the impaired venous flow through the sagittal sinus and the galenic venous system must have been the cause of the increased intracranial pressure that led to hydrocephalus. Another infant has been reported [25] who had a similarly anomalous venous return associated with a nevus angiomatosus involving just the third division of the trigeminal nerve in the absence of glaucoma, seizures, and neurologic deficit.

Intracranial Hemorrhage

Cushing in 1906 reported three patients he surmised had suffered spontaneous intracranial hemorrhage from a "trigeminal vascular nevus" [26] although intracranial bleeding was undocumented. Cushing proposed that bleeding led to hemiplegia, hemianosia, seizures, or a combination of these signs.

A recently reported patient with SWS and subarachnoid hemorrhage [27] is probably the only documented case of this association in the medical literature: a 32-year-old woman with a left facial port-wine nevus also had right hyperreflexia, but no abnormal eye findings, and the head radiograph was negative. The angiogram showed rapid shunting through a "capillary angiomatous malformation in the basal ganglia, early filling of the deep veins and dilatation of the great vein of Galen in its proximal end," findings characteristic of SWS.

Eye Findings

Buphthalmos (hydrophthalmia) or glaucoma associated with a choroidal angioma are the characteristic eye findings. Approximately 30% of patients with SWS develop glaucoma and more than 50% of these have buphthalmos ipsilateral to the facial and leptomeningeal angioma [28] (Figure 40.5). The glaucoma may be bilateral even when the facial nevus is unilateral and vice versa. Unilateral glaucoma is rarely contralateral to the facial nevus [28].

Choroidal angioma occurs in about 40% of patients with SWS [9,28] and is usually found at the posterior eye pole temporal to the optic disc. It may be visible with the ophthalmoscope and has been occasionally mistaken for a malignant tumor such as

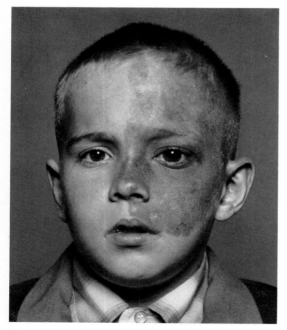

Figure 40.5. Left facial nevus flammeus and buphthalmos. Note the left megalocornea.

a melanoma, unfortunately leading to enucleation of the eye.

The pathogenesis of glaucoma has been explained with one of the following hypotheses: (a) the choroidal angiomatosis results in increased production of aqueous fluid; (b) there is a breakdown of the blood–aqueous barrier in the angioma creating a plasmoid aqueous that blocks the angle; (c) increased permeability of the capillaries allows for greater amount of aqueous fluid formation.

Other eye findings are heterochromia iridis, usually with the hyperpigmented iris ipsilateral [28], and a red discoloration of the ocular fundus that has been likened to "tomato-catsup" also ipsilateral to the nevus flammeus [29].

Laboratory Findings

Electroencephalography

The electroencephalogram is an important tool for the diagnosis and follow-up of patients with SWS.

Two types of findings have been described in the EEG of these patients: epileptiform and non-epileptiform. The most prevalent EEG finding is non-epileptiform: asymmetry of the background amplitude in the waking record, either posteriorly, anteriorly, or in the entire hemisphere. This asymmetry has been found in the EEG recording of patients before they had radiograph calcification. Other non-epileptiform EEG abnormalities that may be found are ipsilateral polymorphic delta activity, decreased hyperventilation buildup on the ipsilateral side, and asymmetric photic driving response with decrease on the ipsilateral side [29].

Epileptiform activity may be focal or generalized and symmetric or asymmetric. In a study of 16 patients, 4 showed ipsilateral focal discharge, and 2 showed bilateral multifocal independent discharges. In both groups the maximal abnormalities were ipsilateral to the decreased background amplitude or to the side of the radiographic calcification [30]. In 3 patients there were bisynchronous or generalized discharges either symmetric or decreased on the side of lower amplitude background activity or radiographic calcification in the skull.

Sleep recordings may reveal a focal discharge not present during the waking state. In 2 patients with bilateral calcification the background activity was asymmetric. The reduced background amplitude is not always proportional to the calcification [21,30]. Focal epileptiform discharges occurred only over the involved hemisphere whereas multifocal abnormalities even though bilateral were more frequent on the involved side [30]. The generalized bisynchronous discharges may vary in amplitude between the two sides, and are lower when the background amplitude is reduced.

Radiographic Studies

Dimitri in 1923 [5] described double-contoured linear images in the head radiographs of patients with SWS. These have been likened to "tram tracks" or "railroad tracks." Characteristically the radiopacity takes the form of two parallel sinusoidal lines that correspond to the calcifications within the cerebral cortex as pathologically proven by Krabbe [6]. The calcium granules deposited in the two cortices along a cerebral sulcus project onto the film two parallel linear "shadows" or attenuated x-ray images. Calcifications are rarely detected before the age of 1 year, although there have been rare instances of calcifications even in the newborn [31,32]. They are found in virtually all adult patients with complete SWS. The calcified lesion appears first or exclusively in the occipital region and over months or years as the calcium accumulation continues and spreads forward the railroad tracks become radiographically more extensive (Figure 40.6) and more opaque. As the disease progresses, the cortex becomes atrophic, demonstrated by the radiographs which show widening of the train tracks and the space between the cerebral cortex and calvarium. In cases of severe atrophy the head radiograph may reveal head asymmetry and in extreme cases microcephaly. Bilateral calcification indicative of bihemispheric involvement generally indicates a poor prognosis.

Computed tomography demonstrates calcium deposits from the first months of life, much earlier than plain radiography. The calcifications are more prominent in the posterior area and may be detected in regions of the brain in which no lesion is suspected, for instance, in the frontal lobe of the contralateral hemisphere, which thus permits the diagnosis of bilateral cerebral hemispheric disease (Figure 40.7). The head CT scan may also display cerebral atrophy better than angiography or the now obsolete pneumoencephalography [33–35].

The original angiographic study reported by Moniz and Lima in SWS [36] did not show any abnormality in the arterial phase. Subsequent studies [37–39] showed a diffusely increased density or stain homogeneously spread over the affected area thought to represent telangiectasias but with no evidence of increased arterial supply or enlargement of neighboring arterioles. Therefore, the persistent stain is caused by delayed cerebral venous drainage and not by increased regional blood supply. This is thought to be due to the basic vascular abnormality in SWS— the lack of cortical venous drainage toward the superior longitudinal sinus through superficial cerebral veins. The lesion may be only occipital, parieto-occipital, temporal, or frontal and, following contrast

Figure 40.6. Extensive intracranial calcification, cerebral atrophy, and microcephaly in a patient with bihemispheric Sturge–Weber syndrome.

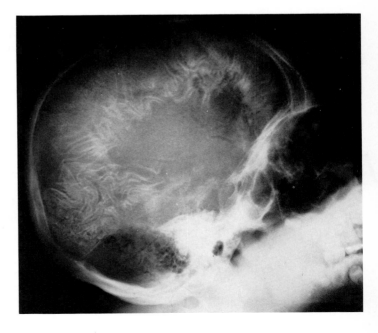

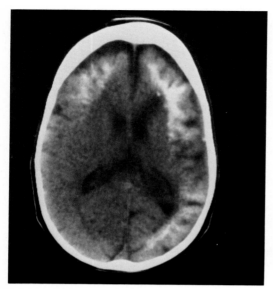

Figure 40.7. Head CT scan without contrast demonstrates extensive cortical–subcortical increased attenuation of the entire left hemisphere and the anterior portion of the right hemisphere in a 1-year-old boy with a left facial nevus flammeus.

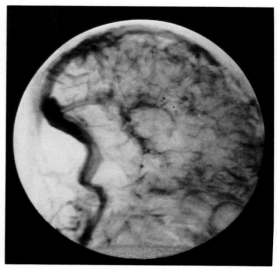

Figure 40.8. Angiogram of a patient with Sturge–Weber syndrome in the venous phase shows the lack of cerebral veins emptying into the anterior portion of the superior longitudinal sinus and scanty veins in the posterior portion of the sinus.

injection, will show that only a portion of the superior longitudinal sinus remains unopacified (Figure 40.8). The deep cerebral veins are enlarged, and the internal cerebral vein and the vein of Rosenthal on the affected hemisphere are most prominent [36] (Figure 40.8). Furthermore, there is enlargement and tortuosity of the deep medullary veins that originate 1 or 2 cm below the cerebral cortex and that run centrally toward the subependymal veins of the lateral ventricles and basal veins. These deep medullary veins usually are not visible in the angiogram of normal individuals but become visible in some pathologic states, that is, SWS, arteriovenous malformations, and gliomas.

Pathology

The facial nevus flammeus is a venous angioma with dilated and tortuous vessels on a region of the skin that embryogenically corresponds to the ectoderm that covers the telencephalon before it enlarges to become the cerebral hemispheres.

The most significant finding on gross inspection of the brain is the regional leptomeningeal angiomatosis, usually occipital, temporo-occipital, or parieto-occipital, either alone or of the entire cerebral hemisphere (Figure 40.9). The pia mater contains di-

lated and tortuous vessels, with the appearance of small veins, that may form several layers in the subarachnoid space but that rarely enter the brain. The profusion of pial vessels gives a purplish-blue color to the leptomeninges.

Microscopic examination often shows subintimal calcification of meningeal arteries [40]. Some of the leptomeningeal veins have a thick muscular coat but no elastic lamina [39]. The angiomatous vessels rarely penetrate the brain. Calcified cortical and subcortical veins may be found. In the cortex underlying the leptomeningeal angioma there is extensive calcification of one or both of the outer (Figure 40.10) and inner layers. When examined microscopically the calcium concretions are small spherules composed solely of calcium. Contrary to what was believed earlier, there is no iron deposited. The concretions of various sizes are confluent with each other and in early stages are found only on the walls of the smaller blood vessels [40]. In an advanced stage the molecular and outer pyramidal layers are largely replaced by calcium deposits. The calcification may be found only at an early stage of the disease, in the deep cortical layers and subcortical white matter, suggesting that calcification begins in the white matter before the cerebral cortex.

Laminal cortical necrosis with calcium deposits are also present, apparently in response to ischemic

Figure 40.9. Leptomeningeal angiomatosis of the occipito-temporal region of the left hemisphere. (From Craig JM. J Neuropathol Exp Neurol 1949;8:305. With permission.)

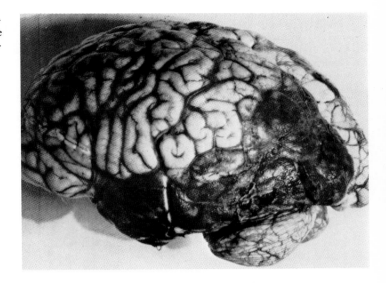

Figure 40.10. Leptomeningeal venous angioma and occipital cortex with cortical calcification (original magnification × 6; hematoxylin–eosin stain).

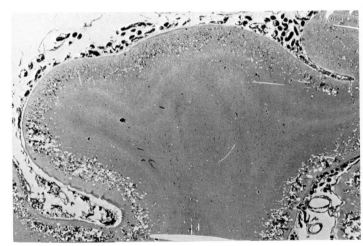

damage that is secondary to the venous stasis in the leptomeninges and in the cerebral capillary bed, which leads to tissue hypoxia, neuronal loss, and gliosis (Figure 40.11).

In some cases, however, instead of calcification the hemisphere, partially or totally, experiences arrested growth, which causes cerebral hemiatrophy or lobar atrophy. This is apparently the result of ischemia prior to cortical development.

The dura mater and the bone overlying the leptomeningeal nevus are rarely involved.

Chemical analysis of the cerebral cortex has disclosed an enormous amount of calcium, largely calcium carbonate, in both the white matter and the cortex. The iron content is the same as in controls [41,42].

A choroidal angioma that caused glaucoma is shown in Figure 40.12.

Pathogenesis

Some of the pathologic findings in the cerebral cortex are explained in part by the abnormal venous return pattern causing blood stagnation, hypoxemia, and impaired neuronal metabolism which must be particularly damaging in the rapidly developing and highly oxygen- and glucose-dependent brain of a young person [43]. The epileptic activity increases the metabolic rate of the cerebral cortex, thus augmenting the tissue demand for oxygen and glucose where there is already blood stagnation and hypox-

Figure 40.11. Leptomeningeal venous angioma and calcification of the superficial layers of the cerebral cortex (original magnification × 20; hematoxylin–eosin stain).

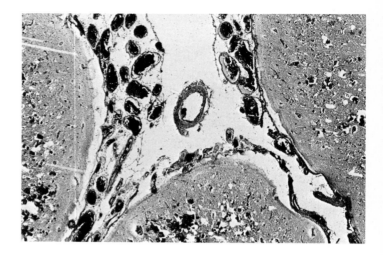

Figure 40.12. Choroidal angioma (original magnification × 20; hematoxylin–eosin stain).

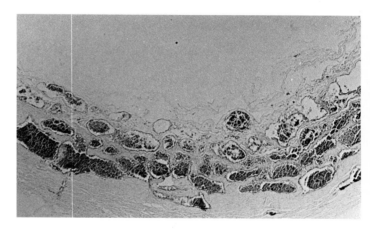

emia that lead initially to post-ictal hemiparesis and subsequently to permanent hemiplegia. The same probably applies to hemianopia and cortical hemi-sensory defects. Thus, in most patients with neurologic deficit a clinical picture of progressive aggravation of the symptoms is associated with the persistent seizures that at first affect only one side. Later, secondary epileptic foci appear in the presumably healthy contralateral cerebral hemisphere. In addition, the partial seizures later become generalized, although in some cases they are generalized from the onset. During this downhill course mental deterioration ensues which is faster and more severe than when the SWS is bihemispheric [14]. The patients who have bihemispheric lesions and seizures are always moderately or severely mentally defective, while those patients with uni- or bihemispheric lesions who never had seizures and some with unilateral or partial seizures, are of average intelligence [14].

The embryopathogenesis of the skin, leptome-ninges, and the choroid and brain lesions of SWS can be explained by a malformation of the primordial vascular plexus that originates in situ within the cephalic mesenchyma between the epidermis and the telencephalic vesicle. These structures are in close proximity to the optic cup from which the eye will develop. As the telencephalon enlarges, the occipital lobes gradually move dorsally, separating themselves from the epidermis of the forehead. The optic cup, however, remains in close proximity to the forehead and to the rest of the face. From the mesenchyma of the forehead a capillary network is formed, in the eye the choroid is formed, and from the same mesenchyma originates the leptomeningeal capillary network. Interference in an early stage with the vascular drainage being formed would then affect the face, the eyes, the leptomeninges, and the brain, including its occipital region.

It is still unexplained why the dura mater and cranial diploë remain for the most part unaffected, and why the pathology is in some cases unilateral and in others bilateral. Also unexplained is the existence of atypical patients with both sides of the face involved and only one side of the brain and vice versa, the combination of unilateral choroidal angioma with bilateral facial lesions and vice versa, and the association of SWS with Klippel–Trenaunay syndrome in some cases but not in others. All these observations serve to argue against a neural factor that affects blood vessel proliferation. Defying explanation too is the excessive amount of intracortical calcification and the sometimes selective calcification of the deeper layers of the cortex and the subcortical white matter that spares, at least initially, the superficial cortical layers.

Although there have been several reports of chromosomal abnormalities in patients with SWS, there is no convincing evidence that the few reported abnormalities are more than incidental findings not necessarily related to the pathogenesis of this disease.

Genetics

Koch [13] and Waardenburg [28] have reviewed the published genetic data and have addressed this aspect of SWS in detail.

The majority of the reported cases of SWS are sporadic. A few families have been reported in which a second member is affected with a similar vascular malformation or with an incomplete form of SWS. Although such cases are uncommon, they give some credence to the hypothesis that a hereditary factor plays a role in the development of angiomatous lesions in different parts of the body.

Monozygotic twins with concordant nevi have been reported [28,44]. A facial nevus flammeus in two family members without the complete SWS syndrome has also been recorded [28]. It is inconceivable that this syndrome is inherited in an autosomal dominant, recessive, or X-linked form since there are no two cases of complete SWS in a family among the hundreds of patients with complete SWS that have been recorded over a greater than 100-year period. One thus concludes that SWS is either not a genetic disorder or at most is multifactorial in origin and that one (or more) of the involved factors is (are) hereditary.

Associated Disorders

The association of SWS with developmental anomalies of the eyes, the central nervous system, or with other neurocutaneous diseases is rare and probably fortuitous.

Of particular interest is the association of the Sturge–Weber with the Klippel–Trenaunay syndrome (see Chapter 40). The patient reported as early as 1860 by Schirmer [1] apparently had the two syndromes. Nakamura pointed out this association in 1922 [45]. The soft tissue hypertrophy in patients with SWS involving the face (Figure 40.12) suggests that the pathology of SWS and the Klippel–Trenaunay syndrome is similar.

Prognosis

The prognosis depends on the degree and extent of brain and eye involvement and, only for cosmetic reasons, the facial nevus flammeus.

Early development, intractability, and generalization of seizures indicate a poor prognosis. Also, the more extensive the lesion, the greater the focal neurologic deficit. There is possibly a kindling effect from early life in some patients leading to persistent partial and generalized seizures. The result may be disturbance of cerebral organization, interference with learning, and mental subnormality. Patients without seizures are never mentally subnormal.

Treatment

Treatment of seizures is the essential ingredient for the proper management and the welfare of patients with SWS. The anticonvulsants used are the same as in other disorders associated with seizures. According to the seizure type, generalized or partial, phenobarbital, phenytoin, primidone, carbamazepine, valproate, or benzodiazepine derivatives may be necessary. Adrenocorticotropic hormone is used in patients with infantile spasms. Despite adequate treatment, many patients continue to have seizures, and there is often mental and physical deterioration. Complications include secondary medical problems, trauma from the seizures, and social, educational, and psychological maladjustments. Accidental falls, injuries, status epilepticus, and aspiration pneumonia should be prevented. Psychological counseling, special education, or training toward independence are other goals for the epileptic patient.

A small minority of patients with intractable seizures originating only in the affected hemisphere, the other hemisphere being normal, may be good surgical candidates. An occipital or parieto-occipital lobectomy or complete hemispherectomy could render the patient seizure-free. A complete hemianopia and hemiplegia [26] will result if not already present according to the extent of the surgical resection but this is a small price to pay for the control of seizures and the prevention of mental deterioration that will develop if seizures persist. The possibility of education and an independent life is an option that may be offered to some hemispherectomized patients with SWS but even if this is not possible, seizure control alone can make this treatment worthwhile.

References

1. Schirmer R. Ein Fall von Teleangiektasie. Graefes Arch Ophthalmol 1860;7:119–121.
2. Sturge WA. A case of partial epilepsy, apparently due to a lesion of one of the vaso-motor centres of the brain. Trans Clin Soc London 1879;12:162–167.
3. Kalischer S. Demonstration des Gehirns eines Kindes mit Teleangiectasie der linksseitigen Gesichts-Kopfhaut und Hirnoberfläche. Berl Klin Wochenschr 1897; 34:1059
4. Weber FP. Right-sided hemihypotrophy resulting from right-sided congenital spastic hemiplegia, with a morbid condition of the left side of the brain revealed by radiograms. J Neurol Psychopath 1922;3:134–139.
5. Dimitri V. Tumor cerebral congénito (Angioma cavernoso). Rev Assoc Med Argent 1923;36:1029–1037.
6. Krabbe KH. Facial and meningeal angiomatosis associated with calcification of the brain cortex. Arch Neurol Psychiatry 1934;32:737–755.
7. Van der Hoeve J. A fourth type of phakomatosis. Arch Ophthalmol 1937;18:679–682.
8. Jennings Milles W. Naevus of the right temporal and orbital region: naevus of the choroid and detachment of the retina in the right eye. Trans Ophthalmol Soc UK 1884;4:168–171.
9. Rosen E. Hemangioma of the choroid. Ophthalmologica 1950;120:127–148.
10. Kalischer S. Ein Fall von Teleangiectasie (Angiom) des Gesichts und der weichen Hirnhaut. Arch Psychiatr 1901;34:169–180.
11. Hebold O. Hemangiomen der weichen Hirnhaut bei Naevus vasculosus des Gesichts. Arch Psychiatr Nervenkr 1913;51:445–456.
12. Gorman RJ, Snead OC. Sturge–Weber syndrome without port-wine nevus. Pediatrics 1977;60:785.
13. Koch G. Neuere Betrachtungen über die Erblichkeit der Sturge–Weberschen und von Hippel–Lindauschen Krankheit. Med Welt 1960;38:1955–1961, 40:2104–2108.
14. Bebin EM, Gomez MR. The intelligence and social achievement of patients with unilateral and bihemispheric Sturge–Weber syndrome (in preparation).
15. Pascual-Castroviejo I. The association of extracranial and intracranial vascular malformations in children. Can J Neurol Sci 1985;12:139–148.
16. Lichtenstein BW, Rosenberg C. Sturge–Weber–Dimi-

tri's disease. J Neuropathol Exp Neurol 1947;6:369–382.
17. Alexander GL, Norman RM. The Sturge–Weber syndrome. Bristol: John Wright and Son, 1960:95.
18. Pascual-Castroviejo I, Roche Herrero MC, Lopez-Terradas JM, et al. Síndrome de Sturge–Weber, Hallazgos en 22 casos infantiles. Ann Esp Pediatr 1978;11:281–294.
19. Peterman AF, Hayles AB, Dockerty MB, et al. Encephalotrigeminal angiomatosis (Sturge–Weber disease): clinical study of thirty-five cases. JAMA 1958; 167:2169–2176.
20. Chao DH. Congenital neurocutaneous syndromes of childhood. III. Sturge–Weber disease. J Pediatr 1959;55:635–649.
21. Alexander GL. Sturge–Weber syndrome. In Vinken PJ, Bruyn GW, eds. Handbook of clinical neurology. vol. 14. New York: American Elsevier, 1972:223–240.
22. Hoffman HJ, Hendrick EB, Dennis M, et al. Hemispherectomy for Sturge–Weber syndrome. Childs Brain 1979;5:233–248.
23. Stephan MJ, Hall BD, Smith DW, et al. Macrocephaly in association with unusual cutaneous angiomatosis. J Pediatr 1975;87:353–359.
24. Fishman MA, Baram TZ. Megalencephaly due to impaired cerebral venous return in a Sturge–Weber variant syndrome. J Child Neurol (in press).
25. Shapiro K, Shulman K. Facial nevi associated with anomalous venous return and hydrocephalus. J Neurosurg 1976;45:20–25.
26. Cushing HB. Cases of spontaneous intracranial hemorrhage associated with trigeminal nevi. JAMA 1906; 47:178–183.
27. Anderson FH, Duncan GW. Sturge–Weber disease with subarachnoid hemorrhage. Stroke 1974;5:509–511.
28. Waardenburg PJ. Genetics and ophthalmology. vol 2. Assen: Van Gorcum, 1968:1333–1424.
29. Susac JO, Smith JL, Scelfo, RJ. The "tomato-catsup" fundus in Sturge–Weber syndrome. Arch Ophthalmol 1974;92:69–70.
30. Brenner RP, Sharbrough FW. Electroencephalographic evaluation in Sturge–Weber syndrome. Neurology 1976;26:629–632.
31. Alonso A, Taboada D, Ceres L, et al. Intracranial calcification in a neonate with the Sturge–Weber syndrome and additional problems. Pediatr Radiol 1979;8:39–41.
32. Kitahara T, Maki Y. A case of Sturge–Weber disease with epilepsy and intracranial calcification in the neonatal period. Eur Neurol 1978;17:8–12.
33. Welch K, Naheedy MH, Abroms IF, et al. Computer tomography of Sturge–Weber syndrome in infants. J Comput Assist Tomograph 1980;4:33–36.
34. Wagner EJ. T-angiographic correlation in Sturge–Weber syndrome. CT 1981;5:324–327.
35. Simmat G, Lelong B, Morin M. Aspects cliniques et tomodensitométriques particuliers de la maladie de Sturge–Weber. J. Radiol (Paris) 1984;65:279–283.
36. Moniz E, Lima A. Pseudo-angiomes calcifiés du cerveau. Angiome de la face et calcifications corticales du

cerveau (maladie de Knud H Krabbe). Rev Neurol 1935;63:743–750.

37. DiChiro G, Lindgren H. Radiographic findings in 14 cases of Sturge–Weber syndrome. Acta Radiol 1951; 35:387–389.

38. Poser CM, Taveras JM. Cerebral angiography in encephalotrigeminal angiomatosis. Radiology 1957; 68:327–336.

39. Bentson JR, Wilson GH, Newton TH. Cerebral venous drainage pattern in Sturge–Weber syndrome. Radiology 1971;102:111–118.

40. Norman RM. Malformations of the nervous system, birth injury and diseases of early life. In: Blackwood W, McMenemey WH, Meyer A, et al., eds. Greenfield's Neuropathology. 2nd ed. Baltimore: Williams & Wilkins, 1963:324–440.

41. Wachswulth N, Lowenthal A. Détermination chimique d'éléments minéraux dans les calcifications intracéré-brales de la maladie de Sturge–Weber. Acta Neurol Psychiatr Belg 1950;50:305–313.

42. Tingey AH. Iron and calcium in Sturge–Weber disease. J Ment Sci 1956;102:178–180.

43. Probst FP. Vascular morphology and angiographic flow patterns in Sturge–Weber angiomatosis: facts, thoughts and suggestions. Neuroradiology 1980;20:73–78.

44. Koch G. Genetic aspects of the phakomatoses. In: Vinken PJ, Bruyn GW, eds. Handbook of clinical neurology. vol. 14. New York: American Elsevier, 1972:507–512.

45. Nakamura B. Angeborener halbseitiger Naevus flammeus mit Hydrophthalmus und Knochenverdeckung derselben Seite. Klin Monatsbl Augenheilkd 1922; 69:312–320.

Chapter 41
Klippel–Trenaunay Syndrome

GUNNAR B. STICKLER

The Klippel–Trenaunay syndrome (KTS) is a congenital anomaly of skin, underlying soft tissue, blood vessels, and bone. The typical findings are angiomatous skin nevus, bony hypertrophy, lymphangioma, or varicosities. The extremities are most often affected, but the hypertrophy and vascular abnormalities may be limited to the trunk. One or more limbs or just a few toes or fingers may be affected. Rarely, there is atrophy of the affected limb. The hypertrophy may be contralateral to the nevus.

Patients with the characteristic skin changes of KTS, but without significant hypertrophy or atrophy of the affected limb, may be said to have a forme fruste, but this term is best reserved for some patients with only two of the three characteristic findings of the complete syndrome, specifically hemangioma and varicosities or just varicosities and hypertrophy. These do not include patients with hemangiomas and hypertrophy alone, who should be classified as having typical KTS.

Among the synonyms used for this disorder are naevus variqueux ostéohypertrophique, Klippel–Trenaunay–Weber syndrome, angiomatosis osteohypertrophica, haemangiectasia hypertrophicans, telangiectasia and angioelephantiasis, angioplastic macrosomia, and angio-osteohypertrophy. The last term is the preferred one if eponyms are to be avoided.

History and Epidemiology

The syndrome is named after two French physicians, Klippel and Trenaunay [1], who described it in 1900, although these authors mentioned that in 1869, Trelat and Monod [2] described the same in six patients. Geoffroy Saint-Hilaire [3] on discussing hemihypertrophy advised not to overlook extensive hemangiomas. Friedberg [4] in 1867 described a 10-year-old girl with hypertrophy of the right leg, phlebectasias, and varicosities.

Weber in 1907 [5] reported patients with hypertrophic limbs and in a later publication [6] pointed out their association with arteriovenous (AV) anastomoses. Kramer [7] discussed the historical aspects in greater detail.

The separation of a Weber syndrome from the KTS has been justified because the former are "hemodynamically active arteriovenous fistulas," which were not included when described by the first author [1]. Today, however, most authors agree that KTS and Weber syndromes are clinically indistinct entities or variants of the same disease. Yet, May and Wiedemann [8] felt that patients with hemodynamically active AV fistulas are to be excluded because their progression beyond puberty may lead to "loss of life or at least an extremity." Van Bogaert and Kegels [9] pointed out that large hemangiomas in KTS patients function as AV shunts. If such hemodynamically active AV fistulas are present in patients with KTS, it may be well to use the term "Weber variant" for a more accurate classification.

The prevalence of the KTS is unknown, but at least 400 to 500 patients have been reported. In our initial series of 40 patients, the male to female ratio was equal [10]. There is no known predilection according to sex, race, or geographic location.

Clinical Findings

The skin lesions and hypertrophy are usually noted at birth, but may not be recognized before school

Table 41.1. Findings in the Klippel–Trenaunay Syndrome

Skin Lesions	**Limbs**
Capillary hemangioma	Ulceration of legs
Cavernous hemangioma	Syndactyly
Pigmented verrucous lesion	Clinodactyly
Papulonodular lesion	Polydactyly
Hyperhidrosis	Lobster-claw hand
Hypertrichosis	Webbed toes
	Metatarsal and phalangeal agenesis[a]
Vascular Abnormalities	Melorheostosis[a]
Varicose veins	Osteolysis[a]
Phlebectasia	Congenital dislocation of hip[a]
Lymphangiectasia	Peripheral neuropathy[a]
Lymphangioma	
Lymphedema	**Head and Central Nervous System**
Arteriovenous malformations, at times with significant shunt (Weber variant)	Macrocephaly
Pulmonary vein varicosities[a]	Intracranial angioma
Chronic disseminated intravascular coagulation[a]	Intraspinal angioma
	Acrocephaly[a]
Trunk	Microcephaly[a]
Angioma of gut, bladder, pleura[a], and retroperitoneal space[a]	Atresia of external ear canal[a]
	Temporal lobe astrocytoma[a]
Hypertrophy[b]	Pneumosinus dilatans[a]
Long bones (legs more often than arms)	
Face	**Eyes**
Gynecomastia	Conjunctival telangiectasia
Abdominal wall	Retinal varicosities
Genitalia	Choroidal angioma
	Glaucoma or buphthalmos
	Coloboma iridis[a]
	Heterochromia iridis[a]
	Intraorbital varix[a]
	Marcus Gunn pupil[a]
	Enophthalmos[a]
	Oculosympathetic palsy[a]
	Optic disc anomalies[a]
	Optic nerve meningioma[a]

[a]Very rare (1 to 2 cases).
[b]There may be atrophy (30 patients reported).

age. Prenatal diagnosis has been made by ultrasound examination at 32 to 34 weeks of gestation [11,12].

Capillary hemangiomas or port-wine nevi are commonly present in 75% and cavernous hemangiomas in 40% of patients. Other skin changes include varicose veins, phlebectasias, lymphangiomas, cherry red papulonodular or pigmented varicose lesions, hyperhidrosis of the skin, hyperthermia, and hypertrichosis. The hemangiomas are often quite large and deep and may function essentially as AV shunts, although their hemodynamic effect rarely leads to cardiac failure. They may give the hypertrophic limb a spongy consistency. Lymphedema is often present. The various degrees of involvement are illustrated in Figures 41.1 to 41.3. The hypertrophy can be mini-

mal and involve only soft tissue, but more often there is moderate to extreme hypertrophy of one or more limbs. The greatest leg length discrepancy in any of our patients was 12 cm.

The legs are more often affected than the arms. Both the leg and arm may be enlarged, but the disease is usually unilateral, as happened to 85% of our patients. The hypertrophy may involve any body part including the breasts and genitalia. Hypertrophic limbs do not always coincide with vascular abnormalities. Instead of hypertrophy, atrophy may be present; 30 such patients were reviewed by Ippen [13].

In our updated series of 42 patients, 16 had involvement of the trunk, that is, the thorax, especially

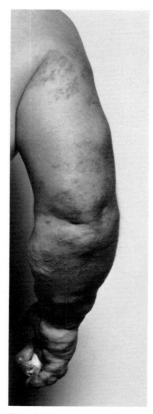

Figure 41.1. Klippel–Trenaunay syndrome involving the right arm with hemangiomas and hypertrophy.

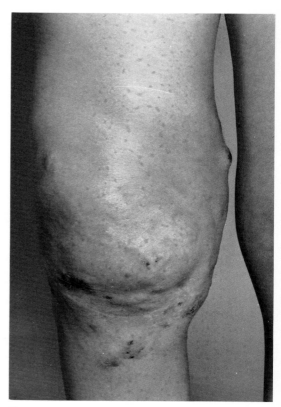

Figure 41.2. A more localized form of the Klippel–Trenaunay syndrome involving the right knee, including varicosities.

the pleura, the abdomen, and the pelvis. If the rectum is involved, the patient may present with rectal bleeding, and if the bladder is affected may present with hematuria [14]. Lesions of the labia and scrotum are common. Unusual manifestations include retroperitoneal hemangiomas or lymphangiomas, chronic disseminated intravascular coagulation and massive osteolysis [15], melorheostosis leri [16], pulmonary vein varicosities [17], micro- and acrocephaly, gynecomastia, syndactyly, polydactyly, lobster-claw hand, hammer toes, webbed toes, and clubbed feet [18].

Abnormalities involving the eye, summarized by O'Connor and Smith [19], include conjunctival telangiectasis, retinal varicosities, choroidal angioma, orbital varix, heterochromia iridis, iritic coloboma, abnormal discs, oculosympathetic paralysis, glaucoma, buphthalmos, Marcus Gunn pupil, and strabismus.

Among the neurologic manifestations is mental retardation, found only in patients with face and head hemangiomas, most of whom also have Sturge–

Weber syndrome. Vascular malformations of the brain have been recorded. Alberti [20] described a 25-year-old man with right-sided extremity lesions of KTS who died of an ischemic infarct of the brain stem. He had an intracranial aneurysmal dilatation of the terminal part of the basilar artery and of the junction of the right vertebral artery with the basilar artery. A review of the medical literature prior to 1976 disclosed 5 additional cases of KTS and angiomatosis of the cerebellum and medulla oblongata. The first description of this association was given by Den Hartop Jager [21], who reported one patient with angiomatosis of the diencephalon, medulla, and spinal cord; and two patients each with involvement of the lower brain stem and the cerebellum and venous angiomatosis of the skull vault. The resemblance of some of these patients' lesions with those seen in von Hippel–Lindau syndrome is striking, particularly Den Hartop Jager's patient, who had, in addition to KTS and angiomatosis of the cerebellum and medulla, what he called "choroiditis," but not the usual angiomatosis of the retina.

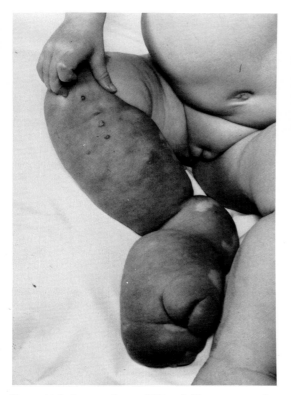 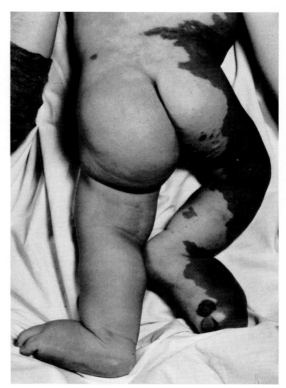

Figure 41.3. A severe form of Klippel—Trenaunay syndrome with an extensive nevus, verrucous lesions on the lower leg, and grotesque hypertrophy of the foot.

Vascular malformation of the spinal cord has also occurred. Den Hartop Jager [21] also described a 27-year-old man with KTS lesions of the right extremities and involvement of the penis, who developed spastic paraparesis and was found to have an intradural venous angioma at the levels of T9 and T10. Djindjian et al. [22], on reviewing 150 patients with AV malformations of the spinal cord, found 5 with KTS. The patients with this combination were between 13 and 22 years old and presented with subarachnoid hemorrhages. One of them had developed left-sided spasticity that was attributed to a bleeding episode at the age of 4 years. Another patient was previously reported by Devic and Tolot in 1906 [23]. Gourie-Devi and Prakash [24] reported a 25-year-old man; Eber et al. [25] a 31-year-old woman; De Mattos [26] a 33-year-old man; Vajda and Brozmanova [27] a 10-year-old boy; and Forster and Kazner [28] a 12-year-old boy, whose bleeding episodes at levels between T2 and L2 led to paraplegia. A similar patient included in our series [10] was a 49-year-old man with hypertrophy of the left jaw,

left arm, and both legs, widespread port-wine nevi and hemangiomas, and varicose veins, who at age 20 years had hematuria that required transurethral excision of a bladder lesion. Subsequently he had a spontaneous hemothorax from a thoracic hemangioma requiring thoracotomy and pulmonary decortication, a retroperitoneal hematoma requiring nephrectomy at age 28 years, and at 49 years developed paraparesis with sensory loss below T11 and bowel and bladder dysfunction.

Radiologic Findings

In patients with leg length discrepancy, scanograms are indicated to determine its degree and to allow judgments to be made about the best time for epiphyseal stapling procedures. Arteriography is indicated only if a significant shunt is suspected or if surgical incision of a larger angioma is contemplated. Arteriograms should be considered if there is a reason to suspect an intracranial or spinal angioma. Magnetic resonance imaging (MRI) scans give the most detailed information about the extent of lesions, particularly in the abdomen.

Venograms are rarely needed, but if they are done, the expected findings in lower limbs are extrinsic obstruction of the superficial femoral vein; large dilated tibial veins without valves and no filling of the deep femoropopliteal veins; deep venous insufficiency; or just anomalous dilated superficial veins. Lymphangiograms are not indicated.

Pathology

With light microscopy the findings are those of capillary or cavernous hemangiomas. There are no specific morphological changes for KTS. Subcutaneous tissue, muscle, synovium, and other tissues contain blood-filled "cavernous" spaces lined with a single layer of endothelium. Vessel walls contain collagen and sparse smooth muscle. The rare arteries are of small caliber and seem to float in the midst of the cavernous spaces. With the electron microscope Leu et al. [29] found the ectatic capillaries and venules to have a thin endothelium, thinned out or even absent in some places. Some lack a basal membrane. Although the vascular wall is altered, there is no cellular extravasation of either erythrocytes or leukocytes, but there is perivascular edema. Lymphangiectases are also present. Schwann cells accompany the nerves within the lesion.

Genetics

Koch [18] made a detailed analysis of the genetic aspects of KTS. He noted four instances in which the complete form of KTS appeared in more than one member of a family and in one of them, mother and son were affected. Lindenauer [30] added an observation of brother and sister with identical lesions. In our experience, a patient's mother had an angioma of the forehead and a patient's sister had a hemangioma of the right lower leg. Koch also reviewed families in whom the proband had the classical triad of KTS and other family members had only the typical skin lesions or some other feature like isolated hypertrophy of a toe. Based on these observations, Koch concluded that "dominant or irregularly dominant genes, acting in association with 'peristatic,' that is, environmental factors, may be the cause of this syndrome." This author suggested that in certain families the mode of inheritance was recessive and speculated that one major gene functions in un-

ison with a modifying gene to give such a high variability of expression. The genetic nature of the disorder is not well established as of yet; environmental prenatal factors such as trauma, infection, or even nutrition may play a role [18].

Pathogenesis

The Sturge–Weber syndrome is evidently due to an embryopathy. The pathogenesis of the lesions has been the subject of much speculation. Various hypotheses propose vascular or neural teratogenic factors that have been reviewed in great detail by Kramer [7] without reaching definitive conclusions. Although it seems plausible to explain the development of KTS on the basis of a transmitted dominant gene or an acquired form of a new mutation, it is unclear how this affects early embryogenesis.

The association of KTS with the Sturge–Weber syndrome (SWS) is more frequent than could be expected from chance alone. Among the 400 to 500 patients reported to have KTS, 40 also have SWS. The reported patients with KTS associated with tuberous sclerosis, neurofibromatosis, or von Hippel–Lindau disease are too rare to believe they have not occurred by chance alone [31].

Course and Treatment

There is considerable variation among patients on the amount of hypertrophy and this discrepancy increases with age. Complications are more common with angiomas involving the trunk, chest, or bladder. Among our 42 patients, only 2 have died: One was an 11-year-old girl with massive involvement of her left leg and trunk who became cachectic and nonambulatory as the thoracic and abdominal hemangiomas grew larger. The other was a 10-year-old boy who succumbed to pneumonia and glomerulonephritis, seemingly unrelated to KTS. Thromboses in the affected venous system can occur.

Patients with minor involvement require no treatment, but if there is leg length discrepancy of more than 2.5 cm, epiphysiodesis is indicated. Elastic support may decrease the lymphedema. Recurrent episodes of cellulitis require antibiotic therapy. In certain instances partial or total excision of deeper angiomas is indicated since there might be reason for performing a varicectomy. In patients with grotesque hypertrophy of all or part of the lower limb, amputation may be the only solution.

Associated Disorders

Sturge—Weber Syndrome

An association between KTS and Sturge—Weber syndrome (SWS) has been reported in more than 40 instances [32]. Long after Sturge's description of this syndrome in 1879 [33], Weber, on describing its radiological features, the intracranial calcifications [34], reported a patient with a combination of signs of KTS and SWS. This was a 28-year-old woman with an extensive facial capillary nevus or port-wine stain, right facial hypertrophy, limb hypertrophy, seizures, mental retardation, and a right spastic hemiplegia. Nakamura [35] was the first author to point out the not extraordinary combination of KTS and SWS.

Sturge—Weber syndrome consists of the characteristic uni- or bilateral nevus angiomatosus of the face, buphthalmos or glaucoma, and meningocortical angiomatosis. The skin lesions of SWS often involve regions other than the face, which are accompanied by abortive or complete KTS involvement with soft tissue or bony hypertrophy. Enjolras et al. [36] reviewed 106 patients with facial port-wine stains and found that only patients with facial angioma involving at least the ophthalmic division area of the trigeminal nerve, that is, only those with true SWS, are at risk for association with KTS. Pietruschka [37], after reviewing 13 patients with combined KTS and SWS, concluded that they are types of dysembryoplasia different only in the location of the lesion and the degree of severity. This idea fits with the generally accepted hypothesis that KTS is a mesodermal dysembryoplasia.

Rivera-Reyes and Toro-Sola [38] reported two Puerto Rican children, offsprings of two sisters who had married two brothers with consanguinity two generations before. One child was a retarded girl, 2 years 9 months of age, with angiomatous nevus on the upper two-thirds of her face, eyelids, neck, back, and arms, who had suffered left-sided focal seizures at the age of 10 days and had asymmetrical macrocephaly, a prominent parietal region, and left spastic hemiparesis, all compatible with SWS. Her double cousin was a 3-year-old boy with bulging of the left parietal region, slight asymmetry of the body, and hyperpigmentation on the left side of his body that spared his face. The hyperpigmentation was classed as nevus unis lateralis. This boy possibly had KTS. While these familial cases suggest a genetic relationship between KTS and SWS, more observations on the association of the two syndromes are needed to make definite conclusions.

Macrocephaly

Association of KTS with macrocephaly was reported by Stephan et al. [39] in three patients and with KTS and SWS in another three unrelated patients. One additional patient with macrocephaly, extremity hypertrophy, and angiomas, that is, KTS, and with features of SWS was reported by Nellhaus et al. [40]; another one, who had hemimacrocephaly, was reported by Meyer [41]; and one more was reported by Matsubara et al. [42].

Tuberous Sclerosis

The association of KTS with tuberous sclerosis and macrocephaly was noted by Laxenaire [43] in a 14-year-old girl. Gomez [44] discussed the association of tuberous sclerosis and KTS in his monograph in which he summarized the findings on three previously reported patients and added a fourth one. A previous observation by Louis—Bar and Legros [45] is without details. The well-documented observations are in four females, age 7 to 41 years. All of these patients had hypertrophy of one leg in addition to the hemangiomas and the findings of tuberous sclerosis. Only one of the three patients had a positive family history for tuberous sclerosis, and none for KTS. Since the association of these two conditions has been reported no more than six times, one could venture the opinion that it is a chance association. However, it is not uncommon to find a large finger or toe in patients with tuberous sclerosis.

Neurofibromatosis

The association of neurofibromatosis with KTS has been described twice. One was a 65-year-old woman with hypertrophy and a cavernou hemangioma in the right leg who also had neurofibromas of the face and left arm [46].

Brechot and Gasne [47] reported a 6½-year-old girl with KTS and numerous café-au-lait spots, but with no other manifestations of neurofibromatosis.

Other Associations

On rare occasions KTS has been associated with central nervous system disease. Howitz et al. [48] reported the clinical findings in an 8-year-old boy who had a port-wine nevus on the right half of his body but not of the face, right facial hypertrophy, and right-sided gingival hyperplasia. The angiomatous areas were hypoplastic. He had developed focal seizures on the left; later at the age of 5 he developed psychomotor seizures. At the age of 8 he was found to have a right temporal lobe astrocytoma. Spoor et al. [49] reported an 18-year-old woman with right blindness and constricted visual field on the left; Adie's pupil (also present in her maternal grandmother, her mother, and three siblings); hemangiomas of the right temporal region, the left leg, and buttock; and left leg hypertrophy. Her twin sister had "similar hemangiomas." A CT scan disclosed bilateral optic nerve meningioma, which was confirmed by needle biopsy. The patient also had sphenoidal pneumosinus dilatans (large sinus containing only air and no hyperostosis or other bone changes). This association with KTS was not found in a series of 67 cases of pneumosinus reviewed by these authors [49].

Finally, a 52-year-old patient with peripheral neuropathy and KTS; has been reported [50].

There are a number of syndromes with features overlapping KTS; the Cobb syndrome, first described in 1915 [51], or cutaneomeningospinal angiomatosis is one [52]. The definition used by Kissel and Dureux [53] includes a vascular skin nevus and angiomas in the spinal canal. The size and the appearance of the skin lesions may vary, but its segmental level must correspond within a segment or two to that of the spinal angioma. No familial cases have been described so far. The best evidence of a relationship between the Cobb syndrome and the KTS would be finding both entities in two or more members of a family (see also Chapter 44).

Also to be considered is the possible relationship to the Ullmann syndrome or "systemic angiomatosis," the angiomatosis affecting the nervous system, skin, and viscera. No hypertrophy of soft tissue or bones has been described in this entity [53]. The overlapping features between the Ullmann syndrome and the KTS include skin lesions varying from vascular nevi, cutaneous cavernous hemangiomas, and telangiectasias of the skin, to the visceral involvement of vascular lesions involving the liver, spleen, kidney, heart, larynx, and, of course, the central nervous system angiomata (see also Chapter 44).

References

1. Klippel M, Trenaunay P. Du naevus variqueux ostéo-hypertrophique. Arch Gen Med (Paris) 1900;185:641–672.

2. Trelat U, Monod A. De l'hypertrophie unilatérale partielle ou totale du corps. Arch Gen Med 1869;13:536–558.

3. Geoffroy Saint-Hilaire E. Histoire générale et particulière des anomalies de l'organisation chez l'homme et les animaux. Paris, 1942.

4. Friedberg H. Riesenwuchs des rechten Beines. Virchows Arch 1867;40:353–379.

5. Weber PF. Angioma: formation in connection with hypertrophy of limbs and hemihypertrophy. Br J Dermatol 1907;19:231–235.

6. Weber PF. Haemangiectatic hypertrophy of limbs. Br J Dis Child 1918;15:13.

7. Kramer W. Klippel–Trenaunay syndrome. In: Vinken PJ, Bruyn GW, eds. Handbook of clinical neurology. New York: Elsevier, 1972;14:390–404.

8. May R, Wiedemann HR. Klippel–Trenaunay–Weber syndrome. Med Welt 1977;28:1045–1046.

9. Van Bogaert L, Kegels C. Syndrome de Klippel–Trenaunay avec communication artérioveineuse. Arch Mal Coeur 1947;40:93–98.

10. Gloviczki P, Hollier LH, Telander RL, et al. Surgical implications of Klippel–Trenaunay syndrome. Ann Surg 1983;197:353–362.

11. Warhit JM, Goldman MA, Sachs L, et al. Klippel–Trenaunay–Weber syndrome: appearance in utero. J Ultrasound Med 1983;2:515–518.

12. Hatjis CG, Philip AG, Anderson GG, et al. The in utero ultrasonographic appearance of Klippel–Trenaunay–Weber syndrome. Am J Obstet Gynecol 1981;139:972–974.

13. Ippen H. Quadrantendystrophie mit Gefässanomalien. Dtsch Med Wochenschr 1973;98:682–686.

14. Telander RL, Kaufman BH, Gloviczki P, et al. Prognosis and management of lesions of the trunk in children with Klippel–Trenaunay syndrome. J Pediatr Surg 1984;19:417–422.

15. Damico JA, Hoffman GC, Dyment PG. Klippel–Trenaunay syndrome associated with chronic disseminated intravascular coagulation and massive osteolysis. Cleve Clin Q 1977;44:181–188.

16. Kumar B, Singh S, Lamba G, et al. Klippel–Trenaunay–Weber syndrome with melorheostosis. J Assoc Physicians India 1983;31:313–316.

17. Owens DW, Garcia E, Pierce RQ, et al. Klippel–Trenaunay–Weber syndrome with pulmonary vein varicosity. Arch Dermatol 1971;108:111–113.

18. Koch G. Genetic aspects of the phakomatoses. In: Vinken PJ, Bruyn GW, eds. Handbook of clinical neurol. vol. 14. New York: Elsevier, 1972:488–561.

19. O'Connor P, Smith JL. Optic nerve variant in the Klippel–Trenaunay–Weber syndrome. Ann Ophthalmol 1978;10:131–134.

20. Alberti E. Ischaemic infarct of the brain stem combined with bisymptomatic Klippel–Trenaunay–Weber syndrome and cutis laxa. J Neurol Neurosurg Psychiatry 1976;39:581–585.

21. Den Hartop Jager WA. About two new forms in the group of the phacomatoses. Folia Psychiatr Neurol 1949;52:356–364.

22. Djindjian M, Djindjian R, Hurth M, et al. Spinal cord arteriovenous malformations and the Klippel—Trenaunay—Weber syndrome. Surg Neurol 1977;8:229—237.

23. Devic E, Tolot G. Un cas d'angio-sarcome des méninges de la mœlle, chez un sujet porteur d'angiômes multiples. Rev Med (Paris) 1906;26:255—269.

24. Gourie—Devi M, Prakash B. Vertebral and epidural hemangioma with paraplegia in Klippel—Trenaunay—Weber syndrome: case report. J Neurosurg 1978;48:814—817.

25. Eber AM, Streicher D, Dupuis M, et al. Syndrome de Klippel—Trenaunay—Weber et angiôme médullaire. Rev Otoneuroophtalmol 1976;48:239—241.

26. De Mattos JP. Sindrome de Klippel—Trenaunay—Weber com angiomatose medula. Arq Neuro Psiquiatr (Sao Paulo) 1975;33:278—285.

27. Vajda P, Brozmanova M. Klippel—Trenaunay syndrome with a developmental defect and hemangioma. Cesk Neurol Neurochir 1983;46:114—119.

28. Forster CH, Kazner E. Spinales Angiom mit Querschnittslähmung bei Klippel—Trenaunay syndrome. Neuropaediatrie 1973;4:180—186.

29. Leu HJ, Wenner A, Spycher MA, et al. Ultrastrukturelle Veränderungen bei venöser Angiodysplasie vom Typ Klippel—Trenaunay. Vasa 1980;9:147—151.

30. Lindenauer SM. The Klippel—Trenaunay—Weber syndrome; varicosity, hypertrophy and hemangioma with no arteriovenous fistula. Ann Surg 1965;162:303—314.

31. Schull WJ, Growe FW. Neurocutaneous syndromes in the M kindred: a case of simultaneous occurrence of tuberous sclerosis and neurofibromatosis. Neurology (Minneap) 1953;3:904—909.

32. Deutsch J, Weissenbacher G, Widhalm K, et al. Combination of the syndrome of Sturge—Weber and the syndrome of Klippel—Trenaunay [author's transl]. Klin Paediatr 1976;188:464—471.

33. Sturge WA. A case of partial epilepsy due to lesion of one of the vasomotor centers of the brain. Trans Clin Soc Lond 1879;12:162—167.

34. Weber FP. Notes on association of extensive haemangiomatous naevus of the skin with cerebral (meningeal) haemangioma, especially a case of facial vascular naevus with contralateral hemiplegia. Proc R Soc Med 1929;22:25—36.

35. Nakamura B. Angeborener halbseitiger Naevus flammeus mit Hydrophthalmus und Knochenverdickung derselben Seite. Klin Monatsbl Augenheilkd 1922;69:312—320.

36. Enjolras O, Riche MC, Merland JJ. Facial port-wine stains and Sturge—Weber syndrome. Pediatrics 1985;76:48—51.

37. Pietruschka G. Zur Symptomatik der Syndrome nach Sturge—Weber und Klippel—Trenaunay. Klin Monatsbl Augenheilkd 1960;137:545—557.

38. Rivera-Reyes LR, Toro-Sola MA. Brief communication: nevus unins lateris and Klippel—Trenaunay—Weber syndrome with the Sturge—Weber anomaly in a consanguineous Puerto Rican family. Bol Asoc Med Pr 1979;71:69—71.

39. Stephan MJ, Hall BD, Smith DW, et al. Macrocephaly in association with unusual cutaneous angiomatosis. J Pediatr 1975;87:353—359.

40. Nellhaus G, Haberland C, Hill BJ. Sturge—Weber disease with bilateral intracranial calcifications at birth and unusual pathological findings. Acta Neurol Scand 1967;43:314—347.

41. Meyer E. Neurocutaneous syndrome with excessive macrohydrocephalus (Sturge—Weber/Klippel—Trenaunay syndrome). Neuropaediatrie 1979;10:67—75.

42. Matsubara O, Tanaka M, Ida T, et al. Hemimegalencephaly with hemihypertrophy (Klippel—Trenaunay—Weber syndrome). Virchows Arch (A) 1983;400:155—162.

43. Laxenaire M. Les gigantismes partialles. Paris: Doin, 1961:156.

44. Gomez MR. Tuberous sclerosis. New York: Raven Press, 1979:197—205.

45. Louis-Bar DL, Legros J. Les hypertrophies partielles avec angiôme (syndrome de Klippel—Trenaunay) et leurs rapports avec les phakomatoses. Conf Neurol 1947;7:245—263.

46. Van der Molen HR. Angiopathie à retentissement osseux ou dysembryoplasia à la fois vasculaire et osseuse. Rheumatologie 1954;4:161—173.

47. Brechot AH, Gasne E. Deux cas de naevus variqueux ostéohypertrophique. Arch Med Enfants 1931;34:320—334.

48. Howitz P, Howitz J, Gjerris F. A variant of the Klippel—Trenaunay—Weber syndrome with temporal lobe astrocytoma. Acta Paediatr Scand 1979;68:119—121.

49. Spoor TC, Kennerdell JS, Maroon JC, et al. Pneumosinus dilatans, Klippel—Trenaunay—Weber syndrome, and progressive visual loss. Ann Ophthalmol 1981;13:105—108.

50. Petschelt E. Zur Klinik, Symptomatologie, Lokalisation, Alters- und Geschlechtsverteilung des Naevus vasculosis osteohypertrophicus (Klippel—Trenaunay—Parkes—Weber syndrome). Arch Dermatol Syph (Berl) 1953;196:155—169.

51. Cobb S. Haemangioma of the spinal cord associated with skin naevi of the same metamere. Ann Surg 1915;62:641—649.

52. Kissel P, Dureux JB. Cobb syndrome (cutaneo meningospinal angiomatosis). In: Vinken PJ, Bruyn GW, eds. Handbook of clinical neurology. New York: Elsevier, 1972;14:429—445.

53. Kissel P, Dureux JB. Ullmann syndrome. In: Vinken PJ, Bruyn GW, eds. Handbook of clinical neurology. New York: Elsevier, 1972;14:446—454.

Chapter 42
Wyburn–Mason Syndrome

BRIAN R. YOUNGE

The Wyburn–Mason syndrome is one of the rarer neurocutaneous syndromes. It is nonhereditary in nature. It involves an arteriovenous malformation that variably affects the retina, optic nerve, orbit, optic chiasm and tract, facial angioma, and similar malformations of the midbrain; not all of these sites are necessarily involved in each case. Magnus described the retinal condition in 1874 [1]. It was described in 1937 in association with intracranial vascular malformations in the French literature by Bonnet et al. [2], and in European literature is known as the Bonnet–Dechaume–Blanc syndrome. The association of retinal and intracranial arteriovenous malformations was described in detail by Wyburn–Mason [3] in a review of 27 case reports.

Archer et al. [4] revealed by means of fluorescein angiography the basic nature of the retinal lesion: one or more abnormal communications between arteries and veins, with a wide clinical spectrum. This has led to various descriptive names, but the primary defect is an arteriovenous communication. There have been no well-documented hereditary patterns in this disorder, as compared to the dominant inheritance of the von Hippel–Lindau disease.

Clinical Features

Archer et al. [4] subdivided their cases into three groups: group 1, a less severe type involving an interposing arteriolar capillary bed between arteries and veins, usually localized to one sector of the retina. It was their impression that these were stable and were not associated with cerebral anomalies. Their group 2 patients had direct arteriovenous communications, with the tendency to higher flow rates and pressures, and some decompensation of the involved vessel walls

and surrounding tissues. Shunting of highly oxygenated blood past poorly perfused capillary beds was evident. Hemorrhages, leakage of fluid with edema, and exudates may cause decreased vision in some of these cases. With a few exceptions these, too, seem unassociated with cerebral lesions. Group 3 had much more severe retinal involvement, with a higher likelihood of intracranial and other site involvement. In these the retinal vessels have very large communications; they are of large caliber and are intertwined, convoluted, and highly arterialized in blood content. There is considerable retinal degeneration and generally poor vision. Varying amounts of exudation and pigmentary migration occur, and there are often ghost vessels and sheathed vessels in parts of the retina (Figure 42.1). This is the group that corresponds most closely to those described by Wyburn–Mason in 1943. There are many case reports of associated cerebral and facial arteriovenous anomalies, although in not as high a proportion as that reported originally [5,6]. Taken from the other viewpoint, the number of patients with cerebral arteriovenous malformations that have concomitant retinal findings is rather low, 4 in 90 reported by Yaşargil [7], and in about 10% of those reported by others [5,6].

In our own 4 cases there was visual loss in 2, and cerebral manifestations in only 1 case. We have not studied angiographically 2 of these cases, but have detailed knowledge of the other 2, illustrated here.

Case 1

When first seen in 1968, a 16-year-old boy had been suffering slowly progressive weakness on his left side for about 7 years. His hearing was reduced on the right, and his right eye had been blind for some years. An outside angiogram showed an arteriovenous lesion of

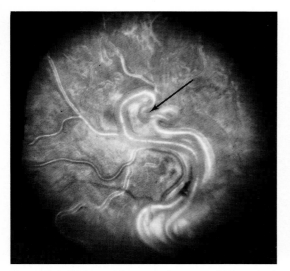
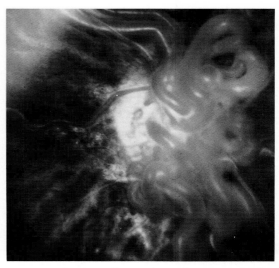

Figure 42.1. Wyburn–Mason syndrome. *(Left)* Note in the superotemporal retina a direct end-to-end anastomosis of retinal artery and vein with sclerosed and gliotic vessels nearby *(arrow)*. *(Right)* Grossly dilated arteries and veins at the disk. The dark background belies the pigment migration of the choroid near the disk.

the right side of his brain that involved multiple areas, including the thalamus. Hollenhorst described the retinal lesion: "In the disk region of the right eye there is a massive vascular anomaly, with huge tortuous vessels, mostly carrying arterial blood, although obviously some of these vessels are veins anastomosing with arteries. Away from the disk most of the vessels are empty" (Figure 42.1). The cerebral lesion was considered inoperable at that time, and the patient has not been seen since.

Case 2

A 14-year-old girl had been noted at age 5 to have an esotropia, which did not respond to optometric treat-

ment with patching and prisms. Referral to an ophthalmologist revealed a massive anomaly of the retinal vessels (Figure 42.2), normal vision, and no other signs of cerebral involvement. When studied at the Mayo Clinic there was no evidence of an intracerebral vascular anomaly either on computerized tomography scan or digital subtraction angiography. Her local ophthalmologist continues to follow her, and there has been no change since 1982.

Walsh and Hoyt [8] described involvement of the orbit and optic nerve, the maxilla, mandible, and pterygoid fossa, the basifrontal region as well as the sylvian fissure, and the posterior fossa, including the

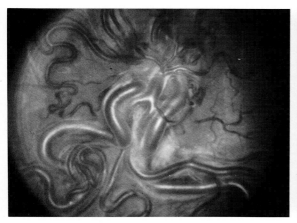
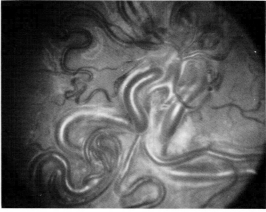

Figure 42.2. Stereo pair of the left optic disc showing considerable elevation of the anomalous vessels and the inferior artery emerging between two grossly dilated veins filled with highly oxygenated blood.

rostral midbrain. There are two cases reported by Brown et al. [9] in which the syndrome was encountered without retinal involvement. There is an additional case of the coexistence of the Wyburn–Mason syndrome plus Sturge–Weber syndrome [10]. Wyburn–Mason described in his original series facial involvement, and others have found the entire visual tract involved, from retina to orbit, along the optic nerve to the chiasm, the tract, the geniculate area, and along the optic radiations. From a review of the various literature it would seem that about 25% of the cases with retinal lesions are found on further examination to have concomitant cerebral lesions.

Pathology

Brock and Dyke [11] reported in 1932 a necropsy case of associated cerebral and retinal arteriovenous malformations. Krug and Samuels described in the same year a venous angioma of the retina, optic nerve, chiasm, and brain [12]. Most of these malformations are a grossly tangled mass of convoluted vessels that histologically are neither arteries nor veins, with direct continuity from the arterial side to venous side. The vessel walls are ectatic; show hyalin degeneration, hemorrhage, and calcification; and may be of such size as to occupy more than the entire thickness of the retina. Nearby tissues are often gliotic and have loss of neurons. This is evident in the retina [13], presumably because of the great mechanical distortion and compression of the neurons, although optic atrophy can occur from compression elsewhere on the optic nerve or chiasm, even in the absence of the retinal lesion [14]. Thrombosis and organization may be present to a variable degree.

Pathogenesis

Danis and Appen [14] have summarized the embryologic literature [15,16], and described the anomaly to be the result of a persistent primordial stage of vascular development without separation of arteries from veins in that part of the circulation shared by the optic cup and prosencephalon. The various systems that are affected in the head likely represent the effect on the particular stage of differentiation at the time of the insult. This has resulted in a plethora of names and syndromes for the multitude of arteriovenous malformations that affect the head, brain, and eye. Although the malformations have an effect upon the neighboring structures either

by shunting and thus compromising the vascular supply or by direct compression, they are often stable for long periods of time. Intracranial lesions may produce pressure symptoms, seizures, or sudden intracranial hemorrhages. Because the visual pathways are located in close proximity to the vascular lesions, visual field defects are common and may be progressive. Change over a long period of time has been recorded in the retina [17], and the dynamic nature of the intracranial vessels results in changes that usually become apparent before the end of the second decade of life.

Radiologic Features

The most important studies to undertake in a patient harboring a retinal vascular malformation involve contrast studies of the cerebral circulation, most safely by means of digital subtraction angiography (Figure 42.3), or when surgical treatment is anticipated, cerebral angiography (Figure 42.4). A screening computerized tomographic scan is useful, and plain head films might show whorl-like calcifications and an enlarged optic canal. In the study by Théron et al. [18] lesions always were found ipsilateral to the retinal lesion.

Treatment

With the use of fluorescein angiography several authors have studied the anastomotic connections, which range from small connections of a near-capillary caliber to huge shunts with very rapid transit of dye at high pressure [4]. In many of the advanced cases there is considerable leakage of dye, and retinal edema, exudations, and hemorrhage may be evident. In these more advanced cases, visual loss may be progressive, or in the case of vitreous hemorrhage, sudden. Thus, treatment of such cases by photocoagulation is a consideration, provided that spontaneous resolution of the vitreous hemorrhage permits visualization of the leaking areas. There are no reports of significant success with this treatment, however; this is understandable when one views the retinal vessels involved, as the risk of hemorrhage is considerable.

Various surgical and radiologic approaches to cerebral angiomas have been attempted with some success. Pool and Potts [19] reported good results in 74% of subjects with surgical excision and in 44% with medical treatment and irradiation. Carotid ligation and ligation of efferent vessels, as well as co-

Figure 42.3. Digital subtraction angiogram of an arteriovenous malformation.

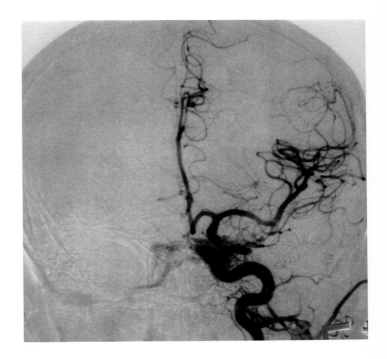

Figure 42.4. Cerebral angiogram of left carotid artery showing the arteriovenous malformation extending from the posterior orbit. The choroidal blush (C) indicates the position of the eyeball in relation to the sella turcica (S). (From Dannis and Appen [14]. With permission.)

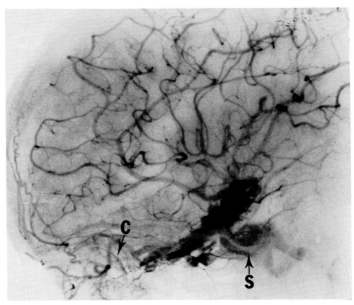

balt radiation, all have their advocates, but have proved to be worthless, and extirpation should be performed whenever possible [8]. Treatment is important if hemorrhages occur or if growth of the lesion produces pressure symptoms. Often the depth of the cerebral lesions makes operative removal impossible. In most cases it seems wise to watch these patients until something forces definitive treatment. Treatment of the orbital, maxillary, mandibular, or surface vascular malformations is usually by excision, although some success has been obtained with selective embolization and intravascular balloon occlusions. Comprehensive review of surgical management of these malformations is beyond the province of this chapter, and neurosurgical texts should be consulted. The most recent articles on the Wyburn–Mason syndrome contain excellent reviews along with case studies [14,20].

References

1. Magnus H. Aneurysma arteriosovenosum retinale. Virchows Arch Pathol Anat 1874;60:38–45.
2. Bonnet BP, Dechaume J, Blanc E. L'aneurysme cirsoïde de la rétine (Aneurysme racémeux). Ses relations avec l'aneurysme cirsoïde de la face et avec l'aneurysme cirsoïde du cerveau. J Med (Lyon) 1937;18:165–178.
3. Wyburn-Mason R. Arteriovenous aneurysm of midbrain and retina, facial nevi and mental changes. Brain 1943;66:163–209.
4. Archer DB, Deutman A, Ernest JT, et al. Arteriovenous communications of the retina. Am J Ophthalmol 1973;75:224–241.
5. Bech K, Jensen OA. Racemose haemangioma of the retina. Acta Ophthalmol (Kbh) 1958;36:769–781.
6. Cagianut B. Das arterio-venöse Aneurysma die Netzhaut. Klin Monatsbl Augenheikd 1962;140:180–191.
7. Yaşargil MG. Quoting Unger HH, Umbach W. Kongenitales okulozerebrales Rankenangiom. Klin Monatsbl Augenheikd 1966;148:672–682.
8. Walsh FB, Hoyt WF. Clinical neuro-ophthalmology. vol. 2. Baltimore: Williams & Wilkins, 1969:1694–1713.
9. Brown DM, Sadek KH, Tenner MS. Wyburn–Mason syndrome: report of two cases without retinal involvement. Arch Neurol 1973;28:67–68.
10. Ward JB, Katz NN. Combined phakomatoses: a case report of Sturge–Weber and Wyburn–Mason syndrome occurring in the same individual. Ann Ophthalmol 1983;15:1112–1116.
11. Brock S, Dyke CG. Venous and arteriovenous angiomas of the brain: clinical and roentgenographic study of 8 cases. Bull Neurol Inst NY 1932;2:247–293.
12. Krug EF, Samuels B. Venous angioma of the retina, optic nerve, chiasm, and brain: a case report with postmortem observations. Arch Ophthalmol 1932;8:871–879.
13. Cameron ME, Greer CH. Congenital arteriovenous aneurysm of the retina: a post mortem report. Br J Ophthalmol 1968;52:768–772.
14. Danis R, Appen RE. Optic atrophy and the Wyburn–Mason syndrome. J Clin Neuro Ophthalmol 1984;4:91–95.
15. Langman J. Medical embryology. 4th ed. Baltimore: Williams & Wilkins, 1980.
16. Dibony P, Lessel S, Wray S. Chiasmal syndrome created by arteriovenous malformations. Arch Ophthalmol 1982;100:438–442.
17. Augsberger JJ, Goldberg RE, Shields JA, et al. Changing appearance of retinal arteriovenous malformation. Graefes Arch Klin Exp Ophthalmol 1980;215:65–70.
18. Théron J, Newton TH, Hoyt WF. Unilateral retinocephalic vascular malformations. Neuroradiology 1974;7:185–196.
19. Pool L, Potts DG. Aneurysms and arteriovenous anomalies of the brain: diagnosis and treatment. New York: Harper & Row, 1965.
20. Hopen G, Smith JL, Hoff JT, et al. The Wyburn–Mason syndrome: concomitant chiasmal and fundus vascular malformations. J Clin Neuro Ophthalmol 1983;3:53–62.

Chapter 43
Maffucci's Syndrome

W. EDWIN DODSON

Maffucci's syndrome (dyschondroplasia with hemangiomas) is a disorder of multiple mesenchymal neoplasms [1–3]. Most of the tumors are benign but an estimated 30% of patients develop malignancies [4]. The clinical hallmarks are cutaneous hemangiomas and skeletal tumors, most commonly enchondromas, but any body tissue may be affected. Vascular mesenchymal tumors are widespread. When there are macular melanotic spots, the name Maffucci–Kast syndrome has been applied [2].

The major differential diagnosis includes Klippel–Trenaunay–Weber syndrome, the blue rubber bleb nevus syndrome [5], and Ollier's disease (multiple enchondromatosis) [6]. Superficially Maffucci's syndrome has features of both Ollier's disease and Klippel–Trenaunay–Weber syndrome, but there is more. The tumors in Maffucci's syndrome and Ollier's disease have a high propensity for malignant degeneration, especially to chondrosarcomas [4,7–9]. Maffucci's original report described a 40-year-old woman who died of osteosarcoma arising from dyschondroplasia. A variety of systemic neoplasms besides sarcomas have been reported [10,11], indicating the widespread potential for neoplasia in Maffucci's syndrome. Examples of other visceral tumors include pseudomucinous cystadenocarcinoma, teratoma of the ovary [20], and multiple endocrine adenomas [12,13]. Patients with Maffucci's syndrome are also at high risk to develop gliomas [9,12,14–17].

Maffucci's syndrome is sometimes congenital but most patients appear normal at birth. Neither a chromosomal basis nor a mendelian inheritance pattern has been defined [18]. Chromosomal analysis has been normal but for a single exception [9,18]. No clearly familial case has been reported, and the risk of recurrence in a family is very low. Although more than 100 cases have been documented in the world's literature, the condition is rare. Earlier reports suggested a preponderance of males; more recent reviews indicate that males and females are afflicted with equal frequencies [3,16]. The disorder has been reported in all races. It has been speculated that dysplasia of the centrally situated mesoblastema during embryogenesis is the unifying defect that contributes to lesions of both the skin and the skeleton [4].

Clinical Features and Course

Maffucci's syndrome may be detectable at birth but it is usually recognized in early childhood, largely because of skeletal problems [3]. The cutaneous and osseous lesions appear and progress during the first two decades. Osseous tumors and abnormal skeletal growth can lead to severe skeletal deformity. The tumors often grow in proportion to the somatic growth rate. Some, but not all, patients experience stabilization of tumor size after puberty, when growth ceases. Malignant transformation of tumors and development of brain gliomas occur predominantly in older adolescents and adults [8].

Skin

The most common cutaneous lesions are cavernous hemangiomas [9]. These are soft, blue, and compressible, but usually do not blanch completely on compression [9]. Lymphangiomas are soft and flesh colored. Other cutaneous abnormalities include vitiligo, café-au-lait spots, and pigmented nevi.

Besides cutaneous cavernous hemangiomas, other vascular tumors include hemangiomas, phlebectasias, lymphangiomas, angiofibromas, and combinations of venous and lymphatic lesions. Any organ may be affected, but brain arteriovenous malformations are not a feature. A meningeal angioma was an incidental finding in a single patient treated surgically for a hemispheric glioma [4]. An angiolipoma of tendon sheaths was also reported in a single patient [18]. Vascular tumors affecting the upper gastrointestinal tract may cause obstruction but gastrointestinal bleeding is less frequent than expected, given that polypoid hemangiomas in the gut are fairly common [6,19,20].

Bone

Bony tumors develop independently of vascular lesions. They arise autonomously, not as secondary manifestations of vascular tumors [6]. Long bones of the hands and feet are affected most frequently [18].

Dyschondroplasia refers to the abnormal accumulation of cartilaginous cells that fail to regress normally in the progression to ossification [6]. Enchondromas originate in regions of abnormal cartilaginous persistence. At the epiphyseal plate the results are irregular growth and limb deformity with bowing, often described as rachitic. Metaphyseal enchondromas cause vulnerability to pathologic fracture and more limb deformity. Limb deformities that accrue from the combination of disturbed growth, pathologic fracture, and bone tumors may be severe enough to warrant amputation. Disrupted vertebral growth causes scoliosis. Large osteochondromas of the sphenoid and clivus cause compressive cranial nerve palsies and other problems.

Metaphyseal osteochondromas typically present as rock-hard swellings of the digits. Radiographically the lesions are characterized by expansion or swelling of the bone and variable, sometimes mottled, radiolucency. Next most commonly affected are the lower extremities, the tibia, fibula, and femur, and the upper extremities, the radius, ulna, and humerus [18]. Although virtually any bone can be involved, tarsals and carpals are rarely affected.

Rapid enlargement and development of pain in the absence of trauma may indicate malignant transformation. Sarcomatous change of bony lesions occurs in 15 to 20% of patients and most commonly results in chondrosarcoma [16]. All told 30% of patients develop malignancies. Other malignant tumors that have been reported include cerebral gliomas, hemangiosarcomas, and lymphosarcomas.

Nervous System

Neurologic dysfunction in Maffucci's syndrome has several pathogenetic contributors. Brain compres-

sion by osteochondromas and intrinsic glial brain tumors may coexist or occur singly. Although vascular tumors are common in other tissues, symptomatic parenchymal brain vascular lesions or arteriovenous malformations have not been reported. Brain tumors have been described in several patients [12,14–17]. There is one report of a leptomeningeal angioma found incidentally during operation for a frontal lobe astrocytoma [4]. There is also a single report of thoracic neurilemoma [13].

Local or systemic visceral disease may mimic neurologic abnormalities. For example, polypoid hemangiomas of the posterior pharynx may cause dysphagia [6]. One patient who also had multiple endocrine adenomas had hypercalcemia due to an associated parathyroid adenoma [13]. That same patient later developed a chromophobe adenoma. Localized skeletal deformity can also make neurologic assessment difficult.

Because of the multiple pathologies involved in Maffucci's syndrome, the neurologic abnormalities may be quite complicated [9,13,14,20]. Cranial nerve dysfunction is common among those patients who have enchondroma of the base of the skull [17,21]. Anosmia, optic atrophy and blindness, proptosis, palsies of ocular muscles with diplopia, facial palsies, facial sensory disturbances, and abnormal hearing have been reported. Cranial nerve palsies may also result from intrinsic tumors of the brain stem. One previously reported patient [9] was later found at autopsy to have apparently multicentric gliomas arising both in the brain stem and in the left cerebral hemisphere. A sphenoid osteochondroma nearly obliterated the pituitary and compressed both optic nerves. A clivus osteochondroma deformed a grossly enlarged brain stem in which a grade 3 glioma that extended into the cerebellum and rostrally into cerebral peduncles was found. The hemispheric tumor was a pilocytic astrocytoma. Multiple tumors of the thyroid, kidney, and lung were also present.

Laboratory Findings

Imaging procedures are the mainstay laboratory tests for evaluating intracranial pathology. Osteochondromas may exhibit either radiolucency or irregular calcification on plain radiographs. Radionuclide brain scanning may reveal vascular lesions or cerebral neoplasms. Computerized tomography may be preferable to magnetic resonance imaging because of the superior visualization of bone that it provides. Patients with hypothalamic or sphenoid lesions may require endocrinologic assessment for hypopituitarism [7,9,13].

Patient Management

There is no specific therapy that prevents or arrests the progression of neoplasia in Maffucci's syndrome, but the range of symptomatic or palliative therapies that may be required is extensive. Typically multiple specialists are involved because of the multisystem nature of the disorder. Virtually all of these patients require long term orthopedic attention because of their numerous and potentially handicapping skeletal abnormalities. The services of neurologists, dermatologists, radiation therapists, and oncologists may also be needed. Because so many specialists may be involved simultaneously, the coordination of care by a knowledgeable primary physician can enhance the patient's overall quality of care.

References

1. Maffucci A. Di un caso enchondroma ed angioma multiplo: Contribuzione alla genesi embrionale dei tumori. J Movimento Napoli 1881;2:399–412.
2. Liebaldt GP, Leiber B. Cutaneous dysplasias associated with neurological disorders. Synopsis and differential diagnosis. In: Vinken PJ, Bruyn GW, eds. Handbook of clinical neurology. The phakomatoses. New York: Elsevier, 1972;14:101–131.
3. Toomey K, Hollister DW. Enchondromatosis and hemangiomas. In: Bergsma D, ed. Birth defects compendium. New York: Alan R. Liss, 1979:393–394.
4. Cremer H, Gullotta F, Wolf L. The Maffucci–Kast syndrome. Cancer Res Clin Oncol 1981;101:231–237.
5. Sakurane HF, Sugai T, Saito T. The association of blue rubber bleb nevus and Maffucci's syndrome. Arch Dermatol 1967;95:28–36.
6. Laskaaris G, Skouteris C. Maffucci's syndrome: report of a case with oral hemangiomas. Oral Surg Oral Med Oral Pathol 1984;57:263–266.
7. Anderson IF. Maffucci's syndrome: report of a case with review of the literature. S Afr Med J 1965; 39:1066–1070.
8. Banna M, Parivani GS. Multiple sarcomas in Maffucci's syndrome. Br J Radiol 1969;42:304–307.
9. Loewinger RJ, Lichtenstein J, Dodson WE, et al. Maffucci's syndrome: a mesenchymal dysplasia and multiple tumour syndrome. Br J Dermatol 1977;96:317–322.
10. Bean WB. Dyschondroplasia and hemangiomata. Arch Intern Med 1955;95:767.
11. Bean WB. Dyschondroplasia and hemangiomata. Arch Intern Med 1958;102:544.
12. Kuzma JF, King JM. Dyschondroplasia with hemangiomatosis (Maffucci's syndrome) and teratoid tumor of the ovary. Arch Pathol 1948;46:74–82.
13. Schnall AM, Genuth SM. Multiple endocrine adenomas in a patient with the Maffucci syndrome. Am J Med 1976;61:952–956.
14. Ashenhurst EM. Dyschondroplasia with hemangioma (Maffucci's syndrome): report of a case complicated by brain tumor. Arch Neurol 1960;2:552–555.
15. Carleton A, Elkington JStC, Greenfield JG, et al. Maffucci's syndrome: dyschondroplasia and haemangiomata. Q J Med 1942;11:203–228.
16. Lewis RJ, Ketcham AS. Maffucci's syndrome: functional and neoplastic significance: case report and review of the literature. J Bone Joint Surg 1973; 55A:1465–1479.
17. Strang C, Rannie I. Dyschondroplasia with haemangiomata (Maffucci's syndrome): report of a case complicated by intracranial chondrosarcoma. J Bone Joint Surg 1950;32B:376–383.
18. Das P, Gupta SC, Keshwani NK. Dyschondroplasia with hemangiomata (Maffucci's syndrome). Ind J Pathol Microbiol 1976;19:261–264.
19. Kennedy JG. Dyschondroplasia and haemangiomata (Maffucci's syndrome): report of a case with oral and intracranial lesions. Br Dent J 1973;135:18–21.
20. Lowell SH, Mathog RH. Head and neck manifestations of Maffucci's syndrome. Arch Otolaryngol 1979;105:427–430.
21. Nielsen JL. Ollier's disease: report of first case with involvement of the optic nerve. Bull Los Angeles Neurol Soc 1941;6:104–114.

Chapter 44

Rare and Questionable Vascular Neurocutaneous Diseases

MANUEL R. GOMEZ

Cutaneomeningospinal Angiomatosis (Cobb Syndrome)

The association of an angioma of the spinal cord with a skin angioma was probably first reported by Berenbruch [1] on a 16-year-old boy who rapidly developed a paraplegia and at autopsy was found to have an angioma extending from C5 to T3. Cobb described an 8-year-old boy who developed a flaccid paraplegia, analgesia below T9, and loss of sphincter control [2]. He had a flat vascular skin nevus on the right side of the back at the level of the analgesia. Cushing [2] suggested the patient had an angioma of the cord in the same metamere as the skin nevus and confirmed this diagnosis at surgery.

There are not more than 20 patients reported with this syndrome although there are many patients with disorders resembling it, having the spinal cord angioma and the cutaneous angiomatous nevus at different segments or metameres [3].

The majority of patients were in the first or second decade of life when symptoms appeared but a few were in the third or fourth decade. The first symptom is often abdominal, lumbar, or lower limb pain or weakness of sudden onset. These symptoms may be progressive or intermittent. The patients rarely present with sphincter disturbance or with a subarachnoid hemorrhage. The skin lesion is a flat nevus (port-wine stain) that may not be recognized right away [3]. The Valsalva maneuver has been recommended to enhance the skin lesion that is converted from a faint reddish-brown to a deep-red crimson stain [4]. All reported patients had developed a flaccid or a spastic paraplegia, and an intradural or epi-dural venous angioma or angiolipoma was found at surgery or autopsy.

Selective arteriography with catheterization of the intercostal vessels demonstrates the arterial feeders that supply the spinal vascular malformation. The posterior branch of the intercostal artery may supply both the spinal and the cutaneous angioma when the latter is dorsally located. A more ventrally located cutaneous angioma may be supplied by the anterior branch of the same intercostal artery that supplies the spinal angioma through its posterior branch [4].

Among spinal cord angiomas the incidence of cutaneous lesions corresponding to the same segment as the spinal cord angiomas is probably not higher than 10% [3]. Familial cases have not been reported. There are many doubts as to whether cutaneomeningospinal angiomatosis constitutes a different clinical entity. Vascular nevi of the skin are not uncommon and when taken as an entire group very few must be associated with a spinal cord angioma. On the other hand, spinal cord angiomas are not necessarily associated with cutaneous vascular nevi. If one considers only those angiomas within the same segment or metamere, the association is indeed rare, and thus it could be proposed that this is just a coincidence. This is not the case in Sturge–Weber syndrome, a true nosological entity, because the vascular malformation in the brain is unique and can be pathologically recognized as such even when there is no cutaneous angioma. The spinal angioma in the so-called cutaneomeningospinal angiomatosis is not different from other spinal angiomas. This is not to say that the spinal and cutaneous angiomatoses do not have a common embryopathogenesis.

Ocular Neuroangiomatosis (Brégeat Syndrome)

An 11-year-old girl reported by Brégeat in 1958 had angiomatosis of the oculo-orbital vessels, an ipsilateral thalamoencephalic angioma of the choroid plexus, and a contralateral angioma of the skin of the forehead.

The ocular angiomata were round tumor-like subconjunctival masses several millimeters in diameter situated around the limbus. They were smooth, regular, and interconnected by vessels. The superficial conjunctival vessels were not involved. The patient also had mild nonpulsating exophthalmos without associated bruit. Examination of the fundi did not reveal retinal or choroidal angiomatosis. Corneal sensation was normal. External carotid angiogram showed the opacified superficial temporal artery and the vascular tumors.

Symptoms began in the first year of life with excessive lacrimation, photophobia, and headache. Neurologic symptoms included seizures and mental subnormality. Head radiograph showed lacunae and increased orbital diameter ipsilateral to the lesion. The EEG disclosed high-voltage waves ipsilaterally. Arteriography showed a thalamoencephalic angioma in the arterial phase that consisted of a dense network of small vessels. The venous phase showed large-diameter veins with an atypical course [5].

Systemic Angiomatosis (Ullmann Syndrome)

Van Bogaert gave the name systemic angiomatosis of Ullmann to the association of cavernous and telangiectatic cerebral angiomas with visceral or cutaneous vascular malformations. In a review of the subject, Kissel and Dureux [6] pointed out that the concept of a systemic or universal angiomatosis as proposed by van Bogaert would require ruling out von Hippel–Lindau disease, Sturge–Weber syndrome, and hereditary hemorrhagic telangiectasia. This would leave patients with telangiectasia or cavernous angioma of the nervous system and similar lesions in the eye, skin, bone, or viscera. These authors found only 16 cases with such association: 7 had cutaneous angioma, 1 had a facial angioma, 2 had angioma of bone, and 11 had visceral anomalies including cavernous angiomas, telangiectasia, and cysts or tumors. In total there were 19 anomalies in the 16 patients, either telangiectasias, cavernous angioma, or venous angioma of the cerebrospinal axis. Clinical and pathologic studies did not support the

concept of "systemic angiomatosis" as a definite entity since the visceral involvement did not differ either in incidence or in type from the visceral involvement in other forms of angiomatosis of the nervous system. In brief, systemic angiomatosis does not constitute a morphological entity because it lacks precision. Nevertheless, the idea that vascular malformations may also be found in other organs when present in the central nervous system may have clinical or didactic value.

Oculocutaneous Melanosis Associated with Sturge–Weber Syndrome

Under this name [7,8], and also under the name phakomatosis pigmentovascularis [9–11], a few patients have been described with a typical facial nevus flammeus that is often bilateral and that also involves the trunk and extremities, seizures, hemiparesis, and bilateral oculocutaneous melanosis similar to the nevus fuscoceruleus of Ota [12].

References

1. Berenbruch K. Inaugural Dissertation, Tübingen, 1890, p 24; cited by Kissel and Dureux (see Ref. 3).
2. Cobb S. Haemangioma of the spinal cord associated with skin nevi of the same metamere. Ann Surg 1915;62:641–649.
3. Kissel P, Dureux JB. Cobb syndrome: cutaneomeningeal angiomatosis. In: Vinken PJ, Bruyn GW, eds. Handbook of clinical neurology. New York: Elsevier, 1972;14:429–445.
4. Doppman JL, Wirth FP, DiChiro G, et al. Value of cutaneous angiomas in the arteriographic localization of spinal cord arteriovenous malformations. N Engl J Med 1969;281:1440–1444.
5. Brégeat P. Brégeat syndrome. In: Vinken PJ, Bruyn GW, eds. Handbook of clinical neurology. New York: Elsevier, 1972;14:474–479.
6. Kissel P, Dureux JB. Ullmann syndrome: systemic angiomatosis. In: Vinken PJ, Bruyn GW, eds. Handbook of clinical neurology. New York: Elsevier, 1972;14:446–454.
7. Noriega–Sanchez A, Markano NO, Herendon JH. Oculocutaneous melanosis associated with Sturge–Weber syndrome. Neurology (Minneap) 1972;22:256–262.
8. Ortone JP, Floret D, Coiffet J, et al. Syndrome de Sturge–Weber associé à une mélanose oculo-cutanée: étude clinique, histologique et ultrastructural d'un cas. Ann Dermatol Venereol 1978;105:1019–1031.
9. Ota N, Kawamura T, Ito N. Phakomatosis pigmentovascularis. Jpn J Dermatol 1947;57:1–3 [in Japanese].

10. Kitamura W, Iwai M, Sakamoto K. A case of phaco-matosis pigmentovascularis. Rinsho Hifuka 1981; 35:399–405.

11. Ruiz-Maldonado R, Tamayo L, Laterza AM et al. Pha-comatosis pigmentovascularis. A new syndrome? Report of four cases. Pediatr Dermatol (in press).

12. Helmick ED, Pringle RW. Oculocutaneous melanosis or nevus of Ota. Arch Ophthalmol 1956;56:833–838.

Index